SIXTH EDITION

MODERN CLINICAL PSYCHIATRY

ARTHUR P. NOYES, M.D.

Late Director, Psychiatric Education, Pennsylvania Department of Public Welfare. Formerly Superintendent, Norristown State Hospital, Norristown, Pennsylvania

LAWRENCE C. KOLB, M.D.

Professor and Chairman, Department of Psychiatry, College of Physicians and Surgeons, Columbia University. Director, New York State Psychiatric Institute and Psychiatric Service, Presbyterian Hospital of New York

W. B. Saunders Company

PHILADELPHIA

LONDON

Reprinted August, 1963 and June, 1964

Modern Clinical Psychiatry

PREFACE TO THE SIXTH EDITION

THESE PAST FIVE YEARS have brought again a large publication of new learning that has both enriched our knowledge and clarified those concepts that pertain to personality, its development and pathology. The pressure of this knowledge urged the preparation of the sixth edition. It is reflected in the revision and reorganization of the earlier chapters. Here are included consideration of the consequences of deprivation of all kinds upon the growth and later integrative functions of the personality demonstrated by the studies of social isolation as well as by various laboratory investigations.

New sections will be found on the brain syndromes associated with hepatolenticular degeneration, hepatic insufficiency, the headache syndromes, and genitourinary disorders. Those many cytogenetic and biochemical discoveries that have illuminated the etiology of mongolism and led to the discrimination of a number of specific metabolic defects upon which defective brain growth and later intellectual retardation depend demanded expansion and rewriting of the chapter on mental deficiency. The clinical success of the new antidepressant agents and certain other pharmaceuticals required their inclusion in the chapter on pharmacological therapy. Elsewhere the text has been thoroughly up-dated in keeping with the dynamic and developmental orientation of earlier editions. The index reflects these additions in over a hundred new headings. It is a pleasure to acknowledge indebtedness again to the many writers whose contributions these past years have offered the rich harvest of new understanding that we trust is reflected in this edition.

We are indebted especially to Professors Harlow D. Dunton, Arthur Carr, Sidney Malitz, and Shervert H. Frazier for their critical reviews of various portions of the text, to E. D. Baskerville for editorial assistance, to John Balkema for bibliographic corrections, and to Margaret Neubart and Sara Klein for their assistance in the preparation of the manuscript. Also we are grateful to Drs. Maurice E. Linden and Samuel B. Hadden for a revision of the section on Group Psychotherapy.

THE AUTHORS

CONTENTS

Chapter One

THE BEGINNINGS
OF PSYCHIATRY

"Those who fail to know the past are doomed to repeat it."

Santayana

Modern psychiatry is that branch of medicine which is concerned with the manifestations and treatments of the disordered functioning of personality which affect either the individual's subjective life or his relations with others as well as his capacity to adapt to life in society. Psychiatry is directed, as well, to the origins and the dynamic interactions of the personality which contribute to the development of mental disease. "Origins" include the genetic determinants, whether of chromosomal derivation or arising as the result of family and social patterns which often underlie the specific selection of forms of behavior. "Dynamic" refers to the motivations that direct the behavior and the adaptive processes and mechanisms utilized to fulfill the requirements for maintenance of personality functioning at the biological, familial, and social levels of one's life. The variations of disturbance include those involving disorders of overt behavior as well as those influencing feeling, thought, and the functioning of various organ systems. Psychiatry's concern is directed to failures

of personality development, expressed in certain persisting immaturities as well as in more severe disorganizations of the individual.

Since disordered behavior touches upon many aspects of life in society, the psychiatrist and psychiatry have interest in knowledge obtained not only from all the biological sciences which contribute information of personality growth and pathology but also from those other professions and institutions which contribute to the management and social control of those with personality disturbances. The latter include psychology, the social sciences, law, philosophy, and theology. In the former, modern psychiatry seeks for explanations in the individual's genetic inheritance. This includes predispositions, the influence of anatomical, physiological, and biochemical processes, and the determining effect upon the maturing nervous system of the recording of the individual's life experiences. The recording begins in the prenatal period and extends through childhood in the family to the later environmental and cultural pressures. To

1

the psychiatrist, the interaction of these factors determines the *personality* of the individual.

Personality has been defined in a multitude of ways; some are concerned only with the outward expressions of behavior, while others consider as well man's subjective experiences. For psychiatrists, both aspects of individual experience are covered by the term "personality." Personality is perhaps best recognized as each individual's characteristically recurring patterns of behavior. These patterns, diagnostic for the individual, are evident in response to both the sudden and persistent stresses of life.

The Beginnings: Primitive Concepts

The origins of the majority of the scientific concepts of psychiatry are, of course, rooted in the past. There are, at best, conjectures as to the manner in which disturbed behavior was viewed by prehistoric man. The study of the primitive tribes of this day lends support to conjectures concerning the concepts of illness held by prehistoric men which are reflected in the myths and records of the early pages of history. Comparative studies also have provided valuable insights into the ranges of behavior of man under varying conditions. They have made evident the modifying influence of culture on the symptom expressions of psychopathology and illuminated the deficiencies in certain theoretical explanations of behavior that come from a study of man in a particular culture during a given time span.

The concepts of disease found among primitive people differ from those held by the scientific communities of today, and remnants of such primitive ideas of illness may be noted from time to time in the general populations of even the most technologically advanced societies. To primitive man, all illnesses are attributed to the influence of forces acting outside the body. Such forces are seen as supernatural; they are the evil spirits, witches, demons, gods, or magicians. These demonological explanations are particularly strong as explanations for ill-

ness affecting behavior. It is pertinent to speculate that primitive man came to such ideas from his own personal experiences and his contacts with the sick. His own dreams of return of the dead and his remembrance of their threats, demands, and affections perhaps fostered the explanation of influence from beyond life. His observations of the nonsensical, impertinent, meaningless, and destructive behavior of the delirious and psychotic, his apprehensions in the face of a convulsive attack, and his efforts to explain the phantom after limb losses must have fostered the concept of demonological possession as the causal means for the peculiar and frightening changes of behavior which fell upon those with whom he was close and familiar.

Primitive societies devised methods of treatment which are used even now almost exclusively in the framework of magical and religious practices. Within these methods (which often were followed by recovery of the afflicted) one may perceive the rudiments of psychotherapy.

Since like produces like to primitive man and since objects once in contact continue to have an influence even at a distance, the use of charms for their protective or healing force is a frequently used measure among such men. Charms may be viewed as homeopathic or imitative magic. Other ways in which imitative magic is used constructively is in the rites of the healers who act out the experience of the person to aid them. Good examples are the healer among the Dyaks of Borneo who plays the role of the parturient woman or the medicine man who enters a state of trance before indicating the treatment. The effectiveness of such methods of treatment may have rested on the patient's identifying himself with the healer and entering into a state of death and rebirth. The therapeutic use of trance states is another widespread measure of the primitive groups. In some tribes, trance states were induced by fixation on objects much as one may induce hypnotic states.

The quest of the medicine man is often

to find the lost or afflicted soul, to drive out the demon, and then return the soul to the body. Exorcism, the forcing of an evil spirit from the possessed, is brought about by many means in different groups and areas and may be easily recognized as a form of psychotherapy in which the ill person is encouraged to speak of those actions and misdeeds which have guilty connotations. The rites of self-punishment appear to have the same purpose. Other primitive ways include the use of spells and incantations with their repetitive offerings, the rituals of silence, and also the applications internally and externally of herbs and other medicines. Throughout one may recognize the primitive methods as beginning with simple cause and effect explanations and empirical observations, without recognition of the operation of internal forces, of either a biological or psychological nature. Nor does the medicine man direct his efforts to the individual but rather to a malignant invading force foreign to his primitive patient. The meanings and aims of primitive rites, while psychotherapeutic, hold no relationship to modern treatments which find the sources of illness within the biosocial organization and development of man.

Greco-Roman Era

References to mental disorders in the early writings of Egypt, India, China, Greece, and Rome disclose the beginnings of those major streams of thought and action which now pervade the growth of psychiatry as a science. The beginnings of the humanitarian attitude, reflected today in the area of social psychiatry, was seen as early as 860 B.C. when Greek priests supplemented incantations and exorcisms for the mentally disturbed with recommendations for kindness and suggestions for the use of physical and recreational activities.

A significant move occurred in the 6th Century B.C. as the Greek healer's interest turned towards observation and experimentation; these were the first scientific steps in biological science. Alcmaeon dissected and noted the connections of the sense organs to the brain, from which he inferred that the seat of reason and the soul were located in this organ.

This early scientific movement is best observed in the writings of Hippocrates (460–375 B.C.). He initiated a classification of mental disorders into mania, melancholia, and phrenites. His descriptions of disease indicate the existence then of knowledge of epilepsy, hysteria, postpartum psychosis, and the acute brain syndromes (delirious states) which occur with infectious diseases and after hemorrhage. He flatly rejected the influence of the gods as causative of mental disease. Hippocrates influenced, as well, the social attitudes of his day. While Athenian courts recognized the rights of the mentally disturbed in civil affairs, they gave no consideration to their rights in a capital offense. Through his influence, if it could be proved that the individual on trial suffered from a condition which Hippocrates designated as paranoia, the court appointed a guardian for the accused.

Although others expanded the Hippocratic approach, undoubtedly the high point of scientific observation was reached in the life of the Roman physician, Galen (130–200 A.D.). Using the scientific approach, he studied the anatomy and physiology of the nervous system and postulated that the existence of symptoms did not necessarily indicate that the organ or part of the body which served as their expression was the affected part. Galen developed a theory of the rational soul as divided into external and internal parts. The former, in his system, consisted of the five senses; the functions of the latter were such things as imagination, judgment, perception, and movement. Galen concluded, as Plato thought and Aristotle denied, that the brain and not the heart was the seat of the soul.

The problem of mental disorders occupied the attention of the Greek philosophers as well. Empedocles spoke of the importance of the emotions and pointed out that love and hate were fundamental sources in determining changes in human behavior. His concepts were incorporated by Plato in his consideration of Eros in the personal life of man. Thus, the third main stream of modern psychiatry, the psychodynamic, had its recorded beginnings in the Greco-Roman period, largely disappeared in the Dark Ages, and occasionally re-emerged in the philosophical writings of the Middle Ages. It is finally recaptured in the modern psychodynamic movement initiated by Sigmund Freud.

With the decline of the Roman Empire and throughout the Dark Ages of Western man, there followed a revival of demonology, spiritual explanations, and tortuous exorcisms, disagreed with only by a few solitary individuals. Beginning with Francis Bacon in the seventeenth century, the philosophers recognized that the functions of "mind" were of concern to the natural order of the universe. These views came to have a profound influence on medical thought.

The Modern Era

At this historical time, there again took place a revival of interest in the humanitarian care of the mentally ill. Led by Chiaruggi in Italy (1759–1820), Philippe Pinel (1745–1826) in France, Daniel Tuke (1827–1895) in England, and Dorothea Dix (1802–1887) in the United States, the shackles of patients were removed and hospital surroundings were developed for their care. Today, with the almost universal acceptance of mental illness as a medical problem in Western European and North American society, these changes continue to expand and are currently manifest in the "open hospital" movement started in England and in the new British Mental Health Act.

More or less coincident with the humanitarian reforms in treatment, there transpired the growth of medical interest in mental illnesses. Following a long series of observations by the brilliant clinicians in Europe, *Emil Kraepelin* (1856–1926) gave to psychiatry the first comprehensive description of what he believed were entities of mental disease. Prior to his time, psychiatric attention was directed to the symptom which was regarded as the illness. Kraepelin assumed that mental disorders were definite disease entities analogous to the physical diseases and defined by etiology, symptomatology, course, and outcome. This led him to stress clinical observations and the search for physical origins for mental diseases. His classificatory system was based on descriptions, symptoms, and outcome, since it was frequently impossible to make the diagnosis by laboratory examinations. Thus the classifications were not based on an understanding of etiologic factors including those of psychodynamic processes. While his system brought clarity to a mélange of psychiatric observations and thereby aided scientific study, yet, in fact, Kraepelin appears to have had limited appreciation of the inner life of his patients. His work did little to promote understanding of mental disorders, particularly the psychodynamic forces operative in them. His name, nevertheless, must be considered among the psychiatric great as he observed with discernment and systematized the results of his observations—a necessary stage through which every science must pass.

The "Mind"

The philosophic interests of Descartes and others on the "Mind" and its function established a dualistic explanation of human behavior. It will be noted that in the definition of psychiatry there was no mention of the word "mind." There need not be, however, any objection to the use of the word provided it is employed as a collective designation for certain functional activities of the organism, particularly those of the organism as an individual personality. As a corollary to this definition of mind, the reactions of parts of the organism would be designated as physiological and mind as the integrated response of the organism to the complex physiological, psychological, and sociological forces that impinge upon it. The "mind," therefore, is merely one aspect—the psychological aspect—of biological functioning of the organism and not a metaphysical entity having an existence parallel to the body. The dichotomy which is implied by "mind and body" does not exist in the organism. They are equivalent and inseparable expressions of life itself—the two aspects of psychosomatic existence. They are different phases of one fundamental unity of biological functioning which we separate only for convenience of discussion. It is in this sense, as a biological manifestation of the organism's responding and adjusting as a whole, that the word "mind" will be used in this book. The expression of this reacting unity of function, or mind, constitutes behavior, which may be defined as the sum of the responses to stimuli arising from both within and without oneself. As we shall see later, behavior is a product of both conscious and unconscious processes acting jointly.

BIBLIOGRAPHY

Ackerknecht, E. H.: A Short History of Psychiatry. New York, Hafner Publishing Company, 1959.

Braceland, F. J.: Kraepelin: his system and his influence. Am. J. Psychiat., 113:871–876, 1957.

Cobb, S.: On the nature and locus of mind. Arch. Neurol. & Psychiat., 67:172–177, 1952.

Hunt, J. McV.: Personality and the Behavior Disorders. New York, The Ronald Press, 1944.

Kluckhohn, C.: The Influence of Psychiatry on Anthropology in America in One Hundred Years of American Psychiatry. New York, Columbia University Press, 1944.

Lewis, N. D. C.: A Short History of Psychiatric Achievement. New York, W. W. Norton & Co., 1941.

Linton, R.: Culture and Mental Disorders. Springfield, Illinois, Charles C Thomas, 1956.

Opler, M. R.: Culture, Psychiatry and Human Values. Springfield, Illinois, Charles C Thomas, 1956.

Schneck, J. M.: A History of Psychiatry. Springfield, Illinois, Charles C Thomas, 1960.

Zilboorg, G., and Henry, G. W.: A History of Medical Psychology. New York, W. W. Norton & Co., 1941.

Chapter Two

DEVELOPMENT OF DYNAMIC PSYCHIATRY

"Now we, like all animals, carry with us vestigial traces of our past ancestry, not least in our mental processes. To develop psychologically we must understand ourselves, and it should help us to do so if we can find ways to investigate those hidden depths in our minds from which we draw our impulses."
Sir Walter Langdon-Brown

That body of knowledge which is directed to understanding the psychological influences and maturations that determine psychopathology is known as dynamic psychiatry. It rests essentially on an evolutionary basis. In its theory, behavior, no matter how abnormal, is the result of needs and drives which are built into the personality through the innately-given biological inheritance. It is complicated and modified by other needs and counter-strivings acquired in the long learning experience of family and cultural interactions that establish the foundations for man's social life. The basic maturational forces or drives are considered often to operate beyond the range of conscious awareness; that is, they are "unconscious." While dynamic psychiatry is oriented in the understanding of *motivations* as determining behavior, it recognizes as well *capacity to function* as a central determinant in eventual adaptation. Capacity to function rests on the genetically de-

termined anatomic—physiologic structure. Its development is influenced through experience and learning but is, in turn, influenced again by the biological and social motivations which determine aspiration and drive intensities. "Psychodynamics" is the generally used term applied to the systematized knowledge and theory of human behavior and its motivations.

EVOLUTIONARY BASIS OF PSYCHODYNAMICS

It is now generally conceded that many of the symptomatic expressions of personality disorders are rooted in modes of behavior which have been manifested earlier in life; that is, they are ontogenetically determined. Either through failure of maturation, which may be the consequence of physical maldevelopment, or an experimental deprivation necessary to

6

foster maturation of a function, there may persist into later life evidences of immature and maladaptive behavior. Another type of failure in the maturational growth of the personality occurs through excessive stimulation or gratification during the sequential stages of personality development. Whether it be through deprivation or excessive gratification, the term *fixation* is applied to the process by which facets of the personality do not progress to maturity.

The recurrence of infantile and childish behavior is noted frequently in the clinic when the patient is unable to solve some emotional conflict. A simple example is that of the six-year old who has long since learned to control his urinary functions but, again wets himself with the birth of a sibling. In this instance, the child, frustrated in his need to hold the attention of his mother, "regresses" to an earlier mode of behavior when it was presumed this need was gratified satisfactorily by the parent. Such regressions explain many of the bits of behavior characteristic of the severely ill.

The evolutionary orientation of modern psychodynamics stem directly from the genius of Charles Darwin and later Herbert Spencer who influenced the great English theoretical neurologist *John Hughlings Jackson* (1835–1911). Jackson set forth an evolutionary theory to explain the functions of the nervous system in health and disease. In so doing, he drew from his careful clinical observations of epilepsy and other diseases of the brain. Jackson postulated that the functions of the nervous system were integrated at progressively more complex levels; with mentation the highest level of function was subserved by the vast cell aggregations of the human cerebral cortex. He viewed the symptoms accompanying disordered brain function as representative of both the loss of more recently acquired functions of the brain and the reappearance of more primitive functions which are submerged in evolutionary growth. According to him, when a brain injury produced a permanent deficit in the functioning of the nervous

system, in addition to the symptoms due to loss of function, the re-emergence of more primitive actions was also recognized by the clinician as symptoms. A classic example of the latter is the Babinski reflex, a primitive toe sign which disappears during infantile life with myelination of the corticospinal pathways to re-emerge again as the result of disease to the pathways from the cortex. Jackson also indicated that the organism tends to adapt to the loss of function by a substitutive or compensatory behavior which sometimes also was viewed as a symptom by the clinician. The Jacksonian theories on evolution and dissolution of function within the nervous system inherently contain the postulate that the understanding of any behavioral disturbance is dependent upon foreknowledge of the progressive development of that behavior in a given organism. While Jackson's attention was directed principally to the functions and dysfunctions at the lower levels of integration of nervous activity, he wrote briefly on higher functions and commented that the study of dreams and jokes would provide an important means of furthering the origins of psychological pathology. Jackson's works and his concepts were known well and were incorporated into the later theories of Sigmund Freud, then a promising neurologist who established the major premises of dynamic psychiatry and also by Adolf Meyer, the proponent of the dynamic evolutionary school of psychobiology.

PSYCHOLOGICAL BASIS OF PSYCHODYNAMICS

European Workers

Anton Mesmer

Over the furor which Anton Mesmer (1734–1815), a Viennese outcast, stirred in Paris by the cures he induced through treating many diseases, including hysteria, by means of his technique of "animal magnetism," the scientific world first took cognizance of the influence of purely psychological processes in , influencing symptoms of illness. Members of the committee of the French Academy of Science, which included Benjamin Franklin among its roster of distinguished members, were impressed by the results of Mesmer's touching of his patients but duly noted the lack of evidence of animal magnetic fluids. While Mesmer's success was short-lived, his technique was picked up and used in both England and the United States. The English surgeon, James Braid (1795–1860), provided a descriptive formulation of mesmerism and introduced the term "hypnotism." The French country physician, A. Liebault (1823–1904), learned to use hypnotism widely in his practice and was responsible for teaching the technique to Jean Martin Charcot (1825–1893), the renowned French neurologist. Liebault's work represents perhaps the first direct use of psychological forces in the practice of medicine—its use in an equivalent sense with other conventional techniques for the relief of suffering of the ill.

Jean Martin Charcot

While Charcot (1825–1893) questioned the growing view that psychological forces could cause hysteria, his eminent position in French neurology brought the study of this disturbance and others directly into the stream of serious medical investigation. From his own studies, Charcot presented a report to the French Academy of Science that the phenomena of hypnotism were manifestations of abnormality and that the hypnotic state only occurred in those with hysteria. Charcot's fame and wide publications brought him numerous students, including Sigmund Freud.

Hippolyte–Marie Bernheim

Bernheim (1840–1919), professor of clinical medicine at Nancy, vigorously disagreed with Charcot's views and maintained that the phenomena observed by the latter took place only when conditions of suggestion were set up by the hypnotist. He stripped the subject of hypnosis of much of its mystery, dispelled ideas of special hypnotic powers and magnetic influences, and demonstrated that patients are also susceptible to suggestion in the waking state. Bernheim advanced the theory that hysteria was of mental origin. He was probably the first to apply the term "psychoneurosis" to hysteria and similar states. Some consider Bernheim's work the first effort to evolve a general understanding of behavior. From his studies came new questions pertaining to the legal responsibilities of criminals and the etiology of criminal behavior. Bernheim challenged the thought that "will" was the agent of crime and evil by advancing the belief that the mechanism of suggestion underlies the endless variety of both normal and abnormal behavior.

Pierre Janet

Another of Charcot's students at the Sâlpetrière was Pierre Janet (1859–1947), who also fostered the growth of the psychodynamic viewpoint. Contrary to his teacher, he recognized the fixed ideas and inner conflict with reality in the hysteric as neurotic and insisted on treatment by psychological means. His therapy was essentially through persuasion and the use of techniques for altering the environment of the patient. Janet evolved a theory of the neuroses as the lack of psychic tension on the part of the patient. By psychic tension, he meant an integrating force which, when abundant, held the stream of conscious activity intact. Through constitutional deficiency or as the consequence of fatigue or stress, the psychic energy became defective. Janet saw the disintegration of the stream of consciousness as the expression of psychoneuroses. He introduced the term "psychasthenia" to include reactions characterized by phobias, compulsions, and anxiety. Psychasthenia, to him, was the consequence of a general lowering of psychic energy, while hysteria represented a limited diminution of energy. Based on this concept, the idea of *dissociation* was formulated. As the result of dissociation, elements of consciousness were considered to take on an independent existence and express themselves clinically in the form of alternating personalities, fugues, anesthenias, and other hysterical expressions. The concept of dissociation has an established position in the field of abnormal psychology. Janet also introduced the idea of subconscious processes occurring independently of the mainstream of consciousness but later rejected Freud's explanation of "repression."

Sigmund Freud

Initiating his practice as a neurologist well acquainted with Jackson and the French school, Sigmund Freud (1856–1939) turned his attention to the psychoneuroses following his studies in Paris with Charcot. On his return to Vienna, he became associated with Josef Breuer who was perhaps the first to recognize that neurotic symptoms had "meaning" in relation to the patient's previous life. Breuer and Freud observed that under hypnosis their patients recalled old ideas, impulses, and experiences which they had found necessary otherwise to put aside or repress. As the patient disclosed and "talked out" his emotional upheavals, his symptoms subsided. Breuer gave up this treatment, presumably concerned over the deep attachment which patients evidenced to the therapist. Freud continued alone and soon found that it was unnecessary to hypnotize the patient. He persuaded his patients to speak freely and to bring up anything that came to their minds no matter how irrelevant it might initially seem. With the use of this "free associational" technique, Freud found that he had a means of widely exploring the earlier experiences upon which the patient's mental processes and current symptoms rested. He was able to analyze the meanings of dreams, slips of the tongue, mistakes and errors in everyday life such as simple forgetting. From his careful clinical observations, he constructed a system of psychology to which he gave the name "psychoanalysis."

Freud's psychoanalytic psychology is fundamentally psychogenetic and evolutionary. It aims to discover the motivational conflicts which determine behavior whether healthy or disordered. It provides as well a concept of personality structure and development not previously advanced by other schools. His clear penetration of the relationship existing between patient and physician with the overdetermined attitudes of affection or dislike, which he termed "transference" and in which he saw the recapitulations of earlier infantile and childish relations to a parental figure, represents a monumental insight. The analyses of the transference relationship and the patient's resistence were to Freud the essential elements in his psychoanalytic therapy.

Freud also insisted that much of mental life occurs beyond the realm of awareness and is unconscious. The concept of the unconscious has been one of the great contributions to psychiatry. While some psychologists dislike the use of such a metaphorical word as "the unconscious" for those impulses, desires and emotional responses which are inaccessible to our introspective observation, such a hypothesis is required for the explanation of many mental phenomena.

Freud's emphasis upon personality as a process developing step by step has given us a clearer understanding of personality manifestations. Many, too, do not accept Freud's concept of infantile sexuality with its uncompleted differentiation and the influence of its persistent hangovers on personality. Freud's demonstration of the importance of inner conflict with its dynamically opposed impulses is the first theoretical system to provide meaning to the genesis of neurotic and psychotic reactions and such other psychological phenomena as the dream, forgetting, slips of the tongue, and various errors. Although some have misinterpreted Freud as referring to the generalized systems of drives and to the structural elements of the personality (the id, the ego, and the superego) as if they were entities, yet the use of such terms for certain dynamic parts or functions of the personality has simplified thinking concerning personality functioning. Freud's emphasis upon a determinism of psychic processes has led to a greater clarity in our thinking. His psychological theory revolves around the problem of the development of infantile drives into adult personality. He contended that psychopathology resulted from a failure of a smooth, scheduled progress through the successive stages of psychosexual development.

Alfred Adler

This Viennese psychiatrist (1870–1937), an early student and associate of Freud, later came to dissent from the latter's emphasis on infantile sexuality and believed that the child's resistance to domination and his drive to self-assertion, domination, and superiority were more important than the sexual drive in the development and structuring of the personality. Adler's psychological formula may be stated as follows: Due to a sense of inferiority—organic, intellectual, social, or the result of past experiences—a will to power is stimulated resulting in compensatory reactions directed to goals of superiority. Adler included these various compensatory activities under the term "masculine protest." He adopted this term on the assumption that the exaggerated "will to power" with its drive to prestige, superiority, and achievement implied a struggle for power which might be compared to what he believed was the reaction of women to their feminine status. He observed that in European culture, women were usually regarded as inferior, a status to which he considered they reacted by a so-called "masculine protest," that is by trying to act like men. The will to power need not have its origin in a patent organ defect but in whatever feeling of inferiority, be it organic, sexual, economic, or social, leads to feelings of inadequacy. Adler gave his psychological movement the name "individual psychology" to indicate that each individual has his own special goals and a unique manner of attempting to achieve them. These methods mark the individual off from others and largely determine the structure of his personality. The various psycho-

logical processes by which he seeks to deny his inferiority and maintain the fiction of achievement constitute the symptoms of the neurosis. Adler's emphasis on power and prestige motivations, on cultural determinants of neurosis and therapy as a re-education have been absorbed to a greater extent than is conceded by adherents to other "schools" of thought.

C. G. Jung

Originating in Switzerland, Jung (1875–1961) became closely associated with Freud during the early days of the latter's development of psychoanalytic theory. In 1911 he broke with Freud over the all-importance of infantile and childhood levels or stages of sexuality development and the effect upon personality of trauma sustained during these developmental phases.

Like Freud, Jung assumed the existence of an unconscious, but he did not conceive of it as containing the same type of material or as acting in the same way in the production of psychopathology. Jung presented the belief that the unconscious is made up of material derived from two sources. He called one of these sources the "personal unconscious" and the other the "collective or racial unconscious." He considered the "personal unconscious" to be more superficial than the "collective unconscious" and therefore more accessible to consciousness. He contended that the "personal unconscious" contains the individual's personal urges and thoughts that developed in his individual history and forgotten impressions and reactions to environmental experiences. To the deeper layer of the unconscious Jung gave the name "racial or collective unconscious." The contents of the latter are not related to personal experience but consist of instinctive impulses and primitive fears, feelings, trends, and thoughts not connected with personal but with racial experience and thought. According to Jung, feelings and desires which belong to modes of thinking and acting which have undergone racial repression and belong to phases of past human cultural epochs belong in the "collective unconscious." To this psychological movement Jung gave the name "analytic psychology."

While Freud attributed the non-organic mental disorders to unresolved, unconscious conflicts, Jung explained them on the assumption that the individual is overwhelmed by the contents of the collective unconscious, and the psychic organization is broken down by its phylogenetic determinants, with the result that its impulses and feelings sweep the individual along, regardless of his conscious will or reason. In such disorders as the compulsion neuroses, the individual, according to Jung, is not overwhelmed by the uncontrolled impulses of the collective unconscious, but the individual's self-imposed rituals and compulsive ceremonials serve as defenses and protections against the domination by the collective unconscious.

Jung contributed many other concepts which have received wide acceptance. Among them was the word association test for investigating hidden regions of personality, which is discussed in Chapter 35. Jung was among the first to emphasize the nature of the child's interpersonal relationships and to point out that neurotic difficulties of parents are decisive influences in the difficulties of children. Working with Bleuler, Jung applied psychoanalytic concepts to the psychoses and was the first psychiatrist to suggest a psychological approach to the study of dementia praecox (1907). He presented a penetrating, analytic description of personality types, developed the extravert–introvert concept, and studied artistic creations, mythological themes, and religion, and their relation to dreams, phantasies, and the neuroses. He greatly stressed symbolism and religion. His critics comment upon the extent to which he combined psychological, philosophical, mystical, and metaphysical elements.

America and Psychoanalysis

In 1909, Freud was invited by G. Stanley Hall, president of Clark University, and by James J. Putnam, a Boston neurologist, to give a series of lectures at Worcester, Massachusetts. In the same year A. A. Brill (1874–1948), a former pupil of Freud's at Vienna, translated the latter's "Selected Papers on Hysteria."

White and Jelliffe

Soon the influence of William A. White and Smith Ely Jelliffe gave an added impulse to the acceptance of psychoanalysis in America. Through the medium of their "Nervous and Mental Disease Monographs" and the *Psychoanalytic Review* founded by them in 1913, they made many original contributions to the theory and therapeutic principles of psychoanalysis. With his inquiring and analytical mind, always eagerly in search of underlying factors in the development of abnormal reactions, it was natural that White should adopt a Freudian orientation toward psychiatry. A facile writer and speaker, interested in the dynamic forces of the personality, White perhaps contributed more than any other American psychiatrist to a recognition of dynamic factors in the causation of mental disease. White also contributed immensely to the understanding of the relationship between psychopathology and the legal problems of patients, and to a scientific basis for the present-day mental hygiene movement.

Adolph Meyer

Slightly younger than Freud but with a similar interest in the basic sciences of neurology, neuroanatomy, and pathology, and having knowledge of the foremost works of the French and British schools, Adolph Meyer (1866–1950) played a prominent role in the development of dynamic psychiatry in the United States through his pluralistic and interactional concepts of human behavior. He insisted that multiple biological, psychological, and social forces contribute to the growth and determination of personality. This approach he designated as "psychobiological." Meyer, as well as Freud, stressed the importance of early parental influences in shaping the development of the child's personality and conceived of mental disturbances as progressive habit formations.

The techniques which Meyer devised for the psychiatric examination form the basis for most of those now used in English-speaking countries. He taught that the understanding of maladaptive behavior requires a comprehensive study of the life history of the individual in which is traced the growth of personality through each unfolding stage to that of the individual's life situation. In his teaching Meyer condemned the focus upon a single complaint or single aspect of the patient's problem or the examination of it from the standpoint of a particular system of psychiatry. He inveighed against the Kraepelinian nosology with its prognostic import and spoke of psychiatric illness as reaction patterns. His own classification of adaptive patterns—the ergasias—has not received acceptance, although generally his tentative approach of defining reactions rather than diseases has been accepted by the psychiatrists in the United States and is applied in the nomenclature of the American Psychiatric Association.

Meyer emphasized that each personality has its assets and liabilities. The existence of faulty habit patterns implies the potentiality for teaching healthy socialization. Psychobiology, then, is the biology of the whole personality—the whole person in the whole situation—which must be accounted for and understood in assessing the personality reactions. Thus Meyer's influence, particularly in psychiatry in the United States, rested upon his insistence on a comprehensive study of the numerous factors that contribute to mental health and disease. This point of view distinguishes American psychiatry with its vigorous tendency to draw upon the knowledge and techniques of many disciplines, both biological and sociological, in its search for the determinants of pathological behavior.

The weakness of the psychobiological school rests in its failure to work through the study of intrapsychic processes and their origins in the dynamic interactions of the life of the individual. It remained for the psychoanalysts to clarify through their work these processes which, nevertheless, were always clearly perceived as important in psychobiology. As the first to emphasize that psychiatry is a biological science and that its practitioners must study the actual and complete dynamic situation in which the patient lives, Meyer has left an indelible imprint on American psychiatry which may now be regarded as a psychobiology extended in depth by psychoanalytic insights.

THE STUDY OF BEHAVIOR

Kraepelin's effort to classify conglomerations of human behavior into identifiable syndromes represents one of the major beginnings of the study of the source of behavior. While his classificatory system has been widely criticized, all subsequent attempts at improvement or modification are essentially grounded upon his system. Nevertheless, the critical attacks upon the classifications that have been established have led to new approaches that warrant some consideration and perhaps point the way to fresh methods of studying the nuclear processes which underlie the various psychopathological reactions.

The comparative studies of behavior in many species make it possible to identify a variety of patterns of activity that are directed to maintaining the life adaptation of each individual in each species. There are those forms of activity which are directed essentially to maintaining the biological needs of the individual: for food, water, oxygen, warmth, and elimination of waste products and protection against attack. These may be classified as (1) ingestive, (2) eliminative, (3) shelter-seeking, and (4) agonistic patterns of behavior, the latter being any activity resulting in contact or contest, whether it results in fighting or flight. The other forms of behavior are concerned with the procreative and social existence of species, the identifiable activities of which are (5) sexual and mating, (6) care-giving and care-taking, (7) mimetic and communicative, and (8) exploratory or investigative.

Man's behavior, whether in times of health or illness, may be examined in one or all of the above contexts. He differs from other animal forms in several ways. First is his outstanding capacity for flexible and intricate manipulatory activity acquired through the freeing of his upper extremities from locomotion by the assumption of bipedal gait. His major adaptive power, however, rests upon the range and versatility of his communicative and investigatory activities associated with the enormous growth of the human brain and its expanded capacities for storing and aggregating experiences. He is able to express through language those thought processes and affective states which accompany the arousal of his needs and the outcome of those drives motivated for their satisfaction. This, in turn, has led to the evolution of the complex symbolizations that he utilizes for communication with his fellows and the capacity to allow perpetuation of knowledge over time through their recording and passage by the cultural institutions. These progressive accretions of knowledge have provided.for the solving of increasingly intricate problems.

Those disorders of behavior now recognized in man involve not only various groupings of defects in his behaviors directed to satisfy his basic biological needs, but, more important, those affecting the essentially human elements of behavior; his social relations, ability to communicate, to act, think, and feel appropriate to his maturational state and his situation. The psychiatrist is a scientist with particular knowledge and interest in ranges of behavior pathology characteristic to man; many of these will not be found in other living species.

Motivation: Drive and Needs

Behavior may be generally recognized as directed toward some goal, some aim that promises or provides satisfaction or a state of well-being. Behavior may be stated to be motivated, that is, activated and also selected as the appropriate means to accomplish a goal. Within the concept of motivation, questions may be asked as to the forces which lead to the activation or inhibition of a particular form of behavior and those forces which select one or another form as the appropriate one at a particular time period.

BIOLOGICAL NEEDS. Each form of behavior has as its goal the satisfaction of a need. Thus, the lack of food, water, or warmth impels the individual to activity which is aimed at satisfying the bodily lack. Needs are determined by the unique biological organization of the species. It is assumed theoretically that a *drive* is induced by the establishment of a need which provides the physiological substrata for the motivation to behavior. In all species, there exist certain biologically primitive or physiological needs necessary for the survival of the individual and the species. The needs for oxygen, water, food, maintenance of bodily temperature, and avoidance of tissue damage exist at birth and persist throughout life. The need to copulate and to procreate the species and care for the young, while innately given with vertebrate life, is activated only after full maturation of the genital apparatus of the organism coupled with appropriate stimulation and later mating behavior with another member of the species.

While these biologically primitive needs are observed early in phylogenetic growth, they are neither psychologically primitive nor simple in their mechanisms of operation. This is particularly true in man who, as a result of his long period of dependency and the influence of socially determined goals, learned many other needs. The satisfaction of the need for food, as one examines behavior from the simple to the more complex organisms, may be found to be an increasingly complex behavioral task. The simple annelid ingests and eliminates earth, removing from it the necessary nutrients by its peculiar physiological processes. A carnivore, stirred by the need for food, must stalk his prey, capture, and eventually devour it. In this action, however, there are elements acquired through repeated experiences and even observations of other animals in hunt. Even in play, kittens hunt with the mother feline and may, through learning, acquire new facilities for satisfying the need for food. With the growing child, the satisfaction of the need for food passes through numerous stages of development from that of making the need known through crying to its satisfaction with sucking and ingesting of milk. With this behavior, there is associated contact with the mother, or food giver, who thus comes to signify a source of pleasure and security. Her care determines further associations and behavior, including all those ways in which men in various cultures eventually obtain, prepare, and finally eat to satisfy hunger. The many patterns of food acquisition and ingestion are learned acquisitions or derivatives of the original need for food.

While the physiological needs are innately determined, those acquired through association are learned and are the products of the unique interaction of one individual with others. The acquired needs of man then develop in particular family cultures and are determined by associations. Needs for social status, whether acquired through power or prestige and whether or not they are satisfied by the different means of birth, material wealth, creativity, conformity or capacity to gain the confidence or others, are learned.

"INSTINCT." In the past, the term *instinct* was widely used to explain patterns of behavior innately given to the organism. In the description of motivations and drives, it is clear that the existence of an unsatisfied need establishes in the organism a set or attitude which primes it for action in the face of an adequate excitant or stimulus in the external environment. This stimulus leads to arousal of the function and also guides or cues the response to satisfy the need. In the latter instance, it determines whether the response will be one of action or inhibition, fight or flight, leaping or stalking, speech or silence. The same stimulus may lead both to arousal and to determining the response. It may, in terms

of the behavioral scientists, have both "releasing" and "consummatory" properties. For man, the smell of food may excite hunger and also direct his steps to its presence. Often, however, there is required a series of stimuli, each necessary to determine some phase in a chain of behavior required to satisfy the need. A bee-hunting digger-wasp, for example, flies from flower to flower in search of a bee. In this phase, it is indifferent to the scent of bees, as can be determined by making available the odor of bees by having groups of them nearby but concealed. Any visual stimulus by a moving object of the correct size, whether a fly or a bee, releases the wasp's first reaction of turning towards and positioning itself, hovering to leeward of the quarry. From then on, the wasp is susceptible to bee scent. Dummy bees without scent are abandoned, but those with the right odor release the second reaction in the chain, a flash-like leap to seize the bee. The third reaction, the delivery of the sting, is dependent on a new tactile stimulus. Many studies by animal psychologists have demonstrated the necessity for the proper maturation of the organization, its necessary exposure to the appropriate stimuli, and the influence of actual experience in determining the development of effective adaptive behavior. Likewise, the deprivation by experience at a critical stage in the maturational process may result in a continuing deficiency in the evolution of particular behavior sequences.

The accumulated evidence indicates that it is misleading and incorrect to consider "instinctive" behavior as a separate form entirely unrelated to "learned" behavior. The two types blend into each other. If by "instinct" is meant that process in the nervous system which produces innate behavior, it is again misleading, as no special portion or brain process is involved that may be specifically related to innate behavioral activity in contrast to that acquired through learning. Instinctive or innate behavior is carried out for its own sake and not for what it may produce in the future. Neither does it imply knowledge of its ends. What is desirable in the study of behavior of man as well as animals is the eventual isolation and understanding of the various fragments of each behavioral act and also the contribution of the total bodily structure. That of the brain as the integrating organ will be found the most important.

The necessity to separate learned from innate responses in man is most significant from the standpoint of treatment. Learned processes, deficient or disordered, may perhaps be modified by learning or relearning—in other words, by psychotherapy. Those disorders dependent primarily on dysfunctions of primary organization, i.e., "innate," are unlikely to be so modified.

In psychiatry, the term "instinct" is used in a psychological sense and may be considered the innate biological drives which determine motivations. They are the dynamic agents not only for the maintenance of the life of the individual including his social adaptations, but also of the energy for creative purposes in all walks of life.

Affects and Emotion

There is much to suggest that the processes, activities, or patterns which we call "emotion" appear when there is some bar to the smooth and complete satisfaction of a drive. If there is no interference with its satisfaction, all the auxiliary activities stimulated by the vegetative nervous system and felt in consciousness as affect would not take place. When, however, there is interference with the execution of an instinctive activity, the vegetative nervous system initiates those activities of the organs under its control that will assist in carrying out the activity. If, for example, there is obstruction to an action which would serve the instinct of self-preservation, both epinephrine and norepinephrine may be poured into the blood, as a result of which the blood pressure is raised, the heart and lungs work more rapidly, and the arterioles of the skin contract—all being processes which force blood into the lungs, muscles, and brain where, during the emergency, it

will be of maximum service. At the same time, sugar is mobilized for the production of energy in the muscles, the coagulability of the blood is increased so that wounds are less likely to be fatal, and the pupil of the eye is dilated so that the field of vision may be widened. All these changes serve to aid the self-preservative drive and are fused in the fields of sensation and consciousness into an affect which we speak of as fear. The subjectively-experienced feeling aspect of an emotion may be regarded as an affect. The physiological and psychological aspects are, however, integrated and nonseparable.

Affects, which may be defined as feeling-tones, are pain-pleasure accompaniments of an idea or mental representation. By stimulating or facilitating some innate drive, they exercise a strongly determinative influence in giving direction both to thought associations and to overt behavior reactions. The terms "affect" and "emotion" are often used loosely as if these two aspects of mental life were the same. This is because the term "emotion" is used with many and, therefore, ambiguous meanings. Its use should probably be confined to indicate either the complex biochemical, physiological processes or functions concerned with the somatic expression of feeling or else the patterns of behavior that express affect rather than subjectively-experienced feeling phenomena to which the term "affect" is more applicable.

The common affects are those of pain, fear, and rage aroused with experiences attacking the integrity of the individual. Others associated with social existence are those of anxiety, affection, tenderness and love, guilt, shame, and disgust.

Once a drive state is successful in bringing about behavior to satisfy a need, the individual is free to respond to other needs. As we may recognize, there is a drive to maintain a constant internal state devoid of need and the tensions that such needs arouse. This concept is generally referred to by the term "*homeostasis*," first applied by the American physiologist, Walter B. Cannon. As an example, respiration forms a portion of the homeostatic system to maintain a constant level of oxygen and carbon dioxide in the blood stream. Any modulation of these levels quickly leads to change in breathing to return the levels to constant. Also, when changes of body temperature take place, sweating or shivering may occur to correct the modification. When this reflex type of behavior is adequate, the homeostatic process is not motivational. While the term "homeostasis" is often applied rigorously to the corrective physiological functions, it proves a useful concept in psychiatry and psychology. Thus the failure to satisfy social needs also sets up tensions which lead to bringing into play the psychosocial adaptations.

Conation

Containing components derived both from innate drives and affects, and in many ways merely a name for the urge created by these two dynamic agents, is that striving aspect or urge of the personality for expression known as "conation." As conations, we include those intention sets of the personality having motivating urges behind them. Here, too, one would include attitudes or those responses determined with special reference to feeling states. Conation lacks the degree of consciousness which we usually associate with the idea of will or volition, since the individual may not recognize the affective-instinctive sources by which his action was prompted.

Intelligence

In vertebrates, the modifiable and integrative aspects of behavior are greatly increased. In them appears the cerebral cortex, developed for the purpose of providing a mechanism capable of elaborating, integrating, and controlling impulses and functions more perfectly than is possible with a more elementary nervous system. In fact, evolutionary stages in development are traceable in the cerebral cortex itself, associated with a corresponding hierarchy of functions. The older part of the cortex, the archipallium or limbic system, as MacLean designates it, is concerned with self-preservative and self-procreative functions and the basic emotional responses and visceral functions, in contrast to the more recently developed portion, the neopallium, essential for progressively complex discriminations and integrations characteristic of the highest psychic functions. The biological purpose of its development was so that the organism might secure a more flexible capacity for adaptation.

Biological processes have evolved from conditions of simplicity and diffusiveness to complexity, differentiation, and definiteness. Similarly, an imperceptible transition has evolved from innate drive states to cognitive ability of that adaptive attribute called intelligence. Since, from a practical standpoint, the intelligence of an organism is fundamentally its psychological capacity for adapting to, and making use of, its environment, it is quite arbitrary to say where in the phyletic series intelligence was acquired. In fact, intelligence probably was not superimposed on earlier instinctive processes at some definite stage of evolution but was an outgrowth of them. Those, be they species or individual human beings, that possess the greatest capacity in these respects are the most intelligent.

Consciousness

A prerequisite for that degree of adapting to, and making use of, the environment to which we apply the term "intelligence" is that function we know as "consciousness." By this term is meant a sense of awareness of self and of the environment. Its major biological purpose is to permit the organism to adapt itself to novel circumstances.

ORIGIN. How such consciousness develops is unknown, but it seems reasonable to assume that, in common with higher functions in general, it is a specialized development of lower ones. Such an assumption is in agreement with the general evolutionary propositions. Although no conclusions as to the origin or nature of consciousness can be secured by objective observation, one may speculate that it originates in the properties of irritability of protoplasm. When protoplasm—let us assume it to be in the form of an extremely simple organism such as a protozoan—is stimulated, a response occurs. A response, however simple, implies a change, a difference. As evolution progresses and the organism becomes more complex, and as the types of stimuli and of responses multiply, one can imagine that the organism becomes gradually but dimly aware that modifications are induced, that changes occur in itself. Thus a sense of comparison arises until, finally, sensations are produced, an awareness of which constitutes the dawning of consciousness.

DEVELOPMENT. These beginnings of perceptive processes undergo evolutionary expansion from the simple to the more complex until, finally, a conceptual consciousness with ideative and affective components is reached. Whether the dawning phases of consciousness arose in some such way can only be conjectured, but it seems safe to assume that its development was through an expanding process, a successive integration, which has progressed simultaneously with zoological evolution. At the psychological level is to be found the highest phase in integration in the continuity of nature. A consideration of the evolutionary process suggests that there is no sharp distinction between the conscious and the unconscious and that conscious thinking represents the most highly developed and most fully integrated process of organizing and dealing with experience.

DEGREE OF CONSCIOUSNESS. A phenomenon that should be mentioned in the consideration of the dynamics of behavior is that many psychobiological activities which we term "mental" occur without conscious awareness. It was formerly assumed that consciousness or sense of awareness was a prerequisite for all those expressions of the organism we refer to as "mental." While many of these psychic functions are manifested only under conditions of clear awareness, observation of mental processes, particularly of those occurring in states of pathology, reveals that many highly significant

psychic processes operate under widely varying degrees of awareness, and even in the absence of awareness. Most students of man's mental life agree that he is greatly influenced by unrecognized psychological forces and that much behavior originates from motives of which one is not aware in his normal waking state. Psychological motivations are undoubtedly a result usually of combinations of causes, of which those least acceptable socially and morally possess the greatest driving force and are farthest removed from consciousness, whereas those which the individual considers the most acceptable are in the forefront of consciousness and are manifest.

The Unconscious

In order to explain many mental phenomena, the features of which are not manifest, it is necessary to hypothesize the existence of a stratum of the personality referred to as "the unconscious." It includes material that under ordinary circumstances does not enter the conscious part of the personality. For the most part, those drive states determining behavior to satisfy the physiological needs of man operate unconsciously. The diabetic favors foods containing sugar, drinks excessively, and urinates frequently due to his defect in sugar metabolism and its ultimate influence on the body's fluid balance. All this behavior is determined beyond the level of conscious awareness. The individual only knows consciously what he does or must do to remain comfortable.

Various psychological drives exist beyond conscious awareness and are manifested in such forms as dreams, amnesias, purposeful forgetting, mistakes, split personality, and other phenomena. There is abundant evidence that unconscious drives exercise a fundamental influence upon behavior, feelings, decisions, and interpersonal relationships. In psychopathological states, it is particularly apparent that unconscious psychic forces are powerfully active in influencing personality. Emotional forces of which the individual is unaware may be in conflict and act in such a way as to determine his behavior, even though he knows nothing about them consciously.

As will be discussed later, conscious and unconscious forces or motivations may pursue opposite goals. Much behavior, in fact, is a complex of conscious and unconscious motivations. It is only through active repression or through dissociation that any sharp division is produced between the "conscious" and the "unconscious." A great deal of our knowledge concerning motivations has been acquired by the psychoanalytic method of studying the unconscious through free-association technique. Some psychiatrists raise the question whether, instead of speaking of the unconscious, one should not emphasize unconscious mental processes.

The Preconscious

The "preconscious" is a term applied to mental processes which are not conscious but possess the attribute of easy recall to consciousness. Unconscious mental processes differ in that they do not have access to consciousness except under special conditions, such as psychoanalytic therapy or the psychoses.

BIBLIOGRAPHY

Alexander, F., and Ross, H. (eds.): Dynamic Psychiatry. Chicago, The University of Chicago Press, 1952.

Allport, G. W.: The trend in motivational theory. Am. J. Orthopsychiat., 23:107–119, 1953.

Bailey, P.: Janet and Freud. Arch. Neurol. & Psychiat., 76:76–89, 1956.

Bernheim, H.: Suggestive Therapeutics. New York, London Book Co., 1947.

Cannon, W. B.: Bodily Changes in Pain, Hunger, Fear and Rage, 2nd ed. New York, D. Appleton Co., 1929.

Freud, S.: New Introductory Lectures on Psychoanalysis. New York, W. W. Norton & Co., 1933.

Hunt, J. McV.: Personality and the Behavior Disorders. New York, The Ronald Press, 1944.

Hebb, D. O.: A Textbook of Psychology. Philadelphia, W. B. Saunders Company, 1958.

Janet, P. M. F.: Psychological Healing. New York, The Macmillan Company, 1925.

Jones, E.: The Life and Work of Sigmund Freud. 3 Vols. New York, Basic Books, 1953–1957.

Lief, A. (ed.): The Commonsense Psychiatry of Adolf Meyer. New York, McGraw-Hill Book Co., Inc., 1948.

MacLean, P. D.: Contrasting functions of limbic and neocortical systems of the brain and their relevance to psychophysiological aspects of medicine. Am. J. Med., 25:611–626, 1958.

Murphy, G.: Personality: A Biosocial Approach to Origins and Structure. New York, Harper & Brothers, 1947.

Oberndorf, C. P.: A History of Psychoanalysis in America. New York, Grune & Stratton, Inc., 1953.

Scott, J. P.: Animal Behavior. Chicago, The University of Chicago Press, 1958.

Taylor, J. (ed.): Selected Writings of John Hughlings Jackson. Vols. I, II. New York, Basic Books, Inc., 1958.

Tinbergen, N.: The Study of Instinct. Oxford, Clarendon Press, 1951.

Winters, E. (ed.): The Collected Papers of Adolf Meyer. Vols. I–IV. Baltimore, Johns Hopkins Press, 1950–1952.

Chapter Three

PERSONALITY DEVELOPMENT

"During man's growth, mere individuality becomes personality: and the developed individual personality is not only the most complex type of organization known, and one which exhibits a far greater range of diversity among its members than any other single type of organization, but the highest product of evolution of which we have any knowledge."

Julian Huxley

Each organism undergoes a process of development of biological structure from the time of the fusion of the male and female germ cells until adult maturity has been reached. At any time during this biological development, noxious factors may limit the growth of the organism, produce malformations, or impair the functioning of an organ or of the entire living being. Each person, therefore, has an anatomical structure conforming in general to the species pattern yet unique in certain details. Also, he has more or less enduring and consistent patterns of temperament, character, intelligence, beliefs, desires, and adaptational tendencies which give him an individual uniqueness. As defined before, the distinctive whole formed by the integration of these relatively permanent patterns and tendencies of a given individual is spoken of as "personality." In its consideration it will

be helpful to apply the concepts of developmental evolution and functioning.

To a limited extent, certain patterns are already laid down at birth, yet for the most part only the potentialities for the development of personality components exist at that time. Whether the successive stages of the unfolding personality proceed in a wholesome manner and in a normative, harmonious sequence of biopsychological and biosocial maturation through infancy, childhood, maturity, and old age with realization of personal potentialities, subjective satisfactions, and social adaptations, or whether there is an arrest or uneven growth of various personality components depends upon complex genetic, environmental, social, and emotional factors. In personality development, there is normally a maturational sequence, each stage developing as a logical sequel to the previous one—an emergent growth through distinctively different stages, each having its particular needs and problems. If residues of an earlier stage are carried over to later ones, they may serve to produce malformations of the personality and to become a source of psychopathology. Early experiences also continue to exert their influence on the developing personality, even though they are not available to conscious recall.

Genes cannot transmit acquired characteristics. Although the biological development of the fetus may be influenced by the intrauterine environment, there is no reason to believe that personality, as just defined, is largely influenced by prenatal life or even that it exists in the newborn infant. This statement does not deny a genetic anlage or congenital aspects of biochemistry and reactivity which create biological predispositions to the temperamental components of personality in later life. However, while extreme abnormalities in vegetative, central nervous, and endocrine systems may have a demonstrable relation to personality characteristics, there seems to be little relation between them and persistent features of the normal personality.

It is difficult to state just when evidences of personality formation appear. However, it is certain that maturity of personality is attained only through successive stages of maturation. The processes of maturation and personality development involve several steps or phases which are not separate and distinct but may be distinguished for purposes of discussion. There is a process of repeated relinquishment and supersedure of an earlier pattern of functioning or conduct by another pattern more appropriate to the growing, developing, aging individual. Personality development is, therefore, an ongoing process of maturation which may be stunted, distorted, or even prematurely developed. Issues at one level must be dealt with fairly conclusively before those of a higher level can be managed. Each stage of development, too, should be characterized by patterns of thinking and feeling appropriate to it.

PERSONALITY STRUCTURE

It is convenient to think of personality as having parts or divisions which perform specific functions—as having structure. Such a concept facilitates the idea of dynamics in the functioning of the personality. However, these parts must not be considered as concrete realities or self-acting entities but as groups of forces and functions. The concept of personality structure now generally followed is that proposed by Freud who postulated three psychic segments in the structure of the personality. While these structural divisions are hypothetical, they offer a useful classification of the systems of drives. Many of the terms used in describing their dynamic interrelationships are highly figurative.

The Id

The "id" is a collective name for the primitive biological impulses. It represents the innately given portion of the personality. The physiologically determined drives for air, food, water, and other nutrient substances, maintenance of bodily temperature and physical integrity, and procreation are thought of as id functions. Thus dependent longings, aggressive and flight tendencies, rage, and sexuality are thought of as id drives and affects. When ego functions are maldeveloped or impaired, id impulses may erupt into consciousness either as fantasy or in more overt expressions.

The Ego

The "ego," or reality-testing self, is that part or function of the personality which establishes a relationship with the world in which we live. The ego, of course, is a group of functions for which a metaphor is employed for ease of conceptualization. The ego deals with the environment through conscious perception, thought, feeling, and action and is, therefore, the consciously controlling portion of the personality. It contains the evaluating, judging, compromising, solution-forming, and defense-creating aspects of the personality. The ego organization concerned with such important functions as perception, memory, evaluating and testing of reality, synthesizing of experience and of acting as intermediary between the inner and outer worlds, may be regarded as the integrative and executive agency of the personality. The ego develops by a gradual learning process and is determined largely by the individual's interactional processes occurring between himself and others. Its functions are to deal rationally with the requirements of reality, to adapt behavior to the environment and other reality situations, and to maintain harmony between the urges of the id and the demands and aspirations of the superego.

For normal development and functioning of the personality, the ego must be able to modify both the id drives and the superego's demands for acceptable conduct without extreme sacrifice either of satisfactions of emotional and instinctive needs or of ethical ideals. In this way the ego serves as mediator and directs behavior into acceptable compromises between the blind drives of the id and the inhibitions of the superego. The guiding role of the id is that of the *pleasure-principle*, but that of the ego is the *reality-principle*, i.e., the demands of the external world to which practical adaptation must be made.

The ego directs instinctual energy into channels which will, in the long run, bring the maximum pleasure and satisfaction. Its processes take place largely, but not entirely, at the conscious level. It constructively integrates impulses and thus secures mastery over them. If, through conscious control, it deals effectively with inner and outer stresses, and through reason and circumspection it deals rationally with the requirements of reality and of society, the ego is said to be "strong and healthy."

A "strong ego" achieves an integration of the demands of the id, the superego, and reality. It modifies or sublimates primitive urges into socially acceptable patterns. The individual with a "strong ego" shows flexibility in handling the various stresses of life without resorting to inflexible and repetitive defenses that distinguish neurotic or psychotic symptoms or to characterological defects. If the ego is "weak" and dominated by unconscious factors, it may undergo disintegrative processes. It may be unable to withstand the strain of continued repression with the result that mental symptoms or characterological defects appear.

The Superego

The third hypothetical segment of the personality structure is the "superego" or inhibiting and conscience-including component of the personality. The superego functions to sustain the internalized moral and social values. It is a conceptualized advisor, admonisher, and threatener with both conscious and unconscious aspects. The basic process of organization of this function of the personality is advanced by the age of five, but it continues to develop through adolescence and probably through young adult years. During this period, figures of authority capable of punishing or rewarding become incorporated into the personality to form the distinguishable part known as the "superego."

It is derived particularly from identification with parents and their substitutes. The prohibitions and obligations noted in these identifications are internalized and incorporated into the unconscious psychological structure of the child. Later, the injunctions and prohibitions of other authorities and of cultural influences are absorbed into the superego, the whole acting as censor. The ascetic and moral demands of one's social group become introjected and organized into an uncompromising, unconscious, internal inhibitory law of which the superego is the personification. It acts as the supervisor of the ego and of inner, unconscious tendencies and, therefore, as the repressing part of the personality. It criticizes the ego and causes pain to it whenever the latter tends to accept impulses from the repressed part of the id. The superego may contain irrational and even sadistic elements. It may threaten and punish and thereby seek to maintain its authority. It does this by creating anxiety and by producing guilt and remorse. If the superego is severe and inflexible, the resulting fear of it will lead to a rigid, inhibited, unhappy, anxious, and often neurotic personality.

A closely related aspect of superego function is that of the ego ideal, the internalized picture of what one desires to become, the idealized image toward which the ego strives. Thus the superego pushes toward the aspirations sustained in the ego ideal of the individual. Such ideals again are gained through the identifications imposed by the growing child's contacts with parents, teachers, and others significant to him in both elder and peer groups.

Balance of Segments

In the well-adjusted person, his behavior simultaneously and successfully meets the demands of the id, the ego, and the superego. On the other hand, the behavior of the neurotic, the psychotic, and the pathological personality with serious and repetitive social maladjustment may be conceived of as resulting from a disturbance in the dynamic checks and balances of the id, the ego, and the superego.

PERIOD OF INFANCY

While the physiological needs of the human infant are innately determined, their satisfaction both in the prenatal period and for a prolonged period after birth is dependent entirely upon maternal care-giving. The ongoing dependent relationship of the infant establishes from the very beginning of extra-uterine life the association with others from which derive the forces that mold his personality and his eventual capacities for social adaptation.

Maternal Dependency

"Objects relations," that is, relations with others, are no longer considered to exist only after a year or so of life. They are initiated with the first acts of mothering which are centered on satisfying the infant's needs for food and warmth. They demand from the mother constant attention to maintain the child's comfort through avoiding the irritations caused by wet and dirty clothing or exposure to other damaging forces around him. Thus maternal care is directed to much more than satisfying the "oral" needs of the infant who, in turn, must be envisaged as sensing in the early days not only just through the oral mucosa and perioral musculature but also by means of the general tactile–kinesthetic sensory systems which are known to be myelinated at the time of birth. The early interactions between most mothers and infants extend beyond that of satisfying these basic physiological needs, since the infant is stimulated by the play of the mother, by the fondling he receives, and also by the attempt to gain from him by facial gestures and verbal signs some indications of response. As early as three or four months the infant responds differently to people; he is in contact with those upon whom his life depends.

In the first several years of life, the responses to the immediate discomforts of the infant dominate his behavior. He demands, through his crying, immediate help in relief of his tensions, whether they are induced through external discomfort or from internal unrest. The infant may be described as directed by the "pleasure principle," unable to delay his demands. Until he is several years old, he will not be able to delay the urgency of his need for relief and to accept delay in response for some future gain or greater satisfaction of desires in terms of the perceived problems and goals and the problems of others—that is, to be guided by the "reality principle." The persistence into later life of emotional states characterized by dependency and the immediacy and urgency of demands, with absence of responsibility for or consideration of others and associated with stages of rage when the need is not met, may be identified then as *infantile*.

This early mothering process, if warm

and consistent, lays the groundwork for a continuing sense of satisfaction, security, and trust in others, while its absence, as Erickson suggests, may establish the early roots of mistrust and insecurity. These are the origins of ego attitudes significant for carrying the infant through later stages of growth.

It may be surmised as well that the intermittent contacts with the mother, alternating with states of discomfort and comfort, establish those varying sensory experiences that set down the infant's slowly growing discriminations of self from another, the basis for a sense of space, and also the rhythms that establish time as a modality.

The descriptions given before of the transactions between growing infant and mother as providing the sensory experiences and thus the basic percepts making for personality emphasize the current interest in precise study of development. They contrast with the early psychoanalytic theories of growth with their greater reliance on answers based upon instinctual urges and drives centered around certain libidinous zones.

The period of infancy is described in psychoanalytic terms as the *oral stage*, which is conceived of as progressing from an essentially "receptive" to an "aggressive" phase. Prior to birth, the infant is fed through the maternal blood stream and has never experienced the satisfying pleasure provided by the gratification of an instinctual need. With birth, however, a biological need for food arises and he receives satisfaction through sucking. Not only is the discomfort from hunger relieved by this sucking, but, as other and more complex tensions arise, the infant turns to the most available substitute as a source of security and satisfaction and therefore sucks his thumb. The mouth becomes, accordingly, the part of the body in which interests, sensations, and activities are centered and through which gratification is secured. The second phase (from about eight to eighteen months of age) of the oral stage is that in which the pleasure of biting is added to that of sucking, and when one may hypothesize that aggressive drives appear.

AUTO-EROTISM. It is conceivable that the oral satisfaction secured from nursing may be the first primitive manifestation of what through many subsequent stages of development will ultimately become adult heterosexuality. At this stage, however, the pleasure seeking is related to the mouth and contains no discernible relation to the genitals as in the adult. To speak of this oral phase as the first stage of psychosexual development is figurative and not actual, but has become an accepted term in psychoanalytic terminology.

Because of its pleasure-giving potentiality at this stage of psychosexual development, the mouth is spoken of as an erogeneous zone. Satisfactions thus secured from such pleasure-giving zones are called *auto-erotic*. Too little or inconsistent "psychological mothering" is apt to promote auto-erotism in the form of prolonged or excessive thumb-sucking, constipation, or early and excessive masturbation. On the other hand, consistent and healthy emotional satisfactions in the child's relationships to his parents shorten the auto-erotic period of development and promote a natural sublimation of the instinctive drives—a wholesome progress in the successive stages of these aspects of personality development and differentiation.

ORAL PERSONALITY. If the individual, far beyond the age when the mouth should have ceased to be a focus of satisfaction, continues to be mouth-centered, he is said to be of an oral type of personality. Although this stage of personality development is one of dependency, in which the child gives nothing, it is a normal one unless it is pathologically prolonged.

Sexuality

Since the pleasure derived from the satisfaction of psychological and physiological impulses is a matter of much importance in personality functioning and the means of securing this satisfaction an indicator of the degree of personality development, Freud attributed a predominant place to this phase of personality to which he applied the term "sexuality." The selection of this term for pleasure-seeking impulses was unfortunate since it erroneously carries the implications that have become associated with the word through its usual application to adult genital sexuality and pleasure.

In using the term "infantile sexuality," Freud never attributed to infants and children the complex pattern of adult sexuality. If the restricted, even figurative, use of the term sexuality is borne in mind, one may, following the terminology of Freud, trace an orderly and step-by-step development of the psychosexual aspect of personality from its earliest expression to a mature, heterosexual, socially approved mating upon the basis of which the family is founded. These psychoanalytical concepts have laid the basis for, and stimulated, the later studies of personality development.

Aggression

As mentioned in the foregoing discussion, the initial manifestations of aggression may be thought of as taking place during the oral stage of psychosexual development. Even at a very tender age, the nursling is not a mere passive recipient of his mother's milk. On the contrary, the milk is secured by a surprisingly vigorous activity. According to this point of view, aggression makes its first appearance in personality traits characterized by energy, application, and determination and is of a constructive nature. Some stress that aggression arises relatively later in personality development and only as a reaction to frustration, particularly to the frustrations which the child inevitably feels that he suffers at the hands of parents during the process of being brought up. Undoubtedly, there are many occasions in the child's life for developing resentments and aggressive impulses against a frustrating parent.

Body Ego or Image

The maturing infant gives evidence by his responses to others of his perception of the world about him by the third or fourth month. He perceives smiles and returns them, showing the beginning of learning of the expressions of emotion through gestures. By the sixth month, the child is capable of binocular vision and the appreciation of vision at a distance. Also co-ordinate activity is possible between several parts of the body; earlier, eyes turn toward sound, and now so does the body. At the same time, hand and arm movements are well co-ordinated, and the hand brings objects to the mouth easily. This is the beginning of the infant's exploration of his own body, first with the mouth and then the hand. These perceptions, largely tactile and kinesthetic sensations in the early months, establish for him the integrated percept of his physical wholeness which has been designated psychoanalytically as the *body ego*.

BODILY PERCEPTIONS. It must be recalled that the child not only develops bodily perceptions over time which are modified gradually and extended in the course of growth so as to conform with the current body structure, but also takes unto himself the attitudes of others toward his body and its parts. He may develop a satisfying body concept or come to view his body and its parts as unpleasant, dirty, shameful, or disgusting, by which he reflects the interaction between himself, the parental figures and, later, other significant persons. The child's concept of his body will form a nuclear structure of his later personality and will, to a large part, determine his capacity to adapt successfully to the stress of illness, trauma, and physical changes. It is worth while to discriminate those percepts of the body surface and parts which establish the image of the body. These are largely unconscious and function not only to position the body in space and as to the manipulative objects it may control but also to allow knowledge of its surface from those attitudes which one develops towards one's body. The former is best designated as the *body percept* and the latter as the *body concept*. Both are constituted in the commonly used term *body image*.

EARLY SENSORY EXPERIENCES. That a body percept exists is fully demonstrated by the persistence of sensing a limb after amputation or the hallucination of other external parts after their loss—the phantom phenomena. Also the failure to experience over time early body percepts, due to surgical or accidental dismemberments performed in infants and young children, is associated with absence of "phantoms." One must know a body part, experience it through perceptions, in order later to have hallucinatory images of the body or its parts.

The importance of early infantile sensory experiences in effecting the functioning growth of various integrative systems in the brain is established by other clinical and experimental observations. The most convincing illustration has to do with the permanent defects in vision which occur in children with congenital cataracts but intact retina and visual apparatus who fail to have the corneal defect repaired by implanting of a healthy transparent cornea before five years of age. Such children are unable to develop adequate vision, while others with earlier transplants go through long periods of learning before they can perceive accurately and recognize formed images. Artificial blinding of infant chimpanzees with later uncovering of the eyes has reduplicated these findings.

There appears, then, to be a critical period in infancy for experiencing certain sensations and establishing the neural patterns required for later functional maturation of various sensory systems. Much more knowledge is needed of the nature of deficits caused by infantile sensory deprivations, critical periods of growth in various systems, and capacity and means for correcting the functional impairments. Undoubtedly, this information will influence our appreciation of the etiology of many personality problems as well as the treatment of such defects.

The focus of maternal attention gradually shifts from the giving of food to assisting the child develop his maturing capacity for motility, the manipulation of objects with his hands, and later walking and speaking. Coincident with this phase of maturation, the interaction between the child and mother centers over the effort to have the child learn to control his eliminative activities; it is bladder and bowel centered.

Special meanings are supported by the maternal attitudes that dictate the manner by which the mother attempts to instruct her child in these first efforts at personal autonomy. If, for example, urinary or bowel control is attempted before physiological maturation with myelination of the necessary pathways in the spinal cord has made the child capable of recognizing, announcing, or controlling his need to eliminate, or before the child can walk to the toilet or manipulate his clothing, and if the child is punished for his failures, rage or fear will be directed toward the controlling parent. The child then centers his attention on the power struggle between himself and the parent. He may respond with fear of the parent and gradually evolve a pattern of cleanliness, orderliness, submissiveness, and punctuality sometimes referred to as the "anal character." Or again, his subjective response may be one of rage with the evolving defiant reactions of dirtiness, obstinacy, and unreliability. Most frequently the response to the usual mothering process is vacillating, and most often the fear-dominated complex gains in ascendency.

From the experiences in this period of interaction, the beginnings of the capacities for self control, personal independence, and a sense of autonomy and pride may be envisaged. With them arise the learned affects of shame and disgust which are incorporated in response to the parents' attitudes towards the child's excretory functions and are communicated to him through various means. Shame must be recognized as an important infantile emotion, learned by early training—a feeling of being exposed, looked at, and being the object of disgust. Too much shaming may lead to defiant shamelessness as a character trait.

Psychoanalytic theory describes this period as the *anal stage* of psychosexual development. With the termination of the nursing period, the mouth begins to share its pleasure-giving role with that of the organs of elimination. Not until that age does the child's ever-widening awareness extend to and include this function. The interest in excrement and excretory functions which appears at this stage of maturation is probably an illustration of the fact that the exercise of primary body functions is a source of pleasure. The retention and passage of feces leads to pleasurable irritation of the anal zone. The child becomes as much interested in his excretory functions as the parent is in controlling them. The mother, on the other hand, has the usual adult's feeling of revulsion for excreta, not yet at all shared by the child.

Probably conscious cortical control of the rectal sphincter is not fully developed until after cortical development makes standing and walking possible. This period of interest and gratification in the processes of elimination is one of normal physiological and psychological development. If the mother, unmindful of these pleasurable elements and unaware that toilet training is not possible until a certain stage of nervous system development has occurred, and before the child has a sign language with which to make his wants known, attempts to enforce training by severe and punitive repression of the pleasure-giving impulses, conflictful emotions are aroused in such intensity as to influence permanently personality development.

ANAL PERSONALITY. Thus an extremely rigid and severe toilet training combined with special pleasures secured through the child's control of excretory functions may produce the fixation in personality development mentioned earlier as the anal type of personality. It is in a fixation at this stage of personality development that are thought to exist the roots of the adult compulsive neurosis with its uncontrollable impulse to perform certain obsessional acts and the ambivalence of personal attitudes.

PERIOD OF CHILDHOOD

For purposes of descriptive analysis and study it is useful to make the distinctions between various periods of growth. Yet these distinctions are arbitrary and it must be clearly kept in mind that stages of maturation gradually melt one into another; there are no real distinctions. Childhood is here conceived as beginning with the capacity to speak—sometimes between the end of the first year and during the second year of life. Of course, it runs coincidently with those processes of maturation concerned with increasing motility of the child, his growing capacity for elimination and control of excrements, but also marks a major shift in his interpersonal relations as he now grows beyond signalling by means of cries or those early gestures learned in later infancy.

As has already been intimated, the child's emotional growth is dependent upon the existence of a consistent and warm "psychological mothering" which promotes the gradual unfolding of healthy, emotional, social, and ethical development, free from irreversible anxiety and tension. A wholesome mother–child relationship is as vital for emotional growth and personality development as vitamins are for physical maturation.

Since the earliest experiences of the child occur in the family setting, his perceptions and interpretations of these experiences will determine his attitudes toward and evaluations of later, even adult, experiences that contain some apparent similarities. Such a *transference* of an attitude derived from some personal relationship in the family to others in the larger world will exert either favorable or unfavorable influences on his relations with others and thus upon ability to reach his ultimate social goals. Persistent attitudes of resentment of hostility built into personality structure through the early experiences may form the repetitive responses of the neurotic in later life and the focus upon which paralyzing reaction-formations are built. For example, if a young child sees a comforting and protecting mother repeatedly hurt or made to cry by a cruel father, he may acquire a lasting hatred for the father and later transfer this attitude to all men who resemble him in some way. Again, if the mother is vacillating in her care, sometimes comforting and at other times cruel, the child will be unable to make clear discriminations from which ambivalent attitudes of love and hatred will emerge.

A major determinant in personality development is the unconscious modeling of the growing child upon the parents, spoken of as *identification*. The child "identifies" with the perceived aspects of the behavior of the parent; included are those which arouse tension or pleasure, the overrated body parts, actions and capacities which, in the child's growing fantasies, probably give the parent the strength and power he wishes for himself. If the parents are emotionally mature persons, the adaptive process of identification promotes healthy growth.

The widening ability of the child to care for himself now brings him greater relationship with the father and other siblings in the family; his social development extends beyond that of the primary relationship with the mother. With this period of expanding social contact there evolves the necessity to share. In these experiences with others, the associated emotions of jealousy, rage, envy, and guilt develop. His greater activity provides him the opportunity of exercising his exploratory tendencies, his curiosity and initiative at solving simple problems. Differences are discerned between the sexes, and the foundations for eventual sexual identification are laid down. The striving for the first place in affection and acquisition, from the mother against the father and in a struggle with brothers and sisters establishes competitive rivalries that stimulate those wish-fulfilling dreams and fantasies of overwhelming strength and reward, or later, the fear of retaliation, of harm and attack from others.

With the striving initiative of the child and the arousal of the emotions, of jealous rage and anger, there also emerges the super ego, *conscience*. In the face of his struggles the child is curbed by one or both parents, often the father, and in turn develops both feelings of hatefulness and those adaptations of escape from retaliatory attack that may be retained in some form to adulthood—sulking, withdrawal, and finally the internalization of the prohibitions against his expressions of anger.

For psychoanalysis, this period represents the *phallic stage*. Attention has already been called to the theory that at about one year of age the source of pleasure shifts from the oral to the anal region. Similarly, at about three years of age there appears another stage in the development of pleasurable interest with a shift of source from the anal to the genital region. This phase continues until about the seventh year. With the advent of this phase, there is a concern with the difference between sexes and the size, presence, or absence of the phallic organs. There is a predominance of genital sensations, and masturbation may become a source of psychosexual pleasure. The interest is not a sexual one in the adult sense of the term. The boy merely comes to realize that his penis is important and devotes narcissistic attention to it. The girl may become aware that she has no penis and believes she had one but lost it, with the result that she develops feelings of inferiority and jealousy. The oral, anal, and phallic stages of libido development are often spoken of as the pregenital stages.

OEDIPUS COMPLEX.   Continuous throughout the phallic stage up to the fifth or sixth year there exists a period of attraction to the parent of the opposite sex accompanied by jealousy and rivalrous hostility toward the parent of the same sex. To this situation between father, mother, and child, Freud gave the term *Oedipus complex*. Various anthropologists reject the universality of the Oedipus complex. That it is, however, a basically correct psychological feature of our own culture is generally accepted. Some suggest that the Oedipus reaction is determined by the behavior of the parents, not of the child. It is certainly frequently true that fathers are more severe with their sons and more indulgent with their daughters. That mothers frequently reverse this relationship is constantly observed by psychiatrists. In either case, the rivalry and hostility associated with the Oedipus reaction would follow quite naturally. Others regard the Oedipus period as a convenient and expressive metaphorical term for designating the phase of personality development in which the child feels and expresses hostility against one of the parents because of the frustrations experienced.

Normally, this potentially pathogenic relation is resolved by the mechanisms of identification in which the boy identifies with his father and incorporates the father's goals and standards into his own pattern of behavior. Likewise the girl identifies with her mother, advances toward a healthy emotional maturation, and finds gratification and security in a feminine role.

From clinical observation, it is frequently recognized that when the Oedipus complex is inadequately resolved, the individual may introject some of the qualities of the parent of the opposite sex, with the result that the development of "normal" relationships with persons of the opposite sex is precluded. Familiar examples are the adult son who lives with a widowed mother and is oblivious to the charm of women of his own age, or the young man who falls in love with a woman much older than he and who in some way resembles his mother. Psychoanalytically it is said that such fixation occurs at the homosexual stage of personality development.

Socialization Period

Later childhood, that period from six or seven to twelve, is one in which the child's socialization is relegated to others outside the family in our Western culture. The influence of teachers as authority figures outside the home, of older and younger playmates, of other relatives and friends provide important opportunities for new identifications and discriminations which allay, modify, or intensify the patterns of behavioral reactions established in the family and also offer opportunities for the acquisition of new skills and roles. The child is eager to do things; he has the opportunity to learn habits of industry. Yet, if he fails to gain the patterns and otherwise measure up to his peers in school and on the playground, a sense of inferiority is instilled. His play activities provide him the opportunity for gaining pleasure in mastering tasks and, for some, that of prestige in accomplishment. Group play activities allow the gradual growth and pleasure in the companionship of others, in sharing their problems. The era carries with it as well the learning of other patterns of group behavior, those of teasing, disparagement, and ostracism. If the juvenile suffers as a consequence of group actions, his responses may seem to deepen the already existing personality reactions to frustrations at home.

At this time in the child's life, his sexual curiosity is limited; this is the latency period of psychoanalytic psychosexual development. While sex interests and activities do not disappear, there are no such marked and significant psychosexual changes as are seen in both the preceding and following periods. The child does, however, identify more strongly than before with the parent of the same sex and begins more differentiation along masculine and feminine lines. Therefore at this time it is important that there be close association with a parent or some other satisfactory person of the same sex with whom the child may identify in establishing masculinity or femininity. This period is notably one of training in the customs and attitudes of society. There is a progressive development of the ego as a result of growth on the one hand and of education and experience on the other. It is a period during which ideals are formed. The child is exposed to more complex social pressures; also environmental opportunities play an important part in directing individual interests and capacities. In the latter part of the latency period, a quest for status becomes a strong motivating force. It is, too, the period when inner control of aggressive–destructive impulses should be attained.

PERIOD OF ADOLESCENCE

With growing group relations, the juvenile often develops an intense interest in one other child, usually of the same sex. This interest extends to consideration of the feelings and sensitivities of the friend. It represents the first efforts at those intimate contacts which occur in adulthood. This interest in the friend extends to satisfying his wishes as well as being moved and interested in his successes and failures. Groups of juveniles get together and the learning of the roles of leader and supporter occur. These social interactions provide satisfaction and security for the growing youngster.

Adolescence, proper, sets in with puberty, with its rapid physiological development of the sex organs. The maturation of sexual and reproductive capacities stimulates genital and heterosexual interests and activities in the genital stage of psychosexual development. Sexuality is no longer diffused throughout the body as in the pregenital phases of personality development but becomes focalized on the genital organs. The sexual area, however, is only one aspect of the personality in which there is an inherent drive toward maturation.

The growing adolescent is now preoccupied with the manner in which he appears to others and how he perceives himself. He is in search of a *personal identity*, a sense of self. Since the adolescent stands midway between personal independence and continuance of dependence on the parents, many acts of emancipatory behavior occur. Of these the effort to establish a sexual identification leads the boy to seek reinforcement with men or other older boys who are over-idealized, while the girl finds similar sources for her growing femininity. Over-aggressive and competitive attitudes, exhibitionistic poses, or the engaging in cynical and antisocial acts may represent these struggles for a masculine independence from authority at home. There now usually occurs a searching out of members of the other sex with courting as a preparation for eventual intimacy and mating. These adolescent interests break up the more juvenile friendships and call upon the adolescent to relive the experiences of early life with both pleasure in the affection of another and also the emotions of sadness and jealous hatefulness when his friendships break up. Concomitant with his sexual drive, the adolescent develops a fantasy life filled with fulfillment of his desires, yet finds himself in conflict between the latter and the prohibitions of his family and society.

ADULTHOOD AND MATURITY

While chronological age may be recognized legally as an indication of responsible maturity, it is no guarantee of the emotional growth of the individual. The mature adult will be one who has developed a clear personal identity, demonstrated by an ability for an intimate, satisfying, and loving relationship with a mature member of the opposite sex and a personal assumption of the responsibilities of rearing children. He is able both to assume personal responsibilities when necessary and to accept the decisions of those with competent authority for the general good. He independently pursues his own goals, with recognition of his limitations and with willingness to seek advice from others when indicated, and is able to maintain and enjoy his personal relations with others, making due allowances for their deficits with an understanding tolerance. The healthy adult is one who is absorbed and satisfied in achievement relative to his family, vocation, and avocations rather than in personal self-assertions. He functions well at home and at work in terms of developing gratifying relations with others as well as in being generally free of symptoms of illness.

Problems of Maturity

In all periods of adult life, the conflicts that come recapitulate those of earlier life. For the young adult, these struggles center largely over the necessity for making decisions relative to the selection of a mate and then of vocational choice. In each instance the young adult may find himself in conflict between his personal drives and estimates of capacity and opportunity and those expressed by his parents or their representatives. Anxieties that develop in arriving at these decisions may adversely affect both marital and vocational life. Undue dependence upon the parents, if marriage is consummated, will deprive the marital partner of the needed tenderness and attentiveness required to establish a satisfying and growth-promoting home. Attitudes of unusual submissiveness or defiance, originating in the relations to parents and teachers, are likely to be transferred to those in authority in the vocational world. In turn, these may lead either to derogatory attitudes toward the defiant young adult or to failure of associates to recognize potentialities of the submissive person that might lead to advancement. The birth of children often rearouses the sibling rivalries of earlier years in one or both parents with either reappearance of inappropriate hostilities or resurgence of infantile demands.

In middle adulthood, with advancement to senior positions, the rearousal of sibling rivalries leads to paralyzing anxieties over envy and hostility suspected in peers, or to overbearing attitudes of revenge for their assumed earlier punitiveness. Failures to be advanced also bring forth hostilities and resentments that can lead to sulky withdrawal, depression, or accusations of favoritism or influence. Women are exposed to the conflicts centered on a waning sexuality and inability to bear children through their arriving at the menopause. Later life poses again the problems of resurgent dependence with surrender of personal responsibility due to increasing physical weakness or relinquishment of positions of power and prestige, with consequent recurrence of drives of rivalry and the anxieties consequent upon impending death.

Separation and Death

One of the major emotional problems of the elderly, but one to which men are exposed throughout all periods of life, is that of separation from those whom he loves and upon whom rest residual dependencies. Mourning, the period of grief that follows loss through death, an important separation, or even the loss of a body part such as in amputation, must be regarded as a process of anxiety with restitution and re-establishment of the personality in the face of the loss. During the mourning process the intensity of grief leads to both physiological and psychological disturbances which are evidenced in the personal withdrawal from others and the preoccupation with the loss. The process of mourning provides the psychological effort to maintain the lost object by fantasy reviewing of the experiences, meanings, and emotional significance of the relationship and the eventual taking in of certain qualities derived from the association.

Older people frequently suffer this process and may defend themselves against it by adopting attitudes of personal omnipotence and pride in self-sustenance or may be recurrently overcome by overt anxiety and other defenses against it.

For the infant and child, death of another upon whom they are dependent leads to profound emotional disturbances as Spitz, Bowlby, and others have demonstrated.

The growing child's appreciation of death is not that of the adult's, however; until the age of five or thereabouts death is perceived as a departure, a further existence under other conditions, without finality, to which the separated child responds by asking for the lost person. The child at this time interprets the loss frequently as a malignant, premeditated act to which he responds with the emotions of both sadness and rage. He is taught to repress these emotions. Later, between five and ten, children tend to personify death as someone who carries others off, a fearful person. It is only after this age that death is recognized as a universal process with final dissolution of life.

Deaths in the family through suicide or illness or threats of suicide occurring in the life of young children may be perceived by him as hateful or manipulative acts and, in turn, lead to retaliatory fantasies, which form the basis for later suicidal thoughts and acts that have as their motive revenge.

Thus mourning and separation anxiety must be recognized as regular emotional responses to a loss with a recognizable course of development and resolutions. Mourning for adults runs a course of six to twelve months and is differentiated from depression.

FACTORS INFLUENCING EMOTIONAL RESPONSE

Early Environment

While the *only child* may develop well and has often been reported to be superior to others in terms of health, physique, intelligence, and facility at school, his emotional position in the family exposes him to the full intensity of any emotional disturbances that may exist in the parents. As an only child, he may represent the parents' single effort to appear as sexually mature adults and thus he represents a denial of interested and wanted parenthood. The parents' exploitative drives are channeled into the only child, and their over-solicitude leads to an excessive protection, which further isolates him from his peers. He is shorn of the learning experiences of living and sharing with siblings, which is followed frequently by the arousal of fantasies of brothers and sisters. With others of his own age, he may be shy and awkward, thus leading to teasing and rejection, which induces either further withdrawal or over-compensatory efforts for gaining attention and prestige. Such efforts may be expressed either in exhibitionistic activities, boastfulness, or bribery of others

if the means exist. His isolation often leads to the persistence of childish dependency on others, which impairs his capacity for adult relations.

The *institutionalized child* is often exposed as well to an environment unfavorable to emotional maturation. Deprived of a close, continuing, and warm emotional contact with an interested mother substitute and later paternal figure, the child reared in an institution lacks the personal stimulation and the opportunity for the growth of affection and trust that permits development later of the capacity for successful relations and identifications with others. Thus impairment occurs in the maturation of both ego and superego functions. It has been found that such children show a greater frequency of problem behavior characterized by lack of control, anxiety, and aggression, and an affective impoverishment. Specifically, they are more restless, overactive, and limited in concentration; others have temper tantrums and may be impudent, cruel, and destructive. More frequently they show impairment of speech and mental activities which resemble retardation and lead to difficulty in school.

Twins, both identical and nonidentical, as well as those born in other multiple sibships, have special problems in personality growth. The maternal attitude to twins is sometimes one of shame and rejection followed later by efforts to explore and differentiate the siblings as a means for the mother to direct appropriately her responses to one or other of the children. The care of twins demands much of the mother; each receives less attention than the single child. Yet this drives the pair together and establishes the matrix which makes it difficult for them to establish independent self-identities. Their constant closeness interferes with their independent learning of social functions. Twins develop more intense rivalry problems to which they may adapt by attaching themselves to one or other parent or, more commonly, by assuming similar desires and thereby repressing their individual drives. The strong jealousy for the parents generated in the relationship intensifies hostile drives toward the other twin which, in turn, require compensatory efforts at repressions that again bring the twins together. While these pressures are not inevitable, they are of frequent occurrence in twin development and make the individual both insecure in his own identity and extremely vulnerable to the loss of his sibling on whom he is usually excessively dependent.

Biological Constitution and
Personality Types

Although not strictly relevant to the subject of development and structure of personality, there are other factors that have been considered as determinative of personality.

Ernst Kretschmer, professor of psychiatry at the University of Tübingen, emphasized the morphological-physiological-psychological unity of the individual. He maintained the hypothesis that a common constitutional matrix links the phenomena of the mind not only with the functions of the brain and endocrine glands but also with the general body structure. According to Kretschmer, the individual's life "style," his attitude and temperamental reaction tendencies are reflections of his physical make-up. Most American psychiatrists do not accept Kretschmer's emphasis on a somatotype approach to personality with its constitutional predestination of the form of mental phenomena, even though he concedes that the content of these phenomena is conditioned by individual experience.

Kretschmer describes four types of physique into which the configuration of the body may often be observed to fall: pyknic, leptosomic, athletic, and dysplastic. The person of *pyknic physique* is characterized by short stature, short, large neck, and stocky, round figure. Persons of this type frequently accumulate superficial fat, particularly on the abdominal walls. Kretschmer states they tend to be of the outgoing, energetic type known as extrovert (page 33). The *leptosomic* is described as a spare, angular, narrowly built person with flattened chest. Visceroptosis is not rare. Leptosomes seem predisposed to be introverts. The secondary sex characteristics are usually not pronounced. Many writers prefer the term asthenic to Kretschmer's designation of leptosomic. The *athletic type* is characterized by strong development of the skeleton and muscles, particularly of the trapezii and those of the lower extremities. Many consider the leptosome and the athletic but extreme varieties of one group. The *dysplastic type* of physique is characterized by aberrations. Among these physical aberrations one finds the myxedematous product of hypothyroidism, growth disorders of pituitary disturbances, infantilism, and eunuchoidism. A large percentage suffer from disturbances of the endocrine glands. Some dysplastics are biological inverts, while other personality anomalies are not rare. In the opinion of some psychiatrists, the incidence of manic-depressive psychosis is higher among pyknics, and schizophrenia is more common among the leptosomic, the athletic, and the dysplastic types. The conclusion is open to question.

Extroversion and Introversion

Psychobiological constitution and personality types have been discussed from the standpoints of physique and of emotional characteristics. The personality may be classified according to psychological type. One of the most widely followed classifications is that of a Swiss psychiatrist, C. G. Jung. This classification is based on the direction toward which the individual turns his fundamental energy-tendencies (libido*). Jung did not, like Freud, regard libido as a drive solely pleasure-striving and sexual in nature but extended it to include all the psychic

* In Freudian theory, libido is conceived of as a force working in the organism to bring about a pleasurable and satisfying state of affairs. Pleasure-strivings, Freud believed, exist from the beginning of extrauterine life and are comparable to the appetite in the nutritional system. About the fourth year this pleasure-striving appears to have, for a period, a relation to adult sexuality; then for a time its sexual goal is not apparent (latency period). At adolescence it again manifests itself as a maturing form of genital activity.

urges of life. Depending upon the direction of this life energy and of interests, Jung spoke of extroversion and introversion. It is usually difficult to formulate the processes of their development.

EXTROVERT. The extrovert is one who concerns himself with objects, persons, and the realities and activities of his environment. He has a pragmatic outlook and his values and activities are governed by the objective facts of his environment. He is more interested in persons than in abstract ideas. He is characteristically energetic, aggressive, enthusiastic, friendly, emotionally responsive to his environment, sociable, and self-confident, and freely expresses his feelings. Often he is an adventurous spirit whose reactions tend to be immediate rather than logical. He is frequently a leader, although more through comradeship and humanism than through creative thoughts. His emotional expression is spontaneous and natural but lacks the delicacy of feeling of the introvert.

INTROVERT. The interest and attention of the introvert are directed, not toward objects and persons about him, but toward himself and his subjective life, although he need not be selfish in the sense of regarding his own advantage at the expense of others. He is reserved and is unable to form the free and easy contacts of the extrovert; in fact, he often seems cold and aloof. Introversion should be regarded as a matter of direction of energy rather than as one of deficient facility in making social contacts, although the introvert's herd instinct is usually less developed than that of the extrovert. The introvert tends to be contemplative, serious, studious, and sensitive. He is usually lacking in self-confidence and boldness of activity. He may become an artist or a philosopher. He has a less practical mind than does the extrovert and often reacts in fantasy to failures and conflicts.

SUBTYPES AND MIXED TYPES. Jung concluded that to divide people into extroverts and introverts was not sufficiently discriminative, since individuals were further characterized by the relative degree to which the fundamental psychological functions, such as thinking, feeling, sensation, and intuition, also determine personality type. He therefore described four subtypes of extrovert: extroverted thinking, extroverted feeling, extroverted sensation, and extroverted intuitive types. He described four subtypes for the introvert in the same manner.

Jung's classification has considerable usefulness, yet most people are not habitually extroverted or introverted in type or reaction. The factors governing the development of personality are too complex to permit such a simple dichotomy. Personalities tend to be distributed between extreme extroversion and extreme introversion, with a majority falling in the middle zone. This is not to say that each individual does not have a certain pattern of inner psychological forces which cause him to develop a characteristic personality.

SUMMARY

The behavior of the individual, whether normal or abnormal, reveals recurring patterns partly determined by constitution but, on the basis of current knowledge, much more by feeling-experiences dynamically built into the personality during childhood. The type and degree of personality development depends on the stability of the family and on the dynamics of the relationships which exist in it. All too often emotional disturbances in the family are perpetuated from generation to generation, thus becoming familial rather than hereditary in nature.

Progressive Maturation

Thus the development of personality has been presented as a complex evolving process in which there occurs a progressive maturation in the emotional, social, intellectual, and physical spheres. This maturation is affected by the interplay of various forces, particularly hereditary, somatic, cultural, and interpersonal ones. In many aspects the maturational process is guided, promoted, or restricted by the progress and degree of emotional development.

Doubtless biologically innate tendencies, including intelligence, have a marked and continuing effect on personality growth, yet this effect is extensively modified by the individual's feeling-experiences and the influence of his culture. It must be remembered that the significance of any experience is special or peculiar for each developing personality. It is certain, however, that an understanding knowledge of the personality and its pathology must be largely based on data that go back to, and include, the beginning of the psychological and social career of the individual. It is usually assumed, therefore, that the unique individuality of a personality is to a considerable degree developed and directed by psychologically dynamic interactionisms as they have been consciously and unconsciously stimulated through social and cultural influences, but perhaps most of all by effective mechanisms prompted by interpersonal relations.

The stage in personality growth which an individual attains depends in no small part upon the degree to which he has been deprived of such wholesome interpersonal emotional experiences as tenderness in infancy, participation with others in the activities of childhood, the sharing of experiences with peers in the juvenile period, and a close relationship with a member of the opposite sex in adolescence.

Defenses

The type of personality pattern the individual works out for himself in his effort to meet the stresses of life will be influenced by many things. Among them will be the nature and number of the defenses which he constructs against unacceptable strivings, against aggressive tendencies and, against socially unacceptable feeling-attitudes toward persons who have occupied key positions in his life, particularly during childhood. If one develops a multiplicity of such defenses designed to reduce tension and anxiety, a constricted type of personality characterized by rigidity, narrowness, and lack of spontaneity results. If these defenses become pathologically exaggerated or disorganized, they eventuate in the neurotic or psychotic personality. One's basic personality, the kind of person one really is, continues to be the same throughout both prepsychotic and psychotic states. This remains true even though during a psychotic break-through it may appear to be quite at variance with the prepsychotic personality.

BIBLIOGRAPHY

Adler, A.: Individual Psychology. London, Routledge, 1946.

Brown, G. G.: Culture, society and personality: A restatement. Am. J. Psychiat., *100*:173–175, 1951.

Burlingham, D.: Twins: A Study of Three Pairs of Identical Twins. New York, International Universities Press, 1952.

Clark, R. A., and Capparell, H. V.: The Psychiatry of the adult only child. Am. J. Psychotherapy, 8:487–499, 1954.

Dollard, J.: Frustration and Aggression. New Haven, Yale University Press, 1939.

Erikson, E. H.: Identity and the Life Cycle. New York Psychological Issues. Vol. I, No. 1. Monograph. New York, International Universities Press, 1959.

Frank, L. K.: Play in personality development. Am. J. Orthopsychiat., *25*:576–590, 1955.

Freud, S.: The Ego and the Id. Translated by J. Riviere. London, Hogarth Press, 1927.

Idem: Collected Papers. London, Hogarth Press, 1924.

Goldfarb, W.: Effects of psychological deprivation in infancy and subsequent stimulation. Am. J. Psychiat., *102*:18–33, 1945.

Hurlock, E. B.: Child Development, 2nd ed. New York, McGraw-Hill Book Co., 1950.

Jacobi, J.: The Psychology of C. G. Jung, 5th ed. New Haven, Yale University Press, 1951.

Jung, C. G.: Psychological Types. New York, Harcourt, Brace & Co., Inc., 1923.

Kardiner, A., Karush, A., and Ovesey, L.: A methodological study of Freudian theory. J. Nerv. & Ment. Dis., *129*:11–19, 133–143, 207–221, 341–356, 1959.

Murphy, Gardner: Personality: A Biosocial Approach to Origins and Structure. New York, Harper & Brothers, 1947.

Nagy, M. H.: The Child's View of Death. In Feifel, H., ed.: The Meaning of Death. New York, McGraw-Hill Book Co., 1959.

Saul, L. J.: Emotional Maturity, The Developmen and Dynamics of Personality. Philadelphia, J. B. Lippincott Co., 1947.

Sullivan, H. S.: The Interpersonal Theory of Psychiatry. New York, W. W. Norton & Co., 1953.

Chapter Four

ADAPTIVE PROCESSES AND MENTAL MECHANISMS

NEED FOR ADAPTIVE MECHANISMS

In the course of evolutionary development, all species have developed various means and mechanisms to adapt to the life conditions which confront them. Some butterflies, for example, develop a protective coloring whereby they so simulate the appearance of the surface on which they rest as to escape detection by their enemies, and members of the same species come to adapt their coloring when the environment to which they are exposed differs from that of their original habitat. Since adaptation is the very essence of life, it is not strange that man as the most highly developed species has developed not only anatomical adjustments which protect him structurally or physiologically in respect to his environment but also that he has evolved psychological devices which assist him in dealing with his emotional needs and stresses. These devices help to meet such needs as those for affection, personal security, personal significance, and defense against perturbing anxiety. By acting without conscious recognition on his part, such devices effect adaptation to inner situations and experiences that would otherwise be sorely, even intolerably, troublesome. The self-conscious personality with its intense need for a sense of security and self-esteem evokes mechanisms of a protective nature as instinctively as self-preservation prompts the avoidance of approaching physical danger. Just as the body through its physical and biochemical processes strives to maintain a physiological equilibrium or homeostasis, so the personality through automatic and unconscious psychological processes seeks to maintain a psychological stability.

The evolution of a healthy personality requires especially the development of those behavioral processes which are necessary for adapting to life in human society. Therefore the development of the communicative and explorative or problem solving behaviors, especially language and the thought processes, must be considered of paramount importance as human adaptive processes. These processes are acquired through learning as are the various mental mechanisms by which the personality attempts to enhance and defend itself, to mediate between its conflicting drives, and to allay tensions. In terms of psychopathology, the definitions of disturbance will be found particularly in failures of the integrative function of the personality—in its ego functions.

Thus disturbances of language, perception, thought, and memory and of the capacity to delay gratifications of needs, discharge tensions, and learn the ordinary social behaviors or the acquisition of inflexible character defenses against such tensions provide the recognizable symptomatic expressions of the personality disorders.

LANGUAGE AND COMMUNICATION

While the acquisition of language as a communicative device distinguishes man from all other living species, it is often overlooked that he retains and uses other forms of communication as well. When communication is accepted as representing all those methods of influencing others which lead to a response on the part of the other, there is that continuing cognizance of non-verbal communication which is necessary for the understanding of conflict and abnormal behaviors.

To return again to the developmental history of man, the infant's original communications consist essentially of vocalizations which signal his distress and need for help. These vocalizations essentially signal emotional states. The responses from the mother set up the pattern for the growth of the later and more complex communictaive systems, the smiles, pointings, and other gesturings between the two which again signal emotional reactions—signs which later may be adapted, as in the language of the deaf mutes, for an elaborate non-verbal symbolic communicative system. The early gestures are the rudiments of the kinesthetic system wherein bodily movements and postures provide information and convey messages to others. Thus the tight-stepped gluteal pressed walk and stiff posture of a young woman signifies her overconcern with the taboos of sexual behavior, while the overt erect, head thrown back, stiff armed gait tells of the condescending haughtiness of a young man and heralds his effort by a disdainful poise to cover up his unspoken feeling of social inadequacy.

Verbal communication, language, has its beginnings between the first and second years when the necessary neuromuscular structures are fully developed. First the child uses interjections to inform of his emotional states. Later he denotes those about him by naming, and still later designates objects with nouns. Next comes the use of verbs, and by the end of the second year simple sentences are formed. The child indicates his ability to separate himself from others clearly by using pronouns and enriches his informational activity by learning the use of adjectives and adverbs. If the child has failed to speak by the end of three and one-half years, some defect almost invariably exists in the neuroanatomical structures concerned with speech—either failure in the auditory apparatus per se leading to deafness, in the auditory nerves, or in those brain pathways and interconnections mediating the reception, cognition, and activations of speech, or there has occurred a failure in the teaching and learning of speech, in the inter-communication processes that structure language through interplay between parent and child. Language does not evolve in non-speaking environments, as various observations have shown.

But even with the development of verbal communication, language continues to reflect the emotional states and attitudes of the speaker in the hidden meanings of accompanying tone inflection, volume, and gesture. Wit and humor especially, as well as various creative efforts, reflect and reveal the hidden and conflicting motivations through their non-verbal meanings. The psychiatrist must observe the discrepancies between the content of language, verbal communication, and the meanings conveyed in the non-verbal accompaniments of language, for here he often detects the conflicts of the individual. It is perhaps convenient to bear in mind that there is not only verbal language but there is also a non-verbal organ and action language.

Communication involves relations between peoples. As has been described in Chapter 3, growth is associated with establishing successively the capacity to communicate well between oneself and one other (the mother), then with the family members, and finally with increasingly varied and complex groups of persons, in the process of which the individual assumes at one time one role and at another time another role.

PERCEPTION AND THOUGHT

Even more distinctive of man than language has been his unparalleled evolution of a system for problem solving which has demanded an organization of neural functions of much greater complexity than that of a simple receptor-effector relationship with the environment. In contrast to the simple organizations of a reflex–stimulus–reflex system, the interposition of the highly elaborate cellular structure of the brain establishes delay in response, storing, and retention of previous experiences and the capacity for increasingly effective discriminations in exploring the environment.

It has been said that man never contacts reality directly; he first reacts with himself and his preconceived emotions, hopes, fears, and aspirations. It is the interposition of this mediating system, the human brain, which has made possible the acquisition of the potentiality for use of symbols. Through the progressive storing of accumulated knowledge and its transmission from one generation to another by the various cultural institutions, modern civilizations have arisen.

Language with its purposive drives made possible for man the designation and categorization of objects and thus the ability to regroup words to form different meanings or to use the same word in different combinations to specify still further meanings. Thus in the development of language the ranges of discrimination and thought were extended far beyond that found in animal species which use only a non-verbal communica-

tive system. Yet, if thought is considered the capacity for problem solving, it may not be stated that verbal language is a necessary precursor. Experimental psychology has acquired a wealth of data to show that animals may solve problems and also use symbols as signs. Nor is problem solving dependent upon learning, as new insights and solutions depend upon recombinations of previous experience. The parts of the old experience used in the new solutions or conceptions nevertheless must have been explored or learned. Thus animals reared in isolation and denied the opportunity of the experiences of those reared in groups prove inferior in problem-solving tests. Man's great capacity for thought as a purposive problem-solving device rests upon his greater capacity for recording past experiences, for remembering—and therefore for making progressively precise discriminations and complex combinations.

Perception and learning are necessary concomitants of the thinking process. Perception is not sensation; it implies the recognition of an object, an image, or a thought. Perceptions then often represent integrations of many sensations recorded in the brain as the central integrating organ. Thus perception of an orange implies the sensing of both color and form visually. The latter requires the kinesthetic sensing of the ocular muscles as they circumscribe the shape, as well as the olfactory and gustatory memories of previous contacts with the orange. Perception, then, is the act of knowing objects, images, and thoughts by sensory experiences or by recollective thought. *Imagery* takes place when some central brain process is set in action which is similar to the process aroused on earlier occasions on sensing the object. *Concepts*, in contradistinction to percepts, are mental images of something formed by generalizations from the particulars.

The acquisition of percepts takes place only through a long process of repetitive experiencing of the object, a learning process which involves the mental processes of discrimination and generalization. The child who perceives the orange has discriminated it from other round objects and is now able to transfer this percept to other images of the orange such as pictures or models. He generalizes the percept. Yet now he again recognizes the orange image and discriminates it from the real object. In the previous chapter, reference has been made to the serious defects which occur if the growing child is prevented before the age of five from experiencing visual sensation that lays down the patterns of arousal in the central nervous system which lead to recall and the potentiality for effective visual perception. In this chapter, also, mention was made of the acquisition of perception of one's body through experiencing it in the sensing and explorations of the early growth process as well as that of other objects external to the body.

Early Perceptual Processes

To return once more to development, the beginnings of perceptual and conceptual processes are hypothesized to commence in the experiences associated with the early mothering of the infant. Through repeated experiences of being nursed, the infant comes to associate discomfort with absence of the nipple and satisfaction with contact with the nipple. Later discriminations separate the nipple from the breast and eventually the face of the mother. It is conceivable that in periods of feeding frustrations the infant develops an image, or hallucinates the presence, of the breast or the mother as a wishfulfilling substitute for food gratification. There is now evidence from electroencephalographic studies of the capacity for dream life in infants as early as the ninth month of life. This suggests the plausibility of this early type of imagery. In this psychoanalytic theory of thinking, failure to satisfy the need for food forces a form of substitutive mental representation, the infantile prototype of ideation. The unsatisfied need also may be thought of as leading to a heightened awareness and attention which establish the set that

determines what eventually appears in consciousness.

Consciousness

Consciousness includes not only percepts and images of current happenings and those of the past, but also the images of the possible future. There is now mounting evidence that conscious percepts and images are influenced not only by consciously available past percepts, but also those that have been *repressed*. More recently there has accumulated some data to indicate, in addition, the registration of external stimuli that go unrecognized, since they are presented by means of stimuli so subliminal that no immediate conscious recording ever occurs, yet such registrations appear to influence other perceptions. Thus the experiments by Klein have demonstrated that subliminal exposures of emotionally-toned words such as "angry" and "happy" given simultaneously by subliminal tachistoscopic projection will modify the percept of a clearly exposed photograph of a man's face to include the subject's report of the associated subliminal affect word.

It appears, then, that of the many stimuli impinging on the human receptor system, many more register and achieve some subjective representation than may be surmised from simple examination of the thoughts or overt behaviors of the subject. Man, then, is much more receptive of his world and its impingements upon him; his senses range actively and restlessly over wide areas that fall outside the range of perception and immediate consciousness. For such "incidental registrations" to reach consciousness, it seems likely that they must be recruited to reality-attuned schemata.

Registration and perception are considered now by many researchers as distinct processes, the former highly efficient but less selective. The barriers to perception of registered stimuli depend upon their endowment with qualities significant to consciousness at a particular time. Accordingly, it may be said that the state of consciousness at a particular time determines the structure of perceptions and registrations; the "set" or "attitude" of mind selects from the vast barrage of incoming sensory registrations, both internal and external, those to which the individual attends and thereby establishes an effective barrier to perception so as to make adaptations to those most significant to the state of the organism at the moment. Recent neurophysiological work has shown as well that stimuli may be blocked from registration centrally by "feedback" which reduces registrations at the peripheral sensory organs, again providing the organism a stimulus barrier. The foregoing discussion is consistent with clinical observations. As an example, frequently noted is the failure of many soldiers to recall perception of pain at the time of impact when wounded in battle. Here other threats and activities preclude attendance to the pain-inducing wound.

Early Fantasies

The psychoanalytic theories of the early beginnings of hallucinated wishes in the infant have been mentioned earlier. Later, waking images or fantasies, thoughts, and dreams also are considered to fulfill the function of damping the tensions of unmet needs. It has been further suggested that these fantasies evolve in relation to the growth of the child. Thus with the period of toilet training and the exposure of the child to efforts to control him, the thought processes are repetitive, oscillating between the wish to excrete and the defiance to withhold. Here one may conceive of establishing the polar thinking of "is it right" or "is it wrong," or "I am good," "I am bad," or "I shall do it" or "I shall not do it"; modes of thought which are fixed characteristically in the obsessive compulsive mind. Later on, with the child's exposure to the emotional interplay between himself and both parents and siblings, there arise those fantasies dealing with the consequences of relations with others. "If I love father, mother will punish me," or pseudo-masochistic, "If I die, you will be sorry." Finally, the child evolves a variety of thought in which he projects himself into the future and attempts to organize his world for satisfactions to be attained at a later time. By using his past, he attempts to organize his future through thought both to avoid dangers and attain pleasures.

Control of Fantasies

The child's capacity to separate himself from the early fantasy world described before and achieve freedom for organizational thought depends not only on his innate intellectual endowment, but also upon the preservation of his curiosity and a limitation of early fears and anxieties. The parental relationship again, through its capacities for guiding the child's exploratory behavior, protecting him from too great arousal of emotions, allows the potentiality for gaining a period of autonomous thought, free from the intrusive and disturbing fantasies of early infancy and childhood just described. Thereby his capacity for the progressive differentiations, generalizations, transfers, and recombinations that constitute new conceptualizations and underlie creative thought and productive human activity are fostered by contact with adults who desire to impart their knowledge and protect the child through their own mature behavior from behavioral sequences that lead to emotional fixations and repetitive intrusion of immature fantasies.

In the next chapter the deleterious effects on mentation due to isolation from others will be described as an etiologic factor in the disruption of personality functioning. However, it must be mentioned that the healthy individual often finds periods of limited isolation highly significant in terms of creative thinking. In such instances it may be surmised that numerous perceptions and registrations from the past are brought to preconscious and conscious states that allow their associations and recombinations for purposes of gaining new insights and solutions of formerly insoluble problems. There are on record numerous instances of sudden insights into highly important scientific discoveries which took place under such circumstances. Kekuli's conceptualization of the benzine ring is one of the best known.

MENTAL MECHANISMS

Through the long period of development the personality acquires various phychological techniques by which it attempts to defend itself, establish compromises between conflicting impulses, and allay inner tensions. These mediating and integrating activities, functions of the ego as described before, are internal mechanisms of control, unconsciously selected and operating automatically. The personality develops defenses designed to manage anxiety, aggressive impulses, hostilities, resentments, and frustrations. All of us make continual use of defense mechanisms. In themselves they are not necessarily pathological. Life would be unbearable without resort to rationalization and similar psychic protections. Neither is it always the goal of therapy to eliminate them. Since at times they may promote the individual's ability to live in peace with himself, it may, in fact, be a therapeutic objective to strengthen them. The type of motivating device unconsciously selected to meet emotional needs and stresses and to provide a defense against anxiety, the extent of its employment, and the degree to which it distorts one's personality, dominates his behavior, and disturbs his adjustment with others determine the measure of his mental health. Processes similar in kind take place, therefore, in both the "normal" and the "abnormal."

Conflict

Unfortunately the conscious desire of the individual, the recognition he craves, and the gratification of biological impulses with which he was endowed are frequently not compatible with the conventionally-sanctioned habits, attitudes, demands, and values of the larger social group of which he is a member, nor with the prohibiting and censoring forces of his personality. Conscious and unconscious forces pursue incompatible goals. A struggle exists between two powerful incompatible response-tendencies— between the attitudes, habits, and values he has absorbed from the family, school, church, and various other carriers of ethical and moral standards and traditions on the one hand, and his unconscious needs and strivings on the other.

The dilemma in which the individual is impelled by mutually incompatible mental forces and irreconcilable, competing impulses and personality needs is known as a psychic conflict. The conflict may be thought of as a clashing—an internal struggle—between different parts of the personality. According to psychoanalytical theory, many conflicts have their origin in the early struggles of infancy and childhood but through repression become inaccessible to conscious introspection. In his dynamic clashing of impulses, the individual is torn between his conflictful drives, his wishes and aversions, his loves and hostilities, between his fears and longings, his urges and resistances. His satisfactions, stability, and peace of mind may be seriously disturbed because of conflict between his drives and wishes on the one hand, and the codes, traditions, beliefs, and loyalties which he has adopted from his social group on the other.

There is, as it were, a civil war within the personality. The individual is driven simultaneously toward behavior of opposite types. The personality becomes divided against itself, and a sense of tension or inner restlessness exists. It is the task of personality, often a difficult and painful one, to establish a compromise satisfactory to its conflictful strivings. Frequently it is not successful, and as a result the individual experiences anxiety, a condition of diffuse apprehension and of heightened and persistent inner tension.

Later we shall see how unwholesome or extreme psychological devices or mechanisms for dealing with conflicts, frustrations, and other anxiety-producing factors may lead to disorders of the personality.

In other instances, the energy-consuming conflicts may not lead to serious disorders of the personality but may limit and distort the fulfillment of the individual's inherent potentialities. As has been stated, many conflicts are established in childhood, and there is reason to believe that much later behavior and the fabrication of many adult personality patterns rests upon conflicts established at that time and upon the psychological mechanisms with which the individual has attempted to deal with them or with the anxiety and other affects which they create.

Anxiety

Conflict induces the affect of *anxiety*, considered central to the understanding of the psychodynamic processes. Anxiety is generally considered now as a state of tension signaling the potentiality of an impending disaster, a warning of danger from the pressure of unacceptable internal attitudes erupting either into consciousness or action, with the consequent responses of the individual personality or society to this eruption. To put it in another way, in the face of emerging aggressive or sexual drives, the tension of loneliness or sadness or the revelation of love or tenderness, which might expose the individual to the suffering of the affects of guilt or shame, anxiety is first felt in the context of the conflict situation.

While anxiety and *fear* have much in common in that both represent signals of danger, there are certain fundamental differences. Fear is the affective response to an actual current external danger which subsides with the elimination of the threatening situation, either by its disappearance through conquest or by escape. The danger most frequently is one to the physical integrity of the individual, whether from the threat of illness or from some external physical attack. Anxiety, on the other hand, may be thought of as the signal of an impending threat to the personality in the context of his social environment. Sullivan has provided a useful operational definition of anxiety in this context. He describes anxiety as a state of tension existing when one apprehends an unfavorable estimate by a significant person. The sufferer of anxiety is at best dimly aware of the conflict, aware only of the state of dread.

During development of personality, various mental mechanisms evolve to protect the individual from anxiety and other affects and their physiological accompaniments. These are described and illustrated in the following paragraphs.

Repression

One of the commonest of mental mechanisms developed for the purpose of dealing with the conflict, i.e., with irreconcilable desires, competing strivings, action tendencies that constitute a threat to the image which we have of ourselves, is that of repression. By this mechanism, desires, impulses, thoughts, and strivings which would be incompatible with, or disturbing to, the individual's conscious self-requirements and motivations are excluded from the field of conscious awareness, being pushed into the unconscious. Here, through a psychological inhibition of recall, they remain inaccessible in order that they may not be recognized and give rise to unbearable anxiety. Repression acts as a defense against drives and memories that cannot be controlled by the ego. It is not produced by a deliberate and conscious effort of rejection on the part of the person in whom it operates. Rather, it is an involuntary repudiation of denial, a non-conscious process acting automatically. Experiences involving guilt, shame, or the lowering of self-esteem are particularly apt to be repressed. In repression there is an elimination from consciousness of unrecognized motives and of all ideas or memories that might tend to arouse a painful anxiety.

Impulses which the ego cannot handle except by repression nevertheless retain their dynamic drive and tension. They continue to lead a subterranean life beneath a conventional surface, yet they are liable to manifest their influence in traits of personality, in special interests, in some system of beliefs or code of values, or in more marked form as neurotic, psychosomatic, or psychotic symptoms. Frequently repressed material may be dealt with rationally if it can be rendered accessible to the scrutiny of consciousness. It is therefore often desirable to make such recall possible. As will later be pointed out, this may be done by the technique known as free association.

Repression, then, is a primary defense against anxiety which is prone to arise when unbearable ideas and impulses threaten to enter conscious awareness. From a different point of view, one may think of repression as having been induced by anxiety rather than the reverse. In either case, the present tendency is to think of repression as the cornerstone of dynamic psychiatry. If repression is unable to prevent anxiety, then other mechanisms, such as projection or symbolization, may be called on to assist in its failing efforts. If repression breaks down the capacity for evaluating, reality may be impaired and defenses disregardful of reality may be called into action. These may, for example, permit the patient to disown an unacceptable impulse or threatening feeling of hostility by having it attributed to a source, perhaps a voice, outside himself. As we come to consider symptoms, we shall find that the patterns of defense against anxiety may be of various and even of changing forms.

By forbidding the undisguised expression of instinctive strivings and socially forbidden tendencies, repression operates to maintain ethical and social conventions, thus assisting the individual in adjusting to the mores and social institutions. Unfortunately, repression is not without disadvantages. Deep-seated drives and urges are not destroyed by repression but, on the contrary, although automatically restrained, they remain unchanged in quality and intensity. These drives and urges are, in fact, unmodified in any respect save that the individual is not consciously aware of the disowned strivings. Though frustrated, they constantly seek satisfaction. To make sure, however, that the undesired awareness and expression

of these strivings and wishes may not be permitted, the mind, automatically and without conscious deliberation, seeks to crush the strivings, wishes, and thoughts and to reverse their effect by the cultivation and promotion of characteristics sharply opposed in nature. These contrasting aims and efforts, designed to reinforce repression, lead to the formation of prejudices and of pronounced character defenses known as *reaction-formations*. These will be discussed later in the chapter. The more repressions a person has, the more prejudices and biases he develops in order to prevent the arousal of his repressed desires. Similarly, intolerance of the wrongdoings of others is often indicative of the effort required to repress similar unrecognized tendencies on his own part.

It must not be concluded from what has been said that repression is always pathological and its results undesirable. It is a mechanism which, if it operates smoothly and without undue effort, may result in a well-adjusted life. In some instances, repression and other mechanisms designed to deal with conflicts and unacceptable impulses may result in the formation of qualities of character that are estimable and yet, because of the sources from which those qualities have arisen, the psychological purposes and needs they fulfill and the uncompromising tenacity with which they are pursued, they must be looked upon as psychopathological products. Since, however, a tree is better known by its fruits than by its roots, we need not be unduly concerned as to the genetic source and psychodynamic function which these commendable personality traits are serving. Such desirable character traits might be characterized as representing the conversion of liabilities into assets. A careful scrutiny often reveals the same psychological theme running through character, personality traits, and the neurosis or psychosis. This is consistent with the principle of scientific thinking—that boundaries in nature are not fixed. One is forced to the conclusion that an unbroken line of continuity exists from normal behavior through neurotic to psychotic behavior. From the standpoint of dynamic development, many personality traits serve the same psychological purpose as do neurotic symptoms. Intolerance, submissiveness, meticulousness, extreme shyness, and other traits may, like neurotic symptoms, be developed as protection against an awareness of early fear, hate, or resentment long buried in the unconsciousness.

Repression should not be confused with *suppression,* in which a conscious effort is made to dismiss repudiated strivings and undesired memories from awareness.

COMPLEX. Because of the important part that repression plays in its origin, that mental product known as the complex* should now be considered. Not only may instinctive strivings and tabooed tendencies and desires be repressed, but also ideas, particularly those imbued with emotionally painful feeling-tones. A group of associated ideas which are thus invested with common affective accompaniments that are highly troublesome in nature and have therefore suffered repression is known as a complex. The affects impart a dynamic element to the complex, as a result of which it comes to constitute a sphere of thought and interest to which great emotional significance is attached. Such a center of emotional disturbance may exercise a strong, non-conscious influence. Even though such associated ideas and their attached emotions be repressed, they continue to possess the capacity for unrecognized activity, with the result that the latent tension in their affectively-toned content may be touched off by some apparently insignificant remark or experience and manifest itself in various forms. A not uncommon manifestation of the complex is in the form of excessive be-

* Psychoanalysts no longer apply the term "complex" in its original sense. They look upon it as a typical attitude connected with certain special inner needs or topics. They particularly stress the so-called "Oedipus complex" and the "castration complex." The term "complex" originated with Bleuler and Jung.

havior reaction or sudden emotional outburst in response to an apparently slight stimulus. A marked disproportion between stimulus and mental reaction suggests that the latter may be complex-conditioned. The disproportionate reaction shows that the external stimulus has added itself to a subconscious situation. Such emotional storms over trivial occurrences will usually be found to be linked with something very personal and significant.

Sometimes the response arising from complexes does not consist of a sudden emotional outburst or of a more or less isolated instance of striking behavior. In some cases, the complex may lead the person to see certain aspects of life in a particular way, or again it may lead him to establish some sustained idiosyncratic pattern of behavior. It may manifest itself, too, in various character traits, mannerisms, or slips of speech or in forgetting to carry out some intended action. When one exhibiting the complex-determined behavior is asked what has prompted his apparently causeless acts, he will reply that they are merely matters of accident or chance.

Conscious Control

From what has been said, it is plain that repression is a mechanism which, when employed, operates without conscious recognition. The most successful adjustment to life conditions is not possible if there are tendencies or feelings of which one is not aware so that they are therefore beyond the reach of control. The motives directing our behavior cannot be guided into desirable constructive channels unless their hidden sources are exposed to the light of full consciousness, permitting us to face all the facts and direct our promptings by the mechanism of conscious control. It enables us to replace automatic adaptations and repressions by conscious and flexible adjustments. Likewise, if we can learn to recognize and understand our mechanisms of escape and defense, we may exercise a greater measure of conscious control. Conscious control requires a realistic and efficient capacity for perceiving, deciding, and regulating a strong ego.

Identification

Identification is the most important of the psychological mechanisms for determining the growth of the ego. As mentioned in the discussion of personality development, the child takes over the attitudes and behavior patterns of his parents and others significant to him. The motivation for identification is wish-fulfilling in that the child admires or aspires to the strength and qualities of his elders and their associates and attempts to gain for himself their patterns of success by acquiring their modes of behavior. Identification contributes also to the growth of the superego functions. Thus a son may identify with his father and mold his personality on that of his parent, following his patterns of behavior and interest and sharing his ways. This mechanism is not one of conscious deliberation but a simple imitation.

Although identification provides a means for constructive influence on personality growth, this depends upon the personality of those to whom the child is exposed. A child may take on, as well, the socially undesirable characteristics of a parent if these appear to him to provide some special strength or merit. This occurrence is sometimes referred to as "hostile identification." The assumptions of brutality of young Germans preceding and during the World War II may be interpreted as hostile identification with the actions of the Nazi storm troopers of that time. Identification is seldom complete, since the personality of the admired person is never perceived in its totality by either child or adult. Certain traits alone may be picked up and assumed.

A young male school teacher was observed by his friends to change in the sense that he developed an erect posture and spoke to them looking over his glasses with a precise and clipped speech. He had moved from one city to another to assist in teaching in schools under an outstanding superintendent of schools. His friends were surprised, on meeting the latter, to note the superintendent's posture and speech which were those assumed by their friend.

Identification may be wish-fulfilling in its psychological purpose. This function may, for example, be observed in the self-gratifying sense of superiority felt by the servant of a distinguished personage with whom he identifies himself, or again it may explain the self-satisfaction of the psychotic patient who believes he is Christ and who, to complete the role, wears his hair and beard in the manner in which Christ is ordinarily represented.

Through this mechanism, certain circumstances, including relationships with certain people, may be selected because they fit into specific personality needs. The exaggerated sympathy at times shown by one person for another (even though the second person may be charged with some serious legal offense) results from identification—from a certain unconscious sensing of a common quality of impulse shared with the second individual. Through this mechanism, some desire may be vicariously satisfied, any fulfillment or even a conscious recognition of which would not be knowingly permitted. The false confessions of crime of which one occasionally reads in the newspapers are the results of identification which is based on a desire to commit the offense which the confessor alleges he has committed.

TRANSFERENCE. As thus far described, identification is an individual's unconscious molding of himself after the fashion of another or a feeling of a sort of affective oneness with a second person. It is more than the conscious modeling of a child after the pattern of a loved and admired parent. In a second type of identification, more properly recognized as transference, the image of one person is unconsciously identified with that of another. The more recent acquaintance becomes the surrogate of the person previously known and is invested with the same emotions with which the individual had come to surround the image of the original party. In this way are to be explained some of our apparently causeless likes and dislikes of persons whom we have unwittingly identified with someone who had once aroused similar emotions. A person representing authority may come to be identified with a tyrannical father and the surrogate may be regarded with the same emotions as was the original image. This is doubtless the dynamic determinant of the activity shown by some persons who constantly struggle against the regulations and institutions of society. Hostile and other negative feelings having their original source in attitudes created in early childhood may be displaced or transferred to others in later life and thereby seriously distort human relationships.

EMPATHY. A healthy form of identification which is limited and temporary but which enables one person to feel for and with another and to understand his experiences and feelings is that known as empathy. By means of this quality, the individual possesses a warm capacity for projecting himself into the situations and feelings of others.

INTROJECTION. *Introjection,* while often considered a separate defensive mechanism, is best thought of as a form of identification. As with identification, a portion of another person's personality is taken in, yet this introject of the other often becomes the focus of hostility directed apparently toward oneself and is thus the nucleus of depressive states and suicidal acts. It is the obverse of *projection* to be discussed later.

A young married woman was referred for treatment by her husband due to her recent crying spells, self denunciation and deprecation, and inability to care for her home and infant. She quickly advised that her mother was a woman who was frequently in tears, only then held her on her lap, constantly denounced the injustices done her. The patient stated she was afraid she was like her mother and she disliked herself for these traits.

INCORPORATION. *Incorporation* is another term used by psychoanalysts which, again, falls into the general area of identification. It refers to the taking in of early qualities through the infantile nursing experiences with the mother and is considered to begin during the oral stage of development.

Reaction-Formation

Another important device for the establishment of character is that known as reaction-formation. Thus is formed a character trait that is usually the exact opposite of that which would naturally have followed from the expression of unfettered tendencies, a trait developed to maintain the repression of these impulses and to deny and disguise personality trends that have existed under cover, and it is known as a reaction-formation. Perfectionistic and uncompromising character traits are often reaction-formations against forbidden tendencies, desires, or impulses. Often such traits unwittingly reveal troublesome aspects of the personality. The defensive character of conspicuous traits and attitudes is betrayed by the very quality of their exaggeration and at times by their inappropriateness. Such overemphasized character and personality traits may be described as constituting the first line of psychological defense. They can scarcely be called pathological unless they disturb adjustment. Feelings of rejection and hostility may be disguised by scrupulous politeness or effusive expressions of gratitude. So far as conscious intention is concerned, a reaction-formation is always honest and sincere. The overtly aggressive person, constantly demanding his rights and ready to fight at any provocation, may be defending himself against a deeply seated sense of insecurity. On the other hand, submissiveness may be a reaction-formation that serves to cover up unrecognized aggressive tendencies. A façade of excessive amiability may conceal intense hostility.

Great concern for a certain person may be a disguise for unrecognized feelings of hostility, jealousy, or even wishes for his death. Beneath devotion there may lurk a concealed wish for the death of a widowed mother for whom a spinster daughter has sacrificed herself and refused an offer of marriage in order to remain with her. Such devotion serves to appease a sense of guilt. If employed within rational limits, reaction-formation may be a desirable choice of defense against anxiety.

The unmarried sibling of an identical twin pair presented himself for treatment due to mounting anxiety over his flagrant promiscuous homosexual activity. His brother was happily married. He described his adolescent hatred toward his mother for her betrayal of the family in a sordid extramarital affair and his conviction that he could only obtain a trusting relationship with another man—like his brother—indicating that no woman could be trusted. Later he revealed his close and tender relationship with his mother during early boyhood and his expressed wish for a similar feminine companionship. The homosexual orientations represented a spiteful reaction-formation against the, to him, fearful wish for a woman.

Compensation

Physiological and physical compensations are phenomena which the internist and the surgeon observe daily. If a valve of the heart is incompetent, the heart muscle hypertrophies in order that additional force may be available to compensate for the impairment in circulation that would otherwise result from the valvular defect. If, from disease or faulty habits of posture, a spinal scoliosis develops, a secondary curve, opposite in direction to the primary one, is produced above or below the former in order that the center of gravity may not be displaced. Such compensations represent attempts of organs to adjust to physiological defects and inadequacies. Similarly the organism as a whole, in distinction from its component organs, by compensating for its inadequacies and imperfections attempts to secure the recognition which it craves.

Such compensations may easily become exaggerated and are often unwittingly betrayed by behavior. The person of small stature but with aggressive and dominating traits is an example of overcompensation familiar to all. His pompous and pretentious manner may have been unwittingly adopted in order that it may indicate a strength and authority which a diminutive size fails to suggest. His deportment may make the undersized person feel more comfortable and secure and help him forget his physical inadequacies.

Prestige seems to be one of the fundamental needs of the personality. Methods of enhancing our self-feeling and of covering up deficiencies are widespread and vary from the simple "showing off" seen daily on the playground or the pretentious display observed in Peacock Alley to the formations of delusions of grandeur. It should not be forgotten, moreover, that socially acceptable degrees of compensation and even admirable personality traits may be an expression of neurotic needs. Their neurotic origin is often betrayed by the striking degree to which they are developed.

Handicaps and limitations, as factors in the production of compensatory products, may be of a widely-diversified nature, in some instances being physical, in others mental. The inferiority, too, which lies at the basis of compensatory mechanisms may be either real or fancied. In persons whose reactions in relation to reality, in general, and to social stimuli, in particular, are well integrated, the existence of a physical inferiority may provoke constructive activities which result in qualities of outstanding social usefulness. Handicaps may spur one on to greater efforts, as in the case of Wordsworth's happy warrior who "turned his necessity to glorious gain." On the other hand, diseases or deformities that thwart normal instincts or ambitions or cause the individual to stand out unpleasantly from the group may fail to promote desirable qualities of the personality but may lead to wishful thinking, unpleasant traits, or even at times to a psychotic sacrifice of reality. In whatever form manifested, the products represent the results of the personality's efforts to attain a satisfying self-esteem and sense of security. All too often, unfortunately, the mechanism leads to over-compensations which, although satisfying to the individual, are fictitious so far as social values are concerned.

A boy who was so tall, angular and ungainly that he had always been extremely self-conscious enlisted in the Army. (It is quite probable that, without consciously realizing it, he had been prompted to enlist because the military uniform and a certain glamour connected with the military life seemed to offer hope of relief from the unpleasant sense of being different, produced in his tall, ungainly figure.) Here he soon became an object of raillery because of his clumsiness in attempting to execute the various drills. After having struggled in vain for adeptness, the boy was placed in the "awkward squad," where he naturally felt even more self-conscious and more painfully aware of his deficiencies. The indignity suffered by his self-esteem was too great; the need of his personality for a more satisfying recognition and for a sense of security exceeded its limited resources and he therefore constructed a fictitious substitute by developing the belief that he was a major general. He was no longer the awkward soldier, unable to compete with his associates, but was their commander and directed affairs of great military importance. The compensatory delusion satisfied the recruit's emotional needs but destroyed his usefulness for the realities of military life and required his hospitalization.

Rationalization

Probably none of us realizes the extent to which the mental mechanisms operative in our everyday lives are defensive in nature. One of the commonest of these devices designed to maintain self-respect and prevent feelings of guilt is that of rationalization, a term introduced into psychiatric literature by Ernest Jones. It is a self-adjusting mechanism by which we first act in response to unrecognized motives, and after the action we offer various supposed "reasons" for our conduct.

We prefer to believe that our behavior is the result of thoughtful deliberation, unbiased judgment, and a full awareness of all the motives prompting it. As a matter of fact, only to a minor extent is behavior the result of such conscious intellectual considerations. After we have acted in response to these unrecognized motives, we formulate presentable reasons which we believe determined our conduct, although they are really but *ex post facto* justifications. This mechanism provides rational, intellectual explanations of behavior that has really been prompted by unrecognized motives. We think we can fully explain our conduct but are deceived by pseudo-rational explanations. Our real desires and attitudes remain concealed and disguised.

At times certain of our rationalizations contain a minor element of truth which, however, is so unduly emphasized that it serves to conceal the essential prompting motive. Those motives which are acceptable are selected and considered to be the only ones. Our thinking defends our feeling. Since we believe that our behavior ought to be determined by certain motives, rationalization through its self-deception leads us to believe that it is. Frequently several motives participate in initiating behavior. In fact, several motives usually combine and are operative in originating our behavior, some of them having a distinctly ethical value. Other components are of a more selfish, emotional, or instinctive nature.

When behavior is determined by such a coalescence of motives, it will be found that the individual selects the most acceptable from the complex group to explain his behavior. The more selfish and instinctive ones are the more dynamic, and these exercise greater influence in determining behavior, yet are not the ones that are recognized in consciousness as determinative of it. The motives which, from an ethical standpoint, are the highest are those that dominate consciousness and are therefore offered as the real motives, although they are of less influence in determining behavior than are those components that are unrecognized.

The student may ask whether the individual is not aware that the reasons he offers for his behavior are not the actual ones and that he is therefore guilty of a falsehood. To this, one must reply that in the case of a lie one consciously knows that the reason is fictitious, whereas rationalization is so thoroughly a non-conscious mechanism that he does not recognize that motives cannot always be taken at face value. To employ rationalization in discussing his behavior does not mean that he is not honest and sincere. The self-deceptions of rationalization are usually defended with great emotional intensity, since their creation was designed to conceal a truth that would be painful to the ego.

Rationalization is a mechanism that

serves a useful purpose insofar as it is conducive to psychic self-protection and comfort. It leads, however, to self-deception and its conclusions are untrustworthy guides for further conduct. Its products, which are often employed deductively as premises, are so fallacious that they may readily contribute to the formation of delusions.

A not uncommon reaction closely allied to rationalization which helps to maintain self-esteem in the face of inadequacy is one of depreciation often spoken of as the "sour grapes" mechanism. In this defensive, devaluation reaction, the individual disparages some particular goal which, inwardly at least, he would greatly like to attain but which, because of some obstacle, often personal inadequacy, he cannot reach. An expression of depreciation for that for which one is unqualified is not infrequent. It is, of course, one form of response to anxiety. Somewhat allied as a defensive mechanism is a blasé indifference in the face of circumstances that would naturally offend self-esteem.

Substitution

Substitution is a mechanism which may be employed to reduce tension resulting from frustration. Through it are secured alternative or substitutive gratifications comparable to those which would have been enjoyed had frustration not occurred. To yield satisfaction and reduce tension, the substitutive action must have certain similarities to the frustrated one. Many psychiatric symptoms represent substitutive and symbolic satisfactions.

In the effort to solve a conflict, the organism has available to itself the options of (1) continuing to strive toward the desired goal; (2) overcoming the obstacle to achievement of the goal by some aggressive drive, or (3) avoiding or fleeing from the obstacle before him. Among the adjustments possible in personality functioning when it is not possible to utilize aggression or avoidance is the acceptance of a substitute goal or insight. Such a potentiality exists when

the committment to the goal or the use of a particular adaptive technique prevents the individual from relinquishing these possibilities. If he is so committed, frustration and the inevitable affective response must follow, although defense against the latter may be achieved with some other mental mechanism.

Displacement

Another anxiety-reducing device which also operates by a process of substitution is displacement. By this defense mechanism, an emotional feeling is transferred from its actual object to a substitute. The feeling originally directed toward a certain person, object, or situation is transferred and attached to another person, object, or situation which becomes invested with the emotional significance originally associated with the former. In a phobia, for example, there is an unconscious transfer of fear and threat from its original hidden and internal unconscious source to another one which is external and apparently unrelated insofar as the patient is consciously aware. In the frequent handwashing observed in certain compulsive neuroses, affect is displaced from an earlier experience with which a feeling of moral uncleanness was associated to the idea of dirt which comes to possess the feeling value originally attached to the consciously repudiated experience.

Feelings and attitudes, such as love and hate, are particularly apt to be displaced from one person to someone else who comes to be a surrogate for the first person. A feeling of hostility toward a parent may, for example, be so intense that it cannot be consciously entertained. By shifting the hatred to someone who has a resemblance to the parent, the person may be protected against conscious recognition of his attitude toward the parent.

In many instances, symbolism is a kind of displacement. An object becomes a symbol of the person or object which originally stimulated the feeling or impulse. Displacement enables the individual to maintain repression of dangerous or unacceptable impulses, wishes, or thoughts. The displacement of anxiety from the significant to the less significant is common. Allied to displacement is the mechanism described by Freud whereby the conscious may defend itself from material in the unconscious by treating it as a joke.

A 30-year-old housewife entered the hospital for treatment of a phobic condition which prevented her from leaving her home. Her condition was initiated after the birth of her third child, when she developed feelings of panic associated with the idea of being sexually attacked. In treatment she proved to have been very dependent since early childhood and to be seductive. She eventually revealed that in her desire to have men care for her she feared loss of sexual control to the point of becoming a prostitute. This anxiety was displaced by fear of street walking.

Restitution

The mechanism of relieving the mind of a load of guilt by restitutive acts (a making up for, or reparation) is not uncommon. Restitution arising from feelings of guilt may become the main motive in life, as exemplified by the indefatigably, almost wearisomely, benevolent person. Operating to a less extreme degree and in a less obvious manner, the restitutive reaction to unconscious guilt may play a large part in a drive toward creativeness.

Projection

This mechanism is, in many respects, a form of displacement, a means of defense which, to a limited degree, one may observe daily among his associates and which is seen to a psychotic degree in paranoia and in other paranoid psychoses. Acting as a defense against anxiety, projection is directed outward and attributes to others one's disclaimed and objectionable character traits, attitudes, motives, and desires. The mechanism enables one to remain blind to important drives in the personality, while their influence distorts his picture of the outside world.

One constantly meets people who severely criticize in other persons the very same faults which are the weak points of their own character, utterly failing to recognize the fact that they themselves possess the despised traits and motives. The material projected might be said to be an echo of the projector's own unconscious. By projection, one's own aggressive designs and id impulses are attributed to others. Through it repudiated tendencies find outlet.

Feelings of guilt which give rise to anxiety may be alleviated if one is able to cast the blame for shameful tendencies or wishes onto the outer world, leaving himself guiltless or even victimized. One may feel less guilty, too, if someone else can be made to feel guilty. As a further defense against anxiety, one may respond with hostility and aggressive behavior toward the external object which is the focus of projection. Some treat others as projections of certain of their own unconscious trends—hate, fear, and similar feelings. Many times they hold others responsible for their difficulties.

It will be noted that projection is closely associated with the mechanism of denial. This is well illustrated by the formula stated by Freud: A, unable to tolerate the anxiety aroused by his hatred of B, unconsciously changes his attitude, "I hate B," to "B hates me." Repression and projection protect the ego from being overwhelmed or disorganized by the effects of aggression, hate, or guilt.

In the discussion of the mechanism of compensation, mention was made of the fact that physical inferiorities may stimulate compensatory reactions. In some instances, such handicaps may be dynamic factors in the development of other defensive reactions, among these being projection. Although the anatomical defect may be of wide variation, malformations or hypoplasia of the genital organs or disfiguring cutaneous lesions seem especially provocative of defensive reactions. Feeling of inferiority arising from defects of organs so highly prized biologically as the genitals, or so valued as a determinant of physical attractiveness as the skin, may give rise to sensitiveness, dissatisfaction, embitterment, and resentment. Such emotional attitudes readily lead to misinterpretations or even cause a person thus handicapped to attach to others any weaknesses in his own personality. Sometimes a striving for supremacy and security by persons who, compared with others, are actually or in imagination at a disadvantage in life may lead to projection as a defensive means. If the ego fails or becomes disorganized, other phenomena—hallucinations, ideas of reference, and delusions—often become associated with projection.

DELUSIONS AND PROJECTION. Material may be projected in the form either of ideas or of perceptions. In the former case, projection may lead to the formation of delusions, particularly ones of persecution.

During World War I an American soldier, in order to escape from a highly dangerous situation in the front-line trenches, shot himself in the foot. He was at first treated in an Army hospital in France and later transferred to the United States, where the self-inflicted wound healed but slowly. The retrospective discomfort or sense of guilt created by his cowardice and dereliction was alleviated psychologically by projection. He believed that the delay in the healing of the wound was a result of neglect on the part of his physician. The soldier felt no self-reproach since it was not he but the physician who was culpable. He was, of course, quite unaware that the attempt he later made on the life of the physician was an effort to destroy *qualities of which he was the actual possessor.*

Such a projection stimulated by a sense of guilt is at times one of the important mechanisms in the production of paranoia. By this mechanism, a patient may persuade himself that his persecutor is so unspeakably evil that he deserves death, and to inflict this, far from being a criminal act, is a laudable one.

HALLUCINATIONS AND PROJECTION. Frequently in the psychotic, the disowned aspects of the personality are projected, not in terms of ideation, but in terms of perception. In such a case, the repressed mental material or unacceptable tendencies, striving, or qualities may be externalized in the form of hallucinated voices accusing the patient of practices which represent the rejected aspects.

The soldier just mentioned, in his effort to kill the physician, naturally did not destroy the sense of guilt produced by the violations of his code of mental honor, nor did his attempt to kill his physician destroy the despised defects of character. Finally, their projection led to a still greater distortion of reality in the form of hallucinations. One day, as he was walking along a city street, he heard accusing remarks that seemed to refer to him. Glancing about, he saw that the person in the direction from which the accusing voices apparently came was the driver of a passing automobile. Without warning, the former soldier shot and killed the man. Thus he killed a person who, by projection, had become the representative and incarnation of his own hated but unrecognized qualities.

IDEAS OF REFERENCE. The symptom known as "ideas of reference" arises through the operation of the mechanism of projection. The individual who utilizes this type of projective mechanism egocentrically believes that he is the object of special and ill-disposed attention by those about him. Casual remarks by others, for example, are understood as relating to him and interpreted as accusatory or vilifying.

MOTIVES OF PROJECTION. Projection is a psychological expedient which, by its defensive process, makes the individual more comfortable. It is less disturbing for him to discover an undesirable tendency in someone else than consciously to admit that he possesses it himself. Protection against disowned impulses and wishes and the anxiety which they would stimulate is secured by their paradoxical denial and reversal.

Even in the so-called normal person, the mechanism of projection may be employed for its protective function, but it readily becomes a danger to peace of mind and to the integrity of the personality. It prevents him from seeing himself as he really is and leads to excessive criticism, sarcasm, pessimism, cynicism, brooding, prejudice, intolerance, and hatred. While defensive against anxiety, it is often highly provocative in producing disturbance of human relations. It is a mechanism which may set in motion a process that leads to a vicious cycle.

The attitude of the projecting person toward those on whom the projection is focused frequently becomes one of suspicion or even of overt hostility. This attitude readily leads to one of mutual estrangement which, in turn, activates in the projector a sense of an increasingly hostile world. This feeling easily promotes misinterpretations and perhaps the formation of delusions which tend to create more problems. Thus the mechanism feeds on itself.

Symbolization

At first men communicated with each other through the use of concrete objects, but with the development of language they used words in place of objects. Gradually words were employed to represent ideas as well as objects. Similarly, objects became the symbols or substitutes for ideas, feelings, and tendencies. Symbolization with its meaning-carrying signs is therefore a mechanism whereby one idea or object is employed to represent some other idea or object. It is characteristic of words or objects used symbolically that they thereby become significantly charged with meaning. This arises from the fact that the displacement of emotional values from the object to the symbol is the essence of symbolization. The symbol may therefore come to represent mental experience heavily laden with meaning. It is a mechanism extensively employed in psychopathology.

We have seen that conflicting drives and ideas, or groups of associated ideas, with which painful emotions are associated may be repressed because they are distressing to the conscious personality. Such repressed material is still too active, too heavily charged emotionally, not to be constantly seeking for expression. Since denied direct, conscious, and frank expression, the repressed impulses and other psychic content break through and obtain expression at the conscious level in direct, disguised form. The wish or drive, therefore, that cannot be acknowledged consciously may be dealt with or satisfied in a symbolic manner.

The resemblance between the symbol and the object symbolized is generally so slight or superficial that the conscious mind will overlook it. The individual is, therefore, quite unaware of the meaning of the symbol he has employed; indeed, he is often unaware that he has used one at all. To his conscious mind, the symbol is not a symbol; it is reality in and of itself. He therefore treats symbols as if they were real and directs his behavior in accordance with the affective value with which the symbols are invested.

In both the normal and the psychotic individual, repressed material may be expressed through symbolism. It is manifested, not in forms of esthetic value, as in the case of the artist, but in forms equally symbolic, although often in disguises more difficult to read. It is frequently said that symbolism is the language of the unconscious. Symbols, therefore, become the language whereby material that may not appear in conscious awareness in undisguised form finds expression. Appearing in the content of dreams, hallucinations, and obscure or apparently meaningless ideas, symbols express particularly those contents of the individual's inner life with which much feeling is connected.

The disguises under which such material may be manifested are numerous. Various affectations of dress, gait, speech, or manner as observed among persons who are never regarded as suffering from mental disorder are often symbolic disguises expressing products of repression.

A recently married woman was admitted to a hospital for treatment because of her unusual behavior. She stood on her head, was mute, and would communicate by using ball point pens which wrote in red ink. Later she explained her behavior as a means of expressing her anger at her husband for taking her money. She was in love with him so could not speak of her rage, yet the red ink symbolized it. Standing on her head represented both a defiant gesture and a wish for help by being found ill.

Dreams, which are products of thinking lacking the awareness and direction supplied by consciousness, involve various processes, one of the most frequent of which is symbolization. Although not all dreams contain symbolic material and not all psychiatrists agree as to the interpretation to be placed upon dream imagery, many of the images and experiences of dreams represent such products of repression as unacknowledged motives and desires.

Fixation

We know that from infancy to maturity there should be a progressive development, differentiation, and maturation in the instinctive, emotional, and other aspects of the personality. There should be a progressive development not only in the psychosexual aspects of personality, but also in methods of thinking, in meeting difficult situations and the frustration of wishes, in dealing with reality, and in the control and expression of emotions and instincts. Unfortunately, the development of some aspect of the personality may be halted at an incomplete stage of its evolution with a resulting persistence of certain incompletely matured elements. Such a personality shows a lack of harmonious integration. Its emotional organization particularly remains at an immature level, and there is a lag between biological status and emotional independence. This cessation of the process of development of the personality at a stage short of complete and uniform mature independence is known as fixation. Certain phases of development are not successfully passed through and left behind. Just as the child may continue his baby talk and his dependence on his mother beyond the period when these characteristics should have been outgrown, so phases of his personality development may be arrested at various stages. The arrest is not in the intellectual but in the emotional, dispositional aspect of personality maturation.

There are many theories concerning the origin of fixation. According to one theory, fixation is the result of experiencing such excessive satisfactions at a given level that this level can only be renounced with reluctance. According to another theory, a similar effect may be produced by excessive frustration at a given level.

An analogy from somatic pathology will illustrate the mechanism of fixation. It will be remembered that before birth the blood of the fetus passes directly from the right auricle to the left auricle through the foramen ovale, thus short-circuiting the pulmonary circulation, the activity of which is not necessary during fetal life. Sometimes the patulous condition of the foramen ovale persists after birth, with the result that the individual suffers from a congenital heart disease. This passage between the auricles is normal for a certain stage of development, but if the fetal arrangement persists beyond the period of its usefulness, its existence constitutes a serious biological handicap. In the same way, the persistence of tendencies and emotional attitudes which should have been relinquished prevents mature development and harmonious integration of the personality.

Regression

Attention has just been called to the fact that certain aspects of the personality may be arrested in their maturative process, with the result that a full and harmonious development never occurs. By another anxiety–evading mechanism known as regression, the personality may suffer loss of some of the development already attained and revert to a lower level of integration, adjustment, and expression. Thus a child who is toilet trained may again wet his bed following the birth of a sibling who now takes the maternal attention from him. He seeks by his regression to regain the gratifications of an earlier period in life. If the individual is unable to deal realistically and constructively with the various problems and frustrations of life, including those that arise from outside himself, but particularly those that arise from his inner mental life—his conflicts, instinctual drives, and emotional needs—a normal progression to successively higher levels of adjustment may be checked and he may retreat to a lower level of personality development characterized by immature patterns of thought, emotion, or behavior. An infantile or juvenile approach to the world which may have been latent for many years may be awakened by some frustrating experience or situation. Regression to the dependence of infancy or childhood allays the fears and insecurities which arise from the necessity that adult existence meet life situations and responsibilities in an independent fashion. While adjustive in its purpose, regression is disruptive and does not promote a desirable adaptation.

The stronger any fixations which may have been established during the course of development, the more readily will frustrating and conflictive situations be evaded by regression to those fixations. Extreme forms and degrees of regression result in a serious disorganization of personality and often constitute an important element in schizophrenia. In the process of regression, the total personality, or the whole of the personality, does not regress from one developmental stage to the next lower in clearly defined stages or as a total unit. Certain aspects of the patient's feelings, thinking, and behavior may be perceived as operating at various levels within various stages concurrently. The patient may, for example, think, feel, and behave partially as an adult but at the same time may manifest infantile needs.

Following a trip abroad with some friends, an 18-year-old adopted child became withdrawn and preoccupied herself with religious matters and fantasies about her own parents. Some few days before her hospital admission she commenced to repeat whatever was said to her (echolalia). This behavior persisted for some weeks after her admission. Later she said she had suffered from other children mocking her early in life through echoing her words but learned that she could satisfy her own angry feelings to her teasers by adopting the same method.

Dissociation

Another mechanism to which the organism may resort in order to secure a measure of satisfaction when the various components of the personality are not well integrated is that of dissociation. A portion of the personality which is a source of emotional distress may be eliminated by this mechanism. In dissociation, certain aspects of activities of the personality escape from the control of the individual, become separated from normal consciousness, and, thus segregated, function as a unitary whole.

DUAL OR MULTIPLE PERSONALITIES. We are accustomed to looking upon our perceptions, ideas, emotions, memories, and wishes as all belonging to a consciousness, a personality, that cannot be divided. Ordinarily a given topic occupies one's consciousness one moment and some other topic the next moment, but it is felt that there is some connection between the two topics, that both are part of awareness, that consciousness has been continuous, and that one's mental life has not been divided. Occasionally, however, in a person in whom there is an active incompatibility between repressed elements in his mental life and the rest of his personality, the repressed components may escape from the forces that are repressing them, become separated from the usual consciousness, organize a personality of their own, as it were, and thus dictate behavior. This new or secondary personality has its own consciousness which has no recollection of the usual or primary personality and carries out acts independent of it. The consciousness possessed by this independently functioning experience was designated by Morton Prince as the co-consciousness.

The disposition and character possessed by the secondary personality may be quite different from that shown by the primary personality. This contrast should naturally be expected, since the secondary personality is made up of material that has been repressed, that is, has been rejected by the primary personality because it was not of a nature to be consciously entertained or satisfied.

Occasionally more than one body of associated repressions and affective experiences may become sufficiently organized to acquire independent activity, in which case there will be more than one secondary personality, each possessing a character and disposition different from the others and from the primary personality. To these independently-acting personalities is given the term "multiple personalities."

A 28-year-old married woman was admitted to a hospital, depressed and retarded, after a suicidal attempt. Several days later she became angry and assaultive, claimed that it was her fault that she was depressed. She then stated that "Mary" was the depressed person; she was Cynthia. As Cynthia she reported frequently leaving home, picking up sailors and lesbians, and acting in a loose and lascivious manner. As Mary she acted as a dutiful, quiet, submissive housewife and mother, angry and depressed over her husband's poor relationship to her. Periodically she abruptly assumed the character of Cynthia and became loud, boisterous, and uninhibited. In the depressed state she accepted the dictates of her superego, repressed the rage toward her husband, and dutifully attempted to assume her responsibilities as a housewife, as Mary. When overwhelmed by rage, she expressed her rage through defiance and acted her aggressive and sexual urges as Cynthia. Only the latter dissociation recognized the former.

SOMNAMBULISM. One of the simplest forms of dissociation is that of somnambulism in which, while the usual personality is asleep, a fragment or some aspect of the personality assumes direction, with the result that, without the awareness of his usual personality, the sleeper arises and executes some complicated act. Other examples of automatisms, or dissociations of personality in which unconscious factors temporarily gain control, act independently and dictate behavior, are automatic writing, fugues, and multiple personalities. In all these dissociated states, the organization of the repressed tendencies and desires into systems has usually been aided by day dreams.

AUTOMATIC WRITING. In automatic writing, the usual consciousness may or may not be aware that an automatism is being executed, but in all others the usual or primary personality is not aware.

FUGUE. Sometimes the organized material that has broken away from usual consciousness to form the secondary personality may initiate activities that lead the patient far from the scenes and efforts of his ordinary life. Stengel defines such a flight or fugue state as consisting of "transitory abnormal behavior characterized by aimless wandering and more or less alteration of consciousness, usually, but not necessarily followed by amnesia." A desire for escape from some intolerable situation is usually the immediately precipitating factor in the production of the fugue. Frequently the prompting desire is escape either from justice or from domestic stress. An accompanying depressive mood is common. In fugues of short duration, the patient wanders aimlessly, is highly emotional, and when found is agitated and confused. In long fugues he travels far, appears self-possessed, and lives in every way like a normal person except that he is not where he should be. The patient may be his normal self when he emerges from his fugue, aware of his identity with full memory of his past life except for the fugue period, or he may be unaware of his identity and of his past life. Clinically most cases fall into a poorly defined psychopathic-neurotic group. Many have shown a previous tendency to lying or to hysterical features.

Resistance

This defensive mechanism produces a deep-seated opposition to the bringing of repressed (unconscious) data into awareness. Through its operation, the individual seeks to avoid memories and insights which would arouse anxiety and be painful for him to face consciously. It is also observed in psychoanalytical therapy when the psychiatrist, through free associations, encourages the patient to bring repressed material into awareness. It was through the difficulties and obstructions encountered in free association—the blocking, embarrassment, silences, and anxieties shown by the patient to which he gave the name resistance—that Freud built up his concept of repression. Resistances afford a clue to repressed material.

Denial

Denial is an intrapsychic defense mechanism by means of which consciously intolerable thoughts, wishes, facts, and deeds are disowned by an unconscious denial of their existence. What is consciously intolerable is unconsciously rejected by a protective mechanism of non-awareness. Reality is regarded as non-existent or is transformed so that it is no longer unpleasant or painful. The term denial used in a psychiatric sense does not include a consciously attempted endeavor to repudiate or disown as in malingering or lying.

Sublimation

We have seen that repression is a mental mechanism designed to deal with conflicting drives and desires. If it is successful in its purpose and there are no accompanying feelings of anxiety, it facilitates a well adjusted life. Since, however, repression is, in effect, the overcoming of one force by another, the energy in the repressed impulse is not available for constructive, consciously directed activity. It would be highly desirable, therefore, if the energy inherent in primitive or unacceptable impulses could somehow be transformed and flow with relative freedom into the conscious mind and there direct the individual's interests and activities. The mechanism by which this energy is transformed and directed to socially useful goals is known as sublimation. Instinctive needs and unacceptable impulses find an acceptable outlet and mode of expression. Anxiety arising from the threat of these needs and impulses is channeled into patterns of social acceptability. Instead of utilizing primitive tendencies and impulses for selfish or forbidden purposes, sublimation transforms and directs them into vocational channels or into art, literature, religion, science, or other activities that promote cultural development and a richer life both for the individual and the social group. Aggressive impulses, for example, may be sublimated through sports and games or other socially-accepted channels. The energy transformation by sublimation may be compared to the transformation of the hydrodynamic energy in such falls as those at Niagara where the electric generator transforms this hydrodynamic energy into highly useful electric energy. The primitive energy of the waterfall is no longer expended in erosion or some other crude form but, refined and disguised, it serves the material and cultural needs of man.

Rarely does the individual recognize that his activity which serves the material, mental, and cultural welfare of himself and his fellows derives its energy from impulses originally developed for biological and selfish ends. The scientist engaged in research on problems of importance to the health or welfare of the entire race does not consciously recognize that his researches are but the disguised and refined expression of a pronounced, innate drive of curiosity.

DEFENSIVE PROCESSES

Conversion

It is doubtful whether conversion should be considered a defense mechanism as it has been in the past. Conversion is a psychological process in which one finds utilized the mechanisms of repression, identification, displacement, denial, and symbolization. Thus a conflict inducing a painful affect is converted to an inhibition of some motor or sensory functions and in so doing neutralizes the affect discharge. With the paralysis or sensory disturbance the conflict is denied, the affect repressed, and yet the inhibition of function symbolizes the repressed wish and the need for its inhibition. It appears as well that those utilizing conversion often select the symptoms on the basis of identification.

Fantasy and Dreams

In mental health, the freely-wandering thought of imagination promptly corrected by reality plays a useful part in constructive thinking. If, however, the gratifications of reality are insufficient, thinking may not be controlled by the demands of reality but may serve as a regressive or substitute satisfaction. Such musing is known as fantasy. Fantasy provides the illusion of a fulfillment of wishes which cannot be satisfied, either because of the frustrations of reality or because the individual's standards of behavior forbid actual gratification of strivings and wishes. Often these strivings and wishes are of such a character that directed reflection on them would scarcely be permitted. Fantasy is a defensive or tension-relieving mechanism offering either solace and an illusionary release from unsatisfying reality or an imaginary satisfaction of wishes, any actual gratification of which has been forbidden by repression. In Freud's words: "The pleasure-principle triumphs over the reality-principle." By the former, he meant the unconscious processes that strive toward the immediate gaining of affective pleasure. By the latter, he meant the conscious tendency of the individual in his attempt to satisfy his pleasure to consider such practical necessities as the outer world imposes and, if necessary, to postpone the satisfaction of these pleasures. Because so seductive and so satisfying in itself, fantasy may replace necessary reality thinking or effective acting and serve as a substitute for directed effort at adjustment to the actualities of life. Fantasy has much in common with dreams, differing chiefly in being more coherent and in occurring during waking hours.

Fantasy is not an isolated function but an integrated synthesis of idea, conation, feeling, interpretation, and memory in which instinctive and affective elements predominate and largely direct it. By disregarding reality and providing a substitute satisfaction, it aids in resolving conflicts and in preventing the development of anxiety. In extreme cases it tends to enlist the aid of delusions and hallucinations; wishes, particularly those that remain unsatisfied and beyond full conscious awareness, are projected and come back realized. In many cases, at least, fantasy may be regarded as a defense against anxiety. The psychotic patient may live simultaneously in two unrelated worlds—one of fantasy and one of reality.

One patient in his fantasy world owned the United States Treasury and its contents; he built and controlled the hospital in which he lived but had just lost the key to it. Almost daily he would hand his physician an order for a billion dollars, at the same time begging for some tobacco and that he be given parole of the grounds.

This coexistence of the consciousness of fantasy and the consciousness of reality is made possible by the mechanism of rationalization and its production of what is known as a "logic-tight compartment." Related ideas exist in each compartment, undisturbed by those in the other, each group pursuing its course segregated from those which are incompatible by a barrier through which no reasoning or argument can force a passage. "Logic-tight" and "affective-tight" compartments produced by rationalization are not confined to the psychotic but may be seen among those who are considered of sound mental health. In such cases, the compartments assure an affective segregation of incompatible strivings and emotional material.

Dreams and fantasy, like conversion, are better considered processes which utilize and combine many of the defense mechanisms in order to allay anxiety, as Freud so beautifully showed in his study of dreams. In the dreams are found united condensation, displacements, symbolizations, regressions, and others.

Dreams are a form of fantasy or imagery by which the ego attempts to resolve problems and protect against affects. Contrary to earlier impressions derived from simple subjective reports on dreaming, it seems established that dreaming consumes 20 per cent of the sleep time. Dreaming takes place in the lightest stages of sleep, judging from the analyses of electroencephalographic recordings. It is associated frequently with rapid oscillating movements of the eyeballs. There is some evidence to show that deprivation of dreaming establishes a tension state. Thus, the dreaming process is a drive state necessary for proper personality functions.

BIBLIOGRAPHY

Aserinsky, E., and Kleitman, N.: Regularly occurring periods of eye motility and concomitant phenomena during sleep. Science, *118*:273, 1953.

Braceland, F. G., et al. (Eds.): The Psychiatrist, His Training and Development. Baltimore, The Lord Baltimore Press, 1953, ch. 2.

Dement, W., and Kleitman, N.: Relation of eye movements during sleep to dream activity. J. Exp. Psychol., *53*:339–346, 1957.

Fisher, C.: The psychogenesis of fugue states. Am. J. Psychotherapy, *1*:211–220, 1947.

Fisher, C., and Paul, I. H.: The effect of subliminal visual stimulation on images and dreams. J. Am. Psychoanalytic Ass., *7*:35–83, 1959.

Freud, A.: The Ego and the Mechanisms of Defense. Translated by C. M. Baines. London, Hogarth Press, 1937.

Freud, S.: Psychopathology of Everyday Life. Translated by A. A. Brill. New York, The Macmillan Co., 1930.

Greenson, R. R.: The struggle against identification. J. Am. Psychoanalytic Ass., *2*:200–217, 1954.

Kant, F.: Investigations into the dynamics of paranoid reactions. Dis. Nerv. System, *11*:268–272, 1950.

Klein, G. S.: Consciousness in psychoanalytic theory. J. Am. Psychoanalytic Ass., *7*:5–34, 1959.

Kubie, L.: Body symbolization and the development of language. Psychoanalytic Quarterly, *3*:1–15, 1934.

Rangell, L.: The nature of conversion. J. Am. Psychoanalytic Ass., *7*:632–662, 1959.

Rapaport, D.: The Organization and Pathology of Thought. New York, Columbia University Press, 1951.

Ruesch, W.: Disturbed Communication. New York, W. W. Norton & Co., 1957.

Solomon, J. C.: A Synthesis of Human Behavior. New York, Grune & Stratton, Inc., 1954.

Chapter Five

PSYCHOPATHOLOGY

Psychopathology, the definition of abnormal personality functioning, has evolved from the recognition of easily discernible and gross disturbances of human behavior in terms of action, thought, and consciousness to an expanding awareness of the variations in the total patterns of reactions to living of the individual which we recognize as personality. The gross symptomatic expressions of disturbed behavior were known centuries ago; their occurrence in more or less persistent and recognizable groupings led to the Kraepelinian elaboration of the various categories of psychotic behavior which still constitute the matrix for the syndromes now recognized in modern clinical diagnostic nomenclature. Further studies of abnormal behavior have established the various forms of the psychoneuroses, the mental deficiencies and personality disorders of both adult and early life.

The so-called "abnormal" is but an exaggerated or unbalanced expression of the normal. It seems most fruitful to look upon most manifestations of psychopathology not as the result or expression of some "disease" but as a mode of behavior or of living which is the logical, although socially maladjusted, outcome of the particular individual's original endowment, of the molding influence of the home, of traumatic experiences which modified personality development, of the stresses and problems springing from within his emotional and instinctive life, of his inability to meet these strains, of the type of self-defensive reactions habitually utilized for minimizing anxiety, and of any bodily ailments which impair the integrity or efficiency of his biological organism. Mental disorders should, therefore, be regarded as patterns of human reaction set in motion by stress. The tendency to look on those who manifest nervous or mental symptoms as being different in their organization from the so-called "normal" is erroneous.

Just as mechanical objects if subjected to stress beyond the limits of their elasticity suffer distortion, so the personality if subjected to anxiety-producing stresses beyond the limits of its capacity for adaptation may suffer disorganization in both overt and symbolic behavior. Doubtless everyone, however healthy his adaptation appears to be, has particular psychological spheres which are vulnerable to stress. If his experiences touch these areas and the degree of their anxiety-producing nature exceeds his ability to deal with their stresses by healthy, adaptive methods, he will be compelled to deal with them by neurotic or psychotic ones. Through repeated or cumulative stress, the individual's "normal" defenses no longer suffice and his adaptive capacity is exhausted. Stress alone, however, should not be considered as the precipitating factor in mental disorder. It must be a particular stress for a particular person and, perhaps, at a particular time.

Criteria of Mental Illness

Since all behavior is but a reaction to personality and life factors, it is not always easy to define criteria of mental illnesses. An unbroken line of continuity exists from normal behavior through neurotic to psychotic behavior. In the mental field as elsewhere, there are no fixed boundaries. Perhaps the criteria are largely the degree to which behavior becomes undesirably substitutive and symbolic and the extent to which one deals with problems in a neurotic manner rather than by rational decision. As Meyer has stressed, however, the form and coloring of mental illness is as wide as life itself.

Like more narrowly biological phenomena, such as fever, inflammation, and other morbid processes, mental disorders are defensive, protective, and reparative in purpose, but as they deal largely with the affective and psychosocial aspects of the organism, the adaptive ends they serve are those of personal situations. The symptomatology of the personality disorder represents either the individual's attempt to effect an adjustment to the interplay of psychological, social, and physiological forces impinging upon him or his failure in that effort. Again, the symptoms may represent an attempt to hide the truth from one's self, to retreat from difficult situations, to deal with anxiety, or to shut out the stresses of life but with the result that one employs substitutive methods of adjustment that lead away from reality which is sacrificed to attain emotional comfort, maintain self-respect, or provide satisfaction in the easiest way. The comforts and compensations, however, are highly egotistic and are often disserviceable or even objectionable to the social group.

Personality Trends

A longitudinal study of the patient's behavior pattern often reveals the psychopathology as the culminate but logical result of the basic mental habits and personality trends of the individual and an accentuation and distortion of the reaction patterns which he has long employed to meet the stresses of life. The same complex forces which determine the psychotic personality also play an important part in determining the clinical picture of the personality disorder. It reveals more sharply both the attitudes which have been subtly developing for years in response to anxiety-producing situations and to deep-seated psychological needs and the manner in which the personality has attempted to meet its stresses.

The formative factors may be detected in the early patterns and responsive tendencies characteristic of the individual personality. An urge for self-assertion, for example, may have been an attitude or personality trend found useful in dealing with certain anxiety-producing situations or persons. So long as such an attitude or trend remains adequately effective in its purpose, the individual maintains a satisfactory personal adjustment. Should, however, such a personality attitude not continue to provide the needed relief from his anxiety, the individual may resort to an exaggerated or unbalanced manifestation of self-assertion in the form of a manic attack.

Various personality traits may have represented compromises with unconscious conflicts and unconscious purposes. Through such compensatory compromises, the individual may have achieved a certain mastery over them, although he is never free from their influence. Finally, under some unusual stress, the compromise fails and the other symptoms of illness appear. When one discovers the significance of the patient's life pattern, his personality disorder comes to have a logical place in the evolution of that particular pattern. Any absence of continuity between the individual's pre-illness personality and psychic characteristics and those existing after the development of the mental disorder is only apparent. There is a definite correlation between the kind of person one is in health and the type of disorder one develops if he becomes mentally ill.

Personality "Sets"

In psychopathology, too, it is possible to see in isolated and exaggerated form many dynamic mechanisms which are easily overlooked in normal behavior and personality development. The mental disease often represents the result of a progressive development of the pre-illness characteristics to a degree which constitutes a caricature of the previous personality or leads to disintegration and breakdown.

The embryology of the illness may be studied in the habitual reaction patterns employed by the patient in his pre-illness life. The psychological process may lead from a long-standing character disorder into the early stage of an acute illness. The person who cannot modify his ways of thinking, feeling, and behaving as his life advances may find that an adjustment is possible only through a personality disorder. The same psychological theme or conflict runs through the personality, character traits, and psychosis. In all, there may be discovered certain attitudes or "sets" of the organism to respond in a given manner. Sir Russell Brain, the English neuropsychiatrist, in an apt selection of characters from Shakespeare, points out certain well-recognized types of personality and the form of mental disease in which they are prone to culminate. On the one hand, he says, is Cassius with his lean and hungry look and his propensity for thinking too much. In him is typified a form of personality calculated to develop a malignant, paranoid type of psychosis. On the other hand is the fat, jovial Falstaff in whom a personality disturbance, if it occurred, would probably be of a benign, affective type. It will thus be seen that mental disease is not a partial expression but one which goes to the very depths of the personality.

Abnormal Development

Although each person has his own particular characteristics which distinguish him from all others, certain general types of personality have been defined as disordered. For the most part the groupings are descriptive; a better understanding of the dynamics of personality development in each instance represents one of the areas of much-needed study.

The task of the physician and psychiatrist in clinical practice is to define the psychopathology of the patient and then attempt to understand the genesis of the abnormal development. As has been pointed out, the personality of the patient determines largely the manner in which he will respond to stress and thereby the specific definitions of the symptomatic expressions of his illness. In the study of the patient, the type of personality organization that the patient has acquired must be defined as well as the symptomatic psychopathology which he brings with him. This chapter therefore commences with a description of the commonly accepted types of personality disorder and then proceeds to describe the recognized symptomatic expressions of psychopathology. The former are the cyclothymic, hypomanic, melancholic, schizoid, compulsive, hysterical, and passive-aggressive personality structure.

DISORDERS OF PERSONALITY

Cyclothymic Personality

Kahlbaum introduced the term "cyclothymia" to designate the predisposition of the individual to alternating moods of cheerfulness, vivacity, and mild depression; cyclothymia also indicates the tempo of the personality, i.e., whether it is lively or retarded. While oscillations are not uncommon, mood and tempo continue to harmonize and the different components of the personality in their reactions and expressions function as a unit. Kretschmer characterized as "cycloid" those people who are subject to cyclic variations of mood which tends to swing between exhilaration and depression but not to pathological extremes. As might be expected, the cycloids or "cyclothymes" are predisposed to the development of manic-depressive or affective psychoses. Christopher Smart (1722–1771), the English poet who on at least one occasion developed what was undoubtedly a manic-depressive psychosis, said of himself, "I have a greater compass both of mirth and melancholy than another."

Hypomanic Personality

The hypomanics are outgoing, cheerful enjoyers of life. They are free from internal inhibitions, many being vivacious and sprightly and showing a sustained buoyant, confident, aggressive, optimistic, perhaps exhilarated reaction. They are usually energetic, gregarious, pleasure-loving, unstable, given to fleeting enthusiasms and easily swayed by new impressions. Some are blustering, domineering, argumentative, and hypercritical. Their judgment often appears superficial and they have a ready excuse for their failures. The hypomanic cannot subordinate himself, resents frustrations and disappointments, and is usually adept at talking himself out of difficulties. The hypomanic woman is often a chatterbox.

Melancholic Personality

Those cyclothymics at the melancholic pole are often kindly, quiet, sympathetic, good-tempered people, lacking in strained eccentricity but tending to be easily depressed. They feel but little of the normal joy of living and are inclined to be lonely and solemn, to be gloomy, submissive, pessimistic, and self-depreciatory. They are prone to express regrets and feelings of inadequacy and hopelessness. They are often meticulous, perfectionistic, overconscientious, preoccupied with work, feel responsibility keenly, and are easily discouraged under new conditions. They are fearful of disapproval, tend to suffer in silence and perhaps to cry easily, although usually not in the presence of others. A tendency to hesitation, indecision, and caution betrays an inherent feeling of insecurity. A few are irritable and paranoid. Many psychiatrists feel that the melancholic temperament of personality has developed its characteristics as a reaction formation against aggression.

Schizoid Personality

The schizoid (Bleuler) or schizothymic (Kretschmer) personality is marked by incongruities of the feeling-life coupled, characteristically, with a poorly socialized personality. It will often be found that the prepsychotic life of the psychotic schizophrenic was characterized by schizoid tendencies. In the schizoid personality the feeling-life lacks the resonance and responsiveness that characterize the cyclothymic. Its contrasting affective poles are sensitiveness on the one hand and dullness or coldness on the other. The sensitive schizoid feels lonely, imperfectly understood, and isolated. Timid, shy, self-conscious, often self-dissatisfied, perhaps stubborn, secretive, and suspicious, he is wounded constantly.

In childhood, he is often teased by his playmates who look upon him as "queer." In school or college, he rarely takes part in rough-and-tumble games but strives for a sense of security through superiority in school work. Silent and unsociable, his love of books is often a substitute for human companionship. He chooses subjects of an abstract, perhaps philosophical, nature rather than those of a concrete, objective type. He may be imaginative and idealistic, perhaps with vague schemes for bettering humanity. Many schizoids of this group attempt art or poetry. Some are successful in transmuting their daydreams into cultural values.

Many of these sensitive persons suffer from a sense of isolation. What their thoughts may be is often unknown, even to friends, since others are rarely admitted into their confidence. Many have feelings of inferiority and of discomfort in interpersonal relations and are aloof to the opposite sex. In speaking of the sensitive schizoids, Kretschmer comments that they close the shutters of their houses in order to lead a dream life. Many have a genuine love of nature, while those who have had cultural opportunities often show a rare esthetic taste, gentle manners, and an uncommon avoidance of the coarse or vulgar.

Frequently, they are ambitious, conscientious, meticulous, and perfectionistic. The overconscientiousness of the schizoid tends, however, to exert a paralyzing effect on initiative or variation, with the result that he often performs his duties in a stereotyped, almost ritualistic manner. Some schizoids are overscrupulous, and by making a virtue of their repression become ascetics or prudes. To a certain number of these frail, sensitive individuals, the harsh realities and frustrating experiences of life become too painful and they retreat into a world of fantasy.

Many schizoids, while retaining an imaginative attitude toward life and its experiences, lack the finer sensibilities shown by the type just described. The most attractive members of this second group are kindly and honest, but they are also emotionally dull, taciturn, unsociable, and given to rites and cults. Because of a lack of spontaneity, they appear to be indifferent, indolent, colorless persons. The less attractive members are often cold, reserved, callous individuals, frequently jealous of those more happily adjusted. Some shrink unhappily away into themselves and become preoccupied with unwholesome ruminations. In adolescence they are usually willful, disobedient, headstrong, moody, passively stubborn, ill-tempered, easily offended, and resentful of advice, supervision, or correction. Such a schizoid may be described as a "lone wolf" who prefers to get along without strong ties to other people. Often his early relationships within the family are disturbed and unsatisfying.

The self-confidence which sometimes characterizes these unfeeling, distrustful individuals will be found to be of compensatory origin and to arise from a sense of insecurity which, in turn, stimulates defensive attitudes and reactions that tend to increase and complicate the problems of adjustment. They have to show the world how tough they are lest they betray their shyness, diffidence, and sense of insecurity.

The mistrustful schizoid who expects and detects disapproval and insult may feel safer to endure in silence with self-restraint and sullenness, retaliating, as it were, in daydreams, fancying how he may punish and destroy his alleged adversaries. In less marked types, the dearth of esthetic sensitiveness may be shown by a neglect of personal appearance, home, and family, or by a lack of tact and other evidences of social sensibilities and amenities. A rigid moral idealism expressed in inflexible rules of conduct and associated with a self-satisfied intolerance is not rare.

Actually but few schizoids belong to the purely sensitive or to the purely unfeeling type. In the majority of them we find characteristics from both groups. Often, to our surprise, we find a sensitive and tender nature hidden beneath a cold and unresponsive exterior. Similarly one must not conclude that the schizoid type always exists in pure form. Often it is not clearly differentiated from the cyclothymic type, in whom there is a sliding scale between it and the schizoid.

Bleuler preferred the term "syntonic" to Kretschmer's "cycloid" to describe a personality tendency opposed in characteristics to the schizoid. The syntonic person is in vital contact with his environment, is emotionally lively and responsive, and his affects are versatile in expression and appropriate to the occasion. Syntonic characteristics reach their greatest development in harmoniously adjusted persons, whereas schizoid elements reach their maximum development in the schizophrenic psychoses.

Compulsive Personality

Individuals of an obsessive or compulsive nature are those whose superego functions are severe. They tend to be punctilious, rigid, fastidious, formal, meticulous, may be in constant doubt what to do, and have to go over things again and again. They are overinhibited, perfectionistic, self-doubting, and are unable to carry on their work if under pressure. They lack a normal capacity for relaxation. They show a tendency to literal obedience, have an exaggerated sense of duty, are harrassed by their responsibilities and scrupulosities, and cannot make decisions. If circumstances require a decision, regret is expressed for the choice which is made. The person of compulsive character is stubborn in his convictions and manifests a tendency to hair-splitting. In contrast to the suggestible, demonstrative, extroverted personality of the hysteric, he is likely to be of a daydreaming, introverted, self-centered type. The compliance and "correct" behavior of the compulsive personality are frequently a defense against hostile impulses.

If the individual is relatively free from anxiety, the existence in the personality of a certain degree of obsessive compulsive drive and persistence adds a desirable quality. Compulsive personality traits are within the range of normal personality variants as distinguished from symptoms of a compulsion neurosis which are pathological exaggeration of these variants. Such traits impart a desire to succeed; the compulsive person, too, is a hard worker. A degree of compulsiveness adds to strength of character. The difference between a compulsive personality and a compulsive neurosis is therefore one of degree, of the amount of anxiety present and of the extent to which the personality habitually defends itself against chronic anxieties by ritualistic devices. The origin of the compulsive personality, like that of the obsessive compulsive neurosis, is to be found in an investigation of childhood factors which played a role in character formation. Frequently the traits are safeguards against hostile impulses, unconscious aggression, and accompanying guilt. Not rarely the chronic tension of the compulsive personality may as a result of stress lead to an obsessive compulsive neurosis.

Hysterical Personality

More clearly defined for women than for men, this type of personality make-up is recognized by the traits of vanity, self-indulgence and self-centered attitudes associated with histrionic behavior, dramatization or exhibitionism sometimes coupled with lying, exaggerations, or play-acting directed either to becoming the center of attention or avoiding shameful exposure by deceit. Affectively the hysterical personality is labile, emotionally capricious, and prone to emotional outbursts. At other times the affective response appears shallow or fraudulent as though put on for display. Sexual behavior in women of this type is provocative and coquettish, with erotization of non-sexual relations. In actuality there often exists sexual fear with frigidity in women who have a pronounced masculine protest. The provocative attention-getting behavior appears to overlie a driving, dependent need, demanding in quality. There is reason to consider that many women of this type have been spoiled and overprotected in earlier years.

The "Don Juan" character represents for men this personality type. Again there is the histrionic display. The drive for sexual conquest and exhibitionism often rests upon a hidden feeling of masculine inadequacy and is coupled with the need to deceive, outwit, and conquer. The "Don Juan" makes evident through the repetition of his conquests the lack of satisfaction in each successful affair.

Personality Variants

The following descriptions of personality types probably represent ill-defined variants of a similar group in which pathological dependency, with infantile and childish emotionality, is expressed in various forms, that is, either by infantile clinging, passive withdrawal, sullenness, or explosive outbursts. Others show limitations in control or appear to have defects in drive, persistence, and judgment. The terms are contained in the nomenclature of the American Psychiatric Association, described in Chapter 7, and are used widely to describe individuals who are found incapable of adaptation in military and civil life but who do not present features or symptoms of a more clearly-defined personality disorder or the psychological or physiological disturbances. By many the continued retention of these types is questioned in their present vague definitions.

Passive-Aggressive Personality

The passive-aggressive personality is thought to result from failure to attain a mature emotional development of the personality manifested in one of three ways.

PASSIVE-DEPENDENT TYPE. In this type there is a frank expression of an absence of mature self-confidence and self-reliance. The individual is overwhelmed by feelings of helplessness and indecision. He is irresponsible and childish and may cling to others as a dependent child does to a supporting parent. He requires approval and assurance. The clinical picture may include anxiety manifestations. The passive-dependent husband may depend on his wife for all major decisions. Individuals of this type shun overt expression of aggression and withdraw from any situation likely to arouse hostility. They are passive, timid, and fearful. The underlying hostility, covered by a rigid shell of timidity and passivity, is entirely unconscious.

PASSIVE-AGGRESSIVE TYPE. In this type the personality contains a considerable element of aggression, doubtless largely defensive in origin, but it is expressed by passive measures, such as sullenness, stubbornness, procrastination, inefficiency, and passive obstructions. Some persons of this type complain and are dissatisfied. They usually work poorly with others and may have a demoralizing effect on a group. Some have been fearful of or have shown a covert hostility to their fathers who have been dominant, rigid, unapproachable, demanding, and difficult to please.

AGGRESSIVE TYPE. In this type, the outstanding manifestation is a persistent reaction to frustration with such imma-

ture measures as irritability, temper tantrums, and even destructive behavior. Sometimes there is resentment of pathological degree. Many persons of this type are hostile, provocative, antagonistic, competitive, and ambitious. They manifest a "chip-on-the-shoulder" attitude. They may be sharp and biting and aggressively resistant. They demand special attention and assume unwarranted authority. Frequently they attempt to lure those in authority into long argumentative discussion. Grandiose fantasies are common. Earlier in their lives these persons have been openly hostile to their fathers. A deep dependency can be discovered below the surface. The aggressiveness here originates in a reaction formation.

Emotionally Unstable Personality

Individuals of this type of personality are characterized by the explosive intensity of their emotions in reaction to relatively slight external stimuli. Between their outbursts they are usually outgoing and friendly, happy and likable. Their relationship to other persons, however, is constantly subject to fluctuating emotional attitudes because of strong and poorly controlled hostility, guilt, and anxiety. Their emotional tension is usually at a rather high pitch and may suddenly and unexpectedly burst out in uncontrolled anger or other disproportionate emotional display. At these times such persons may shout, bluster, threaten, or even become destructive and assaultive. In some, the excitability may be manifested in outbursts of despair, sulky irritability, or obstinate inaccessibility. Suicidal attempts in response to frustration or as an effort to relieve a situation regarded as intolerable are frequent. Jealousy and quarrels with those of the opposite sex are common. Far from being the desired evidence of vigor and strength of personality, the outbursts of the excitable are often poorly concealed attempts to disguise an inherent weakness. Such reactions, characterized by fluctuating emotional attitudes, unstable and explosive feelings, and undependable judgment, are to be regarded as expressions of an immaturity of personality and probably may not be distinguishable from the passive-aggressive personality type.

Inadequate Personality

In spite of average educational and other opportunities and of normal intelligence as measured by psychometric tests, individuals of inadequate personality type fail in emotional, economic, occupational and social adjustments. They are often good-natured and easy going but are inept, ineffective, and unconcerned. Their judgment is defective; they lack ambition and initiative and may be dreamy and seem to lack physical and emotional stamina. When it is clear that effort would be rewarded, they lack sufficient perseverance to achieve the results already in sight. They can neither work nor wait for deferred pleasure or reward. As a result, they are improvident and shiftless. Many of the ne'er-do-wells belong in this group.

SYMPTOMS AS PSYCHOBIO-LOGICAL REACTIONS

The symptoms of mental disorder were formerly thought of as disturbances of different mental faculties. It is now recognized that the mind is not made up of an aggregation of isolated and more or less distinct, independent functions or faculties, such as memory, will, association, et cetera. These are simply convenient names for groups of mental processes which appear to have some feature in common but are in no sense unitary capacities. They are but different aspects of one homogeneous process. Mind is an integral function of the organism and cannot be split up into components. It must not be thought of as a sort of machine, different parts of which sense, perceive, imagine, remember, associate, reason about, desire, and choose. Although the metabolism of an organism is recognized as an integrated process, yet to describe it one must consider one aspect at a time. Similarly, behavior is a function

of the entire personality; yet in discussing what we speak of as mental disorder, it is convenient to look upon the different symptoms as disturbances of distinguishable phases of the mind. A division into disturbances of emotion, association, and memory is artificial.

Origin and Function of Symptoms

Some symptoms, such as impairment of memory in senile dementia, or confusion in a toxic state, are the results of physiological disturbances of neuron activity involved in the process of thinking. Neurotic symptoms, however, in contrast to those due to physiological or biochemical dysfunction, are manifestations of psychological processes of which the patient is little aware. Symptoms, then, are not abnormal functionings of unitary faculties but are psychobiological reactions or expressions of the total organism at the mental level; they are biological and dynamic concepts.

Symptoms are the results of many forces, some of them from without but more of them from within the patient. Such symptoms indicate particularly his problems and the way he is struggling to meet them. His symptoms may indicate his inability to deal with such problems as instinctive drives, with a difficult relationship to parents, wife, or children, with a feeling of guilt or insecurity, or with disturbing residuals from past experiences. Symptoms, therefore, even though they be weird and bizarre and therefore baffling to our understanding, have a cause and meaning.

To discover the meaning of those unusual personality manifestations that are called symptoms and the functions they are performing in the life history of the patient, one must ascertain the needs and meaningful factors or situations that led to their production. It should be remembered that the pathological psychiatric formations termed symptoms represent the patient's attempt, in the face of great difficulties, to maintain his existence in the best possible way. Symptoms, too, may be not only an expression of a mental illness but also an attempt of the patient to fight the illness. Regression, for example, with its withdrawal to an earlier developmental level, may be not only a symptom of mental illness but also an attempt to deal on that level with tasks consonant with his reduced ability.

Relation to Life History

The method of approach to an understanding of mental disorder is to correlate the symptoms with the whole life history of the patient and with forces which have played a part in molding his personality. The psychiatrist attempts to interpret symptoms not only in their relationship to past experiences but also in terms of the known dynamics of behavior. Clearness of thinking is promoted, too, by efforts to explain psychiatric symptoms in terms of methods of adaptation observed in everyday life or of methods allied to them. Through his symptoms and their motivational sources and adaptive functions it is hoped to read the riddle of the patient's inner life, to see the personality back of the symptoms.

The study of a psychiatric symptom requires, if possible, a knowledge of the history of that symptom within the patient himself. The major contributions to this history are not so much a knowledge of the events of the patient's childhood and adult years but of the way in which these events and experiences were understood by him unconsciously. The patient must be considered not only from the standpoint of his symptom but also within the context of his total situation and history.

Symptoms as Defenses

In studying mental symptoms, it is important to remember that their manifestations are specific and intimate life-revealing signs and that they have but little meaning apart from the setting in which they have developed. All symptoms have a fundamental connection of some sort with the life of the individual. Frequently they are expressions of, and a defense against, troublesome repressions and their resulting anxiety. Much mental material that cannot be expressed in frank, conscious form may be neurotically expressed in the imagery of the symptom.

Again, the symptoms may represent the tension-reducing devices or other defenses to which the patient must cling. If the individual's former choice of defenses against anxiety (repression, reaction-formation, symbolization, and others) proves inadequate, his next resort is symptom formation. Symptoms may therefore be regarded as defenses in an effort to compensate or integrate. Delusions, hallucinations, compulsions, and other symptoms should be traced back to their source just as a physical pain is traced back to its source in order that the factors which produced it may be understood and removed. As they are considered in the following pages, disabling compromises should be discovered with threatening situations and harsh reality.

At times symptoms represent the means employed by the patient in dealing with disowned and terrifying tendencies within him. It may be noted that many symptoms are produced through the operation of the mental mechanisms previously described. Anxiety-laden situations will be found to evoke psychological defenses which are labeled as symptoms. Unfortunately, many symptoms, while representing efforts of the personality to satisfy its fundamental needs, do so with results that disturb inner harmony or prevent social acceptance. They represent failures to deal adequately with frustrations, insecurities, and undesirable impulses.

Motives Underlying Symptoms

It will be found that any explanation of symptoms often requires the assumption that material beyond conscious awareness may possess psycho-dynamic or motivating qualities and to varying degrees may dominate the conscious personality; also, that many symptoms express the patient's feelings and problems in a symbolic rather than a direct way and have a meaning of much greater significance than their manifest appearance.

To the psychiatrist, the patient's behavior and reactions are what physical symptoms are to the general medical practitioner. The psychiatrist goes behind the particular deed and tries to ascertain the motive for it since he realizes that a reaction itself is not important unless it is judged in the light of the underlying purpose and motivation. It will be found, too, that in the symptoms of mental illness the dynamic relationships which frequently occur in normal behavior occur in isolated and exaggerated form.

An individual may use a variety of means (symptoms) to achieve the same goal. It will therefore be noted that similar genetic and dynamic factors may lead to symptom formation in psychological, somatic, behavior, and social fields. Also, the same or nearly identical conduct or emotional response exhibited by different persons may be the result of different life experiences or the expressions of very different affective reactions, and the patient may be greatly plagued and distressed by his symptoms. The symptomatic expressions of illness may be categorized into those of disorders of behavior in action, perception, thought, affect, consciousness, attention, memory, apperception, and orientation.

DISORDERS OF MOTOR ASPECTS OF BEHAVIOR

The disorders to be considered under this heading are those formerly described as "disturbances of volition," a hypothetical faculty assumed to be in the nature of a deliberative will. The disorders are those in the action sphere of the personality.

Conation
While the isolation of any aspect of the mind is purely artificial, yet the disturbances to be considered here lie in the field which the psychologists designate as conation, action tendency, or impulse toward action. This term includes an implication of affect and desire as well as the concept of what was formerly included under will. Conversely, all affects have conative elements and impulses.

Conation is really the intention-set or striving aspect of the personality. It represents the purposive activity of the personality but lacks the degree of consciousness which has usually been associated with the idea of will or volition. It is not a special faculty—there are no isolable "faculties"—but is the whole personality in action.

Attitude
Certain other terms dealing with the action sphere of the personality may be briefly mentioned. By *attitude* is meant a continuing set or predisposition to react in a characteristic feeling or manner. Attitudes are determined largely by one's feeling state and may be consciously or unconsciously acquired. They may become ingrained in the character structure of the personality and influence personality functioning. A bitter feeling, for example, may affect memory, judgment, and reasoning.

Disposition
By disposition is meant the sum of one's tendencies or inclinations as determined by the affective and conative components of his personality.

Assertion
Assertion may be defined as a deepseated drive or pattern of the personality to react in a definitely forceful way. The term assertion carries a certain implication of will to power in contrast to aggression with its implication of hostility as explained before.

Disturbance of Activity

Increased Activity
Disturbances of activity may conveniently be classified as those of overactivity (typically seen in mania), underactivity (depression), and dysactivity (schizoid and paranoid). An increase in pressure of occupation is known as increased psychomotor activity. Such activity is purposeful but no objective is attained, as the goal of the activity is constantly chang-

ing. The patient is very busy but his activities are not productive. A new activity is undertaken before there has been opportunity to complete the task already begun. This celerity is often shared by all conative aspects of the individual so that the stream of thought is characterized by a flight of ideas.

Decreased Activity

A distinct slowing up of conative expression occurs in decreased psychomotor activity or psychomotor retardation. Typically there is a prolonged delay before initiating the intended activity and, once begun, it is executed slowly and as if with painful effort. In extreme cases, the patient is mute and motionless and does not spontaneously undertake any activity. As in increased psychomotor activity, the other conative aspects of behavior may participate in the disturbance, with the result that a retardation of the stream of thought is often associated.

Repetitious Activities

In certain mental diseases, especially in the compulsive reactions and schizophrenia, it may be found that, when an activity has been initiated, there is a tendency to repeat it in the same manner for an indefinite period. This persistent and constant repetition of certain activities is known as *stereotypy* and may be of position, movement of body, or of speech. A constantly maintained immobility of position is known as *catalepsy*. A cataleptic form of immobility frequently seen in schizophrenia and probably to be regarded as the expression of a high degree of suggestibility is *cerea flexibilitas,* or "*waxy flexibility.*" This is so called from the fact that the joints of the patient's extremities may be flexed or extended with a wax-like rigidity, continuing to retain the position imposed as do the limbs of a jointed doll. The extremities may thus be placed and maintained in an uncomfortable position for a much longer period than would be permitted by a normal person. Stereotyped movements, known as *mannerisms,* are com-

mon as well in schizophrenia. These may be in the form of grimaces, repeated gestures, peculiarities of gait, or of numerous other types. Sometimes a complicated series of movements may be repeated and constitute a fairly definite ritual. The same rather meaningless word, phrase, or sentence may be repeated. Such a reiteration in which no coherent thought is expressed is known as *verbigeration.* Stereotypies have a definite psychological meaning, the symbolic significance in each case being peculiar to the individual and determined by his complexes or other affective experiences. After a time, their repetition may become a matter of habit, in which case the original affective value is largely lost.

Automatic Behavior

A phenomenological but not psychological counterpart of negativism is observed in *command automatism,* in which suggestions or requests from without are compulsively or automatically followed. Automatic obedience may also assume the form of repeating words or phrases uttered in the presence of the patient (echolalia), or it may be exhibited by the imitation of movements noted in others (echopraxia). Echolalia and echopraxia sometimes represent regressions to childish forms of "mocking" behavior in which hostility and resentment are expressed under the guise of compliance.

Negativism

Negativism is a psychological defense reaction characterized by opposition and resistance to what is suggested. It may be manifested by behavior which is the opposite of what would ordinarily be called for in a given situation. It is frequently expressed in such forms as mutism, refusal of food, non-compliance with requests, and resistiveness to effort to care for the patient. Psychodynamically the negativistic act provides gratification by the acting out of hostile, revengeful feelings toward significant persons; acts which the sufferer has learned are specifically anxiety provoking to the other and lead through the latter's evident concern to an expression of interest in the negativistic person.

Compulsions

A morbid and often an irresistible urge to perform an apparently unreasonable act repetitiously is known as a *compulsion*. The obligatory act may be of a simple nature, such as touching an object twice, walking on cracks, or it may be complex and constitute more or less of a ritual. A compulsion may be regarded as the result of an obsession, as an obsession in action. Such acts are so closely linked with obsession that the combination is often referred to as the compulsive-obsessive syndrome. They are not meaningless acts, but, through the operation of the mechanism of displacement, substitution, and symbolism, serve as defenses against anxiety. A common form of compulsion is that of hand-washing. Frequently the basic force behind this is guilt over masturbation, the repetitious act serving through the mechanisms of displacement and symbolism as an anxiety-relieving measure. Many people whom no one thinks of as suffering from mental disease have various obsessive-compulsive habits which serve as defense reactions for keeping anxiety, feelings of guilt, and unacceptable instinctual drives at a minimum. Among such habits of personality traits is a tendency to exaggerate the importance of carefulness and details and to stress cleanliness and orderliness. Various perfectionistic strivings and a rigid adherence to routine are obvious.

DISORDERS OF PERCEPTION

Illusions

It will be remembered that the various end-organs or receptors are so constructed as to analyze the environmental energy and select certain kinds which are transformed in the receptor and give rise to a nervous impulse. On arrival in the appropriate area in the brain, this impulse produces a visual, auditory, or other sensory image, the interpretation and meaning of which will depend upon one's previous experiences and interpretations.

One of the ways by which the mental life of the individual may express emotional or striving elements that touch it with peculiarly keen significance is through a perceptual misinterpretation of such sensory images. The elements which are particularly likely to lead to misinterpretations of these images are intense affective states, ardent wishes, or urgent drives and impulses. Repressed elements are especially apt to be highly dynamic and produce misinterpretations that reflect some affect or express some wish or drive. A patient with a deep feeling of guilt, for example, may interpret the rustling of leaves as reproaching voices. Such a perceptual misinterpretation is known as an illusion.

The illusion has the same psychological function as a hallucination, but less reality distortion is involved. The nature of illusions is especially likely to be determined by the prevailing trend of the patient's emotional state and needs. Strained expectation or fear predisposes to illusional interpretations. In mental health, but particularly in mental disorder, the emotional life imbues and tends to influence perceptual experience according to the needs of the personality. In confused, toxic states, caused either by ingested poisons or by infection, perceptions may be misinterpreted because the sensory stimuli and impressions are not sharply defined. Such illusions usually possess less psychological significance than do those occurring in fully clear consciousness.

Hallucinations

In an illusion, an image symbol of a real object is formed, but for psychological reasons it is misinterpreted. Arbitrarily hallucinations are generally regarded as perceptions which occur when there is no impulse created by the stimulation of a receptor. Whether the absence of sensory receptor activity actually occurs remains undetermined, since the casual observer has no means of verifying this assumption. The word *hallucination* was introduced by Esquirol (1772–1840), a pupil of Philippe Pinel (1745–1826). He defined it in accordance with its present meaning as a perception without object and clearly differentiated it from illusion.

Although lacking a basis of reality in the sense that the percept is not aroused by a current stimulus in the periphery, hallucinations constitute an actual part of the patient's mental life. They should not be looked upon as mental products which, arising from within and therefore not related to any external stimulus, come to possess the peculiar vividness that is usually associated with impressions derived from the external world. The content of the hallucinations usually suggests their dynamic significance. They may be regarded as representing a breaking through of preconscious or unconscious material into consciousness in the form of sensory images in response to psychological situations and needs. Anxiety often plays an important part in their genesis. These hallucinated images which the patient accepts as reality represent the projection onto the outer world of such psychological needs and situations as wish-fulfillment, enhancement of self-esteem, criticism, censure, a sense of guilt, self-punishment, the satisfaction of repressed and rejected impulses, or the desire for a more satisfying reality. The dreams of normal persons are prototypes of the mental patient's hallucinations. Sometimes in case of internal conflict there is hallucinatory expression of the internal debate; some of the hallucinations express approbation or commendation, while others represent the other side of the issue and express insults and antagonism. It will be seen, therefore, that hallucinations are *never symptomatic* of a given morbid condition.

The way in which escape from a harsh and unsatisfying reality may be secured through hallucinatory perceptual experiences is illustrated in the actions of a woman whose natural biological tendencies had been frustrated and who, because of personality inadequacies, had found economic and social adjustments too great a burden. One day as she was sitting on the bank of the Potomac River, preoccupied with her problems and dreaming of some means of satisfactory escape from them, she heard the voice of a former lover who had ceased his attentions as her personality limitations had become more apparent. In this thwarted and distressing state of affairs, she received from the old admirer a message pointing the way to an enchanting fulfillment of her fondest hopes. Although she could not see him, the patient heard the lover direct her to jump into the water, from which he promised to rescue her and row her to Norfolk, whence they would sail to Egypt, there to occupy a beautiful castle. So convinced by the vividness of the message that reality was ignored, the woman threw herself into the water where she would have perished except for some chance passers. A correct appreciation of her experience would have been too painful and disillusioning, and so she continued to believe in the reality of these autogenous perceptions.

In mental health the majority of perceptions produced by casual stimuli from our environment are ignored. The content of perceptions in hallucinations is so intimately subjective that in their acute phases, at least, they cannot be ignored and therefore not only absorb the attention but require that reality be made to harmonize with them. As a result, the functional capacity of the ego for testing of any reality that does not harmonize with the hallucinations is usually suspended.

In so-called "anticipatory" illusions and hallucinations, a person in a tense emotional state, say of fear, intently expects to see or hear the object which has excited the emotion. The result is that the perception momentarily expected in vivid clearness appears, but in a projected, hallucinatory, or illusional form.

Sometimes various gradations between normal representation and hallucinations may occur, with the result that the patient is uncertain as to whether his mental experience has been of a perceptual (unreal) nature or whether it has been merely a thought.

Hallucinations may occur in diseases associated with toxic or organic states. Although in these cases there is perhaps an irritation of the association centers connected with the special sense hallucinated, the nature of the material hallucinated is doubtless influenced by the psychological experiences of the patient.

Psychological material may be projected in the image symbols of any of the senses, although the images are characteristically of that sense best fitted to symbolize the particular material seeking expression. Feelings of guilt, for example, may best be expressed in spoken language, and so the patient hears accusing voices. Such accusing voices represent the projection of the critical voice of the superego. Fear of some aspect of the personality may well be symbolized by the sight of terrifying objects, and so the patient sees frightful animals. One patient with an experience which he looked upon as one of moral contamination complained of a constant odor of carbolic acid. To him this chemical had always represented a purifying agent, and its hallucination was well adapted to symbolize his desire for a feeling of moral purification.

Hallucinations are more marked during the early and acute stages of a psychotic reaction. This is to be expected, since it is the period when repression is failing and the solution of the conflict is proving unsuccessful. Hallucinations with clearness of consciousness are of much more serious prognostic import than those occurring with clouding of consciousness. Hallucinations occur less frequently when the patient is occupied with reality than when attention slackens or he begins to daydream. They are often associated with delusions to which they add a support or corroboration. At times, they seem to be the concrete symbolic expression of delusional ideas.

The occurrence of hallucinatory experience is not synonymous with that of mental disorder. *Hypnagogic hallucinations* take place in healthy persons in that period between sleeping and waking. Hallucinations and illusions may be induced in the healthy in periods of prolonged isolation or under the influence of certain pharmacologic agents such as mescaline or d-lysergic acid–diethylamide-25. Hallucinations induced by such agents are seldom formed, are usually lacking in ideational content, and are experienced as outside or beyond the self of the subject. In these respects they differ from the usual hallucinations of the psychotic person, who fails to distinguish his experience from reality and as beyond himself. Otherwise these experiences are *ego dystonic*. Again they occasionally occur as transient phenomena and in a benign sense in familiar situations in which the perceiver is experiencing a special need for food, fluids, or some other unrequested physiological satisfaction.

HALLUCINATIONS OF HEARING. As already indicated, hallucinations of hearing are the most frequent form of perceptual disturbance. Sometimes the hallucinations are in the form of various noises but most often in words arranged in more or less complete sentences. Usually these sentences are remarks concerning the patient or addressed to him. The patient may converse or quarrel with the "voices." He may locate them as coming from any part of the body or from a distance. Sometimes the remarks are of a pleasant nature but usually they are unpleasant, derogatory, obscene, or in the nature of accusations. These unpleasant remarks represent the projection of disowned personality aspects or desires which may not be allowed in consciousness in undisguised form. Hallucinations conveying a command are often convincing and compelling. They may therefore lead to direct and dangerous action. Considerations of reality are of little weight in comparison to their influence. Auditory hallucinatory experiences often are associated with movement of the laryngeal musculature, suggesting that the patient is uttering subvocally the words which he perceives in his hallucination just as a child does as he learns to read silently.

HALLUCINATIONS OF SIGHT. These are not rare but are much less frequent than auditory hallucinations. They occur most typically in the deliria of acute infectious diseases or of toxic psychoses. In each of these states the visual hallucinations are apt to be accompanied by some clouding of consciousness. In general, visual hallucinations are confined to acute, reversible organic brain disorders. Visual hallucinations more frequently excite fear in the patient than do auditory ones, since they produce a greater distortion of reality. One of the most frequent forms of mental disorder accompanied by visual images is delirium tremens in which the images tend to be of a terrifying nature.

HALLUCINATIONS OF OLFACTION. Hallucinations of smell are not uncommon in schizophrenic states and with lesions of the temporal lobe. Olfactory hallucinations are usually of an unpleasant or even of a strongly objectionable character. Their repulsive nature is not surprising, since they are particularly apt to represent feelings of guilt.

HALLUCINATIONS OF TASTE. True gustatory hallucinations are uncommon but at times are associated with hallucinations of smell. Illusions of taste are much more frequent.

TACTILE HALLUCINATIONS. Hallucinations of touch occur principally in toxic states, such as delirium tremens, and in cocaine addiction. Hallucinated sexual sensations are observed in schizophrenia and are often associated with grotesque delusions concerning bodily organs.

KINESTHETIC HALLUCINATIONS. Hallucinations of non-existent body parts (phantoms), of changes in their shape, size, or movement, do occur. They most commonly occur after acute loss of limbs, but also in toxic states and schizophrenic reactions.

DISORDERS OF THINKING

The joining of ideas one to another by imagining, conceiving, inferring, and by other processes, and the formation of new ideas by these processes constitute a function we know as thinking. This may be looked upon as a form of internal or implicit behavior. Thought is the most highly organized of psychobiological integrations. In considering this function from the standpoint of psychiatry, attention should be directed to: (a) the production of thought; (b) the progression of thought; and (c) the content of thought. It should be remembered, too, that thought takes place on several levels, ranging from the fully conscious, dealing

perhaps with highly abstract topics, to that on a primitive, emotional level.

Disorders in Form of Thought

As just indicated, thinking is a form of behavior which implies the existence of stimulus and response, the latter serving some psychologic purpose. In mental health, the stimuli for thought come from various sources, including unconscious and affective ones, but thinking is corrected by reason and logic. Such thought is known as rational or realistic thought. It appears to be directed by, and to take place in, conscious awareness. In day-dreaming, thinking is not fully guided by realistic considerations but to a considerable extent by egocentric wishes and instinctual needs. In mental disorder, and particularly in schizophrenia, thinking may be directed even more by unconscious factors and become of the type first designated by Bleuler as *autistic* and later as *dereistic*. In *dereistic*, in contrast to realistic, thinking, complexes, drives, and other affective and conative thought motivations are given free rein and operate without conscious regard for reality. As a result, associations of ideas are no longer logical but assume the nature of "free" associations.

Disorders in Progression of Thought

The rate and manner of associative activity cannot, of course, be learned except through the patient's stream of talk. It is a matter of familiar observation that, as one's thoughts are expressed in language, there is a pertinent association or linkage of each idea with the one that has preceded, that one's thinking moves in a logical progression toward a more or less definite end. This progression of thought is often known as the "stream of thought" or "stream of talk." Normally, there is a logical and coherent sequence of related ideas passing uninterruptedly and without digression from an initial to a goal idea.

Flight of Ideas

In certain mental disorders, there occurs a disturbance in the progression of thought characterized by an increased associative activity, a rapid digression from one idea to another. Ideas follow in quick succession but do not progress toward the goal idea which is therefore never reached. This disturbance of the stream of thought in which the thinking processes appear to run too quickly and in which no idea is completed is known as flight of ideas. Flight of ideas is associated with an accelerated inner drive and distractability, as a result of which the patient is unable to sustain his attention and hold it directed toward a goal idea. Observation will usually disclose an associated relation between the thought and a prompting stimulus springing from either an external or an internal source. Frequently a word similar in sound, but not at all so in significance, calls up the new thought. This is known as "clang association" and may lead to a senseless rhyme.

One patient with a rapid flow of thought, when asked if he were sad, replied, "Yes, you have to be quiet to be sad. Everything having to do with 's' is quiet—on the q.t.—sit, sob, sigh, sin, sorrow, surcease, sought, sand, sweet mother's love, and salvation. This is my first case—I am kind of a bum lawyer or liar—too damned honest to be a lawyer, so had to be a liar."

Retardation

As already seen, the flow of thought in flight of ideas is abnormally rapid. In retardation, on the other hand, the initiation and movement of thought are slow. Often the patient will state that his thoughts come slowly or that he has difficulty in thinking. It will be noted that he speaks slowly and usually in a low tone. Retardation is most frequently observed in the depressive phases of the affective psychoses but may be noted in schizophrenia.

Perseveration

By perseveration is meant an abnormally persistent repetition or continuance in expression of an idea. This clinging to a thought may be observed at times in aphasia, catatonia, and in those with senile dementia.

Circumstantiality

Another disturbance in the flow of thought is that known as "circumstantiality." In this disturbance, the patient finally reaches his ideational objective, but only after many unnecessary and trivial details have led him into tiresome digressions. Circumstantiality occurs largely among persons who do not form sharply defined concepts or are unable to distinguish essentials from non-essentials. In mental disorder, therefore, it is frequently observed among the feeble-minded, epileptics, and cases of moderately advanced senile mental disorder.

Incoherence

Sometimes the progression of thinking is so disorderly that one idea runs into another without logical consecution, and speech is not bound by any law. The result is a disorganization of syntactical structure with a lapse into disjointed phrases or even into parts of sentences and it is known as incoherence.

One schizophrenic patient, when asked how long she had been in the hospital, answered, "Oh, three weeks—since different statements are made —because it is hot—Mr. Smith is a cheap guy— French—how goes about it?"

In incoherence there is a tendency for ideas to arise from a confusion of complexes, viz., repressed material highly charged affectively. As might be expected, incoherence occurs particularly in schizophrenia, a disease in which the thinking is characteristically dominated by complexes. Much of the thinking of the schizophrenic is described as "scattered," which simply means that in the former condition the thinking is a little less disorderly than in incoherence.

Blocking

Another disturbance in the flow of thought is that known as "blocking." In this disorder, sometimes known as "thought deprivation" or "thought obstruction," both expression and progression of thought suddenly cease. To a degree it may be considered as having a prototype in the sudden inhibition of the train of thought sometimes occurring when one is overcome by some strong affect, such as anger or terror. After a time, the apparent obstruction seems to be removed, and the flow of thought is resumed. This interruption of the progression of thought is probably caused by the activity of a dominant complex with its associated unpleasant affect. At first the blocking may be caused by some definite thought, or rather by the disagreeable affect attached to it, but it quickly becomes general so that nothing more is initiated. Blocking to a severe degree seems to be confined to schizophrenia.

Disorders of Content of Thought

Trends and Overdetermined Ideas

There is a tendency for the associative evolution of ideas, and therefore for thought content, to be determined more by affective factors than by logical reasoning. Ideas having the strongest feeling tones tend to dominate. It is because of this fact that thought content may exhibit a trend, viz., a propensity to center around a special topic. In case an idea comes to have an extreme feeling-tone connected with it, it is spoken of as an overdetermined or overvalued idea.

The importance or value and the meaning attached to an idea are directly proportional to the inner need for such a belief. When an overvalued idea exists, it blinds the individual to all else so that only those observations and memories are selected which suit its purpose or confirm it. Anything which conflicts with it is denied admission into consciousness.

The whole personality, including its thinking and feeling aspects, is absorbed by the idea and placed at its disposal, so to speak, with the result that the overvalued idea becomes one of the most important determinants of behavior. Trends and overdetermined ideas, like delusions, to be discussed later, serve to satisfy some pressing inner need of the personality, such as a sense of security, defense, or self-esteem.

Delusions

Everyone is prone to develop comforting and other psychologically useful fictions to afford support and security to the personality. Apparently, mankind has always developed or adopted elaborate beliefs in an effort to satisfy inner needs. The construction of reassuring delusive beliefs as protection against anxiety and insecurity has been universally characteristic. This has been the unrecognized purpose in our fairy tales, in the folk stories of powerful persons, and in our father-image myths, beliefs, and creeds.

Sometimes the demand for the satisfaction of special inner needs of the personality may be so insistent that the claims of reality are disregarded and delusional ideas appear. Actuality is transformed to make it compatible with the emotional needs of the personality. The delusion is usually defined as a false belief. As we consider delusions and their meaning, value, and purpose, we shall see, however, that such a definition is fallaciously inadequate. It is often said that to be considered delusional, a false belief must be one that a person of similar education and experience would consider improbable or impossible and is not corrected in response to reason or logic. Even this definition is inadequate, since it ignores any consideration of the important principle that the incorrect understanding and use of facts and evidence are in response to definite purposes and needs of the personality and that the prevailing factors which control delusional thinking are affective rather than ideative or cognitive.

How inner needs may produce misinterpretations, denial, and misuse of facts in a way to be considered delusional is illustrated in the following:

During World War I, a woman was notified by the War Department that her husband had been killed on a certain date and buried at a certain place in France. Several months later, she visited the Department and expressed the conviction that her husband was alive and that the body of her supposed husband was actually that of no person known to her. The military authorities presented evidence that no error had been made, but the widow remained unconvinced and demanded that the body of her alleged husband be returned to America and examined. This was done and the identification number and the location of wounds were found to correspond to the records of the War Department. Still the woman remained unconvinced. Finally the reason for the delusion appeared. Among the officer's papers collected after his death and forwarded to the widow were affectionate letters from another woman. The patient had protected herself from the painful realization that she was not first in the affections of her husband by developing the belief that the man who had been killed and whose papers had been forwarded to her was someone other than her husband.

We thus see that situations containing highly affective factors are accompanied by a lowering of the critical faculty and of the threshold of beliefs. Attempts through factual disproof to convince the patient that his beliefs are delusional are therefore rarely successful. The patient's experiences are assimilated and the picture of the external world supplied by his thinking is falsified according to his nonadjusted affective and instinctive demands. He acts as if his delusional system constituted reality—as to him it does.

As already indicated, the thinking which we characterize as delusional is quite similar in kind, although different in degree, to that in which we all indulge. Our beliefs tend to be subjectively colored, and doubtless all of us resort to certain fictions of security. Employment of wishful thinking by "normal" persons in their struggle for a realization of their hopes, and of rationalization or projection for defensive purposes, serves the same psychological ends as do the delusions of the psychotic and imperceptibly merges into them. Prejudices, likewise, often arise from intrapsychic conflict and serve as defensive measures.

From what has been said, it will be seen that delusions are attempts to deal with the special problems and stresses of one's particular life situation in which fantasy is called upon to supply what real life has denied. They differ from the beliefs of the healthy, however, in their irrational fixity, even in the face of what would be considered incontro-vertible evidence to the contrary. As Macfie Campbell expressed it, "The fantasies are not woven into a structure which is compatible with a normal social adaptation."

Delusions, therefore, require an individual approach. Their trend is determined by the prepsychotic personality problems and needs of the patient; the content will be found to reveal significant aspects of the patient's personal problems. The sources of these problems may often be found in thwarted trends and drives, frustrated hopes, feelings of inferiority, biological inadequacies, rejected qualities, teasing desires, gnawing feelings of guilt, and other situations which require a defense against anxiety. A deep-seated need for consolation, for example, may be met by self-flattering delusions.

Often the problem-solving value of the delusion and its relation to the situation by which it was produced are psychologically plain. Many times, however, the function of the delusion is far from obvious and its interpretation must remain a matter of speculation. This does not mean that the delusion is without significance or purpose. It possesses a definite adjustment value, but its source and purpose are concealed by its symbolically disguised content. When this central theme is extensively developed and conclusions are so logically deduced from the premises assumed that a coherent and connected organization of ideas is established, the patient's delusions are said to be *systematized*.

Since the psychological purposes and needs for the satisfaction of which delusions are created fall into certain general classifications, and as well-defined mental mechanisms are employed in their creation for convenience of description, delusions may be classified in accordance with certain type-similarities.

DELUSIONS OF GRANDEUR. Expansive delusions or delusions of grandeur arise from feelings of inadequacy, insecurity, or inferiority, any conscious recognition of which is prevented by the exaggerated ideative and affective components of the delusion. The content of grandiose delusions frequently suggests the nature of previous frustrations or insecurities. The patient who insists that he is God has, by the aid of his delusion, escaped from the troubles of reality which are too great a threat to his emotional security. If his distress was one of guilt, he has achieved perfection; if it was one of intolerable inferiority, he has achieved distinction; if it was one of fear, he has gained security and safety. The symbolic meaning of grandiose delusions is not greatly complicated and is fairly easily analyzed.

DELUSIONS OF SELF-ACCUSATION. Delusions of self-accusation are believed to arise because the repression of unacceptable trends and desires weakens and the superego becomes increasingly critical. In such a case, repression is not destroyed, but the threat, as it were, that consciously forbidden tendencies might be permitted expression creates in the patient a vague feeling of guilt. This sense of guilt is then rationalized in consciousness into ideas of remorse and self-accusation. Feelings of guilt may be appeased through self-punishment.

DELUSIONS OF PERSECUTION. Ideas of persecution are among the most frequent forms of delusions, occurring especially in chronic psychotic disorders. The threat of unworthy desires and of troublesome and disowned aspects of the personality is projected as hostility from the environment. Sensitive dissatisfactions with self, arising from unadjusted elements in the personality, may be projected as a dissatisfaction, and therefore as hostility, felt toward one by others.

The formation of delusions of persecution is facilitated by the mechanism of projection which easily leads to misjudgments of reality. The hostile and aggressive motives which the patient attributes to others reflect his own inclinations. High aspirations without qualities necessary for satisfying success accompanied by an inability to accept defeat may lead to brooding, distrust, suspicion, misinterpretations, resentment, and ideas of persecution, coupled perhaps with aggressiveness. Delusions of persecution permit a

shifting of responsibility and otherwise serve to relieve a guilt anxiety.

As a further measure for averting blows to self-esteem, the patient with ideas of persecution may develop compensatory reactions in the form of an exaggerated self-assurance. It will often be found that persons who develop delusions of persecution have, since childhood, been critical, resentful, suspicious, and unhappy. Not a few of them have been lonely, brooding, and insecure, and have lacked friends with whom they could share confidences. Ready to criticize others, they have been unable to tolerate criticism themselves.

It is not uncommon to find delusions of grandeur and of persecution associated. This is not surprising, since they serve much the same purposes, one tending to supplement the other. By his delusions of grandeur, the patient psychopathologically enhances his self-esteem and magnifies his ego. In the delusions of persecution, he repudiates and rejects by attaching to others those aspects and tendencies which self-respect would disavow. The two types collaborate to relieve anxiety.

IDEAS OF REFERENCE. Through ideas of reference, remarks or actions on the part of other persons, although in no way referring to the patient, are interpreted by him as being significantly related to himself and often as expressing accusation or depreciation. In paranoid states, ideas of reference represent a projection of the patient's own self-criticism onto the external world. In depression, feelings of guilt may stimulate ideas of reference, and these, in turn, contribute to loosely organized paranoid delusions.

DELUSIONS OF SIN, GUILT, IMPOVERISHMENT, AND ILLNESS. In depression, delusions frequently represent the ideational expression of rationalization of an affective depression. If repression weakens, material, such as wishes, memories, or ideas, which is of such a nature that it would cause emotional pain if admitted to consciousness is apt to give rise to depression. Depressive delusions often represent the rationalization of a sense of depression that has had its source in unconscious hostile tendencies felt toward persons against whom such feelings and tendencies should not be directed.

Depressive delusions are most frequently expressed in ideas concerning guilt, disease, or poverty. Ideas of guilt and of loss of self-esteem may arise when the repression of unconsciously desired, but consciously repudiated, tendencies is weakened. The patient, in his attempt to rationalize the vague feelings of wickedness rising into consciousness, formulates ideas of self-accusation based on criticisms by the superego. Unconscious hostile tendencies may be projected outward giving rise to fear of punishment. Any psychological factor which makes the patient feel that he stands out in an undesirable or unacceptable way from the rest of his social group may lead to delusions of guilt and therefore of depression.

Ideas of disease have similar meanings. The illness represents punishment for unacceptable and hostile drives to another; they may originate in identifications with the hated person.

Ideas of poverty are often the ideational representation of a subjective sense of loss of social value. Such ideas of poverty may accompany delusions of guilt, the idea of unworthiness being displaced to the most generally recognized symbol of value—money. Appearing at times with depressive delusions are nihilistic ideas expressing the patient's belief that he has no brain, that he has no feeling, that he is dead, or that other sections of reality no longer exist. Such nihilistic ideas probably have their origin in vague feelings of emotional change and in a subjective feeling of unreality and of changed personality. This subjective sense of absence and of change is rationalized into ideas of annihilation.

In passivity feelings or ideas of control, the patient may express the delusional belief that he is controlled or that people read his mind. Such feelings probably represent the denial of an impulse to yield to threatening internal needs or demands which, however, are disowned through the mechanism of projection.

Suicidal Thoughts

Thoughts of self-destruction, as well as suicidal acts, are evidences of psychopathology. Since the detection of suicidal thoughts gives warning of the possible act, the general subject of suicide is worthy of discussion here, although, of course, affect is involved as well as thought and action. Usually associated with suicidal ideation are self-derogatory ideas, delusions of sinfulness, unworthiness, or hopelessness, or at other times ideas of grandiosity or yearnings to be united with some person lost through death. Transient thoughts of dying or even suicide are probably universal, but obsessive ruminations are pathological. Most often the ideas of suicide and the act are motivated by a wish for instilling guilt through revenge, a hostile gesture toward some significant person who has or is fantasied as abandoning the suicidal person. As Stengel has pointed out, both the threat of suicide, however, and the fact that the majority of suicidal acts are planned so that not all is left to chance indicate that those who make a suicidal attempt are striving as well to give a guilty alarm to those close to them and bring about a change in their personal relations.

By far the majority of those who attempt suicide once do not do so again. Stengel's long-term follow-up studies showed that only one in ten did so. Suicidal efforts seldom occur before puberty in the sense of a deliberate act of self-destruction. Some younger children may die when carrying out an act designed to gain them parental attention through injury, but children of this age have not developed the concept of death as an infallible separation from life. Again, the presumed suicide in delerious states is often accidental—an unfortunate attempt to escape from some panic-inducing situation. Suicidal attempts are common in the personality disorders and depressive reactions, and they occur also with frequency in schizophrenia. Clinically and statistically the likelihood of suicide is increased when some other member of the family has committed suicide. In such instances, it appears that the suicidal person both identifies with his family member and has permission to carry out the act. In depressions, clinical observation has shown that the act is more likely to be performed during the period of recovery than when the patient is seriously retarded.

Hypochondria

Although containing important affective elements of a depressive nature, the symptom, hypochondria, with its exaggerated concern over physical health, may perhaps best be considered as a disturbance of ideational content. In hypochondria, the patient's attention is abnormally concentrated on his own body; he is depressed, and his thoughts are obsessively preoccupied with some organ which he is convinced is incurably diseased, although no pathological process can be demonstrated. A changed feeling of self may be present. Probably hypochondria should be regarded as an organ neurosis, in which tensions generated through psychological factors produce disturbances of organs innervated by the autonomic nervous system. Anxiety is displaced from unconscious mental sources to organs which thereby become the center of effective distress and preoccupation. The organ which is the focus of bodily complaint is usually one particularly subject to physiological expressions of anxiety or to the muscular tension of the anxious state. Hypochondria is more frequently manifested by persons who have shown a previous tendency to solicit desired affection or to evade the responsibilities of life through illness. In its milder forms, hypochondria may have its origin in a sense of insecurity which is rationalized as a threat to physical health. Because of the changing psychological outlook on life, as well as the regressive physiological processes and the failing psychobiological security at that time of life, the involutional period may be marked by hypo-

chondria. If hypochondriasis is consistent with the mood, it tends to disappear as the mood does. If it is symbolic or inconsistent with the mood, as in schizophrenia, it indicates a serious disorder.

Obsessions

Thoughts that persistently thrust themselves into consciousness against the conscious desire of the patient are known as obsessions. Obsessions persist in the conscious mind so tenaciously that they cannot be dispelled by conscious processes and are uninfluenced by logic or reasoning. The obsessive thought is strongly charged with the emotions of guilt or depression, is unwanted, and usually plagues the individual almost constantly. The sufferer cannot understand why he is obsessed with the thought. Obsessive ruminations are of various content. Often the constant preoccupation is concerning some metaphysical question. The patient, for example, may be compelled to keep asking himself why he was born. The explanation of obsessive thought is to be found in the activity of the unconscious and of repression. As a defensive device, a guilty anxiety is displaced to an innocuous idea and the anxiety thereby decreased. The obsessive thought which is consciously distasteful may be related to what is unconsciously desired. Obsessive thoughts are closely related to compulsive acts in which, after a distressing resistance to its performance, the patient feels impelled to perform some act which, because of its elaborate and repetitive nature, often seems almost ritualistic.

Phobias

Allied to obsessive thoughts are phobias, or fears, doubts, and indecisions. Like the obsessive idea, a phobia thrusts itself persistently into consciousness. Morbid anxiety always accompanies a phobia, in contrast to the guilt or depression of the obsessed. Among common phobias are fears of dirt, of bacteria, of cancer, or of crowds. In general, one may say that the patient's anxiety becomes detached from a specific idea, object, or situation in his daily life and is displaced to some situation in the form of a specific neurotic fear. The fear that he feels in the presence of a certain object or experience is really the displaced fear of some anxiety-producing component within his own personality. The situation about which he is phobic symbolizes or represents the incidents arousing affects of rage or shame, affects which must be prevented from coming to the surface, usually out of anxiety of rupturing an important relationship. The patient is not, of course, aware of the psychological source or significance of his fear, and while he may acknowledge that his fear is irrational, he is quite unable to regulate his life except as dictated by the phobia. He is constantly attempting to control his anxiety by avoiding the object or situation to which the anxiety has been displaced.

Finally, before concluding the discussion on ideational content, the student should be reminded that the thinking and behavior of the psychotic are just as "rational" as those of the personality usually called "normal," but are called "irrational" because of ignorance of all the experiences and conditioned responses and more especially the conflicts and anxieties requiring defense. In connection with the subject of ideational content, it should be remembered that the conscious thought content concerning any topic may be self-defensive and therefore directly opposite to that which deeper aspects of the personality would dictate.

DISTURBANCES OF AFFECT

By affectivity is meant the feeling-life or emotional feeling-tone of a person. The strong, temporary variations, modulations, and expressions of this self-feeling are known as *affects*. As pointed out earlier, the term emotion is often used loosely as if synonymous with affect, it connotes rather the physiological correlate that accompanies or expresses affect. By *mood* is meant a sustained, constant affective state of considerable duration. Affectivity penetrates and colors the whole psychic life, determining the general attitude,

whether of rejection or of acceptance, in relation to any experience, promoting any tendency in harmony with it, and inhibiting any impulse not in agreement. It, therefore, contains an inherent dynamic component which serves to influence both thought content and conative activity.

Affective factors may interfere with associative tendencies and prevent one from becoming aware of certain strivings or other consciously unacceptable aspects of his mental life. There seems to be reason to believe that profound disturbances of affectivity may even produce disturbances of consciousness, as in the perplexed, bewildered states of deep depression. In fact, as patients are observed while they are suffering from mental disorders and their feelings are largely determined by unconscious factors, it becomes evident that affective factors influence not only all other psychic functions but often physiological ones as well.

The role of affects for psychopathology is well summarized by Bleuler: "Just as those abnormalities which we call psychopathies are practically nothing but thymopathies (disturbances of affects) so affective influences play such a dominant role in psychopathology in general that practically everything else is merely incidental. Only the feeblemindednesses, the confusions and most delirious states are predominantly disturbances of intellect. But even these are colored by affective mechanisms, and often in both their practical and theoretical significance are determined by affective factors."*

Psychiatric literature strongly stresses the importance of psychogenic factors in the production of mental disorder. Although not clearly so denoted, such dynamic etiological factors are really affective in nature. It is not ideas themselves which are the important factors in determining the patient's mental content or his forms of behavior but the affects that are attached to his ideas. One thinks, therefore, according to the nature and intensity of his moods.

---

* Naturgeschichte der Seele, Zweite Auflage, S. 185. Julius Springer, 1932.

In the full evaluation of the significance of affect or feeling-tone in mental disorders, its consideration must not be confined to that of pathological variations, since, directly and indirectly, it exercises profound influence upon the thought and behavior of every individual. Not only is the thought content composed largely of affectively valued ideas, but judgment is constantly distorted and rendered unreliable by those ideas which are over-valued for emotional reasons. Associations are to a large degree directed by affective factors which facilitate those associations that tend to magnify the ego or aid in attaining some objective, while affects inhibit those associations which are unpleasant or opposed to some psychological need. If the tension of his emotional need or conflict exceeds the individual's capacity for evaluating reality, for appreciating its significance and remaining in contact with it, his experiences may be interpreted in accordance with affective needs and become hallucinatory or delusional.

By the mechanism of identification, an affect may extend or irradiate from the subject to which it was originally attached to one associated with or suggested by it. If, for example, a child came to hate a person who chanced to have some particular striking physical characteristic, then the child might always thereafter dislike persons who have a similar physical characteristic. In psychopathological states there is this constant tendency for the transfer of affects from material beyond conscious recognition to conscious thought content. In the psychoses, affective states of great intensity are often determined by unrecognized but highly dynamic factors. All affects possess conative elements; for this reason there is a delicate responsiveness of associations and behavior to affect.

Pleasurable Affects

A moderately pleasurable affect is known as *euphoria*. The euphoric patient is of an optimistic mental "set," is imbued with a subjectively pleasant feeling of well-being, and is confident and assured in attitude. Euphoria is most frequently noted in hypomanic states and in certain organic disorders such as general paresis, multiple sclerosis, and some cases of frontal lobe tumor. In *elation* an air of enjoyment and of self-confidence radiates from the patient, and his motor activity and drive are exaggerated. His circumstances may be such that unhappiness should be produced, yet everything that would normally produce that feeling is lightly brushed aside. It imparts a false sense of reality. Elation is often labile and readily shifts to irritability.

In *exaltation* there is an intense elation accompanied by an attitude of grandeur. A less frequent affective disorder is *ecstacy*. In this the mood is one of a peculiar, entrancing, peaceful rapture and tranquil sense of power. A religious feeling is an essential part of the state. The patient identifies himself with an immense cosmic power. He feels detached from outside things and on a new plane of existence, accompanied often by a feeling of having been reborn. That is attained, beyond which there is nothing better. After having emerged from the experience, the patient retains a vivid recollection of it. Dynamically, ecstacy probably represents the achievement of the maximum of wish-fulfillment. Sometimes ecstacy occurs in persons who have had a strong sense of guilt. It has been observed in dissociative, epileptic, schizophrenic, and affective reactions.

Depression

Depression, an affective feeling-tone of sadness, is probably the commonest type of complaint in psychiatric patients. Depression may vary from a mild downheartedness or feeling of indifference to a despair beyond hope. In the milder depressive syndrome, the patient is quiet, restrained, inhibited, unhappy, pessimistic, and self-depreciative and has a feeling of lassitude, inadequacy, discouragement, and hopelessness. He is unable to make decisions and experiences difficulty with customarily easy mental activities. He is overconcerned with personal problems. Some depressed persons are petulant, querulous, and distrustful. In somewhat deeper depression, there is a constant unpleasant tension; every experience is accompanied by mental pain; the patient is impenetrably absorbed with a few topics of a melancholy nature. Conversation may be painfully difficult. He is dejected and hopeless in attitude and manner. The patient's dispirited affective attitude is projected toward his environment which reflects his dolesome outlook. He feels rejected and unloved. He may be so preoccupied with depressive ruminations that attention, concentration, and memory are impaired.

Associated with this affect, some patients are anxious, perplexed, and complain of a feeling of unreality or of inability to think. Bodily complaints such as headache, tightness in the head, fatigue, loss of appetite, and constipation are common and occur in more than half of all cases of depression. Insomnia, especially that caused by awaking early, is the rule. Since mental content is greatly influenced by affective states, ideas of reference are frequent. Delusions are common and are prone to express ideas of guilt, unworthiness, and self-accusation. Suicidal thoughts are frequently entertained. Events and pecadilloes long past come to receive an interpretation determined by the present mood. Initiative is lost and replies to questions are delayed and often monosyllabic. The facial expression is one of dejection, perplexity, hopelessness, and perhaps of fear; the lower eyelids droop and the skin on the forehead may be furrowed, the corners of the mouth sag, and the eyes are often directed downward. In agitated depression, there are deep furrows between the eyebrows. Antagonist groups of muscles show slight imbalance, the flexors and adductors being moderately contracted, with the result that the neck, trunk, and extremities present the so-called "flexion" attitude of depression. All movements are executed slowly and with apparent difficulty. Depression is often accompanied by poor appetite, loss of weight, coated tongue, foul breath, and constipated bow-

els. Brain metabolism apparently remains normal in depressive states.

Depressions, in respect to their source, may be classified as reactive or endogenous. Reactive depressions are those that arise in reaction to obvious external causes which might naturally produce sadness, such as bereavement, business difficulties, or other adversity. They are not usually of protracted duration and are more responsive to the immediate environment than are the endogenous depressions. Retardation is more unusual in reactive states.

Depression has its roots in unconscious guilt arising from interpersonal issues, perhaps from unconscious ambivalence and hostility with resentful and aggressive impulses directed toward persons who are the objects of an undesired obligation (a mother whose dependency prevents her daughter's desired marriage) or toward persons on whom one is dependent for security. The hostile impulses originally directed against other persons become directed against one's own self.

Depression may arise not only as an affective repercussion to such a psychologically unhealthy method of dealing with aggressive impulses, but it may also become directed toward the individual's self, with a resulting affective reaction of depression. Feelings of remorse and guilt are more common in endogenous depressions than in the reactive ones. In depressions of a simple, retarded type, the anxiety may arise largely from past events, whereas in the agitated depressions common in elderly patients, the anxiety may be relative to future security.

It should be recognized that the affect of depression may include varying degrees of sadness, guilt, and shame simultaneously—sadness because of a loss, guilt over a repressed hostile drive, and shame due to failure to live up to some personal standard. The further study of depressions and the analysis of the pre-potent affect underlying the various forms of this state will go far to providing knowledge as to those types most amenable to alleviation. It is said that states of shame are much more impregnable to change than those in which guilt predominates.

Grief is to be differentiated from depression as an affect of sadness suffered from a loss of a close personal relation and unassociated with the affects of guilt or shame due to some repressed hostility towards the lost person. Grief, while leading to a withdrawal and preoccupation with the lost person, is self-limiting and seldom leads to serious impairment of usual activities, personal derogation, suicidal thoughts, or serious domestic disturbance.

Anxiety

Anxiety is a persistent feeling of dread, apprehension, and impending disaster. It is a response to threats from repressed dangerous impulses deep within the personality or to repressed feelings striving for consciousness, a warning of danger from the pressure of unacceptable internal attitudes. It differs from fear in not being referable to specific objects or events. The patient is ignorant of its source.

Most psychiatrists, in using the word "anxiety" without a qualifying adjective, mean neurotic anxiety arising from self-inaccessible sources as just described. Some speak of "normal" anxiety, meaning thereby that there is an actual danger which is realistically appraised and that the degree of anxiety is not out of proportion to the threat. Such an anxiety does not have to be managed by forcing it out of awareness by such mechanisms as repression or dissociation or by using neurotic defenses.

Anxiety is often displaced from its original, but unrecognized, source to some other situation which appears to the patient to afford reasonable grounds for apprehension, to be the excitant of his diffuse, unformulated uneasiness and painful apprehension. Sometimes the anxiety is not attached to any ideational content but is felt as a morbid fear without apparent source. Anxiety which is directly felt and expressed in this manner is known as *free-floating* anxiety. Again anxiety may be covert. In this hidden form, there is not obvious tension and painful apprehension with their physical manifestations. The various personality traits of the individual, together with the mental mechanisms which he has developed to conceal or displace his anxiety, may serve sufficiently well as defenses to prevent its overt expression. It may still, however, be the fundamental basis for the development of serious personality deviations or disorders. Anxiety is the presenting symptom in the so-called anxiety neuroses and may often be openly manifest in other neuroses. Anxiety, therefore, together with the various defensive mechanisms, such as repression, regression, conversion and displacement, developed to avoid it constitute important factors in the psychopathology of abnormal personalities, psychoneuroses, psychoses, and psychosomatic disease.

Anxiety occupies a position of great importance in psychoanalytical theory, according to which it results from the threat either of uncontrollable id forces or of self-destructive superego forces. According to this theory, anxiety is of significance in two roles: It serves not only as a signal or indicator of conflict but also as a reinforcing agent for repression, reaction-formation, and projection. In fact, the various mental mechanisms and devices which serve a defensive purpose exercise that function through their ability to reduce the strength of anxiety.

Through its effect upon the autonomic system, anxiety is particularly apt to disturb physiological functions and to find expression in psychophysiological symptoms. In acute forms, it may, through stimulation of the autonomic system, produce generalized visceral tension and therefore hyperventilation, spasm of the cardiac and pyloric portions of the stomach, intestinal irritability, hyperchlorhydria, diarrhea or constipation, palpitation, tachycardia, extrasystoles, vasomotor flushing, and respiratory distress. It may be accompanied by fainting, weakness, nausea, and tremor. Hands and face may perspire; the patient may assume a tense posture, show excessive vigilance and fidgety movements of the hands or feet, the voice may be uneven or strained, and the pupils be widely dilated. When anxiety is severe and overflows in this way into the muscular system with its production of gross motor restlessness, the reaction of the patient is spoken of as "agitation."

Tension is sometimes confused with the affect of anxiety. In tension, the patient has a continuing feeling of tautness, both emotionally and in his muscles. He senses a restlessness, dissatisfaction, dread, and discomforting expectancy. He presents a strained, tense expression of the facies, his fingers are tremulous, and he manifests an abrupt haste in movement. The patient may experience difficulty in concentration and complains of tightness or other unpleasant sensations in the head. Tension may arise when a person is torn between contradictory desires and strivings, by a struggle for security, and by various other situations. Its origin may be from either conscious or unconscious sources. It is accompanied by, or more accurately, is a component of, anxiety.

Panic may be considered as a pronounced state of anxiety which is productive of disorganization of ego functions. One of the best descriptions is that of Diethelm: "Panic is not merely a high degree of fear, but a fear based on prolonged tension, with a sudden climax which is characterized by fear, extreme insecurity, suspiciousness and a tendency to projection and disorganization." Misinterpretations are followed by projections that may assume the form of hallucinations having a threatening and accusatory content, and also may have the form of delusions of persecution. The situations giving rise to panic are ones in which some long-standing insecurity of the personality has created tension and become particularly threatening. Homosexual and occasional disowned heterosexual tendencies are the most frequent factors. Because of the underlying sense of insecurity, the patient may react with self-assertion and aggressiveness, may rush about or, in other cases, exhibit dilated pupils and the other usual sympathicotonic manifestations of great anxiety, yet remain immobile because he does not dare move. He often has difficulty in thinking and at times a sense and appearance of bewilderment. Suicide is not uncommon in panic states.

Inadequate Affect

Emotional dulling or detachment in the form of indifference or apathy is a frequent form of affective disturbance and is characterized by an inadequate sensitiveness to those experiences which normally give rise to pleasure or pain. The facies shows an emptiness of expression. Patients suffering from this affective impoverishment show a lack of drive and interest in those matters which have previously appealed to them. There is an indifference to esthetic and other finer sentiments. Such qualities as gratitude, sympathy, hope, anticipation, grief, regret, pride, or shame no longer appear to form part of the patient's subjective experience. This absence of emotional responsiveness may cause the patient to seem out of touch with reality. Apathy may be regarded as a protective, defensive reaction, perhaps against painful perceptions.

Inappropriateness of Affect

Disharmony of affect is a common emotional disturbance, particularly noted in schizophrenia. The patient smiles when the social situation suggests a serious mien as appropriate. He laughs or cries out of context to the interpersonal milieu and apparently in relation to his inner percepts and associations. The affect may be quite appropriate to the latter.

Ambivalence

Recognizing that each feature of the personality has a double aspect, each having a counterpart closely connected with it, Bleuler introduced into psychiatric thought the concept of ambivalence. In affective ambivalence, contradictory feeling attitudes may exist toward the same object. Both of these conflicting attitudes are faces on the same coin; while only one may be visible, the other is nevertheless present. One of the two components of ambivalence remains repressed but may nevertheless give rise to anxiety and feelings of guilt. A common form of ambivalent polarity is a subtle combination of love and hate. A person caring for an invalid member of his family may, for example, have mixed feelings. One feeling may be that of love, of wanting to be helpful, but another, of which he is not conscious, may be that of annoyance and hostility. Affection is linked with a sentiment of rejection. In the confusion of hostile and affectional impulses, there may be an intensification of conscious love in order to repress the fundamental hatred. An expression of hostility toward one to whom a person should be indebted, a parent, for example, is not consciously tolerable. The hostility, therefore, necessarily remains unconscious lest it give rise to anxiety. The ambivalent attitudes of hostility and love are accordingly developed. Often when ambivalance of feelings exists, the repressed component of the dual affective attitude will be projected. The repressed hatred existing in the ambivalent feelings felt toward another person may be projected and, therefore, experienced as hatred directed toward one's self by the other party.

Depersonalization

Depersonalization, a pervasive and distressing feeling of estrangement, known sometimes as the depersonalization syndrome, may be defined as an affective disorder in which feelings of unreality and a loss of conviction of one's own identity and of a sense of identification with and control over one's own body are the principal symptoms. The term was introduced by Dugas in 1898. The unreality symptoms are of two kinds: a feeling of changed personality and a feeling that the outside world is unreal. The patient feels that he is no longer himself, but he does not feel that he has become someone else. The condition is, therefore, not one of so-called transformation of personality. Experience loses emotional meaning and may be colored by a frightening sense of strangeness and unreality. The onset may be acute, following a severe emotional shock, or it may be of gradual onset following prolonged physical or emotional stress. It is more frequent in personalities of an intelligent, sensitive, affectionate, introverted, and imaginative type. The patient may say his feelings are "frozen," that his thoughts are strange; his thoughts and acts seem to be carried on mechanically as if he were a machine or an automaton. People and objects appear unreal, far away, and lacking in normal color and vividness. The patient may say he feels as if he were going about in a trance or dream. He appears perplexed and bewildered because of the strangeness of unreality feelings. He has difficulty in concentrating and may complain that his brain is "dead" or has "stopped working."

Depersonalization is probably not a specific disorder but occurs in various neurotic and psychotic states such as depressions, hypochondria, obsessional states, and hysteria, and in some early schizophrenias. Apparently it may occur in some normal persons after exhaustion or shock. It is more common at puberty and in women. The reaction may be regarded psychopathologically as a form of withdrawal from reality, as a means of escape from an intolerable situation by an insecure and self-observing personality. The syndrome is not influenced by drugs, but a remission follows a course of electroshock treatments.

DISTURBANCES OF CONSCIOUSNESS

Perhaps from a descriptive standpoint the word "clearmindedness" or "awareness" best indicates what we designate as consciousness. The sensorium is clear, i.e., the functioning of the special senses is intact, and the apprehension of external stimuli presented to them is unimpaired. The individual is able to apprehend his environment as to place, time, person, and general setting, to understand questions, and to reflect upon them.

Full consciousness demands attentiveness as well as that complex function known as *apperception,* by which through active, attentive thoughts one analyzes, integrates, evaluates, and absorbs experience. W. M. Wundt (1832–1920) defined it as "the single process by means of which any psychic content is brought to clear conception." By it new ideas are formulated and related to ones already familiar, with the result that one is able to understand or "grasp" new situations, events, and experiences. In *disturbances of apperception,* the patient has difficulty in understanding questions, unaccustomed situations, and experiences. Disorders of apperception occur in psychogenic diseases involving intense preoccupation and in other disturbances of attention, also in toxic and organic states. Faulty capacity for apperception exists, of course, in mental deficiency. The projective psychological tests (Rorschach and thematic apperception) are examinations of this function.

Among the disturbances of consciousness are those imposed by *disordered attention.* The conscious, selective reaction by which the organism examines the external world for useful data is known as attention. Successful examination requires a certain degree of vigilance and a certain length of tenacity. Attention is greatly influenced by conation, affect, and associations. Feeling and attitudes influence attention, not only directly but indirectly, through their effect upon associations. Fatigue, toxic states, and organic lesions strongly modify both vigility and tenacity and so influence attention. Toxic and organic factors, by interfering also with associations, tend to lower attention. Similarly, a poverty of associations is largely responsible for defects of attention in the mentally deficient. Even a normal person who has few associations connected with an object submitted for examination will, in the absence of strongly affective factors, exhibit but little attention. The inability to hold the attention a sufficient length of time to render adequate examination possible is known as *distractibility.* In this disorder, every fleeting stimulus or an abnormal lability of affect redirects the attention, which is lacking in normal tenacity. Profound depression, on the contrary, may cause too great tenacity of attention. No stimulus or experience can divert the attention to an idea or object not related to the patient's depressive mental content or not in harmony with it. Emotional disorganization as seen in the apathetic schizophrenic may greatly diminish the degree of attention.

As indicated in an earlier chapter, consciousness may be considered to exist at varying levels of awareness of one's environment. Thus it is to be suspected that the clinical disturbances of this function roughly describe progressively serious levels of impairment. The clinician defines as successive steps in defects, from the least to the greatest impairments, states of confusion, clouding of consciousness, delirium, dream, and fugue states, to complete stupor.

Confusion

Confusion is a disturbance of consciousness characterized by bewilderment, perplexity, disorientation, disturbance of associative functions, and poverty of ideas. The face of the confused patient presents a distressed, puzzled, and, at times, surprised expression. Confusion is confined largely to conditions in which there is a diffuse impairment of brain tissue function, especially associated with toxic, infectious, or traumatic agents, although it occurs also in dissociative reactions and epileptic dream states. Most psychiatrists believe that the term confusion should not be loosely applied to those subjects, such as retarded, depressive, or perplexed schizophrenic patients, whose replies are neither prompt nor pertinent. Many consider that true confusion is found only in toxic-organic reactions. Certainly clouding of consciousness is the basic feature in the toxic-organic states.

Clouding of Consciousness

Clouding of consciousness is a disturbance in which clear-mindedness is not complete, usually because there are physical or chemical disturbances producing functional impairment of the associative apparatus of the cerebrum. The threshold of consciousness is high, and perceptions are not produced by those sensory stimuli which ordinarily result in clear perceptions. The capacity to think clearly and with customary rapidity, to perceive, respond to, and remember current stimuli is impaired. To make the patient understand a question, it may be necessary to shake him, to shout the question, and perhaps to repeat this procedure several times before he apprehends sufficiently to reply. Attention wanders, and the patient's apprehension of his environment is incomplete and inaccurate. The symptom is frequent in general hospitals where it is often seen in patients suffering from infectious diseases and other conditions affecting cerebral oxygenation and metabolism. Clouding of consciousness may also occur in psychogenic disturbances, such as dissociative reactions. In this the clouding and the subsequent amnesia for events of the clouded period may serve the purpose of excluding from awareness material which deep-seated wishes would shut out. Clouding of consciousness may be of various degrees, ranging from mental hebetude to somnolence, stupor, or coma.

Delirium*

Although involving much more than a disturbance of consciousness, mention should be made of the symptom-complex known as "delirium," now designated as the acute brain syndrome. This syndrome, ordinarily acute in both development and course, consists of clouding of consciousness, bewilderment, restlessness, confusion, disorientation, incoherent or dreamlike thinking, illusions and hallucinations, and apprehension or fear. Its occurrence

* The clinical picture of delirium is well depicted in Shakespeare's description of Falstaff's death: "For after I saw him fumble with the sheets, and play with flowers and smile upon his finger's ends, I knew there was but one way; for his nose was sharp as a pen, and a'babbled of green fields." King Henry V, Act II, Scene iii.

is usually associated with infections accompanied by fever, toxic states, metabolic disturbances (uremia, pellagra, pernicious anemia), cardiac decompensation, or head trauma, which impair cerebral functioning and cause cerebral insufficiency. Some persons develop delirium more readily than do others. Perhaps in some cases this tendency is caused either by an inherently greater vulnerability of the brain to toxins or by a less resistant blood–cerebrospinal fluid barrier. On the other hand, the susceptibility may depend upon the integration and stability of the personality. Electroencephalographic changes are usually found in delirium. Generally, the greater the reduction in the level of awareness, the greater the shift toward slower frequency ranges. The electroencephalographic changes are reversible to the extent to which the clinical delirium is reversible.

Delirium is usually more marked at night when the ordinary background of sensory input is reduced; at times it may be limited to it, the patient being seemingly normal mentally during the day. The most frequent prodromal symptoms are drowsiness, restless sleep, difficulty in grasp, and impaired attention. In very mild cases, the patient may merely appear mentally dull and sluggish and not keenly aware of just what is happening to him. He may show a little "wandering" but become clear when addressed. Attention is impaired, and there is a reduction in capacity for abstract thinking. The patient usually has difficulty in performing tests requiring concentration and sustained attention, e.g., the serial subtraction of 7's from 100. As the delirium becomes more marked, the patient seems dazed, baffled, and bewildered and fails to recognize members of his family.

Important symptoms are fluctuations in grasp or perception of reality, orientation, and consciousness. Shifting degrees of awareness and of orientation should always suggest the possibility of delirium. Moments of rationality often alternate with ones of irrationality. If the clouding of consciousness has been marked, the patient, after recovery, has no recollection of what occurred during the delirium. Frequently the memory is "patchy," varying with the fluctuations of consciousness that occurred during the delirious episode. Other variations in the clinical picture often co-exist and are also suggestive. Comparative calmness, for example, may exist for a period, to be suddenly followed by restlessness or impulsive activity. The patient's mood may shift rapidly or be characterized by doubt, perplexity, irritability, apprehension, fear, and even panic. Frightening dreams and fantasies may arise, and both illusions and hallucinations occur, the former being more frequent. Visual hallucinations are more frequent than auditory ones and at first are often in the form of ill-defined or shadowy figures. The content of thought and of hallucinations is more dependent upon the patient's personality problems and tendencies and his previous life experience than upon the nature of the underlying physical process responsible for the delirium. Frequently the patient shows motor disturbance, manifested in mild cases by tremulousness in writing, but in more severe cases by picking, grasping, and groping. Activity may vary from mild restlessness to intense and uncontrollable overactivity.

Delirium rarely continues for more than a month and in infectious diseases may be of only fleeting duration. Later, delirious episodes tend to resemble any previous ones, both in content and course. Following his recovery, the patient often describes his hallucinations and other delirioid experiences as having been dream-like in nature. Although the delirious syndrome occurs frequently in infectious diseases and in their febrile period, it is by no means confined to such association. Toxic-delirioid reactions occur in old age in a wide variety of physical illnesses. Postoperative psychoses, more frequent in elderly patients than in younger ones, usually resemble those of toxic-exhaustive and infective states and therefore present delirioid features. Puerperal psychoses, even those that are fundamentally affective or schizophrenic in nature, often show delirioid characteristics in their onset. The delirioid reaction may, too, follow the abuse of bromides and other drugs.

Dream and Fugue States

Presenting a somewhat similar but more exaggerated symptom–complex is the disturbance known as "dream state" or "twilight state." Such a state does not, like delirium, arise from toxic–organic condition, but is of affective or other psychogenic origin. Consciousness is usually disturbed, in some cases being so clouded or confused that the patient is not aware of his real surroundings. Visual and auditory hallucinations occur, in response to which the patient may perform complex acts, such as running away or committing acts of violence. These dream states may last from several minutes to a few days.

When normal consciousness is regained, the patient may report that during the twilight state he felt as if he were dreaming and will have little or no recollection of events which occurred during its existence. Such dream states occur for the most part in dissociative reactions and in epilepsy. In dissociative reactions they represent escape from unpleasant reality or the gratification of frustrated wishes. In epileptic dream states the behavior is motivated by more deeply unconscious factors.

Stupor

Stupor occurs both in the toxic–organic and in the psychogenic groups of mental disorders, but the similarity of disturbance of mental processes in the two groups is more apparent than real. Stupor may occur in a diversity of physical and mental conditions, from toxic states, organic brain disease, intense apathy, profound depression, blocking, epilepsy, and dissociative reaction to overpowering fear. In neither toxic-organic stupor nor psychogenic stupor does the patient move. In toxic-organic stupor, conscious thought processes are suspended; in catatonic stupor, there is intense preoccupation of thought which is often dereistic in nature, with a loss of reality sense but no real suspension of consciousness. A sudden change from stupor to activity, often impulsive or excessive, occurs in psychogenic stupor only.

DISORDERS OF ORIENTATION

The process by which one apprehends his environment and locates himself in relation to it is known as orientation. If he knows his position in reference to time, appreciates his situation both as to space and circumstances, and understands his relationship to other individuals, he is said to be oriented. If he does not recognize and locate himself in respect to any one of these matters, he is said to be disoriented in the particular sphere of which he has an inadequate grasp. The development of personality identity, which commences with the early exploration of one's body and that of the mother, as well as the exploration of space and the growing awareness of time, established through the periodic experiencing of emerging needs and their satisfactions, lays down the individual's orientation in these spheres.

Disorientation may occur in any mental disorder in which there is extensive impairment of the patient's memory, of the extent or accuracy of his perceptions or of his attention. Disturbances of orientation are the significant symptomatology of acute cerebral insufficiency which are designated as the organic brain syndromes (delirious states) when the physiological functions necessary for memory, perception, and attention are impaired. Less frequently, disorientation is caused by acute conflicts, intense affective factors, distractibility, or lack of interests or attention.

DISORDERS OF MEMORY

The function by which data acquired and presented to consciousness through the observations of attention are stored, later to be summoned and again presented to consciousness, is known as memory. For the purpose of description, it may be con-

sidered as consisting of three processes: the reception and *registration* of a mental impression; the *retention* or preservation of the previously acquired impression; the reproduction or *recall* of the impression. One must not conclude that memory is a special and more or less isolated function or faculty. It is but one aspect of that highly-integrated part of the behavior of the organism known as mental. It is adjustive in its purpose and tends to promote adaptation with the minimum of effort by virtue of its role in assisting the individual to profit by his experience. Largely as a result of the investigation of abnormal psychology, it is known that memory is influenced by affect, the tendency being to modify it in the interests of the emotional needs of the individual.

The disorders of memory are three: abnormally pronounced memory or *hypermnesia*; loss of memory or *amnesia*; falsification of memory or *paramnesia.*

Hypermnesia

Hypermnesia is occasionally seen in mild manic states, paranoia, and catatonia. This excessive mnemonic capacity is largely limited to specific periods or to specific events and experiences, connected with which are particularly strong affects. Impressions arising from emotionally colored events are registered with more than the usual intensity with the result that the patient has a vivid recollection of details.

Amnesia

Amnesia may be produced either by organic or by psychogenic factors. In *organic amnesia*, physiological disturbances of neurons, through chemical alterations, trauma, or degenerative changes, interfere with associative processes. Organic loss of memory is caused both by impairment of registration and of retention, more especially of the latter. In *psychogenic amnesia*, recall, for psychologic reasons, is inhibited. Strictly speaking, forgetting in psychogenic amnesia is not a passive loss of memory trace. The absence of memory is an active defense against experiences which have proved unbearably painful or anxiety–producing. The memory of an actual event is repressed and kept repressed because consciousness finds it too painful to face. Psychogenic amnesia not only may provide escape from the memory of intolerable experiences but may serve as a device for escape from the consequences of an act. If anxiety is very severe, a dissociative reaction may occur with a resulting fugue or flight automatism in which the patient experiences a loss of memory both as to his past experiences and as to his identity. By this escape, the patient's symptoms supply him, without awareness on his part, with a seeming solution for his difficulties.

Another and more frequent form of psychogenic amnesia is that for intended action. This is a result of conflict of wishes. We "forget" to perform some task or keep some appointment because the proposed act conflicts, perhaps unconsciously, with some wish or interest.

The differential diagnosis between organic and psychogenic amnesia is important. To differentiate between these two forms the psychiatrist must determine the nature of the cause. Often this is obvious, but if not readily apparent, a careful history should be secured and a searching examination of the nervous system be made before concluding that the amnesia is of psychogenic origin. Such an origin should not be accepted unless a psychological need for its occurrence is discovered.

If there has been no disturbance of consciousness and no impairment of intellectual functions, the amnesia is probably psychogenic in origin. A selective amnesia in which inconvenient events or topics are forgotten is of psychogenic origin. A sudden and complete recovery of memory is not rare in case of psychogenic amnesia but does not occur if the amnesia has been caused by organic factors. Any recovery of memory which has been lost through organic causes takes place gradually and is often incomplete. A fragmentary type of amnesia with a scattered loss of memory for unrelated details of experience, as noted in general paralysis or senile dementia, is of organic origin.

Amnesias for circumscribed periods of time may be either psychogenic or organic in nature. A generalized failure of memory for both recent and remote events denotes an organic degenerative disease of the brain. A patchy amnesia with a memory for isolated events in a period of confusion is frequent in delirium. An organic amnesia may be followed or widely overlapped by a psychogenic failure of recall, especially in head injuries.

ANTEROGRADE AMNESIA. An anterograde amnesia is one that progresses coincidentally with the passage of time and the stream of experience. It extends forward to cover a period following the apparent regaining of environmental contact. Anterograde amnesia is sometimes observed in boxers who have received a severe blow on the head. The pugilist is hit but continues boxing in an apparently normal manner. Retrospectively, however, he reports a gap in his memory extending forward from the time of the injury and covering the period to the end of the fight or even beyond.

RETROGRADE AMNESIA. In retrograde amnesia, there is a loss of memory extending back over a period prior to the time when the onset occurred. In cases of trauma to the head, there may be a retrograde amnesia reaching back over a variable period prior to the injury with its accompanying loss of consciousness. It may also follow many other forms of organic interference with cerebral function, such as suicidal attempts by hanging or gassing, or following epileptic convulsions. It is often seen after treatment by electric shock.

Recovery from retrograde amnesia is chronological, those memories nearest the injury being the last to return. The amnesia in Korsakoff's psychosis is both retrograde and anterograde. Retrograde amnesia may also be of psychogenic origin and has been known to stretch back over a prolonged period. In psychogenic retrograde amnesia, an experience has been registered but is not recalled except through an association of ideas. As it is recalled in this manner, the recall is accompanied by an emotional response appropriate to the forgotten material.

As the result of precise surgical extirpations it has been found that bilateral lesions of the medial surface of the temporal lobe are followed by severe memory defects, particularly in the ability of retention. There also took place after such operations both anterograde and retrograde amnesia; early memories and technical skills remained undisturbed.

Paramnesia

Paramnesia, or falsification of memory, as well as distortions of memory, also serves as protection against intolerable anxiety. In the form known as *confabulation* the patient fills the gaps in his memory by fabrications which are without any basis of fact, although, when relating them, he accepts them as actual occurrences. These fictions change from moment to moment and may often be suggested and directed by the person to whom they are related. Paramnesia is observed occasionally in the senile psychoses but particularly in Korsakoff's syndrome.

RETROSPECTIVE FALSIFICATION. Of different psychological significance are the retrospective falsifications, or illusions of memory, created in response to affective needs. We all tend to embroider the truth in accordance with these needs or unconsciously to select those memories which suit our interests. Two persons who have intense but different emotional attitudes relative to a certain event or experience will relate quite different accounts of the circumstances. Both persons may be honest but each will remember details in harmony with his emotional needs and forget those not consistent with his affects. In paranoid psychoses, one meets with exaggerations of this tendency. Here one finds that the patient misinterprets an actual event, appends imaginary details to it, or even relates experiences that have little or no basis of fact. Such falsifications of memory serve the purpose of supplying supporting evidence for the patient's delusions, which, too, are products of affective needs.

Defensive distortions of recall may serve to avert threats or to enhance self-esteem. Early childhood memories reported by patients sometimes represent such distortions. Whether distorted or not, they are worthy of note as are first and repetitive dreams. It has been reported that the early memories of psychotics are more frequently of being lost, being threatened with death, or of losing control. The psychoneurotic more frequently reports self images. Memories of sickness and death in the psychotic are often those of neglect; in the neurotic, of overdependency.

"Déjà Vu"

Mention should be made of the illusion of memory known as *déjà vu*. In this phenomenon, there is a feeling of familiarity on observing something—a new scene, for example—of which there has, in fact, been no previous observation, or of having previously lived through a current experience. It arises when the present situation has an associative link with some past experience or occurrence for which the patient is amnesic.

Various explanations have been offered for the phenomenon, but it seems to occur when the forgotten experience has been the center of psychological conflict and consequent repression. Several psychodynamic explanations have been offered. For instance, there is a drive for a repetition, a second chance to solve a conflict, so that the outcome of the incident may coincide with the wish. Again, the déjà vu both symbolizes and stimulates the revival of an anxiety producing wish or fantasy which is then defensively dealt with as unreal and projected onto the current external situation which is offered as a substitute for the past. Thus repression is maintained. It may occur in normal people, especially in young people who are given to daydreaming. In the phenomenon of *jamais vu* there is a false feeling of unfamiliarity with situations which have actually been experienced. These phenomena may occur in schizophrenia, psychoneuroses, lesions of the temporal lobe including epilepsy, and states of fatigue or intoxication.

Functions of Psychogenic Memory Disturbances

It is apparent from what has been said that memory loss, in the absence of structural or toxic changes in the higher cortical neurons, is a selective process and not a matter of chance. It plays an important part in promoting the comfort and self-esteem of the individual.

Largely through the observations of Freud and of Brill it has become realized that slips of tongue and pen, such as use of a wrong word, of one opposite to that consciously intended, the loss or destruction of objects consciously valued, little forgettings, and various erroneous acts of everyday life that are ordinarily regarded as merely "accidental," are determined by unconscious motives. Since these apparently unmotivated errors resemble symptoms in their relation to repression, they are often spoken of as *symptomatic acts.*

DEMENTIA

In any structural disturbance or degeneration of the higher cortical neurons, such as those caused by prolonged intoxication or malnutrition, there results a permanent, irreversible loss of intellectual efficiency known as dementia. If of but slight degree, the impoverishment may be manifested by defective self-criticism, and by impairment in capacity for fine discriminations, in decisions involving delicate moral issues, and in ability to employ abstract ideas.

As dementia progresses, there is an increasing poverty of initiative, a restriction of interests, and a blunting of concern; impressions are taken in and assimilated slowly, with difficulty and often inexactly. There is therefore a failure to profit from experience. Aptitude and learning capacity are reduced. It becomes increasingly difficult or even impossible for the patient to understand and follow conversation.

Questions are not answered or are answered only after several repetitions. Memory is defective and disorientation and confusion may exist. There is a poverty of the imagination necessary for productive thinking. The content of consciousness is reduced in both number and variety of associations, with the result that new ones are formed with difficulty, imperfectly, or even not at all. The individual's capacity for integrating his past experience with his present is reduced, and judgment becomes defective. Emotions are unstable or inadequate.

Care must be taken not to mistake for dementia the temporary inhibition of interest caused by preoccupation, or the dulling of consciousness caused by external or internal toxins. One must not mistake the acquired dementia of organic lesions for the innate oligophrenia of the feeble-minded.

The causes of dementia may be grouped as follows:

1. Atrophic changes of the brain resulting in senile dementia
2. Vascular disorders of the brain, including arteriosclerotic dementia and hypertensive encephalopathy
3. Inflammatory disorders of the brain, particularly syphilis and epidemic encephalitis
4. Degenerative diseases of the brain, notably Alzheimer's disease, Pick's disease, and Huntington's chorea
5. Deficiency diseases, including Korsakoff's psychosis, Wernicke's encephalopathy, pellagra, and pernicious anemia or vitamin B_{12} deficiency.
6. Neoplasm
7. Trauma.

BIBLIOGRAPHY

Arlow, J. A.: The structure of the déjà vu experience. J. Am. Psychoanal. Ass., 7:611–631, 1959.
Brosin, H. W.: Panic states and their treatment. Am. J. Psychiat., 100:54–61, 1943.
Chodoff, P., and Lyons, H.: Hysteria, the hysterical personality and "hysterical" conversion. Am. J. Psychiat., 114:734–740, 1958.
Forrer, G. R.: Benign auditory and visual hal-

lucinations. A.M.A. Arch. Gen. Psychiat., 3:
95–98, 1960.

Friedman, A.: Early childhood memories of mental
patients. J. Child Psychiat., 2:266–269, 1952.

Grinker, R. R.: Growth, Inertia and Shame. Int.
J. Psychoanal., 36:242–253, 1956.

Hoch, P. H., and Zubin, J.: Anxiety. New York,
Grune & Stratton, 1950.

Kennedy, A., and Neville, J.: Sudden loss of memory. Brit. M. J., 2:428–433, 1957.

Lhermitte, Jean: Visual hallucination of the self.
Brit. M. J., 1:431–434, 1951.

Milner, B.: The memory defect in bilateral hippocampal lesions. In Psychiat. Research Rep., Am.
Psychiat. Ass., 11:43–58, 1959.

Parfitt, D. N., and Gall, C. M. C.: Psychogenic

amnesia: the refusal to remember. J. Ment. Sc.,
90:511–531, 1944.

Piers, G., and Singer, M. B.: Shame and Guilt.
Springfield, Illinois, Charles C Thomas, 1953.

Prince, M.: The Dissociation of a Personality.
New York, Longmans, Green, 1906.

Idem.: Miss Beauchamp—the theory of the psychogenesis of multiple personality. J. Abnorm.
Psychol., 15:67–135, 1920.

Riss, E.: Are hallucinations illusions? An experimental study of non-veridical perception. J.
Psychol., 48:367–373, 1959.

Scoville, W. B., and Milner, B.: Loss of recent
memory after bilateral hippocampal lesions. J.
Neurol. Neurosurg. Psychiat., 20:11–21, 1957.

Chapter Six

THE CAUSES AND NATURE OF MENTAL DISORDERS

Perhaps there is no phase of psychiatry which has given rise to so much discussion and dispute as has that concerning the causes and even the nature of mental disorders. With the emphasis in medical education placed on biochemistry, tissue pathology, and other objective and impersonal sciences, it is not surprising that, in the approach to personality disorders, much emphasis has been given to attempting to find their causes in the operation of the same sciences.

The physician must realize, however, that patients may become ill from disturbed human relations as well as from genetic, constitutional, metabolic, or other physical causes. He should recognize that mental disorders are not so much diseases as disturbances of persons. It is increasingly clear that, even when anatomical or physiological disturbances in brain elements are known to exist, they cannot adequately explain the behavior which accompanies them. In varying degrees, this behavior will be colored by, and express, the primitive impulses, affective experiences, and other needs and purposes of the patient's inner life. Stresses in interpersonal relations and in the sociocultural field are no less to be considered than stresses in the biophysical sphere. Behavior cannot be adequately described in the terms of an impersonal disorganization of cellular structure or physiological processes, nor do there seem to be any psychiatric symptoms—except in some cases of toxic organic syndromes—which can be considered as correlates of brain changes, physiological, biochemical, or electrical.

Communication theory provides a framework for considering the interrelationship between the structural organization of man and his immediate relationship to his environment as well as the continuing influence of past social forces and experiences upon him which allow for recognizing, selecting, and patterning response and therefore determine his later behavior to a large extent. The brain then functions as a central integrating and communicating system, subserving contact with both man's inner organ systems, past experiences, and outer world. The latter, today, is largely that with other men. Any disturbances of the brain or other bodily tissues which influence the capacity of man to receive, perceive, and integrate information from his environment with past information will lead to defective psychosocial functioning and thereby disturb personality functioning. Any physical disturbance which upsets man's capacity to communicate with others again will lead to ineffective communication that produces disturbing feedback. The latter, in turn, induces anxiety, conflict, and personality unrest.

Thus one may recognize as etiologic factors in disrupting the communicative activity between men the effects of constitutional defects in the perceptual receptive system, such as deafness or blindness, failures of development or acquired defects in the central nervous system (the integrating organ of communication), or the later dysfunction of this organ due to metabolic or toxic agents. Again, failures to learn language, to understand social codes, or to speak effectively, with resultant interference with later ability to recognize and integrate psychosocial signals, or separations from those who maintain stability or provide guiding signs again may be seen as contributing factors to disturbance in communication or psychosocial illness. Viewed as a disorder in interpersonal communication, the arguments relative to the etiology of psychiatric illness as primarily psychical or psychological become meaningless. One attempts to understand the totality of the personality functioning in a communicative relationship with others and to correct or modify for more effective social adaptation any defects found, or to develop substitutive behaviors if the defect is clearly permanent.

Once the psychopathology has been ascertained, an effort is made to formulate the likely etiologic factors productive of the symptom picture. This chapter considers the many factors in the wide range from the biogenetic to the experiential defect that may influence personality functioning adversely.

Constitution

From the standpoint of psychiatry, constitution may be looked upon as that portion of the individual's organization derived from the genotype and the prenatal and early postnatal influences, but exclusive of the learning acquired through interpersonal experiences. Representing as it does the reactive potentialities of the individual, constitution is important in determining modes of behavior which are considered basic to the personality. Constitutional factors and predispositions must, however, be regarded as highly complex and as yet poorly understood. It is not known to what extent characteristics are gene-carried.

Heredity

To paraphrase a quotation from Compoyré, one may say that both normal and diseased personalities are works written in collaboration where it is hard to discover which parts really belong to each of the collaborators, to nature or to education, meaning by education the sum of the individual's environmental conditionings and life experiences. Each stage of development is determined by the interaction of hereditary and environmental forces. Since the earlier stages influence the character of the development of late stages, the hereditary and environmental factors interpenetrate more and more as development proceeds until finally this interplay becomes so complex and complete that the several factors cannot be separated. Nor is there yet adequate knowledge concerning the relationship between heredity and the psychophysiological processes of development.

Before attributing a mental disorder to heredity, the psychiatrist should recall that parents frequently transmit their emotional difficulties to the next generation, not through their germ cells but through the influence of neurotic parents after birth. In most cases of mental illness in a parent, one can presuppose a prolonged period of maladjustment with difficulties and inconsistencies in personal relationships which preclude the existence of a home atmosphere conducive to healthy emotional growth and future mental health. A failure to find gratification of psychological needs in one generation may, too, be reflected in the behavior of the next, with the result that difficulty of adaptation and social misbehavior may follow through several generations. The patient has been conditioned by his interpersonal emotional experiences with parents and siblings; his parents, in turn, had been conditioned by their experiences with parents. Neurotic patterns have been communicated from one generation to another rather than inherited. A negative and hostile relationship toward parent or sibling may, too, carry over and transfer negative, hostile psychopathogenetic feelings towards persons who stand in a parental or sibling role.

More than formerly, it is held that many instances of nervous and mental disorder once looked upon as inherited or of constitutional origin are in reality due to crippling fixations, to hostile, aggressive, or other attitudes growing out of early family interpersonal relationships. The individual's conscious and unconscious defenses against these difficulties may lead to a wide variety of personality disturbances. Whatever, therefore, may be the contribution of heredity in relation to mental disorder, the postnatal influences and growing-up experiences have been of importance in determining personality structure and pattern. It is well recognized that a parent accelerates or blocks the developmental processes of the child's personality.

Up to the present time, therefore, knowledge as to a hereditary or constitutional predisposition to mental disorders is incomplete, and opinions must remain subject to revision. It must be said, however, that the investigations of Kallmann as to the familial occurrence of schizophrenia and manic–depressive psychosis are suggestive. Kallmann found that schizophrenia occurs much more frequently in families which include a known case of schizophrenia than it does in the general population. He found that the average expectancy in any group of persons who are not characterized by blood relationship to a schizophrenia case is 0.85 per cent but that the children of one schizophrenic parent have a probability of developing the disease which is 19 times that of the general population. Kallmann reported that the morbidity rate among the children of two schizophrenic parents is about 80 times the average expectancy, and that among uni-ovular twins of such parents the expectancy rate is 85.8 per cent. He does not mean that a person is "born" a manic–depressive or a schizophrenic, rather that one inherits a specific capacity for reacting to personality stresses with either a manic–depressive or a schizophrenic psychosis while others do not. He believes that health and adequate adjustment are fundamental biological properties, with hereditary potentiality as the common denominator.

In another area the genetic factor is of significant importance. Many of the inborn errors of metabolism which determine biochemical defects leading to brain maldevelopment and secondarily to mental retardation are determined by heredity. In recent years a number of newly discovered and genetically determined inborn errors of metabolism causing mental retardation have been recognized.

Nor are the genetic defects solely determined through transmission of dominant or recessive genic factors; only recently several varieties of deficiency, of which mongolism is the most important, have been shown to be the consequence of an improper splitting of chromosomes during meiosis, leading to an addition to the usual chromosomal number.

Incidence of Mental Disorder

In the United States in 1904 there were 183.6 persons out of every 100,000 in the general population in state mental hospitals, whereas by 1950 this number had increased to 381. This increase in rate of hospitalization cannot be ascribed solely, or even largely, to an upward trend in the incidence of mental disorders. Rather, it is a result of several factors. Among them is the more adequate provision of facilities for the care and treatment of the mentally ill. There has also been a considerable and fairly continuous increase in knowledge concerning the nature of mental illness on the part of the general medical profession. This has resulted in an increased number of patients formerly not recognized as mentally ill being diagnosed and committed to hospitals. There has, too, been a growing realization on the part of laymen that mental illness is a problem in which the patient requires psychiatrically oriented treatment, and an increasing knowledge that the individual is susceptible of improvement and recovery if treatment is taken in time. In addition, greater confidence has been shown in the management of hospitals for the mentally ill with a resulting increased use of their facilities.

There has occurred a major increase during the past thirty-five years in the number of admissions of elderly persons. During that period the incidence of admissions in New York, and doubtless in other populous states, of persons suffering from cerebral arteriosclerosis has increased sixfold. This because of an increased longevity and the resulting increase of persons in the upper age brackets.

Age

Psychoses are rare until adolescence, when their incidence rises sharply and continues to show a definite upward trend with the advance of age. This rate of increase is especially sharp at the older age levels. In the northeastern part of the United States, over 30 per cent of first admissions to public hospitals for mental diseases are sixty or more years of age. In proportion to the population, more than five times as many persons enter hospitals for mental disorders at the age of eighty as at the age of twenty. As indicated, psychoses are uncommon among children. Those which occur at that age tend to be strongly influenced by situational and psychological tensions.

The critical points in development of adolescence, involution, and senility bring not only physical changes but also new psychological problems. The rapid increase of psychoses in adolescence is due to many causes. As mentioned in Chapter 3, there is an incongruity between various phases of personality growth; there is the new problem of the integration of sex into the personality pattern. There are also social and employment problems and those of emancipation from parents.

The involutional period brings an increase in mental disorders, due, in part, to declining activity of the endocrine and reproductive glands and to other degenerative involutional changes, but more often to the frustrations, threats, and other problems which the patient then meets. It has been suggested that the age at which a person develops mental disorder is an index of his frustration or conflict tolerance. After the age of sixty, there is a distinct increase of emotional disorders, to which insecurity is apparently a contributing factor. The increase in mental disorder at the senium is largely due to the degenerative processes which may occur in the higher cortical neurons in old age; yet in some instances it is due to the fact that the changes in psychological situations which arise at that time cannot be met successfully. Sometimes, for example, the fact that an individual has to be supported by children, or by children-in-law, or by others arouses hostile feelings which are productive of psychosomatic or neurotic symptoms. Since one-half of the population in the United States lives past the age of sixty-five, the incidence of senile and arteriosclerotic mental disease is high. Omitting diseases of the senium, the occurrence of mental disorder reaches a peak in the forties and then drops sharply.

Sex Distribution

More men than women are admitted to hospitals for mental disorders, the ratio among first admissions being six men to five women; however, because of the greater longevity of women, the number of them in public mental hospitals exceeds that of men. General paresis, alcoholic psychoses, traumatic psychoses, psychoses with epilepsy, and psychoses with cerebral arteriosclerosis are more frequent in men. Manic–depressive psychoses, involutional melancholia, paranoia, and psychoses with somatic disease are more frequent in women. Schizophrenia appears to be a little more frequent in women.

Environment: Social and Cultural Factors

The environment in which an individual lives is much more than a physical world; it consists of the close interpersonal interaction within the family group, the pressures imposed upon this group by the wider cultures and its particular value systems, as well as the influence of socio-economic forces depending upon the class structure of the society in which the individual and his family live. In recent years the family unit has become a subject of special study. Ackerman now differentiates eight different types of family structure in American society.

It remains to determine whether there is a specific relationship between variety of family structure to forms of psychopathology. It is maintained that the attempt to understand personality development solely in terms of the interaction of the individual with past aspects of parents or others fails to provide the structure for a comprehension of the development of the social roles which each person plays in his adult life. The social self is expressed in group actions and modified by them; it may or may not reinforce the goals and values the individual has established for the personal self.

From those who are studying families comes the challenge that it is no longer possible to treat patients as individuals. There is no question that therapy of the individual without consideration for the family homeostasis often leads to its rupture, with the appearance of overt psychiatric disturbance in others than the original patient, or that treatment of the individual will be found to founder through interference by other family members. On the other hand, there is much to show from individual therapy, which is fully cognizant of the dependent bonds between family members, that such pathologic bonds are seldom severed while the disturbed individual remains within the family group.

Spiegel and others, in studying the family in relation to mental illness and health, do so by postulating that what goes on between the sick individual and his family takes place within a series of sub-systems which include the individual, the family, the community, and the value systems of each. Within this "transactional system" the interests center more on questions of those processes which occur between the individual and his family which are considered as pathologic in the larger community rather than on the narrower question which involves the interactions of the family members in relation to the pathology. Those working with the transactional method attempt to define strain as it exists in the culture, the family, and the individual and to relate one to the others. Much emphasis is placed on value systems and the conflicts which exist between those within the various units. These new working models remain to be tested as a means of adding to the effective knowledge valued in clinical practice.

That cultural factors influence the etiology and psychopathology of mental disorders is generally agreed on the basis of studies by cultural anthropologists and by psychiatrists who have worked with persons ill in different cultural groups. Within a lifetime, the clinical phenomenology of various psychotic reactions has changed. As an example, the megalomanic delusions of being Napoleon, so common in the nineteenth century, are seen no longer. Now patients who have such a need fall upon a character of this century or develop a Messianic complex. In the United States the manic–depressive reactions are less prevalent than they were a quarter century ago, although they are common in the Scandinavian countries. Conversion hysteria is thought to be less common in Western culture; alcoholic psychoses are frequent in the Irish and uncommon in those of Jewish faith.

Since man learns his patterns of behavior within a family impressed with the codes of a constituted culture, it is not surprising to recognize this important source as a fluctuant factor, determining not only patterns of neurotic and psychotic illness but also their changing symptoms and frequencies over time.

The demands of the social environment with its variable competitiveness, sexual repressions, and contradictory codes bring differing conflicts, individual frustrations, and dilemmas as these factors shape the adaptive capacities of the individual.

It is known that more patients per unit of population are admitted to public hospitals from urban than from rural communities due, in part, to the fact that admissions vary inversely with the remoteness of the community from an institution for mental diseases. Alcoholic psychoses, general paresis, psychoses due to drugs, manic–depressive psychoses, paranoia, and psychoneuroses are more frequent in urban areas. Senile psychoses, psychoses with cerebral arteriosclerosis, involutional melancholia, and psychoses with mental deficiency occur with relatively greater frequency in rural regions. Schizophrenias occur with about equal frequency in urban and rural areas.

In Hollingshead and Redlich's studies on the influence of social class upon the occurrence of mental illness in New Haven, it was found that schizophrenia was found more frequently in families in the lowest socio-economic classes as well as other disturbances indicative of superego defects. (Ninety-five per cent of persons in prison come from these classes.) On the other hand, obsessive compulsive disorders are most common in the highest socio-economic groups and oedipal conflicts in the middle group.

One might expect that anxiety, open and often unopposed aggression including sexual aggression, lowered self-esteem, and limited opportunities for emotional and cognitive growth are more often the ways of life in the pattern personality development in those reared in the lower socio-economic groups. In the higher social classes, in contrast, demands for conformity presumably lead to the expression of compulsive patterns of living.

Marital Status

Statistics show that mental disorder is more common among the single than among the married. While this may be due in part to the more stable and regular mode of life led by the married person with the accompanying sense of domestic responsibility, this is probably only a minor reason for the better mental health among married persons. It should be remembered that the marital association is one of the most important of all human associations. It provides not merely for the satisfaction of sexual urges but for various important securities, the absence or loss of which may be very disturbing to the personality. The feeling that one is desired as a marital partner, that one is appreciated and is the subject of interest and affection contributes greatly to a sense of security. The security from loneliness, the emotional satisfaction of parenthood, and frequently, in women, the added sense of economic security add wholesome satisfactions. With marriage the individual may be compelled to adjust to a very different type of environment and to personal relationships quite foreign to those in which he was reared. Marriage and success in the responsibilities of marriage suggest great interpersonal adaptive capacities and personal esteem. The development of mental disorder before marriage naturally decreases the prospects of subsequent marriage; many whose affective and other personality limitations are so great that they are predisposed to mental disorders are never sought as partners.

Statistics show that there is a marked preponderance of mental disorder per unit of population among divorced persons. There are several reasons for the more frequent occurrence of mental disorders among this group. In many cases maladjustments representing early stages of mental disorder led to domestic discord and divorce before the personality disturbances were sufficiently developed to be recognized as constituting mental disease. On the whole, divorced persons represent a group suffering from conflicts so unusual both in number and intensity that the high incidence of mental illness is not surprising. The same deep-seated mechanisms which tend to lead to marital discord also lead to psychosis or neurosis. It should be remembered, too, that marriage is a relationship which demands a most highly sustained adaptation. The unmarried person may have been unable to achieve the adult toughness necessary to stand the give and take of adjustment to marriage and parenthood. Perhaps she may have been unprepared for this adjustment because her parents before her had not been healthy models for identification as mates and parents. A mental illness may be precipitated by factors concerned with sexual functions such as anxiety with motherhood, pregnancy, or abortion. Parenthood often re-lights conflicts over dependency or early sibling competitiveness which arouses quantities of anxiety, rage, and aggression.

A person who has failed to reach a mature, heterosexual level but remained, even though unconsciously so, with a basic sex interest in persons of the same sex may be unable to establish an abiding harmonious partnership with one of the opposite sex. Usually there will be no physiological interference in the exercise of sex functions natural to his or her sex, but the emotional, dispositional tendency of sex expression is directed to a homosexual partner. The attempt to meet this conflict between emotionally determined and biologically determined impulses may be made by projection or other psychopathological mechanisms which eventuate in mental disorder.

Pregnancy

Mental disorder may be associated with pregnancy or the postpartum period. There are, however, no specific mental disorders related to either of these periods. Latent or repressed psychological material may, under the stress of maintaining physiological homeostasis and of the emotionally significant situation, prove too great for the patient's ego resources with the result that psychopathological reactions occur. What her pregnancy unconsciously means to the mother is of significance as is the birth of her child. Doubtless, it reanimates the patient's old attitudes toward her own mother and may revive old complexes of bodily harm or injury. Sometimes the patient expresses delusions indicating hostility for either the husband or child, thus reflecting a conflict about married life or motherhood. Rejection of the child may be expressed by a delusion that it is dead, by abusive treatment of it, or by fear that something will happen to it.

Psychotic illness in association with pregnancy is rare; the expectancy is about 14 cases in 10,000 confinements. About 50 per cent of the mental illnesses associated with pregnancy or the postpartum period are schizophrenic, about 25 per cent are manic–depressive, and 20 per cent are psychoneurotic reactions.

The occurrence of such a reaction does not predispose to a similar reaction in a subsequent pregnancy. Almost one-half of such illnesses occur with the birth of a second or a later child, and the outlook for recovery is similar to that of the general reaction type. These disorders occur with the same frequency in the postpartum setting as they do in any other setting.

Occupation and Work Load

Aside from brain syndromes due to toxic substances to which individuals may be exposed as a consequence of the occupation (lead, particularly), occupation does not determine or precipitate personality disorders.

Overwork was formerly ascribed an important place in the etiology of mental disorders. It is now generally held, however, that so far as unusual application to work constitutes exhausting effort it is a symptom of mental disorder rather than a cause. The compulsive neurotic may work excessively hard, his job serving as a means of reducing anxiety and of support. Work may be the only outlet for an otherwise creative person. It may also in some instances serve as a neurotic outlet for aggression. It may give strong ego support through success or prestige to a person besieged with feelings of inferiority. For the withdrawn person, work may be his chief means of contacting others in a non-threatening manner. Finally, satisfying work is important for mental health. It brings such healthy gratifications as creative expression, companionship, and a feeling of accomplishment.

The mental disorder, as recognized by the patient's family, may have been preceded by unaccustomed effort, but if a complete knowledge of the motivating forces is available, we should discover that the unusual assiduity represented an attempted flight from conflicts and problems for which satisfactory and successful solution had not been reached. It should undoubtedly be conceded that fatigue may at times weaken the controlling strength of the ego. Probably the factors in modern life productive of nervous and mental disorder lie less in overwork, in the speed and stress of work, distraction of noise and the like than in dissatisfaction, insecurity, distasteful work, and lack of incentive. Those anxiety-inducing situations of inability to accept the authority of competent superiors, to suppress dependent longings and demands often lead to breakdowns or failures at work in groups. The competition for advancement with the mobilization of envy, or the fear of it in the dependent person advanced to a position of responsibility sometimes precipitate emotional disturbance as in the case of a dependent vice-president advanced to presidency and fearful of facing the envy and loss of acceptance by his former peers. Failures to receive advancement also mobilize aggressive fears that may precipitate disorder. There is evidence that mental effort in the presence of emotional stress and tension can produce either neurotic or psychotic reactions. There is no justification for the pessimistic suggestion frequently made that the pace of modern life conduces to mental breakdown. Again, retirement from an occupation is now known to produce anxiety in many. Here, with the giving up of work, stress arises from the loss of prestige, of being valued by others, and from the frequent isolation from old companions.

Alcohol

The role of alcohol in the production of mental disease contains many complex elements and, while in some respects our ideas are becoming clarified, there are still many unknown and variable factors. That there is a direct relation between the amount of alcohol drunk in a community and the incidence of psychoses classified statistically in the alcoholic group is certain, as shown by experience in the United States during the past third of a century. In 1920, immediately following the enactment of the prohibition amendment, the number of first admissions of alcoholic psychoses to New York State hospitals for mental diseases per 100,000 of general population fell to 1.2. This rate gradually increased to 7.1 in 1941, decreased until 1945, and has again continued to rise since World War II. During the three years (1919 through 1921) of relatively successful observance of the prohibition amendment to the Constitution there were 720 first admissions with alcoholic psychoses to all hospitals for mental disease in New York State. The total of such first admissions increased to 2,013 in 1929 through 1931 and reached 3,132 in 1939 through 1941, since which time there has been no appreciable change per unit of population. The more carefully the history of a patient suffering from a chronic form of mental disorder is studied, the more frequently it will be found that any associated alcoholism is either a symptom of the psychosis or another method of dealing with the same personality problems which contributed to the mental disorder rather than an essential cause of it. The role of avitaminosis in producing a psychosis in the chronic alcoholic must be borne in mind.

Physical Defects

Physical anomalies or disturbances not caused by endocrine dysfunction, yet ones which occasionally provoke resentment and other undesirable psychological reactions, particularly of a compensatory, aggressive, or other defensive nature, are genital deformities, clubbed feet, scoliosis, kyphosis, and congenital defects of vision and hearing. Cleft palate, also, tends to create a sense of inability to meet social situations and to lead to feelings of inferiority and insecurity again expressed in derogatory attitudes to one's self and body. Children with congenital or acquired defects develop feelings about the defects partly because of the way they see other people reacting to them. If others about them react with repugnance, revulsion, or abhorrence, so too will the child regard his deformity. Adolescence is the period in which physical defects are most apt to evoke unwholesome psychological reactions. It must be said, however, that the personalities of individuals having physical defects are not always affected by such handicaps.

PHYSICAL ILLNESSES

Acute physical illnesses with an associated toxic state frequently lead to an acute brain syndrome with an accompanying delirioid state but are rarely directly responsible for neuroses or the so-called functional psychoses. Chronic illness, however, with its handicaps, frustrations, and unhealthy methods of attempting to surmount them, is a severe neurosis-producing stress. The patient with an organic illness is confronted with two types of problems for which he must mobilize a variety of defenses and mechanisms of adaptation: (a) problems, largely conscious, related to the realities of the pain, inability to make a living, and handicaps imposed on or by his family, and (b) problems arising from emotional needs and from the activation of hitherto repressed, unconscious conflicts. These are discussed in Chapter 28 in the section on Disturbances of the Body Image. There will be noted, however, a relationship between the psychological symptoms released by the ego-weakening effect of the illness and the pre-morbid personality of the patient.

General Cerebral Dysfunction

It was formerly assumed that every mental disease was due to cerebral disease and that a psychosis without disease of the brain did not exist, also that spe-cific brain lesions were accompanied by special mental symptoms. While in some instances of mental disorder an associated disease of the brain is known to exist, in most instances there is not, so far as our present knowledge goes, any cerebral pathology. Even when mental symptoms accompany disease of the brain, they cannot be explained by considering the location of the brain pathology alone.

Mental symptoms arising from general dysfunction of the brain are dependent to a large extent on whether the brain disorder is of an acute or chronic nature, and, if chronic, whether the involvement is diffuse or circumscribed. The resulting symptom pattern tends, therefore, to fall into one of three types: (a) an acute organic syndrome; (b) a chronic syndrome due to a diffuse lesion; and (c) a chronic syndrome due to a localized lesion. The acute organic reaction is the result of temporary, reversible, diffuse impairment of brain tissue function and is characterized by a disturbance of consciousness, difficulty of apperception, somnolence, coma, and cloudy and delirious states. The disturbance of the sensorium may release hallucinations and poorly organized transient delusions.

Chronic organic brain syndromes result from relatively permanent, usually irreversible, diffuse impairment of cerebral tissue function. The chronic brain syndrome may vary in degree of progress but usually some disturbance of memory, judgment, orientation, comprehension, and affect persists permanently. Frequently the organic syndrome is colored by the patient's individual personality with its particular conscious and unconscious impulses, fears, and wishes. It should therefore be remembered that structural changes in the brain may release symptoms of a neurotic or "functional" nature. The causes of general brain dysfunction are trauma, infection, toxic states, metabolic disturbances, and various deprivational states.

Trauma

Trauma of the head, with lesions ranging from a diffuse but minute separation of neuron structure through edema and hemorrhage to destruction of brain tissue with subsequent scar formation, may be followed by varying defects of mentation. The clinical picture is usually at first that of an acute organic syndrome. If the impairment of brain function is persistent, the clinical picture becomes that of the chronic organic brain syndrome with a permanent impairment of mental function. Trauma of any part of the body may be reacted to, usually after a latent period, by a traumatic neurosis.

Infections

Of all infections, syphilis still plays the most active part in causing mental disease. The most common psychosis resulting from such infection is that associated with syphilitic meningoencephalitis (general paresis) which accounts now for about two per cent of all first admissions to public mental hospitals. During the past twenty-five years there has been a constant decrease in the relative prevalence of syphilis with a resulting decrease in general paresis. Also, the treatment for general paresis is now begun much more promptly and carried out much more efficiently.

Toxic Agents

Certain chemicals and drugs may give rise to acute brain syndromes, not infrequently in the nature of a delirium of brief duration, although occasionally a delirious state of such an origin may continue for several weeks. The most frequent agents producing mental symptoms are bromides, barbituric acid derivatives, sulfa drugs, morphine, cocaine, marihuana, thiocyanates, and lead.

Endocrine Disturbances

Abnormal functionings of the endocrine glands will undoubtedly influence personality functioning through disturbing bodily functions. Such disorders, for example, may lead to changes in general efficiency of bodily functions with resulting feelings of frustration or insecurity. Occasionally neuroendocrinal dystrophies produce biological defects which cause the individual to appear conspicuous in physical appearance, and lead to a disturbance in his body concept or image. The dissimilarity between the patient's concept and the change in his body induced by the endocrine disturbance contributes to self-consciousness, which favors the development of defensive and compensatory mechanisms that distort the personality and render adaptation more difficult. The question, however, whether minor or major mental symptoms are related to any specific endocrines is highly debatable.

Deprivations and Deficiencies

Lack of the basic bodily needs (oxygen, nutrition and fluids, sleep, perceptual stimulation), if sufficiently great or prolonged, may lead to serious constitutional deficits if they occur in the developmental period. Later in life such deprivations act as important etiologic factors in the determinations of various brain syndromes and in precipitating or complementing the primary psychogenic disorders.

OXYGEN DEPRIVATION. Beyond all other bodily organs and tissues the brain is the most susceptible to dysfunction and structural damage as the consequence of oxygen lack. Developmental defects and later behavioral changes are a regular accompaniment of hypoxia from whatever cause. Cerebral hypoxia in the perinatal period, inferred on the basis of clinical observation and now established by experimental studies, leads to profound defects in development from which result both mental retardation and personality disorder as well as physical defects.

In later life, transient or chronic hypoxia, as the consequence of acute oxygen lack at high altitudes, asphyxia, cerebral ischemia following arteriolar spasm, infarction, or cardiovascular failure, chronic pulmonary disease such as emphysema, anemia, or poisoning by carbon monoxide and other cellular poisons, if severe, produces the symptomatology of general cerebral insufficiency (the brain syndrome).

A drop in arterial oxygen saturation to 85 per cent which persists over a period of two or three hours has been shown to lead in otherwise healthy persons to hyperpnea, fatigue, headache, and lassitude followed by difficulty in concentration and impairment of emotional control. Depending upon the personality of the individual, the oxygen-deprived individual may become over-confident and elated and demonstrate judgmental defects in interpersonal contacts expressed in undue irritability and aggressive behavior toward others. Others become increasingly dull and depressed. Impaired emotional control is one of the finer indices of cerebral anoxia; evidence of it occurs long before difficulties in performance of routine tasks, psychological tests, or changes in the electroencephalogram. Under ordinary conditions of stress, healthy men exposed to hypoxia at the level of 85 per cent arterial oxygen saturation lose emotional control without warning and respond with unexpected truculence to verbal challenges directed to their superego values in the sexual or aggressive areas.

Prolonged ischemic anoxia is probably the major etiologic factor in the organic brain syndromes associated with arteriosclerosis. Whether the diminution of oxygen utilization found with the senile psychosis is representative of a primary anoxic defect or is secondary to the neuronal loss found with this condition is not known.

Cerebral hypoxia occurs with the use of convulsive therapy. It is known that the structure and probably the function of the most recently developed areas of the brain are most impaired through oxygen lack; thus the frontal lobe cortex often shows pathological damage when other areas appear healthy on examination with cellular stains.

LACK OF NUTRITION. Nutritional deprivation has profound effects on personality in terms of drive states, mood, and performance. The consequences of primary nutritional deprivation may come to the attention of the physician as in the case of those starved during the great wars or those suffering from brain syndromes as the consequence of vitamin deficiencies. More frequently encountered are the secondary states of semistarvation which occur in depressives, some schizophrenias, and anorexia nervosa. The studies of experimental semistarvation in man have shown well the subjective changes which this state induces and which may complicate the primary phenomenology of any illness. In addition to the weight loss, fatigue increases steadily. There takes place an increasing preoccupation with food, including frequent simple wish-fulfilling food visions and dreams. Increasing appetite, muscle soreness, irritability, apathy, and sensitivity to noises gradually appear, with feeling of loss of drive and ability to control oneself associated with a diminution in attentiveness and ability to concentrate. The sexual drive becomes progressively weaker with eventual lack of interest in the attractive sex partner, disappearance of masturbation, seminal emissions in men with diminution of the sperm count, and amenorrhea in women. Recovery of these functions in previously healthy men semistarved on a 1600 calorie diet for 24 weeks has required a full six weeks of re-feeding.

As observed, during wartime starvation leads to personality changes; meanness, secretiveness, and suspiciousness emerge associated with social withdrawal. In the early period of starvation there is a general lowering of moral standards and a drive for other gratifications. Some wished to be cared for like children, became emotionally labile and impulsive, developed enuresis and interest in feces and anal functions. If food deprivation continues, aggressive impulses, sucking activity, and oral interest appear to be subsequently superseded by apathy and eventually the symptoms of general cerebral insufficiency.

LACK OF VITAMINS. Specific vitamin deficiencies are known to produce encephalopathic syndromes resulting from metabolic or organic disturbances in the cerebrum. Pellagra and Wernicke's syndrome are among the most clearly recognized of the deficiency reactions. Brain syndromes rather than disorders of psychogenic origin usually occupy the foreground in personality disturbances associated with these deficiencies, although trends that have been developed for dealing with anxiety-producing situations may be revealed.

SLEEP DEPRIVATION. Continuous lack of sleep, as has been demonstrated by numerous studies on healthy young people, produces deterioration in personality functioning, expressed both in unpleasant subjective experiences as well as changes in appearance, speech, mood, perception, and thought. Whether these changes are due solely to lack of sleep or to the associated muscular fatigue or even associated dream deprivation is not known. When a person is deprived of sleep, his prolonged attention to any task gradually diminishes and is associated with increasing restlessness, apathy, and inability to concentrate. Lapses of ongoing behavior or periods of extreme drowsiness or sleep take place in which delays or actual breaks occur in the performance of tasks, even though the situation is perceived by the non-sleeper as requiring action and a response. He may lose his contact with the immediate situation and confuse external and internal events. Thus a dream or intrusive thought becomes attached to the outward situation, and the faulty sleeper suffers a distortion of perception. Over a period of time, lack of sleep leads to misperceptions which range from changes in the shape, size, movement, texture, or color of objects to misbelieving and misperceiving them. Such misperceptions at times appear to be hallucinations. Temporal disorientation gradually appears. Initially time seems to pass slowly, while later the sleep-deprived subject makes first occasional and then frequent errors in designating time to the point where eventually he is unshakingly deluded. His cognitive process suffers as well, as evidenced by infrequent lapses of thought or speech with limited lack of sleep; these lapses extend over time to loss of the train of thought, incompletion of statements, forgetting, and eventually rambling and incoherent verbalizations, with inability to recognize errors or make corrections. Lack of sleep gives rise frequently to a bandlike sensation about the head, "the hat illusion," while there are often other subjective experiences reflecting feelings of change in the self or the body—feelings of not being one's self, of strangeness, which may be classified as depersonalization.

Associated with sleep lack, physiological depression takes place in muscle tone, body temperature, sweating, and capacity to respond to noxious stimuli. Thus, prolonged wakefulness may be interpreted as leading to decreased capacity for arousal. Increased pulmonary ventilation takes place as a means of removing the greater blood carbon dioxide and lactate.

LACK OF DREAMS. Dream deprivation also has been examined recently. While it is not possible to separate the consequences of sleep from dream lack today, the effects of the latter are of significance psychologically.

In a typical night's sleep, there occur four or five periods of dreaming which account for 20 per cent of the total sleep time. In experiments performed by Dement in which the subjects were awakened briefly on four to seven consecutive nights when they were observed to show the eye movements and characteristic accompanying low voltage, non-spindling electroencephalographic pattern discovered only during the dream period, it was observed that the amount of dreaming increased during nights after dream deprivation. Also, the healthy experimental subjects became anxious and irritable and showed difficulty in concentration in performing daytime tasks during the period of nightly dream deprivation. Some were noted, as well, to develop an increase in appetite associated with weight gain during this period. Dreaming, then, appears to represent a psychological drive state of importance.

SENSORY DEPRIVATION. A series of clinical investigations during recent years gives strong support to the hypothesis that a steady state of sensory stimulation or "input" is necessary to support the usual ego functions. As early as 1819 Dupuytren described delirious reactions with hallucinatory and emotional disturbance which occurred in the period of covering the eyes following cataract extractions. Since the experimental studies of Cameron, it has been known that one factor in the causation of senile nocturnal delirium is the loss of vision consequent to darkness.

The factor of lonely immobilization is thought to be responsible for the states of anxiety, disturbances in time sense, and delusional and hallucinatory experiences of some patients immobilized in respirators. It has been suggested that similar symptoms associated with alcoholism are caused, in fact, by isolation and reduction in sensory input. The factor of social isolation now is thought to contribute to "brain washing" or "thought reform" programs used by the Chinese with their war prisoners, to the prison psychoses, hallucinatory states of the shipwrecked and lost person, and perhaps also the elaborations of the chronically hospitalized and isolated psychotic.

Healthy persons with no previous experimental experience, isolated with vision and hearing diminished by the use of patches and ear plugs and with mobility limited after several hours, experience anxiety, a desire for external stimulation and motor activity as well as progressive difficulty with directed thinking. After seventy-two hours they develop delusional and visual hallucinatory experiences. Following such experiences, visual disturbances continue for some time. They are reported as fluctuations, driftings, and swirlings of objects and surfaces in the visual field, associated with difficulty in fixing objects in space on eye or head movement, with distortions of margins, and exaggeration of contrasts and colors. During the deprivational experience, the electroencephalogram shows slower rhythms and slow wave activity.

It it not known whether the series of events is the simple reduction of the level of sensory stimulations and of its patterning, the occlusion of specific sensory modalities, or the limitations of interpersonal contact. The perceptual phenomena and other ego disruptions seem less likely to occur when some meaningful stimuli are present and when the deprived subject is allowed kinesthetic and tactile stimulation through movement. Personality plays a factor in determining the characteristics of the response, with exaggeration of the usual adaptations and defenses.

It appears that sensory deprivations during early life impose permanent developmental defects which impair later learning. As far as perceptual and kinesthetic learning is concerned, the proposition seems well established for man; the clinical observations on the children who failed to evolve good visual perception after corrections of congenital corneal defects by late transplantation of the cornea are fully supported by studies of artificial blinding of growing chimpanzees.

SOCIAL ISOLATION. Social or experiential deprivation in early life may well play a major role in many of the adult personality disorders. A mass of observations reported by child psychiatrists and animal psychologists shows that capacities for exploratory behavior, control of fear and anxiety, perception of pain and recognition of threat, somatic response to stress, effective sexual and child-rearing behavior, and affectional relations are impaired by isolation of developing young from others. As yet undetermined for the growing child and the young of other species are the critical maturational periods during which appropriate experience must take place in order to allow maturation of structure and related function. There exists now a scientific void relative to such questions as the quantity of experience required to allow full evolution of function and the ultimate capacity of the growing or adult organism to repair deficiencies or develop them through later learning.

Psychogenic Causes

Mental disorder is the maladapted and disordered psychobiological functioning of a social organism and not a disturbance in the function of a single organ, the brain. Impersonal disturbances of tissue do not alone explain disturbances in belief, mood and behavior. In the majority of mental disorders, no functional imperfection has been found in the brain tissue; rather does the mental disturbance represent the reaction of an individual personality to his special life situation, including his interpersonal and emotional experiences. Much mental disorder and many maladaptations can be understood only in terms of lifelong dynamic interactions between the individual and all the forces—internal and external—which have impinged upon him. Such disturbances are described as psychogenic, i.e., they are life-experienced or "mental." They are usually associated with unmet emotional needs, conflicts, disturbing interpersonal relations, guilt-producing situations, and other antecedent psychological determinants. The mental and emotional factors, the meaningful situations, are numerous.

In the psychogenic mental disorders, we deal with concepts of genetics and of dynamics. Genetics refers to anxiety-producing sources, the predisposing determinants for the reaction type or symptom expression. Dynamics refers to the psychological forces which have evoked pathogenic defenses against the anxiety. While genetic factors tend to represent certain general themes, they are uniquely individual in each case. Generally speaking, the emotional and unconscious aspects of personality with their unrecognized motivations are the ones which are of significance in mental disorders and other disturbances of personality. No mental illness, psychoneurotic, psychotic, or psychosomatic, can be understood without taking into account the unconscious dynamic mechanisms designed to deal with anxiety.

Interpersonal Relationships

The earliest and some of the most dynamic stresses, which perhaps can later be met only by psychopathological techniques so disturbing to the happiness and efficiency of the individual or so disrupt-

ing to his social adjustment as to be regarded as mental disorder, arise from repetitive, early interpersonal relations and their stresses within the family. This is not surprising, since human relations are the sources of those powerful affects of pain, pleasure, love, hate, loneliness, sadness, guilt, jealousy, envy, security, and happiness. The arousal of certain of these affects is so impelling that the individual can neither repress nor accept them without anxiety or emotional disturbance.

Of all interpersonal relations, that with the mother is frequently the most determinative of the future mental health of the individual. A strangling, perhaps guilt-ridden, over-protection on her part may prevent the development of a mature, independent personality by the child. Again, the maternal relationship may fail to give him the warmth, security, and support necessary for the emotional and social growth of his personality. Instead, for example, of providing a healthful emotional climate of affection, acceptance, and approval, the mother may to varying degrees reject or overprotect the child, with consequent misshaping of his developing personality. Such attitudes, which exist particularly among mothers who have been damaged emotionally by their own life experiences, are usually unconscious ones. Other attitudes, often covert or ambivalent, which may also be manifested by psychologically important persons, are hostility, aggression, dominance, sadism, and dependence. Out of such relations are established patterns of personality which are culturally so unacceptable that they are repressed and give rise to conflict and anxiety. Ambivalent attitudes, i.e., confusions of hostile and affectionate impulses, which had their origin in some childhood intrafamily relationship often continue to influence the personality pattern throughout later life and constitute unconsciously a conflictful problem which cannot be met except by psychopathological methods.

Much of adult behavior is determined to a considerable degree by events which took place in the pre-verbal age period or through later unresolved childhood conflicts. The *anlage* of many neuroses and of other personality difficulties and characteristics is found in the prolonged experiences of early childhood. Early tension-laden relationships with parents seem to be particularly apt to become pathogenetic. Their interpersonal situations in later life awaken previous feelings and unresolved difficulties and lead to the re-enactment of problems generated in prior relationships. Difficulties in these relationships are therefore both expressions and sources of personality disturbances. Not only may aggression and hostility arise out of family relationships, but many other fixed emotional reactions, such as feelings of insecurity, rejection, guilt, dependency, overprotection, and jealousy, are acquired in response to repetitive early interpersonal experiences.

Bereavement

Through the close and intimate contact of the infant and young child with the mother, there is laid down the basic sense of security and trust upon which the child is able to face separation and its attending loneliness and to seek an autonomous identity. Meeting the early dependent needs of the child through the mothering process lays the groundwork for a healthy personality. Loss of the mother in the first years of life might be looked upon as a deprivation of a significant need for the growing child. Statistical data now show that loss of a mother by death in this period of life occurs in 7 to 10 per cent of those who later become psychotic or neurotic, a much higher occurrence than in the general population. The figures are much more striking for these conditions when one considers loss by separation or divorce. The most critical period of bereavement, in terms of its relation to personality disturbance, is certainly before the age of five. Thus early bereavement by death or prolonged separation may deprive the child of those experiences necessary for sound ego development. In addition, the loss sets in train a series of personality reactions which have psycho-dynamic importance in terms of separation or losses later in life. A bereavement by separation or death is followed by a train of events which are well known. Initially the young child protests by crying or other aggressive behavior, only after some hours to pass through a phase of hopelessness and withdrawal with inactivity. This is succeeded some time later by behavior characterized by detachment, with an unwillingness to resume again the relationship if the lost person reappears. While detachment may be superseded in time, repeated separations lead to an effort at personal isolation from others, motivated, perhaps, as a protection from recurrent anxiety. In older children it is clear that the first phase of anxious protest is accompanied as well by rage. Children deprived early in childhood of mothering either suffer inordinately when separated from significant people due to paralyzing nostalgias, or later may be hungry for dependent relationships. They sometimes develop a protective, isolated defense as a form of pseudo-independency to prevent further repetition of despair and hopelessness.

ANNIVERSARY REACTION. These outbreaks of anxiety or their symptomatic defensive expressions, which occur regularly on specific dates, often represent a symbolic re-enactment of an earlier important bereavement. Such reactions sometimes inaugurate the onset of a psychosis in which the emotional upheaval is observed to coincide with the parent's age at death or sometimes with the birthday of a child coincidental with the age of the patient when the parent was lost. Again, one occasionally sees recurrent attacks of anxiety coinciding with the day of death of a parent. Overbearing anxiety and grief appear to precipitate the ego break which then leads to the effort at restitution through emergence of pathological, neurotic, or psychotic defenses.

Aggression

In recent years there has been emphasis on aggression as a participating factor in the psychogenic production of personality disturbances. Aggression may be defined as a goal-directed self-assertion with an associated implication of attack, of hostile, destructive intent, and attached to an affect of rage. Undoubtedly the learning of control of aggression is one of the major socializing functions of the family. Its arousal and placation are frequent in interpersonal reactions of the family nucleus.

Theories of Aggression

There are two contradictory theories of aggression. The first, stemming largely from the later writings of Freud, holds that aggression is a primary, instinctual drive (more accurately a component manifestation of Freud's death instinct). According to this view, each individual requires a certain amount of gratification of this destructive impulse which, if not attained in one way, will be achieved in some other.

The second theory may be characterized as the "reactive" theory in contrast to the more speculative "death-instinct" theory. According to the "reactive" theory, aggressive behavior is provoked through emotion aroused by thwarting, frustrating experiences. If an individual's habitual modes of action lead most frequently to gratifications, a limited impulse to aggression will be generated, but if obstacles arise in the habitual paths to establish goals, there will be correspondingly strong instigation to ever-pressing aggressive behavior. The sequence, then, is frustration-rage-aggression, the latter aiming to remove the source of frustration and thereby clear the path to the desired goal. Thus the formation of the aggressive personality pattern is frequently established by frustrating forces applied too early, too harshly, or too intensively in the family, with the result that an unconscious aggressive and hostile attitude evolves. Such unconscious hostile impulses stimulate anxiety in those with well-developed super-ego which, in turn, gives rise to neurotic guilt, depression, displaced hostility, and other psychopathological clinical expressions. The fact that the child is dependent on the very persons, the parents, who are the chief frustrating agents further psychologically complicates the situation.

Mental Conflict

One of the major psychogenic factors in the production of mental disorder is that of reconciling discordant desires and conflicting psychological needs and of dealing with incompatible response tendencies. Conflicts may be of the greatest variety. Frequently the conflict is between bodily drives on the one hand, and cultural values on the other. Physiological urges may be beyond the capacity of the ego to handle at the time. Conflicts at a deep level may present themselves on the surface in the form of far-removed symptoms. For example, an unwillingness to accept a feeling of hostility toward a parent may cause the patient to focus his attention upon a local manifestation, such as a difficulty in swallowing. Sometimes an apparently insignificant experience may set off a chain reaction of deeper emotional conflict within the individual, with conflicts spreading from one situation to another. Some situation, specific to the individual, may be so highly charged with symbolic content that it may touch off a major psychotic explosion. Caught in a tangle of attitudes, the unification of the personality has been disturbed. Unless opposing impulses are blended, one is constantly prompted by contradictory drives and disconcerted by the tensions of his emotional dilemmas. Faced with highly charged emotional issues, the individual is unable to attain a working harmony in his personality. Since the most important conflicts take place at levels outside awareness, one may not apply reason, reality, and common sense to their solution.

The personality, if confronted by conflict and by the fact that the repression of forbidden wishes and of instinctual tendencies is in danger of giving way, tends to develop *anxiety*, a persistent fear arising from threatening factors deep in the mental life accompanied by a vague but disquieting anticipatory feeling of prospective harm or disaster. In the sources of this anxiety, whether it be overt or hidden, are to be found many of the causes of mental disorder. The personality devices designed to serve as defenses against anxiety constitute the symptoms of the neuroses, of many of the psychoses and even of personality traits, particularly those known as reaction-formations.

The ways of dealing with anxiety are various and range from those which have social value to those which disorganize the personality. Which of the various defenses are used depends on the personality structure of the individual. As mentioned earlier, both behavior which is socially useful and constructive and character traits which are desirable may be the products of neurotic drives unconsciously directed to the prevention or relief of anxiety. The degree of anxiety from which one suffers, its manner of expression, and the types of defenses which one utilizes against it largely constitute the difference between mental health and mental sickness. When the defenses are limited, repetitive, and incapable of modification by learning and experience, they often function psychogenically. The methods of dealing with anxiety may so disturb personality functioning that social adjustment is destroyed. The more the individual is threatened and the less his tolerance for conflict, the more he is driven to defend himself. Among the less malignant devices for minimizing anxiety are the phobic, conversion, and compulsive reactions—neuroses which do not seriously disorganize the personality. Devices which may serve a similar purpose but disorganize the personality and produce a serious break with reality are called psychotic. In the former, the patient attributes hostile or aggressive motives to others, and thus, by blaming the other fellow, he relieves his own guilt and anxiety for possessing such attitudes. In the latter, the defense against anxiety may be through a delusional and hallucinatory pre-occupation that disorganizes the personality and disregards reality.

BIBLIOGRAPHY

Ackerman, N. W.: The Psychodynamics of Family Life. New York, Basic Books, Inc., 1958.

Ax, A., and Luby, E. D.: Autonomic responses to sleep deprivation. A.M.A. Arch. Gen. Psychiat., 4:55–59, 1961.

Barach, A. L.: Physiologic Therapy in Respiratory Diseases, 2nd ed. Philadelphia, J. B. Lippincott & Co., 1948.

Barry, J. Jr., and Lindemann, E.: Critical ages for maternal bereavement in psychoneuroses. Psychosom. Med., 22:166–181, 1960.

Bleuler, M.: Endokrinologische Psychiatrie. Stuttgart, George Thieme, 1954.

Bowlby, J.: Separation anxiety. Int. J. Psychoanalysis, 41:89–113, 1960.

Dement, W.: The effect of dream deprivation. Science, 131:1705–1707, 1960.

Farnsworth, D. L.: Mental Health in College and University. Cambridge, Harvard University Press, 1957.

Foundeur, M. C., et al.: Postpartum mental illness. A.M.A. Arch. Neurol. & Psychiat., 77:503–512, 1957.

Grunebaum, H. U., Freedman, S. J., and Greenblatt, M.: Sensory deprivation and personality. Am. J. Psychiat., 116:878–882, 1960.

Harlow, H. F., and R. R. Zimmermann: Affectional responses in the infant monkey. Science, 130:421–432, 1959.

Hebb, D. O.: The mammal and his environment. Am. J. Psychiat., 111:826–831, 1955.

Hemphill, R. E.: Psychiatric disturbances in pregnancy and childbirth. Med. Illus., 10:527–531, 1956.

Hilgard, J. R., and Newman, M. F.: Anniversaries in mental illness. Psychiatry, 22:113–121, 1959.

Hollingshead, A. B., and Redlich, F. C.: Social Class and Mental Illness. New York, John Wiley & Sons, 1958.

Hooker, D., and Hare, C. C. (eds.): Genetics and the Inheritance of Integrated Neurological and Psychiatric Patterns. (Assoc. for Research in Nervous and Mental Diseases, Vol. 33.) Baltimore, Williams & Wilkins Co., 1954.

Kallmann, F. J.: The Genetics of Mental Illness. (American Handbook of Psychiatry, pp. 175–196, ed. S. Arieti) New York, Basic Books, Inc., 1959.

Idem: Heredity in Health and Mental Disorder. New York, W. W. Norton & Co., 1953.

Lejeune, J., and Turpin, R.: Somatic chromosomes in mongolism in mental retardation. Assn. Res. Neur. & Mentl. Dis., 39:67–77, 1959.

Lemkau, P. V.: Prevention of psychiatric illnesses. J.A.M.A., 162:854–857, 1956.

Levine, S., and Lewis, G. W.: Critical period for effects of infantile experience or maturation of stress response. Science, 129:42–43, 1959.

Malzberg, B.: Important Statistical Data About Mental Illness. In Arieti, S., Ed.: American Handbook of Psychiatry. New York, Basic Books, Inc., 1959, pp. 161–174.

Martin, M. E.: Puerperal mental illness. Brit. Med. J., 2:773–777, 1958.

Meerloo, J. A. M., and Klauber, L. D.: Clinical significance of starvation and oral deprivation. Psychosom. Med., 14:491–497, 1952.

Mendelson, J. H., Siger, L., and Solomon, P.: Psychiatric observations on congenital and acquired deafness: symbolic and perceptual processes in dreams. Am. J. Psychiat., 116:883–888, 1960.

Morris, G. O., Williams, H. L., and Lubin, A.: Misperception and disorientation during sleep deprivation. A.M.A. Arch. Gen. Psychiat., 2:247–254, 1960.

Oltman, J. E., McGarry, J. J., and Friedman, S.: Parental deprivation and the "broken home" in dementia praecox and other mental disorders. Am. J. Psychiat., 108:685–694, 1952.

Riesen, A. H.: The development of visual perception in man and chimpanzee. Science, 106:107–108, 1947.

Schiele, J., and Brozek, B. C.: "Experimental neurosis" resulting from semistarvation in man. Psychosom. Med., 10:31–50, 1948.

Seitz, P. F. D.: The effects of infantile experiences upon adult behavior in animal subjects. Am. J. Psychiat., 110:916–927, 1954.

Solomon, P., Leiderman, P. H., Mendelson, J. H., and Wexler, D.: Sensory deprivation. Am. J. Psychiat., 114:357–363, 1957.

Spiegel, J. P., and Bill, N. W.: The Family of the Psychiatric Patient. In Arieti, S., Ed.: American Handbook of Psychiatry. New York, Basic Books, Inc., 1959, pp. 114–149.

Stainbrook, E.: The Community of the Psychiatric Patient. In Arieti, S., Ed.: American Handbook of Psychiatry. New York, Basic Books, Inc., 1959, pp. 150–160.

Ziskind, E., Jones, H., Filante, W., and Goldberg, J.: Observations on mental symptoms in eye patched patients: hypnagogic symptoms in sensory deprivation. Am. J. Psychiat., 116:893–900, 1960.

Chapter Seven

EXAMINATION
OF THE PATIENT

PURPOSE OF EXAMINATION

The purpose of the psychiatric examination is to discover the origin and evolution of such personality disorders as may be interfering with the happiness, satisfactions, efficiency, or social adjustment of the patient. One seeks therefore, to secure a biographical-historical perspective of the personality, a clear psychological picture of the living person as a specific human being with his individual problems. It will be found that there is a logical continuity in any personality manifestations, whether the manifestations be those that are called normal* or those that are called abnormal. The fundamental, dynamic laws of behavior and of personality development are the same for both. By securing the maximum knowledge possible concerning the personality of the patient, the forces that have determined it, and the problems of living which he has found anxiety laden, it should be possible to understand the function of the illness and the meaning of the symptoms.

All phenomena of behavior, including those of mental disorders, are natural

* Normality is, of course, a vague concept, since everyone projects his own ideal of perfection into it.

events and should be studied like any other object of natural history investigation. This requires that an attempt be made to reconstruct the patient's behavior, to unravel the story of his neurosis or psychosis in the light of the fullest information possible concerning physical, chemical, anatomical, physiological, pathological, social, psychological, and educational factors and influences. It will be seen that the mental examination should be a clinical study of personality and aims at a comprehensive appraisal of the patient. Such a study must be made by a genetic and dynamic rather than by a cross-sectional method. Only by a genetic–dynamic investigation, with its emphasis on developmental sequence, can one ascertain how the individual came to express himself in his particular form of behavior—that of the neurosis, psychosis, or behavior disorder. The examiner does not seek to make a "diagnosis" in terms of some disease entity.

After an analysis of the concrete circumstances of the individual life and of the complicated forces that have entered into the organization of the personality, the examiner will re-formulate the patient's particular difficulties and behavior and reconstruct his inner life history.

111

This formulation will include statements as to the significant personal relationships during various periods of the patient's life with special emphasis on the patterns laid down during childhood. The formulation should include experiences that have been important in the development and persistence of personality traits, types of conflict present, the development of various adaptive processes and defense mechanisms. The formulation of the patient's clinical picture is in the form of probable facts and not in diagnostic labels. These facts must be orderly and intelligible. The formulation will include a discussion of the processes responsible for the behavior of the individual patient, will trace the complicated but significant sequences of cause and effect, will, through their dynamic relationship, reconstruct past and present events and to a considerable degree predict future ones.

Although the elucidation of symptoms is important in establishing the evidence of psychopathology, they should be looked upon as surface phenomena, and one should attempt to determine the needs, feelings, and motivations manifested in them. On the other hand, study of the personality will reveal certain themes or recurrent life issues or conflicts running through the individual's life history—topics or problems to which he may at times respond in the patterns known as mental illness. It will be found that a dynamic thread of continuity runs through both the previous personality organization and the ill personality. An examination of the patient's history usually will show that the same anxiety–relieving mechanisms, the same psychological themes which are revealed in the illness have been active in determining his personality type and character traits long before the illness appeared, going back usually, in fact, to early life.

THE PATIENT–PHYSICIAN RELATIONSHIP

While much has been said of the importance of the history in arriving at a diagnostic formulation, it needs to be emphasized that the psychiatric interview consists of significantly more than the verbalized account by the patient of his illness and the sought-for elaboration of his developmental history by the physician. From the beginning, the patient's behavior in relation to the physician is revealing in terms of his personality functioning, and its careful observation in connection with the verbal statements made and questions applied is most important. The relationship between the patient and physician influences to a large extent his motivation to reveal the nature of his problems and their sources in his past experiences. If the physician is perceived as helpful and tolerant, the course of history taking and personal revelations will be facilitated. When the patient thinks of the physician as critical, hostile, or demanding, he will be unlikely to unburden himself and will not reveal his innermost thoughts.

The majority of patients conceive of physicians as persons with whom they discuss their physical ailments, although in western culture today a growing number recognize the psychiatrist as someone to whom one attempts to reveal his feeling states, thought processes, and personal intimacies, generally subjects of less interest to the practicing physician.

Conventionally it is not customary for most persons to discuss openly their intimate relations and thoughts with strangers in the first meeting, nor should the interviewing psychiatrist expect such a full revelation. Much is withheld and perhaps distorted on first contact with the patient, and one should consider as abnormal too open and precise details of usually suppressed and repressed information during an initial interview.

Largely determining the patient's behavior and the attitute he exposes in his relationship to the interviewer are the patterns of behavior he has learned in his relationships with parents and other persons significant to him earlier in life. Thus, he often projects his expectations of how others respond to him to the physician and perceives him in a distorted manner other than that of the special role of a medical aid. In other words, from its inception the relationship is shaped by a transference, and such transference distortions vary considerably, from person to person. The psychotic person is most likely to misperceive the physician, while the person with a neurosis respects more closely the reality role of the psychiatrist.

With the concept of role misperception or transference available to him, the interviewer should carefully notice the attitude of the patient toward him throughout the course of their contact. Does the patient deal with him openly and frankly as an ill person seeking aid? Is the patient unusually dependent, requiring magic reassurance from the beginning or soliciting support for his actions and thoughts? Is his approach one of surliness or suspicion, or is there a seductive or provocative or exhibitionistic trend in the contact? On some occasion, the patient may attempt to ingratiate or bribe the physician for special attention or, on others, openly attack him or become sarcastic, jocular, or tearful. The type of behavior and the immediate sequence of verbal interchange in which it occurs are the important correlations that the skilled physician duly notes.

From these observations, the psychiatrist should infer similar behavior on the part of the patient in the past, an interpersonal approach perhaps revealing evidence of the personality disturbance, and he should question as well in what family setting and circumstance this behavior was learned and from what early sources of identification.

An awareness and appreciation of the dynamics of the patient–physician relationship and its potentialities for transference distortions of the physician by the patient is of major value in allowing the physician to maintain a necessary objectivity and detachment. From such a position, he may remain patient, tolerant, and sufficiently free from personal anxiety so that even the most suspicious and frightened patient will sooner or later perceive him as a non-threatening

aid. To put it more concretely, the physician, knowledgeable of the transference, will not be misled by unwarranted flattery in the initial interview or later nor will he respond either with guilty defensiveness or hostile rebuff in the face of bitter criticism presented by an embittered and suspicious newcomer to his office. He will not succumb to immediate reassurances or provide promises to the magic-seeking dependent person and, in the face of a seductive approach, his information of the transference will hold him aloof since he knows that the same deceptive contact, covering hostility, has been applied to others before him.

It is the function of the psychiatrist, uninvolved in the nuances of the patient's behavior, to arrange and conduct the interview in such a way that the patient, who finds himself in a strange and unaccustomed situation with an individual who often fails to meet his expectations of the role of a doctor, is relieved of as much anxiety as possible. The success of this endeavor to ease the patient's discomfort determines the potentiality of the examiner to provide the information needed to reconstruct and understand the former's illness.

THE CONDUCT OF THE INTERVIEW

It is preferable at all times to interview the patient, when he is accompanied, prior to discussion of his illness with the family member or friend. Furthermore, the patient should be advised of the psychiatrist's wish to discuss his illness with the accompanying person. By this means the relationship with the patient is benefited. He is provided the dignity of the responsibility of presenting his history prior to conversations with others who he may feel are motivated to distort his story. To be interviewed first may, too, allay a suspicion which sometimes exists that the physician is an enemy or is submissive to the wishes of a hostile family. The accompanying family member or friend should be seen on all occasions and, if additional information is provided that the patient has failed to present, he may again be interviewed to determine his conception of the unreported events or factors. The discrepancies between the report of the patient and of any other informant should be carefully noted.

The relative usually brings with him certain fears, misapprehensions, and feelings of guilt concerning the patient's illness. His attitude, too, may vary from acceptance and understanding to intolerance. He may be protective, demanding, condemnatory, or unrealistic. Often the relative, in an attempt to be helpful, may unwittingly contribute to the patient's illness.

It is important that the initial interview be conducted under circumstances that allow for an unheard contact with the patient. This makes for fairness and also leads to further investigation, as the patient often speaks more freely at this time than subsequently. The ease of a patient and his capacities for communication depend to a considerable extent on the manner of the physician's approach. The psychiatrist must be frank and courteous, show that he is genuinely interested in the patient, and, by the implicit elements of his character, be able to command the patient's respect. Rarely does the patient talk revealingly unless the psychiatrist shows signs of interest and understanding. The patient must be made to feel that he is being taken seriously, is being treated with dignity and as an equal, with due consideration for his opinions and statements. Also the psychiatrist must scrupulously seek to maintain the patient's self-esteem and allow him considerable initiative in relating his history.

In order that the optimum rapport and maximum information may be secured, the examiner must be flexible and the interviewing situation must be characterized by spontaneity. A spontaneous unveiling of the patient's account of himself will usually expose more informative material than the patient realizes. The physician, whether visited in his office or seen in an institution, is a stranger to the patient and often is representative to him of a new and perhaps what is regarded as a hostile environment. It is, therefore, too much to expect that the patient will confide extensively his feelings in the first interview. The psychiatrist will gradually seek to gain the confidence of the patient so that he will not hesitate to mention life experiences and desires which are so private that he has not referred to them to his intimates. The patient usually feels that he is understood and his point of view appreciated if the physician permits him to tell his own story, with only an occasional tactful, courteous, and guiding question. Judicious questioning of a patient with an emotional disturbance in such a way that psychopathological mental content will become manifest is a fine art. If the psychiatrist manifests a genuine interest and understanding, the patient will rarely hesitate and will often be eager to make known any problem.

A physician who has placed his patient on the defensive has usually blundered in his technique and has perhaps greatly impaired his future usefulness as a counselor. This does not mean that a sense of delicacy should prevent a search sufficient to describe what is going on behind the scenes but, that having gained the confidence and co-operation of the patient, the questions should be put with discretion and with respect for the patient's feelings and intelligence. Care should be taken not to frame questions in such a way that they will be interpreted as accusations. Skillful questioning should enable the psychiatrist, without arousing undue anxiety, to touch upon the most intimate aspects of the patient's life and open up subjects for exploration that might otherwise remain untouched. Oftentimes the patient is not able to respond affirmatively to certain topics suggested by the questioning. However, the fact that the psychiatrist has intimated through his questioning his acquaintanceship with and availability for discussion of such problems is of utmost importance. The patient has been made aware that he has available to him a person to whom he may reveal himself at an appropriate time.

The psychiatrist will never permit himself to become involved in an argument with a patient. The beginner is apt to think that the principal object of the examination is to ascertain the existence of abnormal ideas and to forget the significance of the social circumstances under which symptoms became apparent. He is often more interested in gross disturbances of behavior or in delusional material, with the result that he overlooks deviations in affect and mood, not to mention those of the sensorium. To become a successful psychiatrist, it is necessary to acquire a penetrating insight into personality dynamics, a procedure which necessitates understanding that the patient is more than a bundle of psychological mechanisms. He must also possess the clinical sensitivity and subconscious summation of knowledge and experience that we know as intuition.

The patient is initially often eager to discuss his symptoms, complaints, and present illness. While it is the custom in many hospitals and clinics to record these data at a later stage in the formal documentation of the patient's history, it will be found most satisfactory to allow the patient and the relatives to discuss these matters spontaneously and initially. To insist on a presentation of material relative to the patient's family and his life history is often regarded by patient and the family informant as irrelevant and irritating.

Although the diagnostic interviews with the patient and his relatives and friends are to be conducted in a flexible manner, the recording of the data for analysis or future reference is best done in accordance with a definite schema. Such a schema is followed in describing the psychiatric examination, and the information to be considered or arranged is detailed under the various headings. In examining a patient, the error is often made of following such a schematic history with its various subdivisions in an obsessive manner, drilling the patient for information on each point. Such an ef-

fort is bound to be unrewarding, as patients are usually too anxious initially to provide pertinent material and therefore will respond to a routine staccato type of questioning only by withdrawal or irritation.

There follows a schematic representation of the headings which are customarily contained in the recorded history. Under these headings are mentioned appropriate areas of life experience upon which the psychiatrist should, at some time, gain knowledge. It is just as imperative to realize what has not been mentioned and discussed in a spontaneously-flowing interview and the extent and affect attached to each area as to record what has been gained. One may then question the existence of some special suppression or repression of experience or even a deprivation that has particular significance to the patient. Later these "missed" areas may arise either through direct probing, or spontaneously, when the patient's anxiety has lessened.

THE PSYCHIATRIC HISTORY

A brief initial description of the patient's status is to be obtained which will include a statement as to his age, sex, marital status, racial background, and occupation. His address and means of direct communication with him (telephone) are also obtained.

Reason for Consultation or Commitment

With the widespread extension of psychiatric services into the areas of private practice, outpatient clinics, courts of law, welfare agencies, schools and the general hospital, as well as the private and state institutions, a patient with a psychiatric disorder presents himself for examination under a variety of circumstances. The patient may come personally for examination or be referred to a private office or clinic by a physician or by a social agency or school. In other instances, he may be required by a decree of court or by certification to be examined or admitted to a hospital. Under all these circumstances, a brief statement of the manner and circumstances which led to examination or treatment should be obtained. This should include a record of the referring physician or agency and the reason for requesting the examination, if this is offered or is available. In the private office or clinic, the patient often comes alone, and the account of his illness, as he sees it, and of his life history is available only through him. This may also be the circumstance when a patient is committed to a hospital. However, if the patient is accompanied by a relative or some close friend, this person, or others with an intimate knowledge of the patient, may be able to impart knowledge of significant import in regard to the illness and the patient's life experiences beyond that immediately available from the patient. The accompanying family member or friend may thus verify or elaborate the information provided by the patient. The name and relationship of such persons should be placed in the record appropriately.

The Problem

A clear statement of the complaints and problems of the patient should be obtained from the patient. If possible, it is best to record statements made by the patient in verbatim form.

Present Illness

A detailed account of the development of the present illness of the patient should be obtained. This account should not only include the patient's statements in regard to the symptoms he has observed but also the acute or insidious changes in character, interest, mood, and attitude toward others, as well as modifications in his dress, personal habits, and physical health. It should provide, as well, a careful description of the social circumstances in which the symptoms evolved. The psychiatrist should attempt to ascertain what relationships with others may have been significant. He should seek to learn what has taken place in the lives of these persons and in their contacts with the patient which may have had an effect upon his emotional and psychological state. The psychiatrist should ascertain whether there have been deaths, separations, conflicts, or losses suffered by the patient in relation to his parents and other members of his immediate family or to relatives or friends who are not initially identified. The interweaving of these data and the patient's emotional responses to changes in his relations with others as chronologically related to the development of his symptoms often provides major clues as to the psychodynamic factors influencing the illness and its prognosis.

The relationship of symptom development to periods of stress induced by interpersonal conflict or significant loss is seldom to be obtained through the process of direct questioning. It is necessary for the psychiatrist to define the potential temporal relationship and then elaborate the problem.

While the search for the emotional disturbance has been emphasized as one of the most important parts of the story of the present illness, the patient and the family or friends usually tell their story by describing the symptoms that preoccupy him. It is important to obtain a clear description of each symptom, when it was first noticed, whether it is episodically observed or persistently present, its severity, the circumstances that influence each symptom for better or worse, and their effect on the patient's life—his social, sexual, and vocational adaptations must be explored.

The psychiatrist should seek to ascertain what changes were first noticed in the patient's behavior and how they developed and progressed. He should secure information concerning changes in emotion and mood and when undesirable emotional and other personality attitudes were first overtly expressed, and determine whether the patient has appeared increasingly tense and anxious or displayed obsessive or compulsive symptoms. Details as to changes in work efficiency, degree of activity, conduct, attention, speech, and memory are important as indicators of illness. Inquiry should be made as to whether the patient grasps questions and new situations as quickly as formerly and whether his judgment is impaired. Specific instances are necessary. Has he mentioned peculiar experiences? Has the patient said or done anything that suggests that he has heard imaginary voices or has had other sensory deceptions? Has he had expansive or depressive ideas, ideas of sin, unworthiness, persecution, jealousy, or infidelity? Have suicidal or homicidal tendencies existed?

All accounts of the current illness must consider the general areas of necessary biological functioning. Therefore, an exploration must be made of the changes in the patient's zest for life, his social drive, and the physiological indications of general anxiety exposed in his sleeping and eating habits, his bowel functions, and his usual sexual activities and gratifications.

Equally rewarding as the previous areas of interest in the account of the present illness will be inquiries which are concerned with the patient's concept of the origins of his illness, its meaning and significance, both now and in the future, for himself and his important relations with others. Is the illness one to which he responds with overt anxiety or sadness, or does it provoke shame or guilt?

The attitude toward the illness is revealing as well. Does the patient deny its significance and seem to be gratified by his symptomatology and the effects upon those upon whom he is dependent? In other words, is there an emotional gain from the illness? In some instances, the matter of material gain demands inquiry when insurance payments or litigation may be pending.

In contrast to the gain from illness, one will wish to consider as well the urge to recover. Some understanding of this urge may be ascertained by studying the patient's response to his previous illnesses. The duration of the dependency induced by illness in the past in relation to the specific disease and his understand-

ing of his present illness and his expectations for its outcome may give clues to his drive for improvement.

All accounts of the present illness should contain a statement as to the reason for the request for help at the particular time that it is sought. Often patients give histories of long-continuing and unchanging symptomatic disturbance without medical consultation. The precipitating event is unrelated in some cases to symptom change and, frequently, is found in some sudden change in the interpersonal life situation. An inquiry must be made of previous illnesses of the same kind, of treatment given for the current illness and any preceding attacks, and of those who provided therapy so that both additional information may be obtained from them as well as an estimate made of the value of the therapy. In some instances, it will be of value to explore the patient's collaboration in previous treatment regimens.

From the present illness, the psychiatrist should distinguish as far as possible the precipitating stress situations from those that predispose. For the most part, the latter will be discovered in the account of the family and personal life of the patient.

Family History

From the family history one may obtain information as to the genetic, familial, economic, and social forces to which the patient was exposed throughout his life. In addition to an account of the parents and siblings with whom the patient lived, which should provide a picture of their personalities, ills, strivings, and other defects, it is important to learn as well of the other persons who resided in or frequently visited the home. By inquiring as to the patient's impression of his parents and other family members and associates, their methods of rearing, and the social mores of their group the examiner may infer much of the familial customs, conflicts, emotional control, and opportunities for identification offered in early life. The methods of enforcing obedience used by the parents and their substitutes are particularly revealing in this aspect. A careful account of the reactions of the family and the patient to illnesses in other family members may reveal the sources of reactions to illness or patterns of symptom expression used by the patient and others. The influence of a powerful or domineering grandparent who has set certain ideals for the family or even of the offsetting factor of training by some domestic helper are worthy of note. The patient is usually able to indicate whether he or some sibling was the favored child of either parent and to comment upon his emotional reaction of pleasure, fear, envy, or jealousy relative to his position in the family as compared to that of his siblings.

Here one should note the response of the patient to events such as loss of a parent by death, divorce, or desertion. The age of the patient at the time that the separation took place is much more important to note from the psychiatric viewpoint than the age of the parent at the time of death or desertion. Whether mourning—or a sense of relief—took place should be learned, as well as the duration of this response to the loss and the response of other family members to the same event.

Specific information should be obtained as to the occurrence of mental illness, suicide, alcoholism, delinquency, or eccentricity in direct or collateral lines, and whether the patient was of legitimate birth, adopted, or a foster child.

Throughout, it will be found that information is more easily elicited by making an effort to obtain specific descriptions of action and interaction with related report of the concomitant emotional response rather than by attempting to elicit responses to questions framed in terms of adjectival descriptions of behavior.

Personal History

It is convenient to think of the personal history as a record of the maturation of the individual and thereby to divide the written report into areas concerned with infancy, childhood, adolescence, and maturity. A report only of maturational development will be inadequate; again, the able historian attempts to define the concomitant interpersonal reactions and their possible influence on the growing person.

INFANCY. Infancy poses a particular problem, since much of the available material is beyond the range of the patient's conscious memory and thereby represents hearsay or the reports available from other family members or observers. Here one wishes to learn whether the patient was a wanted or unwanted child and what expectations the parents might have held for his sex and future development. If he was born with a physical handicap or failed to conform to the family expectations and hopes, the parents' response should be a matter of interest. The nature of the birth itself and the mother's reaction to it often determine mothering attitudes for long periods thereafter and are worthy of discussion.

An account should be obtained of the ages at which sitting, walking, talking, and bowel and bladder control took place. This information provides indications of maturation of functions of the nervous system. The mother's response should be sought to delay in these events and failure of the child to live up to her beliefs in evolving such activities. Important information may be elicited here, too, relative to the patient's infantile patterns of eating, sleeping, and playing and the parents' methods of participation in such activities.

CHILDHOOD. Childhood as a developmental period offers the opportunity to review the earliest aspect of the patient's active relationship with others than himself. It is usually possible to obtain some expression as to his reported personality traits at this time of life. Was he thought of as affectionate, trusting, generous, and active, or as shy, irritable, distant, easily frightened or suspicious, selfish or aggressive. The capacity of the child for playing and sharing with others should be studied.

Here an account of the patient's earliest memories and dreams, particularly if repetitive, offer an opportunity to discern a wealth of material concerning his early inner fantasy and emotional life. Since the major interpersonal growth at this time is concerned with the issue of dependency or autonomy, the history should describe the interplay of forces toward independence or dependence. That patient's early efforts at self-expression and assertion should be sought as well as the parental attitudes and reaction to such actions. An evaluation should be made of the response to separations from the parents, such as homesickness. Particularly to be noted are the childish responses toward parental discipline and the accompanying or related emotional responses of fear, shame, or guilt. If the patient had feelings of inferiority early, their source should be sought, and if there occurred attitudes of self-compensatory grandiosity, they should be noted. The early expressions of hostility, anger, and aggression and their chief targets, as well as the methods of coping with stress (flight, fight, or immobilization) should be observed.

Sometimes, one may obtain only reports of symptomatic disturbances in childhood of maldevelopment expressed in speech disorders or stuttering, enuresis, somnambulism, nightmares, or special phobias.

Since schooling commences in childhood and offers an opportunity of defining not only the early intellectual growth but also the initial socialization over periods of time outside the family, the patient's experiences in this milieu are of particular interest. Thus, one wishes to know the age of entrance and leaving, the occurrence of grade failures or evidence of unusual ability, the child's attitudes toward his teachers and classmates, as well as indications of disturbance expressed in school phobias, truancy, or poor deportment.

Again, the historical study of childhood illnesses and injuries with their duration, complications, and residuals must be conducted, as it reveals the origin of important deficits and later character traits.

ADOLESCENCE. Adolescence holds, once again, at this later period of maturation the potentiality for re-experiencing many of the stresses of the earlier periods of life as well as those uniquely characteristic of this time of the developmental phase. Thus once again, the responses to illnesses, relations to seniors and peers, and schooling as experienced in adolescence should be reviewed. The patient's adaptations and reactions to such events should be noted. Of particular importance for the inquiry into the period of adolescent behavior is the response to pubescent development. The family's preparation of the growing boy and girl for such events as seminal emissions and menstruation needs to be known as well as the adolescent's response to their occurence. His emerging sexual interests and his reactions to those of his peers should be noted. Signs of failure to develop a clear psychosexual identity usually are evident by this life period.

Other questions of importance are: those related to the reaction of mother to sexual curiosity and experimentation of early childhood; strong, persistent, dependent attachment to the parent of either sex; preparedness for and reaction to sexual differences; guilt concerning adolescent masturbation; persistence of "crushes"; heterosexual or homosexual attitude toward sex; frankness, prudishness; overt homosexuality.

Since adolescence is a period of emerging personal identity with evident struggles for autonomy and independence, the nature of the patient's adolescent friendships must be ascertained as well as his participation in or rejection by adolescent groups, his predominant sources of idealized identifications, and his complacent or defiant attitudes to authority. In this period, special capacities or talents may be discerned and ascertained.

ADULTHOOD. Since adulthood brings with it the special stresses of marriage and child rearing as well as of vocational adaptation plus the problems of establishing effective relations with those in authority and peers, as well as of establishing adult social relations, the history should contain information pertaining particularly to these areas.

As for the sexual adaptations of the adult, the historian will include an account of the courtship, the role played by the patient and his partner, their areas of agreement and disagreement. As the more common areas of disagreement in marriage center about the sexual relations, rearing of children, relations to in-laws, and the spending of money, detailed information will be sought in all areas. The attitudes toward contraception, emotional reactions to infidelity, illegitimate pregnancies, abortions, or impotence should be looked into. If divorce has occurred, it should provoke special inquiry into its sources. If the patient has failed to marry, the sources of this lack of adult experience may be looked for in the possible over-fixation on a parent, homosexual drives, aversion to the opposite sex, or some physical or social disability preventing the establishment of a heterosexual relationship.

In considering the occupational adaptation and perhaps the military experiences of males, the most significant areas of inquiry are those concerned with the motivations leading to selection of a vocation, the perseverance and performance of the task, and the ongoing relations with working associates. The patient's ability to accept the direction of competent authority or his defiance of it will indicate in some measure his level of emotional maturity. His emotional response to his advancement or that of his peers is also to be carefully searched. Undue fear or envy or incapacity to adapt to envy of others should be of particular interest. Other revealing areas for study are the various occupations entered, positions held, wages received, reasons for changing, periods of idleness and the reason for same; stationary condition or progress in efficiency and in responsibilities; attitude toward work; satisfaction from work; anything in the present position that is especially difficult, threatening, or inadequate in pro-

viding satisfaction; habits of saving or spending money; whether life aims were achieved.

LATE MATURITY. The later years of life bring their special problems. Here one should examine reactions to the menopause, the emerging independence and separation from children, retirement, and death of others. Here one will wish to know of the existence of special interests and avocations, athletic or other recreations, social and community activities. The satisfactions or stresses which they produce represent important facets of the patient's personality functioning. These should be ascertained as well as the need for alcohol and other drugs to relieve tension. An account should be given of the patient's religious interest and practices as well as the satisfactions gained thereby. It is often useful to have the patient describe a typical 24-hour day. One should also inquire about his current dreams, daydreams, and plans for the future; this information gives clues to his aspirations, ideals, and hidden drives.

Personality

On the basis of the developmental history, the interviewer may arrive at estimates of the social adaptability of the patient, his general activity, and his personality traits and characteristics. These estimates may be derived both from the patient's own comments about himself and those made by his relatives and friends, as well as the inferences obtained from the personal history. These statements and inferences should be recorded as a part of the personal history, with references as to their source.

Particularly important here are the references to the prevailing mode of interpersonal relations. Have relations with others been satisfying to himself and them? If not, why not? Has his inner feeling for others seemed to have been one of hatred or of liking? Has the patient enjoyed a degree of affection and respect from others that provided emotional security and self-assurance? Since interpersonal relationships with their positive and negative feelings may be of much significance, inquiry should be made concerning any special attitudes toward parents, siblings, spouse, or others closely associated with the patient. Has filial devotion to either parent been extreme?

GENERAL ACTIVITY AND INTERESTS. Assessment should be made of the degree of initiative and of activity, the fluctuation of activity, the industry or the indolence; intense and poorly balanced devotion to special activities in work or recreation; range of interests; use of leisure; preoccupation, alertness, talkativeness, taciturnity. What have been the patient's dominant interests and activities? What satisfactions and dissatisfactions are experienced from work and environment?

EVALUATION OF PERSONALITY TRAITS AND CHARACTERISTICS. One wishes to have an opinion as to whether the patient is given to emotional fluctuations; cheerful, light-hearted, optimistic; gloomy, pessimistic, worrisome, daring, or timid; overconfident or cautious; self-reliant or dependent. Does he seek support, reassurance, and approval from others? Is he demonstrative or stolid, out-going or shut-in, frank and open or reserved and reticent, bashful or at ease in the presence of strangers, talkative or taciturn, aggressive or submissive? Has aggression been constructively or destructively expressed? Is he generous or stingy, honest or deceitful, suspicious, given to misinterpretations, easily offended, prone to feel slighted, resentful, hostile, cynical, inclined to blame others, argumentative, stubborn, envious, cruel? Is he self-conscious, self-blaming, meticulous, perfectionistic, excessively orderly, overconscientious, overscrupulous, or boastful, overbearing, resentful, arrogant, calm or irritable, preoccupied with bodily complaints? Are his opinions and habits rigid, adaptable, characterized by special prejudices? Does he accept or shrink from responsibility? Does he have feelings of inadequacy? Is he given to daydreaming? What is his attitude toward authority? Does he have a sense of humor? What

are his characteristic ways of handling stresses, failures, and frustrations? What is tendency to evade reality and what methods does he employ? What are sets of reactions and patterns of behavior with which the patient responds to new situations? What tension-relieving devices does he habitually use? It is also helpful to ascertain the persons toward whom the patient manifests any of the special personality characteristics described.

Information concerning the patient's personality organization will be secured by ascertaining the type of interpersonal relationships which he has tended to develop, e.g., those marked by a predominance of hostility or of affection, of aggression or of submission, of projection or of incorporation, of independence or of dependence. What type of emotional disturbance has the patient most characteristically manifested when defenses have broken down, e.g., anxiety, depression, elation, rage, or others?

Expression of the patient's attitude toward himself and his body and an indication of his ideals, goals, aspirations, and the sources of his chief identifications, if obtainable, should be ascertained. In addition, there should be a statement as to his superego function with a note as to the person after whom he has modeled his conscience. Also included should be any past indication of the manner in which he placates feelings of guilt, whether, for example, by penitence, mourning, physical suffering, deprivation, or bribery.

Emotionally Disturbing Experiences

Special attention should be paid to respects in which life has not been psychologically satisfying. Was the need for affection in childhood adequately met? Were there frustrations of hopes and wishes or wounds of pride, vanity, and self-esteem? Were love and sex experiences of emotional significance? What experiences produced pent-up emotional tension or domestic, economic, or social stress? Have family or environmental entanglements been anxiety-producing? The patient should be encouraged to express freely his associations with significant life events and his feelings about them.

Either at this point or in the account of parental relations, the age of the patient at the time of death of a parent or other significant person should be noted. Furthermore, the patient's response to this loss in terms of sadness, depression, guilt, anxiety, or failure to respond emotionally, as well as the duration of the emotional response and its effect on his various activities, should be determined.

PSYCHIATRIC EXAMINATION

An examination must include a thorough physical and neurological examination together with all indicated laboratory examinations. These investigations, which must be sufficient to discover all structural, functional, somatic, and metabolic factors, need not be discussed in this textbook. It should be borne in mind that psychotic patients may utter no word or complaint even though they are suffering from serious organic illness.

General Appearance, Manner and Attitude

One will observe how the patient enters the room and how he shakes hands. He will note the patient's facies and the various psychomotor tensions through which emotions are expressed. The initial interview affords opportunity to note any obvious physiological signs of anxiety, such as moist hands, mopping of perspiration from the forehead, restlessness, tense posture, strained voice, wide pupils, or guarded vigilance. Note should be made of any peculiarities in the patient's physical appearance, including observation of any features suggestive of the opposite sex. Attention should be paid to his dress, gait, posture, gesture, or voice as well as the care of his person and clothing. Dress often reveals much concerning personality. Note should also be made as to whether the patient is accessible, frank, evasive, self-defensive, suspicious, ingratiating, superior, disdainful,

irritable, or otherwise characterized in manner and bearing and in his attitude toward the examiner and the environment. Is he assertive and aggressive, or is he meekly submissive? Is he superior and condescending in speech and manner, or is he self-depreciatory? Is he critical, sarcastic, and verbally abusive? Is he irritable and irascible? Is he opinionated or indecisive? Is he arrogant or obsequious? The patient's general reaction to examination may be significant. Does he welcome, tolerate, or refuse the interview? It will be remembered that surface attitudes are often compensatory or otherwise protective. Aggressiveness or a rugged and rough surface attitude, for example, may be a chronic defense against internal anxiety. While many of the data under this heading may be noted and recorded at the beginning of the interview, they may frequently be modified or enlarged at its conclusion.

After having noted such general observations as those indicated, the psychiatrist examines the patient in respect to the following part-functions of the personality.

Consciousness

Under this heading one notes the sensorium, or functional state of the special senses, especially as it is related to the condition of consciousness, which may be clear or clouded to varying degrees. Deeper states of impairment are confusion, stupor, and unconsciousness. If necessary, the patient is questioned to determine his orientation as to time, place, and person. It is a matter of great importance to determine whether symptoms are presented in a setting of mental clearness or one of clouding.

Affectivity and Mood

By this, the character tone of the patient's feeling-life is referred to. The psychiatrist will note the type of affect, its intensity, depth, and duration. The prevailing mood is often suggested by the patient's facial expression, muscular tensions, and bodily attitude. One usually inquires, too, of the patient as to his emotional state. The question should not be of a leading or inappropriate type. One, for example, would not, of course, impair the confidence of an obviously depressed patient by asking him if he were happy. Frequently, the inquiry, "How are your spirits?" will evoke the desired description. Discreet questions designed to bring out the patient's estimate of self may elicit not only a reply suggesting his mood but one containing other significant information. When the patient has indicated his mood, he may be asked the reason for his feelings, although the reply frequently represents the rationalization of factors not consciously recognized. In addition to the important observations as to the intensity of affect, its appropriateness, modulation, responsiveness, and oscillation, such states as euphoria, elation, exhilaration, exaltation, ecstacy, depression, gloomy irritability, and apathy or incongruity are noted. The patient who is euphoric or exhilarated will often be optimistic, self-assured, friendly, and buoyant. The depressed patient is usually quiet and restrained, often dejected and hopeless in attitude and manner. Affective states readily influence attention, concentration, memory functions, and thinking processes. Somewhat more complex states marked by disturbed affective components are fear, panic, hypochondriasis, apprehensiveness, worry, despair, chronic dissatisfaction, irritability, suspiciousness, anger, hate, and silliness.

Conation and Expressive Aspects of Behavior

In this phase of the examination, observation is made of the patient's general activity with special reference to the urges, drives, tendencies, and habit formations that determine this activity. The examiner notes both the spontaneous and the reactive behavior of the patient. Does he act in a reality-adjusted way? The physician should note whether the patient is ready for effort or whether he avoids it; whether he is overactive and energetic or whether he is slow and retarded and perhaps unable to initiate action. Is he restless, agitated, impulsive, or assaultive? What, if any, activities does he spontaneously initiate? Distinction should be made between pressure of occupation with its eager output of energy and a mere undirected restlessness. Other disturbances of activity are inability to initiate action, reduction of activity, stupor, negativism, stereotypy, catalepsy, mannerisms, tics, posturing, grimacing, silliness, automatic obedience (flexibilitas cerca, echopraxia), playfulness, impulsiveness, combativeness, and destructive tendencies. The apparent stupors designated under this caption do not include those caused by an extreme clouding of consciousness. Among these apparent stupors are those associated with deep depression, those resulting from negativism or resistance, and those resulting from resentment. Note should be made of any compulsive acts or ceremonials. Any evidence of a compulsive personality as shown by scrupulosity or by excessive emphasis on orderliness or cleanliness should be described.

Considerable information can often be obtained by having the patient write a simple sentence from dictation. The handwriting may show tremors, as in the paretic. In the same disease, too, various elisions are common. The manic frequently writes in bold characters, underscoring many words or adding spontaneous productions. Negativism, retardation, or pressure of activity may be demonstrated by the manner in which the patient approaches the task. Note should be made as to the patient's degree of alertness, as to whether or not he is mute, as to whether he eats or refuses food, as to the presence of queer postures or of the sustained immobility of catalepsy.

If the patient is depressed, a careful effort should be made to ascertain any possible inclinations toward suicide. Inquiry should be made as to whether the patient considers life worth living. If his response is in the negative, he may then be asked more specifically as to whether he has considered doing anything about it and what thoughts and plans he has constructed. Note should be made concerning sex attitudes or habits observed, including flirtatiousness, hypereroticism, anaphrodisia, exhibitionism, homosexuality, and overt or covert masturbation.

Disturbances of attention, in the form of distractibility, preoccupation, excessive tenacity of attention, and absence of attention should be included in this topic.

Associations and Thought Processes

In this field of examination the examiner observes not the content of thought but the tempo of associations and the characteristics of thought processes. Note should be made of any unusual rapidity of associations, as in flight of ideas, also of any slowness in associations, as in retardation. Disorders in the logical progression of thought will be shown by the patient's associations as he talks. The examiner should therefore note such disturbances as circumstantiality, incoherence, blocking, or irrelevance. Record should be made of any distortions of thought processes, such as neologisms, word salad, perseveration, echolalia, or condensation.

Thought Content and Mental Trend

In the investigation of this important field, an error is often made by confining it to a search for delusions. The patient's dreams, the content of his fantasies, his ambitions, fears, and identifications afford significant glimpses into his preoccupations and personal problems. The psychiatrist will note the extent to which the patient misinterprets facts and reality in his unrecognized effort to meet his emotional and personality needs. The psychiatrist should be on the watch for a trend or general theme that runs through, correlates, and tends to determine beliefs and conduct. Some patients are eager to express any beliefs that center around such a trend, while others are evasive or suspicious.

In patients who are otherwise accessible but who are reluctant to divulge such content of thought as they fear will be considered disordered, much depends on the experience of the physician and the rapport he establishes with the patient. Sometimes outlines for psychiatric examinations contain a list of fixed questions designed to bring out the commoner types of delusions if they exist. The patient soon discovers their stereotyped, uncorrelated nature and their lack of spontaneity and so may quickly become resentful and assume a defensive attitude. The wisdom of their use is therefore questionable. Usually, while giving the story of his life and of his recent experiences, the patient will have divulged whether he has resorted to delusional beliefs in his efforts to deal with personality problems and difficult situations. If, up to this point, the patient has made no references to material which suggests that it may be delusional, its existence and an intimation of its nature may sometimes be secured by asking him if he has recently had any unusual, strange, or troublesome experiences. If it is suspected that he has resorted to projection as a protective device, the patient may be asked if people have been spreading lies about him or if ill-disposed people have attempted to harm him. Efforts to solve given personality needs are often met not only by projection and delusions of persecution but also by the mechanism of compensation. For this reason, inquiry may be made as to self-flattering beliefs designed to magnify the patient's estimate of self. If the patient's mood is one of depression, he may be asked if he has done anything that is wrong or if he has sinned more than other people. Escape from intolerable reality may be provided by delusional consolations.

A spontaneous development of the patient's mental content should be encouraged, and the narration should be interrupted with a minimum of guiding questions. Such questions as are asked should be carefully individualized, and pertinent to and in logical relation to content that has already been expressed. The construction of the questions designed to search for delusional material must be determined largely by the intelligence and by the educational and social status of the patient. As the interview proceeds, the patient's capacity for discriminating between reality and subjective mental experience is learned and the physician guides his questions accordingly.

Psychopathological mental content includes special preoccupations, overvalued ideas, disproportionate emphasis on certain topics, depressive ideas with expression of self-depreciation or of sin and self-accusation, hypochondriacal ideas, ideas of disease or of poverty, ideas of unreality with feelings of strangeness and unnaturalness in one's self or the environment, nihilistic ideas with denial of the existence of things, misinterpretations and ideas of reference, ideas and feelings of influence, beliefs that one is being persecuted, feelings of jealousy and accusations of infidelity, and expansive and grandiose beliefs with ideas of wealth, power, et cetera. The psychiatrist notes whether delusions are transitory or persistent. By asking the patient if he is troubled by the recurrence of the same thought, the existence of obsessions may be ascertained. Whether or not there is an impoverishment of thought must also be noted.

As the patient reveals his conscious ideational content, the examiner seeks, by the type of delusion, to ascertain what is being symbolically told him, also the relationship of its specific content to the patient's emotional needs as well as why at this particular time he has had to have the protection and support of his delusion. It will frequently be observed that the conscious content of the delusion is the converse of the true meaning. Statements made by the patient are often clues to the psychological realities they conceal. Motives ascribed to others, too, may represent the patient's own wishes and urges. Grandiose delusions often give a clue to previous frustrations.

If the patient is requested to write an account of his life, he will frequently disclose a trend or express material of psychopathological significance. Mental content previously undiscovered is at times revealed in letters or other writings.

Perception

In deeply toxic and in organic states, consciousness may be so seriously disturbed that the mental processes necessary to complete perception are impossible, with the result that imperception exists. In suspected mental disorder, particularly in delirioid or in strongly affective states, the examiner should scrutinize the accounts of the patient's perceptual experiences and his observed reactions to them in order to discover any indications that they are illusionary in nature. Illusional misinterpretations which are not of psychopathological origin are usually, in the face of reasonable evidence, recognized by the individual as erroneous. If, however, the illusions have arisen from a deep-seated anxiety or other personality basis, they are not amenable to reason.

The ease with which the occurrence of hallucinations is ascertained varies greatly. One looks first for auditory hallucinations, the method of inquiring for which will depend upon many factors, particularly upon the apparent integrity of the patient's personality and the extent to which he recognizes that hallucinations are mentally pathological. If the patient's evaluation of reality is considerably disturbed, he may be frankly asked if he hears voices. The subject may often be approached somewhat more indirectly by asking him if he has observed that he has been called derogatory names, or if unpleasant remarks have been directed to him. Frequently some remark of the patient affords a lead which, if pursued, will indicate as to whether or not hallucinations exist. It often happens that the patient will describe hallucinatory experiences if he is asked if he has had any "imaginations." The same inquiry may occasionally reveal delusions when the patient has some realization that his mental content is abnormal. This is not surprising, since the unitary reaction of the individual frequently uses both perception and mental content for the same purpose. Indeed, ideational and hallucinatory content are so intimately reciprocal and complementary that in a guide for mental examination they might properly be considered under the same heading.

In Chapter 6 attention was called to

the fact that both hallucinations and delusions represent an inner falsification of the outside world in accordance with the needs and wishes of the personality. The psychiatrist seeks, therefore, to determine what function the patient's hallucinations are serving in his total psychological experience. When the patient denies hallucinations, a suspicion that they exist may sometimes be confirmed by the nurse, who may observe him in listening attitudes or responding to his hallucinations. Since, in disguised and projected form, the hallucinations express mental material that intimately pertains to his personality needs and problems, the patient is usually much preoccupied during his hallucinatory experience. In toxic states, the patient's behavior may suggest reactions to visual hallucinations; in other instances, an inquiry if he has had any visions may furnish information. For diagnostic purposes, it is a matter of great importance to determine as to whether hallucinations, irrespective of the type of sense expression, occur in a setting of clear consciousness. If consciousness is not clear, it is probable that toxic or organic pathology exists.

Memory

If, as is frequently desirable, the patient is asked, as part of the general mental examination, to give a chronological account of his life, by his success in giving dates of entering and leaving school, the places and dates of employment and the names of employers, a reasonably correct estimate of his remote memory can be determined. Special attention should be paid as to whether the stated activities and dates are properly correlated. The patient's memory concerning events of somewhat less personal interest may be tested by asking him concerning local or national events known to have occurred during the patient's life and concerning which any person in the community would ordinarily have knowledge. Frequently, particularly if there is a history of head trauma, delirium, epilepsy, fugues, or other dissociative reaction, one should ascertain if there is a hiatus of memory for a circumscribed period of time.

Recent memory can easily be tested by asking the patient when he came to the hospital, from what place, by whom he was accompanied, or concerning other events in the immediate past.

If the patient shows impaired memory for recent events, note should be made of any tendency to fill the gaps of memory with pseudoreminiscences (confabulation). Sometimes alleged activities and incidents can be suggested. In paranoid psychoses, especially, it should be determined if the accounts of any incidents are elaborated with details, really fictitious but believed by the patient to be facts. In more exaggerated cases, the entire account of alleged incidents may be a retrospective falsification of memory.

Retention and recall ability may be tested by giving a series of four or five nonconsecutive numbers and asking the patient to repeat them in the same or in reverse order. Another frequent test is to give him a street address or the names of a few objects with instructions that they be remembered. After a given period, e.g., five minutes or an hour, the patient is asked to repeat what he was enjoined to remember.

Fund of Information

This will be indicated by the patient's replies to questions concerning current events, matters of common knowledge, and retention of knowledge acquired in school. The character of the questions will depend upon the opportunities the patient has had for acquiring information.

Judgment

By judgment is meant the ability to compare facts or ideas, to understand their relations, and to draw correct conclusions from them. The correctness of the patient's estimates and interpretations of external objective matters and the degree to which he recognizes the interrelation of significant factors and incidents are indexes of the quality of his judgment. Judgment is integrated in all personality functions but is particularly influenced by the patient's general grasp and by emotional factors. It might readily be extended to include the patient's estimate of his mental disorder, but his subjective judgment in this respect is so important that under the designation "insight" it is considered as a special field for examination. If objective judgment is impaired, one seeks to ascertain if the defect is caused by a toxic disturbance of the sensorium, by degenerative or inflammatory involvement of higher cortical centers, or if it is distorted by emotional influences and confined to matters conflicting with delusional trends and affective needs. In estimating the patient's judgment, an attempt is made to learn if the patient's business affairs are conducted with prudence and if his family obligations are met.

Insight

By insight one refers to the extent to which the patient is aware that he is ill, that he recognizes the nature of his illness and understands the special dynamic factors that have been operative in its production. It refers to the patient's ability to observe and understand himself— the extent of his self-knowledge. One seeks to learn the patient's estimate of the manner and extent to which personality difficulties are interfering with his social adjustment and the successful performance of his usual duties. An endeavor is made to ascertain if the patient recognizes his adaptive limitations.

The patient is asked the reasons for the psychiatric consultation. If he is in a hospital, inquiry should be made as to the cause for his admission, whether he wished to come, his need of treatment, whether he considers himself to be suffering from a mental illness or has so suffered in the past. Frequently it is well to ask him if he has noticed any change in himself or in his outlook on life, or if there has been any change in his feelings, interest, memory, or thinking. One seeks to learn whether the patient desires to be helped and to ascertain what attempts he has made to adjust himself to the situation. Many patients state that they are or have been "nervous" or have suffered from a "nervous breakdown," and yet have no actual realization that they have suffered from a mental disorder. Not a few patients, on recovering, have what might be described as a verbal insight but are quite lacking in any psychological insight, i.e., an appreciation of the presumed motives associated with the illness and the genesis of their symptoms. They are unable to reflect retrospectively on their feelings and experiences or to understand how the past interferes with present functioning. They may readily admit that they have suffered from mental disorder, yet they have little realization as to what their symptoms have been, none as to the significance of their experiences, and no recognition of the factors which were operative in the production of their mental disorder.

Absence of an understanding insight is not surprising, since there is usually great resistance to the uncovering of dynamic tendencies that have been operating beyond the sphere of awareness. The patient is not emotionally prepared to face clearly and appreciate fully the existence of conflicts or the nature of the symptoms to which his symptoms constitute a defense. He is blind to their meaning since he needs his blindness. The patient must, too, avoid realizing that he has adopted delusional beliefs or otherwise disregarded reality in order to attain his ends. An inquiry of the patient as to whether he has had any imaginations will often reveal the extent of his realization of his entertainment of delusional ideas or whether he has had hallucinatory experiences. In hospitalized patients, significant information can often be secured by asking the patient why he has been detained so long in the institution.

The extent to which the patient recognizes any continuing disabilities may at times be learned by inquiring as to what he expects to do when he leaves treatment. It is often well to ask the patient what the various psychopathological phenomena discovered mean to him and why he did this or that, not that he can or will give the real explanation, but that his rationalizations may at times betray significant factors or psychological areas that require defenses. At its best, insight is usually a mixture of self-knowledge and of rationalization. The goal of psychotherapy, frequently not attained, is that the patient gain such insight into and understanding of the unconscious roots of his problems, their genetics, and dynamics, that changes in the dynamic structure of his personality will be promoted. Insight alone, however, does not cure; it must be applied.

Personality Maturity

As the psychiatrist continues his study of the patient's personality through successive interviews, he makes an evaluation of the latter's emotional and personality maturity. He will note whether the patient's interpersonal and other attitudes are appropriate to a stage of personality development consistent with his chronological age. The degree of maturity of personality may be suggested by the perspective in which he sees his life and work. The psychiatrist will observe the patient's pattern of securing satisfaction, also the roles which he unconsciously demands from others. As a confidential rapport is established, the psychiatrist will study the patient's psychosexual development since, through the intimate and pervasive role which it plays in life, it becomes an important and sensitive indication of personality development. The evaluation of the maturity of the patient is important in assessing his capacity for various types of therapeutic endeavor.

While the levels of emotional maturity have been described previously, they are noted again in the following schematic manner. Infantile attitude is evident when the patient expects from others infinite service and tolerance and responds with petulance when his desires are not immediately gratified. Childish emotional maturity is signified in those in whom the psychiatrist finds a limited degree of responsibility with the expectation that, when required, his parents or those upon whom he is dependent will assume his care or excuse his defects. Such individuals also demand a complete trust in another as the basis of any acceptable relationship. The early adolescent stage is epitomized in youths concerned with the problem of independence from parents by their tendency to admire and be devoted to extrafamilial figures. They may be much interested in social organizations and mystic rivalry. Here, then, are consciousness and awareness of sex. In the late adolescent stage, emotional drive at the adult level is for self-advancement through growth and learning.

Those with infantile and childish emotional fixations in their relationship to the physician have expectations that the physician must do all things for them by some magical means, or entirely through his own efforts. The patient does not commit himself to participation in the treatment. A more adult development allows the patient the capacity to work with the psychiatrist and to learn to use his own assets and make full use of his resources. It is important to recognize that the individual's emotional development may not have advanced equally in all respects or in all relationships. An individual may function at different levels of maturity in relation to members of one or the other sex, to those in authority, or to group activities.

Psychometry

Although intelligence* is but one of many functions of a total personality, it is often desirable to determine whether a patient is feeble-minded, and if defective, the degree of intelligence. Facilities should, therefore, be available for psychometric examinations. Since the conclusions reached by such examination are of little value unless it is performed by a trained, experienced individual, no details as to the application and interpreta-

* Kanner excellently epitomizes the prevailing concept of intelligence as "the capacity to think, solve problems and analyze situations in life." He re-emphasizes that intelligence, like emotion and conation, is not a separate area or compartment of mental functioning, but merely one aspect of an integrated function of the organism.

tion of psychometric tests will be given. A brief discussion of their nature will be found in Chapter 21.

From such tests, not only is the subject's native intellectual ability determined but also the level of his functioning in different areas. Frequently the psychotic patient is unable to make use in an effective manner of the intelligence he basically possesses. In such a patient, therefore, the physician should not usually expect to ascertain accurately by psychometric tests his normal level of intellectual development. However, it is desirable to know how much intelligence the patient can now use, also any peculiarities and inconsistencies of intelligence now existing. In spite of the fact that in many psychotic states the patient is unable to demonstrate the intelligence he possesses, considerable interesting and frequently valuable information may be secured by a psychometric examination.

It should not be forgotten that high scores in psychometric tests are not incompatible with serious mental disorder; in fact, patients suffering from paranoia frequently have a high intelligence quotient. On the other hand, some mental disorders are accompanied by an impairment of the original capacity for mental functioning, the deterioration being particularly manifested by difficulties in forming new associations, in making correct associations, in retaining recent memories, and in fixing attention. Certain functions may become impaired more rapidly than others, with the result that there may be a wide variation or "scattering" in the extent of the loss when one compares mental functioning in one area as against that in others. The use of the intelligence test extends far beyond that of simply stating the intelligence quotient of the individual. Modern tests are devised to examine a wide range of functions and mental deterioration as inferred from the variabilities exposed in the capacities of the patient to perform in the various subjects. A brief description of the most commonly employed tests of intelligence follows. The personality tests will be included as well. These examinations may be supplemented by a variety of other test devices for special functions that are available for application under appropriate circumstances by the clinical psychologist. In cases in which particular aspects of the personality deserve study, consultation with the clinical psychologist may provide advice as to methods of examination that are not described here.

The development of these tests all derive from the original work of the French psychologist, Alfred Binet (1857–1911), and Simon, a psychiatrist, in 1905. Since the series of modifications of the original psychometric test are described in Chapter 21, entitled "Mental Deficiency," as well as certain schedules for examining development, the only test described here is that most frequently employed in the examination of the adult and adolescent.

Wechsler Adult Intelligence Scale

In contrast to the earlier tests of intelligence which were largely verbal, the intelligence scale constructed by David Wechsler performs its measurements on suitable verbal and performance material in such a fashion that the age of the subject is taken into consideration. This scale is an individually administered scale which consists of eleven sub-tests applicable to ages 16 to 64 and over. The *verbal scale* consists of six sub-tests which examine general information, general comprehension, digit span, arithmetic, similarities, and vocabulary. The *performance scale* includes picture arrangement, picture completion, block design, object assembly, and digit symbol. In the verbal sub-tests, the responses to verbal stimuli are given orally by the patient. The performance scale includes certain sub-tests in which manipulation by the patient is important and others in which this element operates minimally. In scoring, items of each sub-test are scored separately and the sum of these items yields a raw or unweighted score for particular sub-tests. These scores are then weighted and converted into an IQ in accordance with the average of the individual's own age group. The test is an advance over earlier examinations, since it is standardized and the item selection is arranged by actual examination of individuals in the age ranges described. It provides simultaneously an examination of the verbal and performance testing which was lacking in previous tests of intelligence. The use of the numerous sub-tests provides an opportunity for differentiating an individual, for studying the "scatter" pattern of individuals with various types of personality disorder. From an examination of the scatter patterns, certain diagnostic impressions are obtained, although experience has shown that much overlapping exists between the various groups. A similar type of test has been developed by Wechsler for children.

Personality Tests or Assessments

Although a knowledge of the individual's intellectual endowment often gives the psychiatrist useful information concerning the patient, it tells practically nothing about his personality characteristics or the underlying dynamics of his behavior. Much thought has therefore been given to the development of probing techniques whereby one may investigate factors existing in the deeper levels of the personality and uncover unconscious needs and aspects which have been important in determining its structure and the individual's behavior. Such methods are known as *projective tests* since in them the subject interprets ambiguous stimulus situations according to his own unconscious dispositions, i.e., he reads into his perceptions and fantasied creations covert personality tendencies and processes. He projects out onto the external world the pattern of his own psychological life. The subject's performance patterns and responses, being projections of himself, reveal the personality structure and its underlying dynamics. The tests can also tell much concerning the patient's assets and liabilities. The projective tests have done much to close the gap between psychoanalysis and general psychology.

Rorschach Personality Assessment

This "test," devised in 1921 by Hermann Rorschach, a Swiss psychiatrist, furnishes much information concerning the patient's native intellectual endowment but is particularly valuable as a means of detecting fundamental personality characteristics. It indicates tendencies within the patient that may come to overt expression once the effectiveness of his defenses is diminished. In its application, the patient is shown ten cards on each of which is a complex standard "inkblot" picture with two symmetrical halves. Five of the ten cards are dark gray but with many different shadings; two are in dark gray and red; three are multicolored. The inkblots show a great variety of form, shading, and color, so chosen that they may have suggestive value for the responder. In the test procedure, the patient is asked to state what he sees in the relatively formless blot, what it looks like, what it makes him think of, or what it suggests to him.

By creating meaningful forms out of the apparently meaningless material, he unknowingly reveals fundamental traits and dominant trends in his personality. What the patient perceives becomes an expression of himself. In telling how the inkblots look to him, he tells the examiner about his own attitudes, feelings, conflicts, and significant aspects of his personality. In the apparently meaningless inkblot, the free-running fantasy of the patient discovers and reveals content that symbolizes significant and emotionally-charged elements and problems of the personality. Authority figures and attitudes toward them, identifications, suppressed cravings, the quantum of aggression, conception of life role, sexual identification, the psychosexual level, and specific anxiety-arousing factors and stresses are among the contents disclosed.

From this material, the psychologist may determine the underlying conflicts against which the patient's symptoms have been constructed as a means of defense. He not only acquires an idea of the subject's defense mechanisms and against what impulses they are operating, but also of the rigidity, flexibility, and potentiality of his personality as a whole. By this projective technique, the examiner obtains a psychological portrait of the personality and may discover pointers to underlying psychopathology. The patient's responses are scored and evaluated by means of an elaborate system in which perceptions of and associations to the blots have been correlated empirically and logically with certain personality traits. The test gives indications as to how the patient operates, i.e., anxiously, depressively, obsessionally, and so on.

The Rorschach test cannot explain how the personality happened to develop as it did, but it does reveal the underlying structure which makes the patient's behavior understandable. It should yield information concerning "basic personality configurations," intellectual aspects, and emotional aspects of the personality. The interpretation of the test is a task that requires skill and should therefore not be undertaken by an untrained person. It affords much insight into the personality structure, although its critics say it is difficult to tell where the test results leave off and the personality of the examiner begins.

The Rorschach test is sometimes used in psychotherapy. Its value there is its shortening of the therapist's task of elucidating the patient's personality components and reaction tendencies.

Thematic Apperception Test

Another projective test is the Murray Thematic Apperception Test which was devised by Professor Henry A. Murray of Harvard University on the theory that the need is father to the fantasy and on the well-recognized observation that pictures are significantly provocative in stimulating projective expression of the content aspects of the personality. An analysis of the content will reveal the areas around which the patient's major problems revolve. In this test, the patient is shown, one at a time, twenty pictures of persons in various, rather ambiguous, but dramatic situations. From his imagination, the patient makes up a story about each picture, telling how the depicted scene came about, the relation of the individuals in it, what has happened to them, how they feel about it, and what the outcome will be. The patient usually identifies himself with a character and projects an image of himself and of the significant people in his life. He imagines situations and motives that represent projections of his own predispositions, impulses, feelings, thoughts, frustrations, conflicts, and situations. The fantasies evoked reflect inner feelings and states, latent and repressed material, and covert layers of the personality. The test yields information about the patient's attitudes and opinions in respect to his parents, death, violence, sex, and the like. The stories he tells furnish clues as to his level of intelligence, the range and type of his interests, and his unconscious directional tensions. To some degree, at least, the patient's stories represent a projection and expression of his own present or past personality. Not all the elements and incidents are significant personal references, and so care must be experienced in selecting those that are relevant. The stories, like dreams, may be used as points of departure for free associations.

Bender-Gestalt Test

This is a drawing test consisting of nine geometric designs chosen by Lauretta Bender from patterns first devised by Wertheimer in his study on perception. The nine patterns are presented to the patient one at a time and he is asked to copy what he sees. A frequent modification in the administration of this test is, after a short interval, to ask the patient to recall as many patterns as he can. The organization of the drawings, the page placement, the distortions and elaborations in the form of the individual drawings, any relative differences in pattern size, and other miscellaneous factors are used by an experienced interpreter to make inferences about personality functioning. Because of its dependence on visual-motor functions, the test is often helpful in detecting organic pathology. Although it was conceived of by Bender as a "maturational" test, many workers have in recent years found it more useful as a general projective technique and assign certain symbolic meanings to individual patterns.

Draw-a-Person Test

One of the more recent but now widely used projective techniques for personality analysis is the Draw-a-Person Test. The theory upon which this test rests is the assumption that the body or the self, because of its intimate relation to the individual, serves as a natural vehicle for the expression of his needs, interests, and conflicts when projected by him into his drawing of a "person." In the application of the test, the patient is first merely asked to "draw a person." The examiner may then ask certain questions about the drawing in order to secure associations to the drawing. The patient's concept of body image with its peculiar significance to himself is therefore elicited. This self-projection, arising necessarily out of personal experience, manifests itself in the attention and emphasis in certain parts of the body or in the difficulty in handling them in the drawing. Correlations of clinical observations with analyses of material secured by this technique appear to substantiate it as a legitimate testing device. It is now used to supplement other projective techniques.

Sentence Completion Test

This test consists of giving the subject an incomplete sentence and of allowing him to complete it after his own fancy. It explores various life areas and attitudes of the patient about himself and toward others. Among the areas tapped are fears, worries, aspirations, and regrets.

Minnesota Multiphasic Personality Inventory

This test is a questionnaire of 550 items designed to provide scores on all the more important phases of personality and personality adaptation. As such, it ranges across the areas of investigation explored in the psychiatric interview. The patient is given a box containing the questions printed on separate cards. He is asked to separate these cards into one of three categories, "true," "false," or "cannot say." The questions are distributed into some 26 different categories. From this usage, nine clinical scales have been developed. These are: hypochondriasis, depression, hysteria, psychopathic deviate, masculinity–femininity, paranoiac, psychasthenic, schizophrenic, manic. This questionnaire has the special feature of additional validating scales which identify the test-taking attitude of the individual and provide an index of the degree to which the subject has been guarded and evasive, or overly frank and self-critical; a "lie scale," and finally, a set of items infrequently answered in the score directions by the standardization group and thus indicative of gross eccentricity, carelessness in respondent, or deliberate simulation.

Other studies, empirical in nature, have provided additional scales for social introversion, academic achievement, social satisfaction, and social tolerance. When used, a careful study of the item analysis in conjunction with the patterning scales may yield many unexpected insights concerning the individual.

Clinical Usage of Psychological Tests

While the various techniques of personality diagnosis are of considerable assistance in determining whether the basic personality pattern is one of dependence, submissiveness, self-depreciation, ingratiation, arrogance, grandiosity, resentment, aggression, or other type, it must be recognized that the tests alone are not diagnostic procedures and that they do not form the basis for a formulation of the personality structure and its psychogenesis. The information secured through psychiatric examination, in addition to that yielded by the projective tests, should, among other disclosures, enable the psychiatrist to acquire a diagnostic understanding of the patient's attitudes and relationships to others. As the data from the psychiatric history, the psychiatric examination, and the projective tests are assembled and surveyed, one may discover that a meaningful pattern of the personality of the patient has been reconstructed and that its parts and features fall into place like pieces in a jigsaw puzzle. It is well to recognize that the information derived from initial interviews is seldom adequate to answer all the questions in regard to personality organization. Areas in which information is lacking and a satisfactory account may not be found for certain aspects of the personality should be noted. Here the psychological test may give information not initially available through the psychiatric history or psychiatric interview. Alone, the psychological test is not an adequate diagnostic tool.

Examination of the Inaccessible Patient

The student often feels at a loss how to secure significant clinical data when confronted with a patient who is unable or unwilling to speak or otherwise cooperate in the mental examination. The beginner may not realize that the various stuporous states are characterized by more or less well-defined features possessing much of differential value clinically, or that the patient who fails to utter any word, as well as the one who declines to discuss certain subjects, unwittingly reveals much of psychological significance. The inaccessible states existing when the patient is first seen by the psychiatrist are usually rather acute manifestations and yield data of great value both in themselves and when considered in connection with subsequent symptoms observed at a later stage in the evolution of the mental disorder.

Since the clinical reactions of the inaccessible patient are in certain respects less well defined than in the co-operative patient, their detection and interpretation require a systematic method of study. The following plan of examination may serve as a guide to a study of personality expressions in the inaccessible patient.

GENERAL REACTION, MOVEMENT, AND POSTURE. After having described the patient's reactions in accordance with the plan noted in the paragraph entitled General Appearance, Manner, and Attitude, the following may be noted: Nature and degree of response to greeting: Will the patient shake hands with examiner? Is there any spontaneous speech? Are questions at times followed by replies? Is there apparent effort to reply by vocalization or by whispers, lip movements, or movements of the head? Are replies confined to impersonal questions? Are there special topics that the patient refuses to discuss? If he will not speak, will the patient write when offered pencil and paper?

Does the patient appear suspicious, on his guard, preoccupied, inattentive, evasive? Is patient ever observed talking to himself? If so, what is the accompanying emotional state?

Are bodily positions assumed voluntarily or passive? Are they natural, affected, comfortable, or constrained? Describe any sustained, unnatural postures. Does the patient resist change of posture? Are muscles found to be relaxed or tense as extremities are passively moved? Are responses to suggested or passively attempted movements characterized by negativistic resistance or by movements in the opposite direction? What does the patient do when placed in an uncomfortable position? Any spontaneous activity and its amount and rate should be noted.

Does the patient obey commands? Are reactions influenced by distraction or command? Are movements of defense evoked by painful stimuli?

What are the patient's habits as to eating and dressing? If food has been refused, is it subsequently eaten if left near the patient? Is spoon-feeding or tube-feeding necessary? Attention should be given to excretory needs.

Are the various characteristics of attitude, speech, and behavior constant, or do they vary from time to time? If variable, by what do they seem to be influenced?

FACIAL EXPRESSION AND EMOTIONAL RESPONSIVENESS. Should the patient's facial expression be described as alert, apathetic, vacant, placid, stolid, scowling, sullen, surly, morose, discontented, angry, or apprehensive? Does his face express aversion, hatred, bewilderment, perplexity, or distress? Is there any play of facial expression? Are there tears, smiles, or other signs of emotion? On what occasions do they appear? Does the patient appear worried, anxious, fearful? Is grimacing noted? Describe any mannerisms observed.

Is the gaze fixed? Are furtive glances observed?

Is feeling manifested when the patient's family is mentioned? Is it shown when certain topics or certain experiences are mentioned? If so, what are they?

What reaction is shown to visits of the family? Describe any striking reaction to visits from particular members of the family or to those from certain other individuals.

Examination under Narcosis

If, because of mutism, amnesia, or difficulty in establishing rapport one is not successful in securing significant mental material from the patient, an increase in accessibility can often be effected by narcosis technique. Various forms of barbiturates may be used for the induction of narcosis, but one of the slowly-acting forms, such as sodium amytal, is most frequently employed in this type of uncovering technique. A freshly prepared 10 per cent solution of sodium amytal is injected intravenously at the rate of approximately 1 ml. per minute. The injection is continued until the patient becomes drowsy, but care must be exercised that he does not become stuporous. Usually after the patient has received 3 to 6 grains he will begin to respond to questions. In this lowered state of consciousness, midway between being awake and being asleep, inhibitory processes are released, rapport is produced, and suppressed and conflict material is brought into consciousness. With his psychological resistance thus temporarily reduced, drugs may also be used on the patient who is accessible in order to bring repressed material to consciousness and to find underlying conflicts. The occasion can also be used for psychotherapeutic purposes. Since overdoses of sodium amytal produce a fall of blood pressure and respiratory depression, it is wise to have ephedrine sulfate and picrotoxin available.

While accessibility is not increased in patients with organic brain damage and toxic states, the narcosis technique, as shown by Weinstein, may be utilized diagnostically if the patient's attitude toward and recognition of illness and hospitalization is examined. Patients with brain damage explicitly deny their illness, become disoriented for place, and misidentify the examiners. Those without brain damage fail to respond in this manner.

Diagnostic Formulation

A biographical picture of the person as obtained through a psychiatric history, together with a formal mental examination made as indicated, will serve as a guide in the search for signs and symptoms of personality disturbance and usually enable the examiner to determine the character of the patient's reaction patterns. For medicolegal purposes, this is often all that is necessary, but the physician, in order that he may intelligently attempt to redirect the personality functions, desires to know what the life problems are which have led to a disorganizing and asocialized method of meeting them. Diagnosis, therefore, should be based on a case analysis, a dynamic formulation in which is reconstructed the complex, impelling interplay of psychological forces which have served to disturb personality.

Although in most cases these psychological forces seem to be sufficient to account for the disturbed personality functionings, yet it must be remembered that disturbed brain functions may also alter personality performance. The psychiatrist therefore carefully considers and evaluates all the constitutional, neurological, physiological, social, psychogenic, and other factors which the life history of the patient and the physical, laboratory, and mental examinations may reveal. The object should be to obtain, not a static cross section of the psychosis or neurosis, but a dynamic, longitudinal section of the functioning of the personality. The aim should be both at analysis of the present situation and a reconstruction of the personality development from childhood on.

It will be seen, therefore, that the examination as a whole should not be centered so much on the search for symptoms as for the factors and forces that have been operative in the psychological chain of events of which the neurosis or psychosis is one incident. It will usually be found that the psychic needs of the patient have long been finding expression in his dominant life pattern which he has worked out for himself in his effort to prevent anxiety and meet the stress of life.

Finally, in constructing a diagnostic formulation, an effort is made to coordinate and correlate the various symptoms and behavior manifestations and to articulate them one with the other, with the result that a comprehensive, consistent, meaningful, natural-history picture of the personality is obtained, a dynamic formulation that avoids speculative assumption and makes sensible the patient's life history. It should become apparent that the patient's pattern of behavior represents a biological approach to his total life situation. As a corollary, it follows that the human being is so complex that every human reaction is always a consequence of a combination of factors.

As the previous discussion in this chapter is considered, it will perhaps be readily observed that a comprehensive psychiatric diagnosis is analogous to the diagnosis which the internist aims to construct in order that his treatment may be rationally directed. As a result of his various studies of the patient's organs and their functions, the internist makes an etiological, anatomical, and physiological diagnosis. Through the techniques of his specialty, the psychiatrist makes a comprehensive study of his patient's personality and formulates a genetic, a dynamic, and a clinical diagnosis. In his efforts to reach a *genetic diagnosis*, he searches both for any constitutional factors which may have precluded the construction of a strong and wholesomely functioning personality and for emotionally significant and anxiety-producing experiences which made successful personality functioning difficult or impossible without resorting either to reparative or to morbid measures to facilitate its functioning. These inherent limitations to personality development, its arrests in the maturational process, and the emotionally disturbing impulses and events which have been experienced, particularly in early life, establish the primary source or determinant of the mental illness or, in other words, constitute a genetic diagnosis.

Through a study of the mechanisms and techniques which the individual has unconsciously employed to manage anxiety and enhance self-esteem, the discovery is made as to how psychological forces have operated to produce personality characteristics and how those pathological functionings of personality called symptoms have been formed; i.e., a *dynamic diagnosis* that traces the psychopathological processes and their effects is formulated.

Finally, the general pattern of reaction which has resulted from the operation of genetic and dynamic factors is noted and classified in accordance with accepted clinical nomenclature. The *clinical diagnosis* conveys to the psychiatrist useful connotations concerning the reaction syndrome, the probable course and prognosis of the disorder, and often the methods of treatment that will probably prove most beneficial.

The formulation of the case may be schematized in the following way:

1. Summary of patient's problems

a. Behavioral disturbances including character traits and interpersonal attitudes.
b. Psychological disturbances including conceptual, perceptual activities, thought, awareness, attention, et cetera.
c. Affective disturbances.
d. Physiological (somatic) disturbances.

2. Salient features of genetic, constitutional, familial, and environmental influences as revealed by the history and the various medical, neurological, and psychological examinations.

3. Psychodynamic explanation. Here an attempt should be made to reconstruct the origin of the various problems of the patient in terms of the interplay of the genetic and constitutional background of the individual and the impact upon the growing organism and the influences of the family life and other environmental contacts upon his emotional and psychological development. It will not be possible to provide a complete explanation of the intricate processes of the individual's life. However, where gaps are noted or explanations may not be made, a statement to this effect should be included for further reference.

4. Diagnostic classification. Utilize here the classification of psychiatric disorders as provided by the American Psychiatric Association.

5. Therapeutic formulation. Provide a concise statement as to the form of treatment considered most effective, its availability and its source, the need for indicated adjunctive therapies such as vocational, occupational, or recreational therapies, and the role to be played by the social worker in treatment. The desirability of inpatient or outpatient treatment, the need for certification, and the appointment of a guardian if the individual is considered incompetent to manage his personal or financial affairs should be stated.

6. Transference relationship. The expected repetitive attitudes of the patient toward the physician should be indicated if this can be ascertained from the developmental history of the patient. If psychotherapy is recommended, an additional statement should be provided in regard to the expected countertransference responses of the treating psychiatrist toward the patient.

7. Prognostic evaluation. A statement should be made in regard to the expected modification of the patient's problems as a result of the therapy suggested above.

CLASSIFICATION OF MENTAL DISORDERS

Before concluding this chapter, a word may be said concerning classification of mental disorders. Following the practice of other branches of medicine in which pathological entities are ordinarily demonstrable, psychiatry, usually basing its attempt either on similarity of descriptive facts or on prognosis, formerly endeavored to classify personality disturbances as if these, too, were distinct entities. Unfortunately, in such an attempt one may easily err in mistaking reaction-sets for disease entities.

From a descriptive standpoint, the problem is simplified if mental disorders are divided into groups based on clinical and behavioral differences. It is more important, however, to think of a diagnostic understanding in terms of the patient's intrapsychic processes and how they reflect themselves in the patient's behavior and interpersonal relationships. It is well to avoid thinking in categories or disease entities and seek only to present a factual digest of the origins and types of reaction. Although classifications are necessary for statistical and other purposes, there has perhaps at times been too great a disposition in psychiatry to consider that its objective was attained when a classificatory diagnosis had been made. The principal value of classification is not in the categorizing of a disease entity but in the quick elimination of those considerations which will be least useful in understanding the patient and in directing attention to those which are likely to be relevant.

Except in organic disorders, a classificatory diagnosis is less important than a psychodynamic study of the personality. The psychiatrist should be interested in process, not in labels. He should remember that a particular pattern of behavior may stem from widely varying psychological causes, also that a diagnosis on a purely descriptive level without regard to the patient's thought content and inner life is really no diagnosis at all. Even in such disorders as general paresis, in which undoubted organic pathology exists, a study of the earlier functioning of the personality will clear up many points that cannot be explained by neurohistology. It will frequently be found, for example, that organic brain disease has permitted the release of impulses that were formerly inhibited and repressed. It is not even advisable to think of "neuroses" and "psychoses" in rigid terms, since there is no strict separation between them. So far as possible, the diagnosis should be in terms of the patient's problems, their sources and the methods by which he has attempted to deal with them, and the anxiety they have aroused.

These remarks on classification have been introduced to emphasize the facts that many mental disorders, instead of being disease entities, are really methods adopted by the personality in its attempt to meet its problems and that it is not as important to fit the symptoms into a classificatory scheme as to understand the sick person in terms of his life experience, his motivations and goals, and the obstacles he has met in his attempts to secure satisfaction for his basic needs. "In Nature there are no diseases, there are only sick persons."

Although, as just indicated, the psychiatrist should, through his study of the patient, formulate the many data he has secured into a meaningful psychobiological biography of the patient, yet, for purposes of statistical study and for summarized identification of similarities discovered in the study of large numbers of patients, it is necessary to have classifications of the more important clinical features which persons with personality disorders manifest. If disturbed bodily processes have a common relation to certain types of disordered functionings of the personality, these common factors, too, should be included in the clinical classification. In order, therefore, that there may be an established language reference, it is necessary to have a generally accepted nomenclature and a standardized basis for the preparation of statistical data.

Prior to 1917 there had been little effort to formulate an organized system according to which these data should be recorded. In that year the Committee on Statistics of the American Psychiatric Association (then the American Medico-Psychological Association) formulated, and the Association officially adopted, a classification which could be used both as a basis for preparing standard statistical data and for providing uniformity in nomenclature. The National Committee for Mental Hygiene and the American Psychiatric Association then collaborated in securing the adoption of this classification and statistical system by publishing an informative pamphlet entitled, "Statistical Manual for the Use of Hospitals for Mental Disease."

Gradually, in spite of occasional changes, it became recognized that there were certain deficiencies in this system. Beginning in 1948, the Committee on Nomenclature and Statistics of the American Psychiatric Association began extensive studies in an effort to prepare a nomenclature system that indicated more clearly recognized pathogenetic and clinical facts. In 1952 the results of these studies were included in the "Fourth Edition of the Standard Nomenclature of Diseases and Operations" in a section entitled Diseases of the Psychobiological Unit. This classificatory system as prepared by its Committee was adopted by the American Psychiatric Association as its official system of classification and published by it under the title, "Diagnostic and Statistical Manual of Mental Disorders." The previous classification was doubtless not sufficiently comprehensive and flexible, was limited too closely to mental disorders observed in hospitalized patients, and did not make sufficient provision for the various personality disorders or for transient reactions to special stress. In general outline, the new classification will be followed in this book in its discussion of the various manifestations of mental and personality disorders. It will be noted that in several instances the presentation of material is not in such detail of classification as is set forth in the official nomenclature. It is believed, however, that this abridgement will not prevent the student from acquiring a perspective of mental, behavior, and personality disorders sufficiently comprehensive to prepare him for their more detailed study, if desired.

It will be observed that the general categories recognized by the official classification are quite simple and correspond to recognized principles of organic or mental pathology. Approached from this frame of reference, psychiatric disorders fall into the three groups designated by the Manual. (1) In the first group are disorders caused by or associated with impairment of brain tissue function. The clinical picture resulting from this deterioration of function will vary according to whether the impairment is acute or chronic. (2) The second large group of disorders is that without clearly defined physical cause or structural change in the brain, but of psychogenic origin. This group is, of course, a large one since it includes the psychoneuroses, a major part of the psychotic reactions, the psychosomatic disorders, and the personality disorders. (3) This group comprises the mental deficiencies. Strictly speaking, it includes only those in which the mental defect is of familial origin, has existed since birth, and is without demonstrated brain disease or known prenatal cause. The mental deficiencies which are secondary to or the result of chronic brain disease produced by birth trauma, Mongolian, or other irreversible impairment of brain function leading to a developmental defect of mentation are for statistical purposes classified among chronic brain disorders.

The following is the classification of psychiatric disorders officially adopted by the American Psychiatric Association.

I. Disorders Caused by or Associated with Impairment of Brain Tissue Function

1. ACUTE BRAIN DISORDERS

Disorders Due to or Associated with Infection

Acute brain syndrome associated with intracranial infection

Acute brain syndrome associated with systemic infection

Disorders Due to or Associated with Intoxication

Acute brain syndrome, drug or poison intoxication

Acute brain syndrome, alcohol intoxication

Acute hallucinosis

Delirium tremens

Disorders Due to or Associated with Trauma

Acute brain syndrome associated with trauma

Disorders Due to or Associated with Circulatory Disturbance

Acute brain syndrome associated with circulatory disturbance

Disorders Due to or Associated with Disturbance of Innervation or of Psychic Control

Acute brain syndrome associated with convulsive disorder

Disorders Due to or Associated with Disturbance of Metabolism, Growth, or Nutrition

Acute brain syndrome with metabolic disturbance

Disorders Due to or Associated with New Growth

Acute brain syndrome associated with intracranial neoplasm

Disorders Due to Unknown or Uncertain Cause

Acute brain syndrome with disease of unknown or uncertain cause

Disorders Due to Unknown or Uncertain Cause with the Functional Reaction Alone Manifest

Acute brain syndrome of unknown cause

2. CHRONIC BRAIN DISORDERS

Disorders Due to Prenatal (Constitutional) Influence

Chronic brain syndrome associated with congenital cranial anomaly

Chronic brain syndrome associated with congenital spastic paraplegia

Chronic brain syndrome associated with Mongolism

Chronic brain syndrome due to prenatal maternal infectious diseases

Disorders Due to or Associated with Infection

Chronic brain syndrome associated with central nervous system syphilis

Meningoencephalitic
Meningovascular
Other central nervous system syphilis

Chronic brain syndrome associated with intracranial infection other than syphilis

Disorders Associated with Intoxication

Chronic brain syndrome associated with intoxication

Chronic brain syndrome, drug or poison intoxication

Chronic brain syndrome, alcohol intoxication

Disorders Associated with Trauma

Chronic brain syndrome associated with birth trauma

Chronic brain syndrome associated with brain trauma

Chronic brain syndrome, brain trauma, gross force

Chronic brain syndrome following brain operation

Chronic brain syndrome following electrical brain trauma

Chronic brain syndrome following irradiational brain trauma

Disorders Associated with Circulatory Disturbances

Chronic brain syndrome associated with cerebral arteriosclerosis

Chronic brain syndrome associated with circulatory disturbance other than cerebral arteriosclerosis

Disorders Associated with Disturbances of Innervation or of Psychic Control

Chronic brain syndrome associated with convulsive disorder

Disorders Associated with Disturbance of Metabolism, Growth, or Nutrition

Chronic brain syndrome associated with senile brain disease

Chronic brain syndrome associated with other disturbance of metabolism, growth, or nutrition (includes presenile, glandular, pellagra, familial amaurosis)

Disorders Associated with New Growth

Chronic brain syndrome associated with intracranial neoplasm

Disorders Associated with Unknown or Uncertain Cause

Chronic brain syndrome associated with diseases of unknown or uncertain cause (includes multiple sclerosis, Huntington's chorea, Pick's disease, and other diseases of a familial or hereditary nature)

II. Mental Deficiency

Disorders Due to Unknown or Uncertain Cause with the Functional Reaction Alone Manifest

Chronic brain syndrome of unknown cause

Disorders Due to Unknown or Uncertain Cause with the Functional Reaction Alone Manifest; Hereditary and Familial Diseases of This Nature

Mental deficiency (familial or hereditary)
Mild
Moderate
Severe

Disorders Due to Undetermined Cause

Mental deficiency, idiopathic
Mild
Moderate
Severe

III. Disorders of Psychogenic Origin or Without Clearly Defined Clinical Cause or Structural Change in the Brain

1. PSYCHOTIC DISORDERS

Disorders Due to Disturbances of Metabolism, Growth, Nutrition, or Endocrine Function

Involutional psychotic reaction

Disorders of Psychogenic Origin or Without Clearly Defined Tangible Cause or Structural Change

Affective reactions
Manic depressive reaction, manic type
Manic depressive reaction, depressive type
Manic depressive reaction, other
Psychotic depressive reaction
Schizophrenic reactions
Schizophrenic reaction, simple type
Schizophrenic reaction, hebephrenic type
Schizophrenic reaction, catatonic type
Schizophrenic reaction, paranoid type
Schizophrenic reaction, acute undifferentiated type
Schizophrenic reaction, chronic undifferentiated type
Schizophrenic reaction, schizo-affective type

Schizophrenic reaction, childhood type
Schizophrenic reaction, residual type
Paranoid reactions
Paranoia
Paranoid state
Psychotic reaction without clearly defined structural change, other than above

2. PSYCHOPHYSIOLOGIC AUTONOMIC AND VISCERAL DISORDERS

Disorders Due to Disturbance of Innervation or of Psychic Control

Psychophysiologic skin reaction
Psychophysiologic musculoskeletal reaction
Psychophysiologic respiratory reaction
Psychophysiologic cardiovascular reaction
Psychophysiologic hemic and lymphatic reaction
Psychophysiologic gastrointestinal reaction
Psychophysiologic genitourinary reaction
Psychophysiologic endocrine reaction
Psychophysiologic nervous system reaction
Psychophysiologic reaction of organs of special sense

3. PSYCHONEUROTIC DISORDERS

Disorders of Psychogenic Origin or Without Clearly Defined Tangible Cause or Structural Change

Psychoneurotic reactions
Anxiety Reaction
Dissociative reaction
Conversion reaction
Phobic reaction
Obsessive compulsive reaction
Depressive reaction
Psychoneurotic reaction, other

4. PERSONALITY DISORDERS

Disorders of Psychogenic Origin or Without Clearly Defined Tangible Cause or Structural Change

Personality pattern disturbance
Inadequate personality

Schizoid personality
Cyclothymic personality
Paranoid personality
Personality trait disturbance
Emotionally unstable personality
Passive–aggressive personality
Compulsive personality
Personality trait disturbance, other
Sociopathic personality disturbance
Antisocial reaction
Dyssocial reaction
Sexual deviation
Addiction
Alcoholism
Drug addiction
Special symptom reactions
Learning disturbance
Speech disturbance
Enuresis
Somnambulism
Other

5. TRANSIENT SITUATIONAL PERSONALITY DISORDERS

Transient Situational Personality Disturbance

Gross stress reaction
Adult situational reaction
Adjustment reaction of infancy
Adjustment reaction of childhood
Habit disturbance
Conduct disturbance
Neurotic traits
Adjustment reaction of adolescence
Adjustment reaction of late life

BIBLIOGRAPHY

American Psychiatric Association: Diagnostic and Statistical Manual of Mental Disorders. Washington, American Psychiatric Association, 1952.

Brown, Fred: Contribution of the psychologist to problems of psychiatric diagnosis and therapy. Psychiatric Quart. Supplement, 26:8–21, 1952.

Carr, A. C. (Ed.): Prediction of Overt Behavior Through the Use of Projective Techniques. American Lecture Series. Springfield, Illinois, Charles C Thomas, 1960.

Deutsch, F., and Murphy, W. F.: The Clinical Interview. 2 vols. New York, International Universities Press, 1955.

Diethelm, Oskar: The evaluation of a psychiatric examination. Am. J. Psychiat., 105:606–611, 1949.

Gill, M., Newman, R., and Redlich, F. C.: The Initial Interview in Psychiatric Practice. New York, International Universities Press, 1954, Chap. 7.

Hathaway, S. R., and McKinley, J. C.: A multiphasic personality schedule (Minnesota): construction of the schedule. J. Psychol., 10:249–254, 1940.

Hoch, P. H., and Zubin, J.: Relation of Psychological Tests to Psychiatry. New York, Grune & Stratton, 1951.

Holsopple, J. Q., and Miale, F. R.: Sentence Completion: A Projective Method for the Study of Personality. Springfield, Illinois, Charles C Thomas, 1954.

Menninger, K. A.: A Manual for Psychiatric Case Study. New York, Grune & Stratton, 1951.

Idem: A Guide to Psychiatric Books, 2nd ed. New York, Grune & Stratton, 1956.

Meyer, Adolf: The aims and meaning of psychiatric diagnosis. Am. J. Insan., 74:163–168, 1917.
Also in The Collected Papers of Adolf Meyer, Vol. III, E. E. Winters, Ed. Baltimore, The Johns Hopkins Press, 1951.)

Murray, H. A.: Explorations in Personality. New York, Oxford University Press, 1938.

Idem: Uses of the thematic apperception test. Am. J. Psychiat., 107:577–581, 1951.

Saul, L. J.: The psychoanalytic diagnostic interview. Psychoanalyt. Quart., 26:76–90, 1957.

Stevenson, I.: Medical History Taking. New York, Paul B. Hoeber, Inc., 1961.

Sullivan, H. S.: The psychiatric interview. Psychiatry, 14:361–373, 1951, and 15:127–141, 1952.

Weider, A., and Wechsler, D.: Contributions toward Medical Psychology. Vol. II. New York, Ronald Press Co., 1953.

Weinstein, F. A., and Malitz, S.: Changes in symbolic expression with amytal sodium. Am. J. Psychiat., 111:198–206, 1954.

Zubin, J.: Objective evaluation of personality tests. Am. J. Psychiat., 107:569–576, 1951.

DISORDERS CAUSED BY OR ASSOCIATED WITH IMPAIRMENT OF BRAIN TISSUE FUNCTION

In this and the succeeding chapter, the symptom complex now designated as the acute brain syndrome but formerly known as a toxic–delirious reaction is discussed in relation to the more frequently encountered processes which may induce the disorder. This symptom complex is induced by a general derangement of cerebral metabolism which produces a diffuse dysfunction of brain tissue and thereby impairs those functions most expressive in man of brain action—the positive functions of awareness, retention, memory, and comprehension.

DEFINITIONS

The term *general cerebral insufficiency*, discussed as an etiologic factor in Chapter 5, probably best designates these brain syndromes since this term draws attention to the basic etiology of all such states and relates them to the more familiar concepts of medicine such as renal insufficiency, hepatic insufficiency, and cardiac insufficiency. Thus with failure of the metabolic processes there occurs a general lowering of the function of the organ or the loss through death of the cellular units, or both, so that there ensues impairment of the activity of that organ. It may be recognized, then, that dysfunction of the brain caused by disturbance of the metabolic processes may evolve into permanent impairment of its function if the cerebral metabolism is disrupted to such an extent as to render a sufficient number of cells dead. In other words, the condition may be reversible when the metabolic defect is insufficient to lead to cellular necrosis, or it may become permanent if the metabolic defect is sufficiently severe or prolonged.

The designations of *acute brain syndrome* or *delirium* is associated customarily with the reversible picture of cerebral insufficiency, while the designations of *chronic brain syndrome* or *dementia* are associated with persisting damage to brain tissue. As one may surmise, it is possible to have clinically the symptomatic expressions consequent to both permanent loss of function due to cellular death as well as those due to reversible changes due to ongoing partial impairment of the cellular metabolic activity. When symptoms occur which are consequent to both ongoing metabolic disturbance and the effects of permanent damage to brain cells, it is customary to speak of the *organic syndrome.*

The terms *acute* and *chronic* are hardly useful, since it is possible to produce a widespread irreversible necrosis of cerebral cells such as may 'take place after a blow on the head which will give the picture of delirium but end with a persistent defect later to be termed a dementia. On the other hand, some types of cerebral insufficiency such as those associated with prolonged illnesses, e.g., pernicious anemia, may develop slowly and last for weeks or months and yet be largely reversible when the proper treatment is provided.

Pathophysiology

While it is probably correct to state that the brain derives most of its energy from those cerebral oxidative processes which require glucose as the major substrate, there is reason to believe that this statement is not completely accurate. There is some evidence to suggest that some brain function can take place at times in spite of inadequate glucose supply. For the operation and maintenance of proper cerebral oxidative processes there must be available also adequate quantities of oxygen and the necessary enzyme systems. Recent studies have demonstrated an active amino acid and protein metabolism in the brain in which the glutamic acid cycle may act as a maintenance mechanism controlling carbohydrate metabolism. There is good evidence to show that ammonia, which is known now to be produced in the brain, has a toxic effect on the function of the nervous system in certain quantities. Ammonia, apparently, is removable through the glutamic acid–glutamine system. Therefore, the syndrome of cerebral insufficiency may be expected to occur in circumstances wherein there is a lack of oxygen or glucose, an interruption by toxic means, or a deficiency in the enzyme systems related to carbohydrate metabolism and those of certain of the

amino acids, or in the presence of excessive amounts of ammonia due either to excessive absorption or production or to ineffective removal from the brain itself.

In association with the progressive impairment of cerebral functions, there occurs a slowing of the electroencephalogram. It appears that the degree of slowing is more significant in giving evidence of cerebral insufficiency than is the absolute frequency of the wave forms. Therefore, it is possible to have what appears to be an electroencephalogram with a frequency generally considered to be within normal range in an individual whose premorbid frequency was 11–12 per second. A slowing to 8–9 per second will occur in a person with such a premorbid rate during a moderate delirium, yet both values would be stated to occur within the accepted normal range for the adult population. As an aid in following the course of a case of cerebral insufficiency, the electroencephalogram may be most useful through examination of successive recordings taken over time. On the other hand, the single electroencephalogram has considerable limitations as a diagnostic method to be used to establish the existence of cerebral insufficiency. Since the frequency count for the individual is seldom known beforehand, the existence of slowing of frequency may not be surmised.

A much wider understanding is needed of the complex biochemical activities underlying the normal metabolic activity of the cerebral cortex and its disruption by toxic substances of chemical or microbial origin or the biochemical effects of traumatic injury upon the various substrates and their related enzyme systems and interactions in carrying out the specific functions of particular components of cells. As we come to know more of the necessary substrates for the brain's metabolic activity, the associated enzyme systems and metabolites, it is possible that the effects of the various toxic substances upon the metabolic cycles and activities within different parts of the cortex will become understandable and this knowledge may lead to more rational therapy for the delirious reaction.

Symptomatology

Under the heading of Delirium and Dementia, the symptoms of cerebral insufficiency have been described in Chapter 5. The characteristic symptoms of the delirium usually associated with the acute brain syndromes are those of fearfulness, clouding of consciousness with bewilderment, restlessness, confusion, disorientation, impairment in thinking with sometimes delusions and hallucinations. Thus the acute brain syndrome differs from the so-called functional psychosis in the marked impairment of cognitive functions. It must be emphasized that the recognition of the cerebral insufficiency should not wait until the full blossoming of the previously mentioned symptoms. Long before gross cognitive disorganization takes place the acute observer will note failures in cognition. In the earliest stages, in which the condition might be likened to that of mild intoxication experienced by many persons when drinking, there is a blurring or haziness of perception so that the sufferer notices a limitation in the accuracy of identification and apperception of sensations. He has difficulty in focusing attention on important percepts and in screening out interfering percepts. Again, one with incipient delirium will note a difficulty in thinking clearly and coherently; he may complain of inability to bring forward desired memories and associations. In the milder stages of the delirious process, such difficulties can sometimes be overcome by heightened attention and effort on the part of the affected person. Unless complained about, they may be quite inapparent to the clinical observer, who may note only some vagueness, uncertainty, and hesitancy on the part of the patient.

At a further level of impairment of consciousness, the affected person has difficulty performing correctly in spite of personal effort, and there now is evidence of confusion and bewilderment. In addition to hesitation in responses to questions, it is possible to expose defects in memory, retention, and recall. The heightened effort is sometimes revealed by expression of concentration by the knitted brow and a tendency to glance up and around when asked simple questions. At this level of impairment, the patient usually has some difficulty in dealing with abstract concepts; the earliest expression may be in disturbance of time orientation, initially expressed in giving days of the week and later expanding to confusion concerning the month and the year. Furthermore, an examiner will note problems in retention of instructions, grasping their meaning, and carrying out directions. The patient may complain of inability to read as he cannot retain what has been put before him. At a still later stage of cerebral insufficiency, orientation as to place fails, and misidentification of perceptions with a development of illusions is noticeable. At this time, language difficulties appear, and there develops a defect in a coherent train of expression. Eventually there takes place a deterioration in motor activity with problems in personal writing, eating, and grooming, and finally, incontinence of urine and feces may take place. In the later stage of delirium, complete disorientation exists, with delusory and hallucinatory experiences and severe impairment of motor control. Grasping and groping movements may occur. Delirium of this degree represents a critical impairment of cerebral function and should be recognized as diagnostically serious for life if it proceeds without arrest. The final stages of progressive cerebral insufficiency are those of stupor and coma.

It may be seen that impairment of cerebral functioning leads to progressive loss of the more differentiated and elaborated cognitive functions and a re-appearance of more primitive activity. To put it in other terms, there exists a progressive impairment of ego functions of the individual, with interference in the ability to integrate new and current stimuli with the impressed patterns of older experience and bring them to proper thought and action.

The clinical expressions of cerebral insufficiency vary, depending on the nature of the past experience and the variety of ego defenses available to the ill individual as well as the type of support he receives from his environment. Some delirious patients experience much anxiety due to their frightening thoughts and fantasies; these individuals will present, in addition to the evidences of ego disruption and cognitive impairment, the physiological expressions of anxiety. Others, due to their personality make-up, are able to minimize their concern over the progressive impairment of their faculties through such methods as withdrawal, denial, sleep, or a confiding relationship with their attendant. Some utilize the staff of the hospital for support and present denial with an unusual façade of co-operativeness, humor, and pleasantry, while those few individuals with limited ego development react to cerebral insufficiency with gross anxiety, panic, and periods of hallucinatory and delusional presentation. The individual prone to depressive responses in response to frustrations in the past again may respond to impairment of his mental faculties by an affective withdrawal of the same kind. Others respond with shame when they are unable to maintain their ordinary standards of performance. Yet others may act out aggressive and sexual impulses and respond to these with guilt. Such individuals may have suicidal drives.

One of the important characteristics of the delirious state is the variability in the symptoms over short periods of time. Even in one day the evidences of impaired cerebral functioning are often much greater at one time than another. Frequently the most serious disturbances are seen at night when the patient has available to him fewer sensory cues to aid his orientation in the absence of other persons and when there is lack of light. Thus his disability is aggravated by isolation and deprivation of sensory stimuli as well as by the associated mounting anxiety.

Differential Diagnosis

It is most important to distinguish the acute organic brain syndromes with the delirious state from other psychiatric disturbances. In view both of its threat to life and future cerebral functioning, it is imperative to arrive at early recognition and immediate treatment. Schizophrenic reactions are confused frequently, but usually they may be distinguished by the patient's clear orientation and ability to retain and recall past events, thus demonstrating an effective memory. In acute schizophrenic excitement, in which the patient has been heavily sedated, the diagnosis may be difficult. However, a brief period of observation usually leads to clarification. Depressive psychoses with retardation in thought again do not lead to disturbances of orientation or mentation. In patients with hysterical amnesia, the memory defects are usually either too gross or spotty, with great clarity in certain areas. Amnesia for personal identity is not found in delirium. In all the functional psychoses and neuroses, the electroencephalogram will not show the slowing of frequency as in the acute brain syndromes.

ACUTE BRAIN DISORDERS DUE TO OR ASSOCIATED WITH INFECTION

Acute Brain Syndrome Associated with Intracranial Infection

In their early stages, many intracranial infections are accompanied by mental symptoms typical of an acute organic syndrome. Sometimes the damage to brain tissue is temporary and reversible. However, the impairment of brain function may become permanent, with a resulting chronic organic syndrome.

Meningococcal (Epidemic) Meningitis

Probably the most important form of meningitis encountered by the psychiatrist is epidemic cerebrospinal meningitis. Actually the meningitis is but part of a septicemia caused by infection by meningococci. Delirium with confusion, muttering, rambling talk, disorientation, and restlessness usually occurs early in the course of the infection, but the acuteness of the mental symptoms varies as the disease is fulminating, acute, subacute, or chronic in type. At first the delirium may be nocturnal or exist only when the patient is undisturbed. In the acute cases, the patient is usually restless or even noisy and violent. In unfavorable cases, a terminal coma develops, appearing very early in the fulminating forms. In the subacute case, drowsiness, confusion, and mild delirium occur. Recovery may be complete or there may be special sense deprivations accompanied, perhaps, by various types of motor paralyses and a varying degree of mental defect. The resulting mental change may consist merely in moroseness, inability to concentrate, impairment of memory, and irritability, or, especially when the disease occurs in infants, there may be a serious arrest of intelligence.

The diagnosis is established by the existence of the above signs of diffuse cerebral dysfunction with the presence of signs of meningeal irritation, including a stiff neck, Kernig and Brudzinski signs, and often of a purpuric rash, hyperesthesia, and hyperalgesia. Spinal puncture shows a purulent fluid under increased pressure with a predominance of leukocytes. On Gram staining, the meningococcus may be cultured or tentatively identified as a diplococcus. The sugar and alkaloids of the cerebrospinal fluid are decreased.

Parenteral administration of sodium sulfadiazine, the agent of choice, should be initiated, with an initial dosage of 0.05 to 0.1 gm. per kilogram of body weight (approximately 3.5 to 6.0 gm.). The agent should be given intravenously as a 0.5 per cent solution, preferably in 6M sodium lactate solution. Lactate sustains an alkaline urine and prevents the precipitation of the drug in the renal tubules. If 5 gm. of the drug are dissolved in 1000 ml. of 6M sodium lactate, the proper concentration of the agent is provided. Subsequent doses of sodium sulfadiazine may be given in 500 ml. of 6M sodium lactate. A concentration of 10 to 12 mg. of sodium sulfadiazine per 100 ml. of blood is desirable. Concentrations above this level are to be avoided. If the drug is given by mouth, the patient should receive also 15 gm. of sodium bicarbonate daily, in divided doses. This should be continued for two to five days after complete clinical recovery. It is not necessary to consider intrathecal therapy.

Penicillin has been used, but the results are less satisfactory than with the sulfonamides unless large doses in the neighborhood of 1,000,000 units are given every two hours intramuscularly.

Tuberculous Meningitis

In both children and adults, the onset of tuberculous meningitis is usually insidious. The previously-active child begins to tire easily, appears weary, is irritable, peevish, and disinclined to talk or play. Sleep is often restless and disturbed by mild delirium. As the intracranial pressure increases, difficulty of grasp, clouding of consciousness, and confusion begin to appear, and headache increases. For a time, the patient, if roused, may for a short period be fairly well in touch with his environment, although he usually resents any disturbance. Some adults exhibit an agitated confusion. As the lethargy increases, the patient is no longer capable of recognizing friends and sinks into coma.

A diagnosis of tuberculous meningitis is made in the presence of signs of diffuse cerebral dysfunction as described above, with clinical evidence of meningitis indicated by a stiff neck, Kernig or Brudzinski responses, or both, hyperreflexia, petellar and ankle clonus, and Babinski reflexes. Later such signs may disappear with deepening coma. Cerebrospinal fluid is usually clear, with slight increase in pressure. A thin coagulum will develop if the fluid is allowed to stand. Tubercle bacilli may be found in the coagulum. The cells in the fluid are increased to 25 or more per cubic milli-meter. Protein is elevated while glucose content is diminished.

Current treatment with streptomycin and isoniazid has been most gratifying. Intrathecal medication is unnecessary. With adults, streptomycin in the dosage of 2 gm. may be given intramuscularly in two divided doses in conjunction with 8 to 10 mg. per kilogram of body weight of isoniazid by mouth. This regimen should be continued for periods of six months or more after obvious clearing of the infection. The isoniazid may be decreased by 5 mg. per kilogram as im-provement ensues. The clearing of the infection is indicated by the rise in the glucose content of the cerebrospinal fluid. Para-aminosalicylic acid may be given as well. In children, 1 gm. of streptomycin is given intramuscularly with isoniazid 10 mg. per kilogram daily in divided doses. When the cerebrospinal glucose has increased, the same dose of strepto-mycin is given twice weekly for one or two months, followed by sulfone (Promi-zole) by mouth for several years (0.25 to 8 gm.). The use of intrathecal cortico-steroids is advisable in those cases in which the diagnosis is made late in order to prevent the development fibrinous inflammatory exudates which would has-ten the blockage of flow of the cerebro-spinal fluid.

Close observation is required in order to detect signs of intoxication with isoniazid and streptomycin. The sympto-matology of toxicity with isoniazid is described in the next chapter. Deafness and other disturbances have been ob-served with streptomycin. It has been shown that the prognosis for survival is related to the time of initiation of ther-apy and the severity of the illness. The state of consciousness, the degree of ab-normality detected in the electroencepha-logram, and the increase in cerebrospinal fluid protein with decrease in glucose provide indicators of the latter.

Acute (Sydenham's) Chorea

Sydenham's chorea is now regarded as an infectious encephalitis involving both the cortex and basal ganglia. It is thought that it results from the factors which produce rheumatic fever or from similar factors. It is probably a rheumatic en-cephalitis and represents an exudative stage of cerebral involvement similar to the exudative changes which may be observed in the joints and heart. It seems certain that a streptococcus is involved in the process. The involuntary, jerky movements, the muscular inco-ordina-tion, and the grimaces are important symptoms of the disease, but only its mental aspects will be considered here.

Symptoms. In addition to an easy mental fatigability, many psychic symp-toms may be associated with chorea. One of the most constant of these is an emo-tional instability. The choreic child be-comes preoccupied, sensitive, irritable restless, quarrelsome, and resentful of correction. Insomnia, night terrors, and sleepwalking may occur. Heedlessness and impairment of attention and of con-centration are frequent, there is also an apparent inability to remember. The ma-jority of these children are tearful, cry at the slightest provocation, are peevish and fretful. Many show a lack of concern for ordinary duties and obligations. Oc-casionally there may be considerable de-pression. The facies is sometimes de-scribed as wistful in expression. Selfishness and disobedience are common, and many feel that the somewhat frequent associa-tion of behavior disorders and delin-quency with the disease is more than a coincidence. Sometimes the behavior disturbances are not unlike those follow-ing encephalitis or trauma of the head. Delirious episodes may occur. Unfor-tunately the family may fail to appreciate the seriousness and significance of the disease and therefore may scold and pun-ish the child for the emotional and other rather trying behavior characteristics. Such ill-advised treatment tends to ag-gravate the emotional behavior and re-actions. At best, the disease often leads to undesirable defense reactions. Chorea sometimes occurs for the first time, or recurs, in young women, associated with their first pregnancy.

DIAGNOSIS. A history of rheumatism or of repeated attacks of tonsilitis and the presence of heart disease or of high fever may be helpful in establishing the diagnosis. It must be differentiated from hysteria, tics, athetoid movements, and from a restless, general hyperactivity. Sydenham's chorea usually continues for two or three months and occasionally for longer periods. Relapses are not uncommon. The disease occurs much more frequently in girls than in boys. There is much to suggest that a post-infectious encephalopathy may exist following chorea and that it is accompanied by permanent personality changes in the form of hyperkinetic or neurotic symptoms and peculiarities of character or temperament.

TREATMENT. One of the most essential requirements of treatment is physical and mental rest. The earlier the child is put to bed, the shorter, usually, will be the course of the disease. The disturbing presence of other persons should not be permitted. Treatment in a hospital away from disturbing home influences is often wise. Sodium salicylate and aspirin have long been used. In children over thirteen, fever therapy induced by means of the air-conditioned, thermostatically controlled hypertherm has been recommended by some as a means of shortening the course of the illness. The patient may be given daily treatments for two hours with temperatures from 104° to 105° F. Usually eight to ten treatments are given. Some pediatricians advise against fever therapy if cardiac damage exists. Such sedatives as bromides, chloral, or sodium amytal may be required if restlessness is marked. Since the chorea is merely a symptom of the rheumatic infection, the treatment of the latter must be continued until all criteria indicating its arrest are satisfied.

Epidemic Encephalitis

An infectious disease of the brain which appeared in Roumania in 1915 but was first described and identified in 1917 by Constantin von Economo of Vienna spread to America in 1919 and subsequently attracted much attention both because of its devastating epidemiological features and because of its remarkable symptomatological polymorphism. Von Economo termed the disease lethargic encephalitis, but as it was not always characterized by lethargy, it has become generally known as epidemic or Type A encephalitis. No cases of the acute form have been reported since 1925, but the disease continues to have clinical interest, since chronic forms are still seen.

ETIOLOGY AND PATHOLOGY. It seems to be clearly established that the etiological agent was a filterable virus, although its mode of transmission is not known. The most common pathological lesion existing in this form was characterized by a cuffing or infiltration of the perivascular spaces in the brain with lymphocytes. While this may have existed in the cortex, hypothalamus, or even peripheral nerves, by far the most frequent site was the basal ganglia. Ganglion cells degenerated and many disappeared. In the chronic cases, which are the only ones now being seen by pathologists, the chief findings are loss and degeneration of neurons, especially in the substantia nigra, which may be grossly pigmented, as well as gliosis. The virus probably remained active in the nervous tissue for years, much in the manner of the *Treponema pallidum* in neurosyphilis.

SYMPTOMS. Since the acute form of this type of encephalitis is not now seen, little description of it will be given. Not even excepting syphilis is there a disease involving the central and peripheral nervous system capable of such polymorphic manifestations. Following the general symptoms of any infectious disease, there appeared the evidences of an invasion of the nervous system in which any one of its functions might be disturbed. The acute forms tended to fall into two ambitendent types: the hypersomnic–ophthalmoplegic and the irritative hyperkinetic. In the first or negative type, the most conspicuous symptoms were drowsiness with gradations to lethargy, stupor, and coma, slowness of intellectual function, paralytic phenomena of cortical origin, aphasia, agraphia; as- tereognosis and loss of limb sense caused by paralytic lesions in the parietal cortex; ptosis, strabismus, and other disturb- ances of the ocular apparatus as well as other paralytic phenomena indicative of localization in the brain stem. The leth- argy and other sleep disturbances were often the most striking symptoms of the acute form. The patient might remain in a deep sleep for days or weeks. If aroused, he promptly fell asleep again. In the irritative, hyperkinetic or positive type there were restlessness, irritability, excitability, insomnia, jacksonian or gen- eralized convulsive seizures, and other irritative phenomena. Hyperkinetic phe- nomena resulting from involvement of the basal nuclei occurred in the acute form of the disease and were of a great variety. Among them were tremors, my- oclonias, and athetoid and choreiform movements.

Chronic phase. Following the great epidemic mentioned, many patients who had survived the acute phase continued to show symptoms that at first were ascribed to residual lesions. Gradually, however, it became apparent that these symptoms were not stationary and that a continued, chronic activity persisted. Other patients who had supposedly re- covered began, after intervals of months or years free from symptoms, to develop parkinsonism or other evidence of a con- tinuing process. Also during the years since the epidemic, many persons with a history of some previous infection, per- haps diagnosed as influenza but with no associated acute encephalitic symptoms, developed chronic encephalitis. Others with no history of previous infection insidiously developed an encephalitis that was chronically progressive from the onset.

The symptoms of a chronic encepha- litis of the von Economo type are varied and depend upon the areas in which the progressive inflammatory-degenerative changes take place, although the extra- pyramidal basal motor nuclei are the most frequent sites. The most common syndrome is the parkinsonian (cf. Chap-

ter XXI). Tremors, tics, myotonias, and athetoid and choreiform movements are frequently observed. In addition to these dyskinesias and hyperkinesias, there may be paroxysmal symptoms such as disturb- ances in rate or rhythm of respiration, also gasping or yawning. One of the most frequent paroxysmal phenomena is oculogyric crises in which the eyes are spasmodically turned upwards owing to the periodic activity of certain neural mechanisms. Narcolepsy and epileptic attacks may occur. Excessive flow of saliva, seborrhea, and obesity are not uncommon.

The psychic manifestations of the acute phase of epidemic encephalitis presented the general characteristics of an acute organic type of mental reaction of toxic–infectious origin, viz., clouding of the sensorium and impairment of the capacity for apprehension, for elaborating impressions, and for activizing memories. Most patients showed delirium, although in a considerable number the delirium was easily overlooked because of the more obvious stupor, some degree of which occurred in the acute stage of nearly all cases. In a rather large propor- tion of cases, emotional, alterations con- tinued after the acute phases and often constituted the only evidence of a lack of recovery. Among such mood altera- tions were irritability, explosive reactions, stubbornness, and apathy.

Intellectual defects did not usually follow the disease except when the in- fection occurred at a very early age— usually four years or younger.

Behavior disorders. In children the chronic stage of epidemic encephalitis was often associated with serious altera- tions in character and behavior, the se- verity of which bore no relation to that of the acute stage. In some cases, in fact, it was difficult to obtain any clear history of an acute attack. The restless overactiv- ity, emotional irritability, and impulsive- ness of the early period were followed in a certain number of cases by lying, steal- ing, running away, cruelty, gross sexual offenses, and other behavior comparable in many outward manifestations to that exhibited by the psychopathic child. The troublesome behavior disorders shown by the encephalitic child were of every variety and usually in a setting of constant hyperactivity. The behavior or the adequacy of the social adjustment showed no correlation with the neurological signs. The child's personality, too, might be completely changed, yet his intellectual functions might not be affected.

There seems to be reason for believing that psychogenic factors may have played a certain role in the production of these behavior disorders. Not infrequently, for example, the laity looked upon "sleeping sickness" as something mysterious and was therefore prone to suspect that its victim might somehow be peculiar. Such children soon became aware of this attitude. If, too, the victim suffered from strabismus, tremor, narcoleptic attacks, or from parkinsonism with its absence of expressive movements of the face, its rigidity of posture and gait, and its slowness of speech, other children often called him "crazy," "dumb," or with taunting nicknames made him the laughing-stock of his associates. Under these circumstances the child's feelings of inferiority and insecurity led to all sorts of undesirable defense reactions to his handicaps. During convalescence, in some instances, the child was overprotected, his training was neglected and faulty, and regressive tendencies were permitted or encouraged.

DIAGNOSIS. As already stated, acute cases of Type A encephalitis are no longer seen in the United States. A considerable number of patients, however, who exhibit the sequelae of the disease are still seen. The most common manifestations are tremor, rigidity, and slowness of voluntary movements, which combine to form a neurological picture resembling in some ways the hepatolenticular degeneration of Wilson and, in others, paralysis agitans. Chronic epidemic encephalitis does not, of course, show the corneal pigmentation (Kayser-Fleischer rings), a mixed static and intention tremor, and the evidence of liver disease seen in Wilson's disease.

In degenerative parkinsonism, one does not see the bizarre postures and gaits, the muscular spasms such as oculogyric crises, the coarse tremors, or the behavioral peculiarities frequently seen among the sequelae of epidemic encephalitis.

PROGNOSIS. From 10 to 50 per cent of the patients died during the acute phase of epidemic encephalitis, usually from respiratory paralysis. Of the survivors, roughly 75 per cent, within a period varying from a few weeks to six years, developed signs of a continuing infection manifested by neurological, endocrine, or metabolic disturbances, or by behavior, mood, or other personality disorder.

TREATMENT. Atropine, stramonium, and scopolamine have long been used for post-encephalitic parkinsonism. Artane (trihexyphenidyl), which is similar to atropine in chemical composition, may also be used. The initial dose should be 1 mg. the first day, the amount being gradually increased, according to response, to 6 to 10 mg. daily. Rabellon is also helpful. These drugs are more effective in relieving rigidity and associated asthenia than in controlling tremor. Benzedrine sulfate, administered orally two or three times a day, in doses of 25 mg., is useful in reducing oculogyric crises and for asthenia.

Other Encephalitides

While acute forms of von Economo's disease are no longer seen, one should remember that there are other forms of neurotropic virus infections that may cause such mental and neurological symptoms as drowsiness, confusion, stupor, or coma, and other focal symptoms such as convulsions, hemiplegia, aphasia, ataxia, cranial nerve palsies, tremor, chorea, athetosis, and rigidity. Among such forms of encephalitis are St. Louis encephalitis, equine encephalitis, and the occasional cases of encephalitis associated with mumps, measles, infectious mononucleosis, and vaccination against cowpox. Residual psychiatric effects of infection with both eastern and western types of equine encephalomyelitis have been reported in the United States and Canada; also, residuals have occurred following Japanese B encephalitis contracted by United States military personnel in Japan and Korea since 1950.

In both eastern and western forms of equine encephalitis, infants and children have been more prone than adults to infection. In the former, sequelae have been virtually universal and most severe in infants under one year of age, who suffered persisting mental retardation, spasticities, and hemiplegias. Similar residuals have been observed with the western type in infants as well. In one series, approximately 25 per cent of adults affected who were followed over time showed impairment of higher intellectual functions with difficulty in abstract thinking and planning.

Acute Brain Syndrome Associated with Systemic Infection

In the case of the mental disturbances resulting from, or associated with, the infectious diseases that have thus far been mentioned, the infecting organism is located in the brain or its coverings. In many instances, however, mental disturbance may be associated with infections in which the infecting agent does not invade the central nervous system. Such temporary disturbances may result from many severe infections, such as typhoid fever or pneumonia, and appear especially during the febrile period and most frequently in the form of delirium.

Deliria

Depending on their temporal relation to the febrile stage of the infection, the deliria with infectious diseases are known as initial delirium, febrile delirium, and post-febrile delirium.

PRE-FEBRILE DELIRIUM. Initial or pre-febrile delirium is a delirium that rather infrequently develops during the incubation or prodromal period of infectious diseases before there has been any rise in temperature. The cause of the delirium can naturally not be ascertained until symptoms diagnostic of the infection appear. Such deliria may be marked and often imply a serious prognosis.

FEBRILE DELIRIUM. The delirium occurring during the febrile period of an infection is often spoken of as febrile delirium. The intensity of the symptoms is dependent less upon the height of the fever than upon the integration of the personality and the importance of psychogenic factors. The form of this, as of other delirioid reactions, is determined largely by individual personality factors. In milder degrees, there may be merely restlessness, sensitiveness to light or noise, and disturbing dreams. In the more severe cases, there will be hallucinations, confusion which may become extreme, indistinct muttering, stupor, twitching, carphologia, coma, and death.

POST-FEBRILE DELIRIUM. Post-febrile delirium may be merely the continuation of a previous delirium into the post-febrile period of an infectious disease, or it may be a delirium making its first appearance after the temperature has returned to normal. Consciousness is clouded to a variable degree, sometimes even to the point of stupor. In cases showing great prostration after the fall of the fever of infection, the symptoms may be of an extreme severity, constituting what H. Weber in 1866 described as collapse delirium. In this there is clouding of consciousness or a stuporous state, sometimes marked confusion and great motor excitement that appear to be motivated by fear and may increase even to violence and destructiveness. The stream of talk may be an incoherent flight of ideas. Emaciation and exhaustion progress rapidly, and a typhoid state, followed by stupor and coma, may develop. Death occurs in a few days in most of these malignant types of delirium, although a few patients recover after a prolonged sleep.

Treatment of Delirium

The treatment of delirium is primarily the treatment of the infection, toxic state, or other disturbing factor that led to the reaction. This does not mean, however, that the delirium itself should not be actively treated. Occasionally a beginning delirium may be aborted by reducing environmental stimulation, applying an icecap to the head, the reassurance of the nurse, or the administration of chlorpromazine or a hypnotic, such as paraldehyde. Precautions should be taken to prevent accidental injury or suicide. Unless carefully supervised, the delirious patient, usually disoriented and in some cases in intense fear, may unknowingly wander into danger or may attempt to escape imaginary enemies by suicide. Measures which tend to support his contact with his environment will lessen his fearfulness and anxiety. Such measures are the presence of close family members or familiar articles from his home in the room, a quiet environment with continuous light in the room day and night. Changes of environment or of physicians or nurses are apt to be disturbing. Greatly preferable to mechanical restraint are continuous baths or cold wet packs.

The patient should receive an abundance of nourishment which should include a liberal amount of proteins and of carbohydrates. Chlorpromazine given by mouth or by intramuscular injection in doses of 25 to 50 mg. is often effective. Other phenothiazines may be used as well. Nicotinamide or multivitamin preparations are usually advisable. Sodium chloride, or other salts, and glucose, administered orally or intravenously, should be given liberally, if needed, to restore normal acid–base equilibrium. Caffeine may be advisable as a cardiac stimulant. The administration of sedatives should, if possible, be limited to the night. From 10 to 15 cc. of paraldehyde may be given in ice water, tea, or wine. Bromides and the barbiturates should be avoided. Chloral hydrate (7½ to 15 grains) may be used.

After the patient's recovery, the physician may be able to give considerable retrospective interpretation of delusional and hallucinatory experiences.

Post-infectious Mental Disorders

These disorders differ somewhat from the post-febrile deliria just described. Delirium is not usually a conspicuous symptom, consisting, when it occurs, of a mild confusion and fleeting hallucinations. Rather more typical of the post-infectious mental disorders are states of easy exhaustion, reduced attention, restless irritability, difficulty in thinking, suspiciousness, anxious depression, and hypochondriacal ideas. The patient is frequently easily frightened, over-sensitive to light and noise, morose, complaining, and preoccupied with his physical sense of weakness and debility. A state of physical exhaustion and prostration exists and is doubtless an important factor in the development of the disorder. If there has been a prolonged subvitaminosis, there may be a retrospective falsification of memory suggesting Korsakoff's syndrome, which may be complete even to the existence of polyneuritis. On rare occasions, some degree of mental enfeeblement follows. Although the outstanding symptoms in the post-infectious disorders may be mental, yet their cessation depends upon the recovery of the patient's physical health.

Acute Viral Hepatitis. With the increased recognition of acute viral hepatitis in recent years, the occasional association of mental disturbances with this infection has been observed. In some instances, this is a coincidence, as has been noted in public mental hospitals in which mild epidemics of infectious hepatitis have occurred. Occasionally, however, the infection releases a psychotic disturbance in poorly integrated personalities.

Trichinias. Trichiniasis is scarcely comparable to the infections which have just been discussed, yet mention may be made of the fact that occasionally mental disturbances occur in this disease if the young nematodes invade the cerebrum. The symptoms are those of the toxic–organic syndrome—confusion, cloudiness, disorientation, delirium, hebetude, and, at times, confabulation. Occasionally signs of focal neurological disturbances are noted.

BIBLIOGRAPHY

Adams, R. D., and Weinstein, L.: Clinical and pathological aspects of encephalitis. New England J. Med., 239:865–876, 1948.

Bender, L.: Organic Brain Conditions Producing Behavior Disturbances. In Pacella, B. L., and Lewis, N. D. C. Modern Trends in Child Psychiatry. New York, International Universities Press, 1945.

Engel, G. L., and Romano, J.: Delirium: A syndrome of cerebral insufficiency. J. Chronic Dis., 9:260–277, 1959.

Herzon, H., Shelton, J. T., and Bruyn, H. B.: Sequelae of western equine and other anthropoid-borne encephalitides. Neurology, 7:535–548, 1957.

Krauss, S.: Postchoreic personality and neurosis. J. Ment. Sc., 92:75–95, 1946.

Mulder, D. W., Parrott, M., and Thaler, M.: Sequelae of western equine encephalitis. Neurology, 1:318–327, 1951.

Neal, J. B.: Encephalitis: A Clinical Study. New York, Grune & Stratton, 1942.

Von Economo, C.: Encephalitis Lethargica. Its Sequelae and Treatment. Translated by K. O. Newman. New York, Oxford University Press, 1931.

Chapter Nine

BRAIN SYNDROMES RESULTING FROM DRUG OR POISON INTOXICATION

As described in the previous chapter, toxic substances may interrupt the multiple processes of general cerebral metabolism in a variety of ways. The associated clinical syndrome is that of cerebral insufficiency with various symptomatic expressions, depending upon the degree and suddenness of interruption of ego functions, the extent of permanent cellular damage, and the varieties of adaption to loss of function peculiar to the individual personality.

Such brain syndromes are frequently complications of modern medical therapy or represent the secondary effects of suicidal attempts, self-medication, or industrial poisoning. The sections in this chapter are arranged in more or less the frequency in which the specific intoxicants are encountered as etiologic agents in the production of the cerebral insufficiencies in clinical practice.

Barbiturates

INCIDENCE, ETIOLOGY, SYMPTOMS. According to reports of the United States Public Health Service, there has been a great increase in recent years not only in acute barbiturate intoxication but also in barbiturate addiction. Acute intoxication with barbiturates accounts for about 25 per cent of all deaths of acute poisoning admitted to general hospitals, and more deaths are caused by barbiturates, either accidentally ingested or taken with suicidal intent, than by any other poison.

As in alcoholism and in narcotic drug addiction, the important factor in barbiturate addiction is an underlying personality difficulty. Many psychoneurotics become addicted to barbiturates through their prescription for insomnia. Persons with character disorders ("Psychopaths") begin the use of the drug in order to experience its intoxicating effect. Morphine addicts often use the drug when they are unable to secure morphine or in order to reinforce the effect of that narcotic. Alcoholics may begin the use of barbiturates to relieve the tension following a debauch and continue their use to induce toxic effects. In contradiction to the situation in other narcotic drug addictions, a large proportion of the cases of barbiturate addiction results from administration by physicians. The physician should therefore remember that in prescribing barbiturates he assumes a heavy ethical responsibility. There is a possibility that these drugs may create a dangerous type of addiction. Especial care should be exercised in prescribing them for emotionally unstable persons. Simple insomnia alone is rarely a valid indication for the use of barbiturates.

Not only do the barbiturates induce acute brain syndromes but also they cause chronic delirious reactions in those who use the drug in large amounts over periods of time. In the latter there may occur, on sudden withdrawal of the drugs, an *abstinence syndrome,* again characteristically delirioid but often with an associated convulsive state. It is necessary to differentiate the two conditions (that due to intoxication and that due to abstinence); they differ in their clinical manifestations and their treatment.

Acute barbiturate intoxication occurs frequently in those with suicidal intent and sometimes as an accidental occurrence in some who are using such agents for insomnia. In the latter instance, in partial confusional states from previous doses that have failed to provide hypnosis, the patient automatically takes excessive amounts. Again, accidental overdosage may be observed in persons suffering severe anxiety who self-administer overdoses when the prescribed amount has failed to bring relief. Barbiturate intoxication often occurs in alcoholics or narcotic addicts when this agent is substituted for, or used with, the preferred addicting substance.

DIAGNOSIS. With acute intoxication, there is impairment of cognitive functions as with any form of cerebral insufficiency, lack of emotional control shown in bursts of laughing or crying, garrulousness, and poor judgment, followed later by progressive drowsiness, stupor, and finally coma. While the condition often resembles acute alcoholism, there is no odor of alcohol on the breath. It is characteristically associated with certain cerebellar signs such as a gross dysarthria, a constant nystagmus, ataxia in both gait and stature, and adiadochokineses. With deepening intoxication, absence of the deep tendon reflexes, Babinski reflexes,

and contraction of the pupils develop. Respiration is characteristically slow, and in severe intoxication, is shallow or even periodic. Peripheral circulatory collapse may supervene.

In states of *mild intoxication,* the patient is confused or, if drowsy, is easily aroused, judgment is defective, and the nystagmus is transient, with at best reduction in the skin reflexes (abdominal). Neither respiration nor blood pressure is depressed. *Moderate intoxication* may be estimated in the presence of sleep or drowsiness, with arousal only on vigorous stimulation, constant nystagmus, and dysarthria. There is now depression of tendon reflexes and respiration is slow. *Severe intoxication* is judged when the clinician observes unarousable coma, absence of all reflexes, including the corneal and pharyngeal, periodic respiration, and the symptoms of shock.

The diagnosis may be confirmed by the finding of barbiturates in the urine and blood. Since these tests usually are so time consuming and their reporting so delayed, they fail to aid in terms of diagnosis and treatment of the acute condition. With mild and moderate states, the electroencephalogram shows a characteristic fast wave frequency.

TREATMENT. Treatment should be conservative for all patients with mild and moderate degrees of barbiturate intoxication, since only the severe grades of cerebral insufficiency threaten life. In the former groups, gastric lavage is indicated if the drug has been recently taken. The patient should be kept awake and not allowed to sleep by use of such measures as talking, walking, and the administration of caffeine sodium benzoate 0.5 gm. intramuscularly or 10 to 40 mgm. of amphetamine sulfate by mouth or intramuscularly. Comatose patients who may be aroused by manual stimulation or the use of electro-stimulation with the Reiter apparatus may also be treated conservatively. If stupor deepens, adequate pulmonary ventilation must be maintained and circulatory collapse prevented by intravenous administration of a plasma expander. Oxygen is of doubtful value as it may further depress respiration; artificial respiration with the use of an automatic positive pressure apparatus or a Drinker external respirator should be started. In some instances an endotracheal tube or tracheotomy is required. It is now considered that the use of such drugs as pentylenetetrazol (Metrazol) and picrotoxin do not provide better protection and may actually increase mortality.

It must be recognized that in the recovery phase from coma there again supervenes a delirious state which will require protective nursing until the patient fully recovers.

Addiction to barbiturates may develop; yet such hypnotics may be taken in doses of 0.5 gm. or less daily for prolonged periods without harm. Those who consume 0.8 gm. suffer definite impairment of mental functioning and will develop addiction, as judged by the appearance of an *abstinence syndrome* if the drug is suddenly withdrawn after six to eight weeks of continuous ingestion. Those consuming amounts between these levels of 0.2 to 0.8 gm. daily show variable degrees of deficit.

Chronic cerebral impairment due to barbiturates produces signs similar to those described earlier for the mild states of intoxication and are shown in fluctuations in intensity of the degree of confusion and in impairment in thinking, judgment, and motor activity. There exist persistent nystagmus and various degrees of dysarthria, dysmetria, and ataxia, with loss of the superficial reflexes. Often the condition of chronic intoxication is confused with multiple sclerosis. Again, the blood and urine will show evidence of barbiturates, and the electroencephalogram presents a characteristic fast pattern.

Sudden withdrawal of the drug in the addicted will precipitate an abstinence syndrome resembling the delirium tremens of the alcoholic. Within the first eight hours after discontinuing the drug, the patient appears improved as his confusion subsides. Then he develops anxiety, tremulousness, and severe weakness.

Within a day following withdrawal, muscular twitching and severe shaking of the extremities appear. In 75 per cent of patients, one or several grand mal convulsions take place during the second day of abstinence; they may be noted as late as one week after the drug is discontinued. In about 60 per cent, anxiety increases and complete insomnia follows. Between the third and seventh day of withdrawal, there develops a frank delirious reaction associated with vivid delusions and hallucinations, usually auditory. Recovery ensues some three to five days later with a prolonged bout of sleeping.

Treatment of the chronic barbiturate user requires careful evaluation of the extent of his habituation or addiction, which is often most difficult to assay. Here the word habituation is used to indicate psychological dependence on the drug, and the word addiction, to indicate physiological dependence with propensity for development of the abstinence syndrome on withdrawal. In no instance should abrupt withdrawal of the barbiturate be attempted in the chronic user. Since such patients often distort the amount of drug they consume daily, they should initially receive the maximum amount admitted. Withdrawal should be commenced at the level of 0.1 gm. daily. When half the stabilization dose is reached, reduction should be discontinued for several days before a decrease in the drug is continued again. The appearance at any time of anxiety, tremor, insomnia, or weakness or the development of slow-wave activity in the electroencephalogram heralds the onset of the abstinence syndrome. Such symptoms call for termination of withdrawal and support with additional barbiturates. If the abstinence syndrome appears, a dose of 0.2 to 0.3 gm. of pentobarbital orally usually is sufficient to prevent its full symptomatic expression. Following a convulsion, 0.3 to 0.5 gm. of pentobarbital or amobarbital should be given parenterally or orally, followed by the oral administration of these drugs to the level of mild intoxication.

During withdrawal, patients require careful nursing and observation. With the withdrawal complete, it then is necessary to ascertain the motivating forces which led to dependence and arrange for appropriate treatment of the primary psychopathology of the individual.

Bromides

INCIDENCE, ETIOLOGY, SYMPTOMS. If administered in toxic amounts, several salts of bromide may produce acute brain syndromes. A decade or more ago, with the development of methods of determining the bromide content of blood, it was found that mental disturbances resulting from bromides were more frequent than had been realized. In some psychiatric clinics, 4 per cent of all admissions were found to be suffering from bromide psychoses. The condition is now seen less frequently. About 50 per cent of the cases arise through the prescribing of bromides by physicians, the prescription being repeatedly refilled. All too frequently, additional amounts of the drug are further given in an effort to rid the patient of symptoms already caused by the bromides. Many toxic states arise through self-medication, principally by the use of proprietary preparations containing bromides.

The normal bromide content of the blood serum varies from 0.33 to 1.73 mg. per 100 ml. Intoxication symptoms may be expected if the bromide content exceeds 150 mg. per 100 ml. of blood serum, although there is a wide variation in susceptibility to the drug. The mechanism of bromide poisoning is through the replacement of the chloride with bromide. Elderly or arteriosclerotic patients have a poor tolerance and may develop toxic symptoms, even though the blood content be relatively low. Bromides are excreted slowly, and a mental disturbance may develop within two or three weeks after one begins to use amounts as small as 45 to 60 grains a day. Malnutrition, dehydration, and arteriosclerosis render the patient more susceptible to the effects of bromides. Their use is at times associated with alcoholism.

DIAGNOSIS. In mild intoxication there may be a feeling of tiredness or weakness, irritability, broken sleep, slowness of mental grasp, inability to concentrate, faulty memory, drowsiness, impaired attention, and perhaps even confusion. Physically one notes a dry skin, coated tongue, digestive disorders, impotence or menstrual disturbances, ataxic gait, tremors of tongue and fingers, and hyperactive, sluggish, or absent deep reflexes. Dehydration is common. Protein elevation in the spinal fluid is frequent. Acne, considered an ordinary sign of bromidism, is often absent. In more severe intoxication, the clinical picture is one of delirium with fever, confusion, clouding of consciousness, varying degrees of drowsiness or stupor, disorientation, difficulty in grasp, misidentification, motor restlessness even to the point of extreme excitement, fear, and memory loss accompanied by confabulations. Speech is thick, muttering, hesitant, and slurred, and the face is mask-like and expressionless. The mood is often one of fear or depression. In bromide as in other toxic psychoses, there may be a loss of the usual forces of repression, with a resulting appearance of hallucinations. The ideational content of the delirium may be colored by individual psychogenic factors. Paranoid ideas are common. Occasionally a schizophrenic-like syndrome is observed. Bromide delirium may continue for ten days to two months. Remissions and exacerbations with sudden changes in the mental state are not uncommon.

TREATMENT. The treatment consists of stopping the drug, the forcing of liquids, and the administration of 2 to 4 gm. of sodium chloride every four hours unless gastric irritation forbids such large doses. Most patients can take a total of 4 to 6 gm. a day in divided doses if it is given in enteric-coated tablets. Recent investigations seem to show that bromides are excreted more rapidly following the administration of ammonium chloride than after the use of sodium chloride. Ammonium chloride not only furnishes a chloride for displacing bromide but acts also as a diuretic. In some instances intermittent peritoneal lavage or the use of the artificial kidney might be considered to increase bromide excretion. Cathartics are usually necessary for the obstinate constipation that often exists. Paraldehyde may be advisable at night.

CLINICAL REPORT. The following clinical report of an acute reversible brain syndrome associated with bromidism illustrates not only the type of mental disorder associated with toxic states but also the sensorial and other disturbances often seen in delirium:

C. M., aged 38, was transferred to a mental hospital on October 22 from a hospital to which he had been admitted five days previously. His history prior to the present illness was without particular significance, although apparently he was of a somewhat immature, unstable personality. His wife commented, "He could not sit for five minutes. He had to have the last word in everything. He felt that he was never to blame for any difficulty. He lost his temper easily." For several years he had drunk moderately but was never intoxicated.

In September the patient became tense and greatly concerned because, after a brief and stormy marriage, his daughter had left her husband. About October 1 he began to drink more alcohol. Between October 9 and October 13 he consumed four "large bottles" of a proprietary drug product containing a large quantity of bromides. So far as was known, he took no alcohol during that period. On October 13 he appeared confused and showed a slurring of speech and an unsteadiness of gait. Soon, in addition to these symptoms, he stated that he would shoot his son-in-law, also other members of his family.

On October 17 he was admitted to the general hospital. There he was seen by a consulting psychiatrist who suggested that the patient's blood bromide content be determined. This was found to be 600 mg. per 100 ml. The patient was confused, refused to stay in bed, showed poor motor co-ordination, and one night locked himself in a closet. He thought he had a gun in bed with him. He made such irrelevant remarks as, "I know who shot him. I was behind the curtain." He told his wife that the patient in an adjoining bed had "killed the little girl on B Street," located near his home. No such incident had occurred.

On October 21 he became much more confused; he was completely disorientated and his speech was quite incoherent. He heard gun shots in his room; he said there were dead bodies there and that his wife was sleeping in the hospital with other patients. He attempted to jump from a window, and it was necessary to place him in restraint pending his transfer to a mental hospital.

On arrival at the mental hospital, he was found to be heavily sedated with paraldehyde. After emerging from the effects of this, he was restless and constantly responded to both auditory and visual hallucinations. When asked where he was, he replied that he was at "Mom's and Pop's place." Upon being asked why he was in bed, he answered, "It seems to be a precaution to be parked here to smooch." He pointed to the bedcovers and said, "That's my wife there." He felt about the covers and remarked, "See that stone. It makes me G–d mad." He turned and shouted over his shoulder, "Well, come on, you might as well take it off. Sure going to get hell over that. What do you think of buying that place out?"

By October 26 the patient was more co-operative but still disorganized and restless. A physician introduced himself to the patient, who then said, "Yes, I heard about Hugh Pendleton. I better sleep pretty good tonight. He's got his offices at DeKalb and Jacoby Streets. Do you know it's him?"

On October 29 he knew where he was but gave the date as October 5 and had no recollection of having been in the general hospital. He stated that he had been depressed over his daughter's troubles and had taken triple bromides. For several following days there were periods during which he was noisy and restless and his verbal productions were incoherent and irrelevant. By November 9 his sensorium was fully clear and his apperception was intact. When asked about his experiences, he replied, "I must have caused considerable uproar at home with my antics. They thought I was drunk. I insisted I was not. I took it upon myself to take that bromide medicine for my nerves. My wife tells me I was in C. Hospital for four days. It's a blank wall. It seems I only really started remembering things from last Saturday, when my family saw me. My folks were telling me about some of the stuff that I did. I sure feel like an ass."

On November 10 the patient's blood bromide content had been reduced to 75 mg. per 100 ml. His convalescence continued without interruption and on November 20 he was discharged as recovered.

Cortisone and ACTH

These agents may produce a wide variety of mental disturbances, resulting, apparently, from their direct effect upon the central nervous system, although the precise pathogenetic mechanisms are not yet determined. The total energy exchange of the brain as measured by cerebral metabolic rate does not seem to be altered by ACTH or by cortisone, yet these hormones disturb enzymatic reactions by altering the electrolyte and water patterns of the body. In general, the mental reactions do not exhibit the type of confusion, disorientation, and sensorial disturbance characteristic of toxic psychoses. Nearly all patients receiving the drugs show an increased joviality and optimism. Among the common disturbances are affective ones varying from depression to hypomania, also from apathy to panic, and even inappropriateness of affect. Feelings of depersonalization, or a sense of detachment or strangeness in awareness of one's body image, may occur. Disturbances of speech are frequent and may vary from mutism to flight of ideas. Illusions and hallucinations may occur, as also do delusions of depressive, grandiose or persecutory types. A wide variety of motor disturbances may appear including immobility, pressure of activity and regressiveness. In general the type of mental disturbance produced by the drug seems to be determined by the basic pattern or structure of the patient's personality. Complete spontaneous recovery occurs upon discontinuance of the drug. In prolonged cases, lucid intervals of gradually increasing frequency and duration may occur until a normal state is fully established.

Experience has shown that the occurrence of a psychiatric disturbance with use of the corticosteroids does not indicate that a similar disturbance will take place if the steroid is withheld and then again administered at a later date. Nor is there clear evidence that these reactions are related to dosage.

Isoniazid

With the increasing use of this drug for the treatment of tuberculosis, a number of cases of mental disturbance have been observed associated with its administration. The clinical picture is that of an acute, toxic, confusional disorientation for time, place, person, and situation, restlessness, and auditory or visual hallucinations. It is usually preceded by muscular twitching, hyperreflexia, difficulty in micturition, constipation, and sometimes convulsions. Occasionally this toxic state is followed by signs of an organic cerebral impairment of the Korsakoff type. It has been stated that the toxic mental symptoms are related to the plasma level of the drug and that the majority of psychotic reactions occur in patients receiving more than 8 mg. of isoniazid per kilogram of body weight daily. Pyridoxine in large doses may prevent the appearance of isoniazid neuritis. This agent is not effective in reversing symptoms once they are established.

Sympathomimetic Amines (Benzedrine, Dexedrine and Desoxyn)

Chronic poisoning with the sympathomimetic amines, amphetamine, (Benzedrine), methamphetamine (Desoxyephedrine or Desoxyn), may be brought about by the continuing use of these agents. All have cortical excitant action in addition to their sympathomimetic action. They produce a feeling of well being and exhilaration which may lead to a persistent craving. The stimulation produced by the drug is followed by fatigue and depression. As tolerance is acquired, increasingly larger doses are necessary to produce the desired stimulation. Their abuse occurs commonly in the case of alcoholics and barbiturate addicts. They are popular among thrill-seeking adolescents and inmates of penal institutions. Such drugs are almost always taken as tablets. Amphetamine inhalers no longer constitute a problem since they are not available. Some users have taken individual doses as high as 250 mg. of amphetamine and a total daily intake of 1 to 1.5 gm. The symptomatology produced by the drugs is similar to that of intoxication with cocaine. Tension, apprehension, and jerky and tremulous movements are noted in conjunction with tachycardia, hypertension, mydriasis, insomnia, and anorexia. A hallucinatory psychosis and paranoid delusions may occur in certain individuals. Treatment should include the use of sedation and abrupt withdrawal of the drug, with the institution of a program of psychotherapy to correct the underlying personality defect requiring habitual use of the agents.

Sulfonamides ("Sulfa" Drugs)

The administration of sulfa drugs may

at times cause headache, dizziness, confusion, bewilderment, inability to concentrate, and hallucinosis.

Thiocyanates

The continuing use of thiocyanates in the treatment of hypertensive disease with the occurrence of toxic mental symptoms must be kept in mind. Levels of blood thiocyanate that exceed 15 mg. per 100 ml. are likely to produce toxic reactions. It has been shown that thiocyanates are converted to cyanide in the body, and this cellular poison probably leads to depression of utilization of oxygen by inhibition of cytochrome oxidase. The consequent oxygen lack in the cerebral cortex leads to the production of the delirious reactions as well as to other symptoms, such as convulsions, ataxia, aphasia, and paraplegia. The usual toxic mental symptoms are incoherent muttering, slurring of speech, confusion, disorientation, auditory and visual hallucinations, restlessness, agitation, resistance, ideas of persecution, and convulsions. Several deaths have been reported. In addition to withholding the thiocyanate, a trial with methylene blue or sodium thiosulfate is probably worthwhile. It has been suggested that hydroxycobalamine (vitamin B_{12}) may serve as a potent antidote.

CLINICAL REPORT. The following case illustrates thiocyanate intoxication:

A 59-year-old housewife, admitted as an emergency case, complained of "pain all over." She claimed she was paralyzed, yet tossed restlessly about on the ambulance cot. She was confused and unable to give a coherent story. Her daughter said the illness started with a severe dizzy spell that had occurred two months earlier. Her home physician had found that her blood pressure was "over 300," and had prescribed some red tablets. She had continued to take the medicine until she came to the hospital, although at no time had a blood test been made. Three weeks prior to admission, general weakness, tremor of the hands, somnolence, tinnitus, and blurring of vision had developed. These symptoms had become progressively more severe in the meantime.

On physical examination, the patient complained volubly of unbearable tenderness in all her muscles. Her systolic blood pressure was 150 mm. and the diastolic 80 mm. Hg. There were narrowing and sclerosis of the retinal arterioles.

No neurological deficit was detected, although the weakness she described was confirmed.

The concentration of thiocyanate in the blood was 17.6 mg. per 100 ml., and a diagnosis of thiocyanate psychosis was made. On mental examination, she was depressed, withdrawn, negativistic, and distractible. Delusional, self-derogatory thinking was disclosed by her statements that other patients regarded her as a germ carrier and her physicians thought she was a nuisance and wanted to "fumigate" her. Hallucinations were not evident. She spoke haltingly and cried easily. She was disoriented as to time but not as to place or person. She was unable to repeat more than five digits forward and none backward. Simple multiplication was impossible, and she was unable to subtract serial sevens. Her memory was severely impaired for both recent and past events.

Further studies disclosed a blood urea concentration of 60 mg. per 100 ml. and a normal urine except for albuminuria, grade 1. She had a mild anemia, the hemoglobin measuring 10.3 gm. per 100 ml. and the erythrocyte count being 3,000,000 per cubic millimeter. A blood smear revealed no specific abnormalities. A roentgenogram of the thorax, an electrocardiogram, and an excretory urogram likewise did not disclose any abnormality. A provocative test with histamine did not give any evidence of pheochromocytoma, a possibility suggested by the history that her blood pressure on one occasion had exceeded "300."

With a high intake of fluid, the signs of toxic delirium subsided rapidly. The concentration of blood thiocyanate decreased to 8.7 mg. per 100 ml. by the eleventh day in the hospital, and there was only mild residual tenderness in the calves of her legs. When she was dismissed on the twentieth day, her blood pressure was 150/90, and she was free of symptoms.

Lead

ETIOLOGY. Of the various metallic poisons, lead is the one with which mental symptoms are most frequently associated. Both the source of intoxication with lead and the clinical picture differ considerably in adults and children. With adults the inhalation of toxic lead compounds is the major means of intoxication, while in infants poisoning occurs through the eating or chewing of lead-containing paint, often picked up in flakes peeling from woodwork or painted surfaces. The habit of pica in children is frequently associated with mental deficiency, but it occurs also in children of good intellectual endowment who show some emotional disturbance. In adults the history of exposure in industry or building to paint spraying, burning of lead in salvage operations, the oxygas cutting of red lead, of painted steel, and of older structures during the dismantling, as well as vocational employment in bronze, solder, or type metal or in the modern industrial practices of enameling and glass manufacture should suggest the possibility of exposure to poisonous, lead-containing vapors.

SYMPTOMS. Mental symptoms associated with lead poisoning tend to be of two types: (a) acute delirious episodes; (b) progressive mental deterioration. The delirious type may occur in either acute or chronic poisoning. It is of sudden onset and is characterized by confusion, insomnia, restlessness, tremors, fear, outbursts of violence, visual hallucinations, and delusions which are frequently persecutory in content. Convulsions may occur and may be accompanied by a delirium in which the patient experiences terrifying visual hallucinations. In the chronic form, apathy or depression, speech defect, forgetfulness, and at times confabulations suggesting the Korsakoff syndrome are frequently observed. The progressive mental deterioration may suggest general paresis. Occasionally the clinical picture is one of neurasthenia; the patient is irritable and depressed and complains of weakness, fatigability, and dizziness. In association with the mental disturbances there is usually a history of colic, constipation, and vomiting. The former is frequently more severe in adults than in children. In adults, black deposits may be seen around the gum margins of pyorrheic teeth. This is seldom visible in children. There is usually an associated hypochromic anemia with basophilic stippling. In children there may be a mild renal glycosuria. Coproporphyrinuria commonly accompanies intoxication with lead. Roentgenograms will demonstrate dense radio-opaque bands going into the shafts of long bones in children. The spinal fluid protein content is increased to levels between 15 and 200 mg. per 100 ml.

The chronic encephalopathy of children is characterized largely by failure of cerebral maturation and demonstrates itself in defects in attention, judgment, self-control, and visual learning. For those children who survive, a high proportion suffer irreversible brain damage that limits its maturation. The major threat to the life and mentality of the children is increased intracranial pressure. Such children may be verbally facile but find it difficult to learn the techniques of reading, writing, and arithmetic. In both adults and children, a characteristic peripheral neuritis is frequently seen. The most used muscle groups are affected rather than those supplied by individual nerves. Thus weakness of the extensors of the wrist occurs in adults and of the dorsiflexors of the feet in children. All tendon reflexes are lost, but sensation remains intact.

TREATMENT. Treatment commences with removal of the patient from exposure to and absorption of lead. Since there is no antidote to lead, therapy must be directed to relief of the symptoms and elimination of lead from the body. Increasing the output of water is the simplest method of increasing the output of lead. Treatment with calcium disodium versenate (ethylene-diaminetetraacetic acid, EDTA), a chelating agent, which has the capacity of forming stable, water-soluble complexes with metals, is now recommended to promote the loss of lead from the body. It may be given intravenously and by mouth, 1 gm. to 15 kilograms of body weight per day. One-half the twenty-four-hour dose can be administered at intervals of twelve hours in 250 to 300 ml. of 5 to 10 per cent glucose solution. A test dose of 10 per cent of this amount is recommended. Treatment should be continued for three to four days, followed by an interval of three days, and a total of three or four courses should be given. The level of lead in the blood should then be determined. If the concentration of lead is excessive (0.08 mg. or above per 100 gm.), the course of treatment should be repeated. These interrupted courses of therapy should be repeated until the blood level of lead has fallen below 0.06 mg. per 100 gm. Since lead is stored in the skeleton and may be released later at dangerously high levels, it is recommended that subsequent levels of lead in the blood be taken at intervals of four to six weeks and that further courses be given when dangerous rises are observed. Neurosurgical decompression of the skull may be required in patients with evidence of medullary compression.

In addition to the specific therapy described above, patients with lead encephalopathy will require the general measures used in the care of the acute or acutely delirious states. Those with neuropathy should receive orthopedic protection of the weakened muscles and ligaments. In chronic lead poison, alcohol is to be avoided; a high calcium diet supplemented by vitamin B_1 is indicated.

Mercury

Among the mental symptoms manifested by patients suffering from chronic mercury poisoning are irritability, timidity, discouragement, loss of self-confidence, fear, and occasionally outbursts of extreme anger. Less frequent are apathy, drowsiness, and impairment of memory. Chronic mercury poisoning results from the inhalation of volatile mercury for long periods of time. The hazardous trades are those concerned with the production of mercury and its derivatives, the manufacture of scientific apparatus, preparation of hatters' fur, felt hat making, the extraction of gold from silver by amalgamation, and the application of antifouling plastic paint to the hulls of ships. There is usually a moderately fine but later coarse jerking tremor of the orbits, lips, tongue, fingers, and limbs. Sometimes contractions of the limbs occur. The tremor is often intentional and subsides during rest. Weakness of both flexor and extensor muscles of the hand and forearm has been reported. No specific therapy is available for chronic mercury poisoning, although dimercaprol (BAL) has been used in those with acute poisoning. Recovery results following withdrawal from exposure.

Manganese

Workers in manganese may suffer from permanently disabling mental and neurological symptoms. Among the principal neurological symptoms are those of extrapyramidal involvement, including the basal ganglia. Gait and speech disturbances usually exist, also present are tremors of the tongue and of the extremities and muscular weakness. About 20 per cent of the cases show mental symptoms, including restlessness, elation, and uncontrollable laughter or crying. There is no specific therapy available for manganese poisoning.

Carbon Monoxide

The gas which most frequently produces mental disturbances is carbon monoxide. The deleterious effects of this substance, which is inhaled either intentionally or by accident from the exhaust fumes of automobiles or, more infrequently, in illuminating gas or gas produced through the defective combustion of coal in stoves or furnaces, are caused by anoxemia of the brain. Carbon monoxide combines with hemoglobin to form oxyhemoglobin, a stable compound which prevents the blood from absorbing oxygen. In those patients who die after several days, the central nervous system shows ischemic changes of the nerve cells as well as areas of softening, particularly in the cerebral cortex and the basal ganglia. Serious mental sequelae of carbon monoxide poisoning are infrequent in relation to the number of acute intoxications.

Mental symptoms following acute poisoning occur only in cases in which the intoxication has been extreme and unconsciousness complete. Of persons developing mental symptoms, about two-thirds pass directly from the comatose condition into states of confusion and delirium. In the remainder there exists a clear period of a week or more between emergence from the coma and the appearance of mental symptoms, among which are apathy, lack of initiative, and indifference to duties and responsibilities. Some patients continue to show confusion, bewilderment, and impairment of memory, with Korsakoff-like confabulations. Amnesia lasting from six to nine months may occur. In extreme cases, the patient sinks to the level of vegetative existence, with incontinence, unresponsiveness, and inability to carry on any voluntary activity. Occasionally a patient suffers from auditory aphasia. At times neurological complications may occur, owing usually to degenerative changes in the putamen or globus pallidus. Frequently, therefore, there is a modified parkinsonism, with stiffness of extremities caused by muscular hypertonia. Most patients with mental sequelae of carbon monoxide poisoning begin to improve within a few weeks after exposure and completely recover within two years. Those who have not recovered within that period of time remain in a state of mild or severe mental enfeeblement.

Attention has been called to the immediate and the delayed forms of mental sequelae arising from acute carbon monoxide anoxemia. Persons repeatedly subjected to moderate or minimal toxic amounts of the gas for periods ranging from several months to many years may develop mental and nervous symptoms. Among these manifestations are emotional instability, depression, agitation, anxiety, impairment of grasp and of memory, and at times confusion. Other symptoms are headache, vertigo, neuromuscular pains, digestive disturbances, dyspnea, and palpitation.

Carbon Disulfide

The extensive use of carbon disulfide in the manufacture of rayon has resulted in the production of toxic psychoses through its destructive effect upon the lipid content of neural tissue. Among the most commonly observed early symptoms are insomnia, bad dreams, fatigue, impotence, listlessness, and loss of memory. Neurologically there may be symptoms referable to almost any part of the central and peripheral nervous system. Among them are tenderness of nerve trunks and areas of hyperesthesia followed by loss of touch and pain sensation. Irritative

signs of motor nerves include fibrillary twitching and spasmodic contraction of nerves. Among motor signs are early fatigue, weakness, and flaccid paralysis. Basal ganglia symptoms may include parkinsonism, thalamic syndrome, and choreo-athetosis. Diminution and loss of corneal and pupillary reflexes are common.

Other Drugs

Several other drugs may occasionally produce delirium, particularly belladonna, chloral hydrate, and paraldehyde. Of these, belladonna probably leads most frequently to toxic symptoms. Occasionally patients, especially children, may develop delirium following the introduction of atropine into the eye. In addition to the usual physiological symptoms, the patient manifests a delirium marked by fear, excitement, and visual and auditory hallucinations. Prolonged use of chloral hydrate may lead to a delirium lasting two or more weeks.

Recently there have been noted both acute and chronic symptoms of cerebral insufficiency in individuals exposed to organic phosphorus insecticides which may irreversibly inhibit cholinesterase.

BIBLIOGRAPHY

Angyal, A.: Predisposing factors in bromide intoxication. Arch. Neurol. & Psychiat., 49:359–382, 1943.

Blackman, S. S., Jr.: Lesions of lead encephalitis in children. Bull. Johns Hopkins Hosp., 61:1–61, 1937.

Connell, P. H.: Amphetamine Psychosis. New York, Basic Books, Inc., 1958.

Cumings, J. N.: Heavy Metals and the Brain. Springfield, Illinois, Charles C Thomas, 1959.

Domzalski, C. A., Kolb, L. C., and Hines, E. A.: Delirious reactions secondary to thiocyanate therapy of hypertension. Proc. Staff Meet., Mayo Clinic, 28:272–280, 1953.

Gilbert, G. J., and Glaser, G. H.: Neurologic manifestations of chronic carbon monoxide poisoning. New Eng. J. Med., 261:1217–1220, 1959.

Goolker, P., and Schein, J.: Psychic effects of ACTH and cortisone. Psychosom. Med., 15:589–613, 1953.

Isbell, H.: Barbiturate Poisoning. In Cecil and Loeb, Textbook of Medicine, 10th ed. Philadelphia, W. B. Saunders Company, 1959, pp. 1631–1636.

Idem: Chronic Amphetamine Poisoning. (Ibid., pp. 1644–1645.)

Jenkins, C. D., and Mellins, R. B.: Lead poisoning in children. Arch. Neurol. & Psychiat., 77: 70–78, 1957.

Karpinski, F. E., Rieders, F., and Gersh, L. S.: Calcium disodium versenate in the therapy of lead encephalopathy. J. Pediat., 42:687–699, 1953.

Levin, M.: Toxic Psychoses. In Arieti, S., Ed.: American Handbook of Psychiatry. New York, Basic Books, Inc., 1959, pp. 1222–1229.

Perkins, H. A.: Bromide intoxication. Arch. Int. Med., 85:783–794, 1950.

Pleasure, H.: Psychiatric and neurologic side effects of isoniazid and iproniazid. Arch. Neurol. & Psychiat., 72:313–320, 1954.

Ritchie, E. A.: Toxic psychosis under cortisone and corticotrophin. J. Ment. Sc., 102:830–837, 1956.

Chapter Ten

ALCOHOLISM AND ALCOHOLIC PSYCHOSES

"In the bottle, discontent seeks for comfort, cowardice for courage, and bashfulness for confidence."
Samuel Johnson (1709–1784)

Alcoholism and the disturbances of metabolism often associated with it may lead to both acute and chronic brain syndromes. It seems desirable, however, to include a discussion of both of these syndromes in one chapter as well as that of various other aspects of indulgence in alcohol.

The subject of the use and effect of alcoholic liquors, whether considered from sociological, physiological, or psychiatric points of view, still provokes much discussion and wide divergence of opinion. Unfortunately, moralistic implications have retarded the development of a scientific understanding and rational management of alcoholism. Perhaps there is no group of persons in greater need of understanding than alcoholics. It is estimated that there are about four and one-half million persons in the United States on whose lives drinking has an adverse effect in one way or another, also that at least 12,000 alcoholics die each year from chronic alcoholism. Five out of six alcoholics are men between the ages of 30 and 55—the most productive years. Alcoholism, therefore, constitutes a major health problem.

Psychogenic Factors in Alcoholism

Psychological knowledge and experience show that a practice so universal as that of the use of alcohol must exist because it satisfies some deep-seated psychological need. This need, it often appears, is for relief from the tensions which have been induced by conflicts, resentments, frustrations, and other sources of anxiety. Anxiety is such a constant and universal experience of mankind and alcohol is so effective in alleviating it that its use has been widespread for centuries. A well-adjusted person has anxieties but is able to manage them without resorting to measures that tend to disturb his personality. His personality is mature, relatively well organized, and his tolerance for anxiety, guilt, and frustration is adequate. His need for relief from these factors is small and may be met by a few mildly neurotic traits. In contrast, if the individual is emotionally dependent and immature and his tensions are extreme or his tolerance for anxiety and frustration is low, he may either develop a neurotic reaction or resort to excessive drinking, even to intoxication and its blotting out of reality, as an easy means of relief and of handling his difficulties. Any act that readily results in a reduction of anxiety tends to become a habit. All too frequently, therefore, the use of alcohol as a means of narcotizing anxiety becomes habitual. The strength of the habit depends upon the degree of anxiety which prompts it and the capacity of alcohol to reduce anxiety. At the same time, also, the alcoholic, below the level of conscious awareness, develops an obsessive nucleus of thoughts and feelings that drinking, and only drinking, will effectively quiet the maladjustments that make life uncomfortable or even unbearable. Alcohol serves, too, to create a vicious circle that aids in fixing the habit, since its use lowers the capacity for repression and releases inhibitions. The alcoholic expresses his aggressive, sexual, or dependent tendencies inappropriately; he develops resentments when they are frustrated and later, with sober reflection, presents guilt and remorse. Such feelings and reactions constitute sources of more excessive indulgence. Thus, alcohol defeats the ends for which it is taken.

Why, with the many neurotic, psychosomatic, or psychotic methods of defense or escape equally available, the individual makes use of alcohol is not readily determined. A person with strongly-developed defense mechanisms, although he may acquire a restricted personality through them, often becomes able to protect himself against anxiety through the development of character traits or other internal operation. A person who lacks such automatic protection against anxiety may develop either alcoholism or neurosis. Either or both may be established to deal with similar types of anxiety-producing problems. Somehow the alcoholic is unable to construct as defenses against anxiety the character traits which the relatively well-adjusted person employs or the overt neurotic symptoms which the psychoneurotic constructs. Sometimes, moreover, a patient, after long use of alcohol as an anxiety-reducing measure, finds this expedient inadequate and he resorts also, as it were, to an overt anxiety neurosis, to psychosomatic symptoms or

to a psychosis, as a more drastic measure for dealing with his anxieties, frustrations, and conflicts. The psychopathologic conditions leading to alcoholism vary with the individual alcoholic. It would appear in many instances that the addictive drinker may have been psychologically traumatized very early in life and his personality remained fixated at an early, oral stage of development. Again, alcoholism may occur in persons who, through the absence of a desirable identification figure, never developed a stabilizing superego. Lacking in responsibility and ego strength, they are closely allied to the character neurotic. Sometimes the periodic drinker seems by his alcoholic bout to be seeking for relief from an overly strict superego. In some instances there are presumably unconscious homosexual identifications and tendencies. If his drinking continues and the alcoholic pattern becomes established, the disregard of reality which it brings about begins to operate and serves as a further but undesirable defense.

From what has been said, it naturally follows that an understanding of the psychopathologic conditions associated with alcohol can only be obtained by taking into account the developmental organization of the individual personality and its sources of anxiety rather than by stressing any specifically poisonous properties of alcohol. The particular reaction manifested by the individual is usually, in effect, an unmasking or accentuation of his previous personality, of its conflicts and of its defenses. If excessive alcoholism is continued, a social deterioration and a disintegration of the patient's value system frequently results from his habit.

Social and cultural factors influence the amount of alcoholism. It is, for example, distinctly less frequent among Jews and Chinese. Doubtless in some instances heavy drinking is merely the result of a wish to conform to group mores and represents a needed prestige-giving activity. Broadly speaking, however, the causes of alcoholism are the same as are those productive of neuroses in the nonalcoholic. If an individual with a low anxiety tolerance lives in a social set which imposes heavy social penalties on intoxication, he may take recourse to other and frankly neurotic escapes. In general, anxieties, frustrations, fixations in psychosexual development, and prolonged strain of situational difficulties are other mainsprings of unconscious motivations for alcoholism. While alcoholism is symptomatic of psychopathology, it is a symptom which has become a disease.

Physiological Effects

While alcohol affects all cells of the body, its most marked effect is on the cells of the brain and is therefore manifested in behavior. Since alcohol does not require prior digestion, it may be absorbed directly into the blood. The rate of absorption is much more rapid than its elimination, with the result that with heavy indulgence a considerable concentration may occur. While there is an individual tolerance, it is generally accepted that a person showing a concentration of 150 mg. or more of alcohol in 100 ml. of blood, or its equivalent in urine, saliva, or breath, should be considered as intoxicated. In the opinion of the National Safety Council Committee on Tests for Intoxication, this concentration so impairs judgment and performance in driving an automobile as to render the operation of a car unsafe.

The first stage in the oxidation of alcohol consists in the formation of acetaldehyde. While to some degree this occurs elsewhere, it largely takes place in the liver. The second stage of oxidation of alcohol is from acetaldehyde to acetic acid. This occurs not only in the liver but in other organs as well. With the use of disulfiram, combustion of acetaldehyde is inhibited and may reach toxic levels. Finally, acetic acid is oxidized to carbon dioxide and water.

As previously indicated, alcohol is used for its tension-reducing effect. Since it reduces his anxiety, the alcoholic seeks its use more and more frequently and to the exclusion of more acceptable methods. His addiction is manifested not only by this persistent use but also by the effects of its withdrawal. These results may be moderate, such as increased anxiety, a craving for alcohol, weakness, tremor, and perspiration, but may be even serious and include anorexia, nausea, vomiting, fever, tachycardia, convulsions, hallucinations, and delirium tremens.

Although alcohol has long been known to be a depressant to brain function, its method of action is still uncertain. It is thought that it may be by interference with synaptic transmission. The effect of alcohol on the brain is from above downward. Higher cortical functions such as judgment, memory, learning, self-criticism, and environmental awareness suffer first. With depression of higher functions, lower parts of the brain are released from higher control. Thus the excitement frequently seen in an intoxicated person is doubtless a release phenomenon resulting from a depression of the highest brain functions. With the ingestion of excessively large amounts of alcohol, this gradually descending depressive effect may extend to the entire brain and inhibit not only the supramedullary areas but even the medulla with its respiratory, cardiac, and vasomotor centers.

Alcoholism and Crime

It was formerly stated that alcoholism was directly responsible for a large, perhaps a major, part of crime. There is now an increasing tendency to consider that both alcohol and criminalism are caused by similar social and psychological factors. Emotional instability and other expressions of a poorly integrated personality characterize both the recidivous criminal offender and the alcohol addict. More frequently is the relation of alcohol to crime one of a common cause rather than of cause and effect. It should be added, however, that the drinking of alcohol tends to be accompanied by a release of sexual and aggressive impulses.

Alcoholism and Psychoses

The relation between alcohol and the so-called alcoholic psychoses is not as simple as was formerly assumed. In many instances alcohol serves merely to release a reaction that is primarily psychogenic with factors intrinsic in the personality. In other cases there is such an interplay of psychogenic and metabolic factors that the picture becomes complex. In Korsakoff's syndrome and in chronic alcoholic deterioration, the psychosis is not, as was formerly believed, caused by the toxic effects of the alcohol itself but by thiamine deficiency. Even in this, the structure of the personality influences the picture. It is important to remember, too, that alcoholism may be a symptom—sometimes the most obvious symptom—of another psychosis such as paresis or manic-depressive psychosis.

PATHOLOGICAL INTOXICATION

Occasionally an individual of unstable personality may, on partaking of alcohol, suffer from a transitory mental state much more striking in the nature and severity of the symptoms than ordinary drunkenness, and known as pathological intoxication. The onset is dramatically sudden. Consciousness is impaired, and the patient is confused, disoriented, suffers from illusions, hallucinations of sight, and transitory delusions. Activity is exaggerated, impulsive, and aggressive, even to the point of destructiveness. The emotional disturbances are profound and may consist of rage, anxiety, or depression, perhaps with suicidal attempt. The disorder lasts from a few minutes to a day or more and is usually followed by a prolonged sleep, after awakening from which there is an amnesia for the episode.

There is an increasing tendency to consider that such episodes with their disturbances of consciousness and perhaps crimes of violence are really instances of psychomotor epilepsy released by alcohol in persons predisposed to such seizures.

The behavior observed in "pathological intoxication" is in many ways illustrated by the following case:

N. W., aged 28, was seen in jail while awaiting trial on a charge of drunkenness and disorderly conduct. The patient's father had committed suicide as he was about to be sent to a hospital for mental diseases. The patient himself was described as being a friendly but quick-tempered and restless individual whose marriage had terminated in early divorce. He was said never to have been particularly alcoholic, but on one July 4 he celebrated the holiday by drinking two bottles of beer and a glass of wine. Soon afterward he attempted to fling himself down an 80-foot embankment and was so greatly excited that he was taken to the police station for the night. The next morning he had no recollection of the affair. Ten months later the patient called late one afternoon to see friends who invited him to sample what they considered choice varieties of whiskey and gin. He accepted their invitation and drank somewhat more heavily than usual. Soon after leaving the home of his friends he was observed by a police officer to be acting strangely. As the officer spoke to him he attacked him. While the officer was calling for help, the patient disappeared. About fifteen minutes later two women were startled to see a strange man thrust his head through a closed window of their living room and shout, "Help! Murder!" It was the patient, who then ran on to another house where he rang the doorbell insistently. As the occupant answered the summons he again screamed, "Murder!" and ran to the street once more, where he broke the windshields and headlights of several parked automobiles and tore out the seats and pulled parts from other cars. At this point he was seized and taken to the police station where, on awakening the following morning, he had no recollection of his experiences of the previous night.

Treatment of Acute Alcoholism

In the majority of instances, bouts of acute alcoholism may be terminated by withdrawal to a supportive, non-stimulating environment, with provision to insure adequate sleep and rest. In such circumstances, bodily processes quickly metabolize the excessive alcohol.

In cases of prolonged drinking the patient may be much dehydrated and be vomiting. In such a case liquids containing nutritional elements may be given intravenously. A saline solution containing 5 per cent of dextrose may be given in 1000 to 2000 ml. doses in the course of 12 to 24 hours. This may be repeated every day for three days if necessary. It is well to add an ampule of vitamin B complex and ascorbic acid.

In many ways a satisfactory method of treating severe cases of acute alcoholism is by the use of insulin, which accelerates the metabolism of alcohol in the body. Before administration it is advisable to determine the blood sugar level to make sure that the insulin is not given during a hypoglycemic state. If there is no contraindication to its use, the patient is placed in bed and given 46 to 60 units of insulin hypodermically. If this amount is not sufficient to produce somnolence, thirst, and diaphoresis in one and one-half hours, 20 additional units may be given intravenously. Because of the possibility of convulsions, an experienced nurse should be in constant attendance. If the initial dose produces convulsions or deep coma, the patient should receive 5 to 10 gm. of glucose intravenously or 4 to 6 oz. of sweetened fruit juice by mouth. Treatment, with its relaxation and sleep, is continued for two and one-half hours and then terminated by the administration of 8 oz. of fruit juice to which an ounce of sugar is added. While under the influence of insulin, the patient is given large quantities of water to drink. Following the treatment, he receives a full meal. One treatment may be sufficient, but two, three, or four may be required. More than one treatment in the first 24 hours may be advisable.

If the patient is extremely drowsy and somnolent or depressed as a result of excessive ingestion of alcohol, such effects can be counteracted by the use of caffeine and sodium benzoate, Dexedrine, or Benzedrine.

OTHER DRUGS. The various barbiturates have been widely used. Today, however, the consensus is that these drugs are neither necessary nor desirable in the treatment of the alcoholic. Their habituating properties will often lead the addictive alcoholic to switch from alcohol to barbiturates for relief. Another drug that has enjoyed great popularity is paraldehyde. It is little more than a hypnotic, however, and renders the patient sleepy and drowsy even after awakening. If it is desired to continue this drug with chlorpromazine, it should be remembered that the chlorpromazine has a potentiating effect on the sedative and but a fraction of the ordinary dose of paraldehyde should be given. For a long time the use of the aqueous solution of adrenal cortex

extract was popular and is still used intravenously to some extent. The dosage varies from 10 to 30 ml. in 1000 ml. of saline solution injected over a period of several hours.

Chlorpromazine, or chlorpromazine and meprobamate combined, are now extensively used to relieve the symptoms of acute alcoholism. Used in relatively large doses, they produce prompt control of motor excitement and of nausea and vomiting, permit restful, relaxed sleep, and contribute to the relief of tension and anxiety.

DELIRIUM TREMENS

This is an acute psychosis that may develop in the chronic alcoholic following an unusually severe or prolonged debauch. The term *delirium tremens* was first used by Thomas Sutton in 1813 in what is regarded as the classic description of this disease. The nature of the factors that operate in its production is uncertain. It has long been considered as an acute psychosis developed during drinking. At the present time, however, some psychiatrists believe it is a withdrawal syndrome precipitated in the chronic alcoholic suddenly deprived of alcohol. In some instances, at least, this is probably the case, as delirium has been produced in the experimental laboratory by the sudden withdrawal of alcohol in those consuming 12 oz. or more of the agent for 48 or more days. The withdrawal may be associated not only with delirium and sometimes with convulsions but also abnormalities in the encephalogram. On the other hand, the disorder may arise from metabolic disturbances including faulty carbohydrate metabolism, impairment of the detoxicating function of the liver, disturbed protein metabolism, acidosis, suboxidation of the brain, disturbed water balance, and various nutritional deficiencies, particularly of vitamin B which the alcoholic usually takes in insufficient amounts and may not be able to absorb. Absorption of toxins from the gastrointestinal tract may also be a factor in producing the toxic state. The patient is usually dehydrated and the blood chlorides are low.

Delirium tremens is rare in a person under thirty years of age, or after less than three or four years of chronic alcoholism. The delirium is usually preceded by an aversion for food, restlessness, irritability, and disturbed sleep in which terrifying dreams occur. Occasional illusions and hallucinations are soon followed by more frequent ones, usually of a fleeting, terrifying nature. Figures on the wallpaper become menacing animate objects; inkspots become insects which the patient attempts to seize and destroy. The visual hallucinations are often of objects that appear to be moving, and are particularly apt to represent loathsome animals of fantastic shapes which terrify the patient and from which he may struggle to escape. These imaginery animals may be of diminutive size. At times hallucinations can be suggested; the patient, for example, may be handed an imaginary thread which, in response to instructions, he will carefully wind about his finger. Tactile hallucinations, probably associated with peripheral neuritis, are not infrequent. The patient feels as well as sees the insects on his skin. Olfactory hallucinations may occur. The patient may exclaim with terror that gas is being pumped into his room. While visual hallucinations are most numerous, yet auditory ones are not infrequently added.

As indicated, the mood is usually one of irritability, fear, apprehension, and even of terror. Occasionally, however, it is one of euphoria, amusement, good-natured silliness, or grim humor accompanied by the narration of preposterous confabulations.

Consciousness is clouded, and the patient may be greatly confused with disorientation for time and place. Speech is often incoherent. Persons about the patient may be misidentified. Attention is fleeting and impressions are retained but a moment. Not rarely the delirium is of an occupational type. The motor restlessness is marked. The patient repeatedly gets out of bed to attend to some detail of his supposed occupation or to seize some imaginary object. Sleep is usually impossible.

On physical examination, the conjunctivae and face are ordinarily found to be congested. The pupils are dilated and often react slowly. A coarse tremor is an almost constant accompaniment. It is increased by muscular tension, such as extension of the fingers. The tongue is tremulous, as are also the muscles of the lips and face in well-developed cases. The pulse is rapid and often irregular and weak. The temperature is elevated and in some cases may be high. The skin is moist, the face often showing marked perspiration. The tendon reflexes are usually increased although occasionally absent because of neuropathy. At times the nerve trunks and muscles may be painful to pressure. Albuminuria exists in about half the cases. Epileptiform seizures may occur. The cause of the seizures is somewhat uncertain. At times the patient is an epileptic in whom convulsions were precipitated by alcohol. Again, they may be caused by toxic products in the alcohol or by cerebral damage that has resulted from its use. As mentioned before, convulsions may follow sudden withdrawal of alcohol in the chronic drinker.

Differential Diagnosis

Delirium tremens is to be differentiated from other forms of alcoholic hallucinosis as well as brain syndromes. Among the latter, and particularly pertinent to the group of alcoholic patients, is the delirious state associated with *acute hepatic insufficiency* and referred to sometimes as *impending hepatic* coma. Alcoholic cirrhosis of the liver is the most common cause of the condition, although it may occur with other illnesses which lead to severe disturbance of the brain parenchyma. The importance of its discrimination rests upon the necessity of prescribing quite differing therapy; that for delirium tremens may lead to a fatal outcome in the patient with impending hepatic coma.

While both conditions may follow a

period of heavy drinking, delirium tremens more often has its onset after cessation of drinking. The patient with delirium tremens is consciously responsive unless sedated, often aggressive and destructive, and his hallucinatory experiences are generally visual. The patient with impending hepatic coma more often is dull and lethargic, with diminution of psychomotor activity, and seldom has vividly-formed visual hallucinations. Perhaps the most characteristic differential point is the irregular, "flapping" tremor which presents itself on extension of the arms in hepatic insufficiency. Speech is more often slowed, slurred, or monotonous with perseveration and a mask-like facial expression may be seen. Both flexor muscle tonus and tendon reflexes are increased.

Those with impending hepatic coma usually subside into stupor with little indication of anxiety or fear, and there is more likely to be hypersomnia than the insomnia of the individual with delirium tremens. Hyperphagia exists with liver disorder in contrast to the anorexia of the delirium tremens.

Also, the general medical examination in hepatic coma often shows evidence of jaundice, gross hepatomegaly, fetor hepaticus with elevation of the blood ammonia; these findings are absent in delirium tremens.

Pathology

Changes both of a degenerative and of an inflammatory nature may occur. The brain is usually edematous. There is more or less liquefactive degeneration of nerve cells and an increase of glia with some round-cell infiltration. There is degeneration of myelin sheaths, especially in the cerebellum. Punctate hemorrhages occur and there is a mild degree of leptomeningitis.

Prognosis and Course

Delirium tremens usually runs an acute course terminating from three to ten days. Convalescence is frequently preceded by a prolonged sleep following which consciousness becomes clear and the hallucinations disappear, although brief periods of delirium may occasionally recur at night for a short time. The prognosis depends largely upon the presence or absence of coexisting disease. The existence of myocardial degeneration, which is not uncommon in such chronic alcoholic patients, makes the prognosis much less favorable. The mortality in the type of case that reaches a hospital averages from 5 to 15 per cent, the two most frequent causes of death being heart failure and pneumonia. Occasionally, instead of terminating in death or recovery within the usual period, the psychosis may merge into a Korsakoff's psychosis.

Treatment

It has been customary to withdraw alcohol at once, but this practice is questionable. Gastric lavage is advisable to remove both any remaining alcohol and the mucus and other products of chronic gastritis. It is of great importance that care must be taken to conserve the strength of a patient suffering from delirium tremens. The patient suffering from this disease should be placed in bed immediately, and as he is usually fearful he should be constantly supervised and reassured concerning his fears and hallucinations. Many a patient has died from exhaustion while struggling under mechanical restraint or from the depressing effect of sedative drugs. Restraint should therefore never be employed. Chlorpromazine, given in divided doses either orally or by the intramuscular route and up to 1.0 gm. in a 24-hour period, has proved effective in preventing overactivity, providing sleep, and improving appetite. While it does not modify the delusional or hallucinatory state or shorten the course greatly, the anxiety is much relieved. The agent is contraindicated when serious infection or cardiac disturbance co-exists or following the recent use of other drugs. Cardiac stimulation by means of caffeine is usually to be recommended. It is frequently desirable to give some of the less depressing hypnotics such as paraldehyde in doses of 3 to 4 drams one to three times a day.

Other sedation should be avoided. Morphine should never be given. Corticotropin in 25-mg. doses at four-hour intervals may help to bring about a more rapid recovery. This can be given intramuscularly or intravenously in dextrose and saline solution.

It is generally agreed that the patient should receive large amounts of dextrose, the normal nutritive material of the brain. This may be given in the form of frequent, large quantities of orange juice or as intravenous administration of 100 ml. of 50 per cent glucose repeated, if necessary, every three hours. Thiamine chloride (50 to 100 mg.) and nicotinic acid (10 mg.) should be given immediately and repeated three times daily. These vitamins may be added to the infusions for intravenous use. Alcohol disappears from the blood more rapidly if the patient receives 15 units of insulin three or four times a day. The administration of sodium chloride is advisable both to combat dehydration and to increase the alkali reserve. Capsules containing 2 gm. of sodium chloride should be given every four hours. In those patients in whom delirium and marked tremor exist, the possibility of magnesium deficiency must be considered. With evidence of depression of the serum magnesium (normal 2.0 milliequivalents per liter), magnesium sulfate in a 5 per cent sterile solution may be given in doses up to 2.0 gm. four times daily for three days and then 1.0 gm. per day for an additional two or three days.

Unless the patient is also suffering from cardiac failure or there is some other general medical contraindication, he should receive 3000 to 4000 ml. of fluids a day. Orange juice is by far the most desirable form of liquid, since it combats acidity, supplies certain minerals and vitamin C, and perhaps helps to prevent or overcome infection. Milk should also be given freely. Many physicians recommend the use of high enemas twice a day both for the chronic constipation usually existing and for the additional fluids thus made available. The former practice of dehydrating the patient on the theory that he may have cerebral edema ("wet brain") is no longer followed. Likewise, very few physicians now recommend lumbar puncture for the purpose of withdrawing cerebrospinal fluid. The patient has usually eaten little or nothing for several days. Since his gastrointestinal tract suffers from catarrhal inflammation because of his long indulgence in alcohol, he has little appetite and may even be nauseated. It is, however, exceedingly important that he receive an abundant, soft diet, particularly of carbohydrates. If possible, it should contain from 3000 to 4000 calories a day and should be rich in vitamins. The administration of the entire vitamin B complex would seem especially advisable as a preventive of Wernicke's syndrome or encephalopathy from nicotinic acid deficiency. One should not hesitate to employ tube feeding if necessary.

In contrast to the above treatment, alcoholic patients with the deliria of *impending hepatic coma* must be placed on a protein-free diet and fed with fruit juices and dextrose. Tranquilizers, sedatives, and methionine are to be avoided, while tetracycline, 1-2 gm. daily, and infusions of sodium glutamate (25 to 100 gm. daily in glucose solution) and L-arginine may be given to lower the blood ammonia.

KORSAKOFF'S PSYCHOSIS

Sometimes it will be noted in what, except for the absence of the usual critical sleep, appeared to be an ordinary case of delirium tremens that the hallucinations and acute delirium disappear but the clinical picture merges into one characterized by amnesia, disorientation for time and place, and a falsification of memory, associated with the symptoms and signs of peripheral neuropathy. At other times the syndrome develops in the chronic alcoholic who has not suffered from a preceding delirium tremens but has indulged excessively in alcohol for several years. This syndrome was described in 1887 by the Russian psychiatrist, Sergei Korsakoff. Because of its frequent association with chronic alcoholism, Korsakoff's psychosis has long been classified among the alcoholic psychoses. Strictly speaking, this syndrome should not be classified among them.

Etiology and Pathology

The condition is but one of several syndromes that result from vitamin B deficiency, a form of deficiency to which the chronic alcoholic with his impaired gastrointestinal absorption, his diet largely limited to vitamin-free alcohol, and his increased vitamin requirement resulting from the high caloric effect of alcohol, is especially prone. Vitamin B deficiency may, of course, exist under various circumstances. Although a deficiency of other vitamin B constituents doubtless contributes to these syndromes, thiamine and niacin deficiencies are particularly responsible for them. The variations in these syndromes depend largely upon the parts of the nervous system in which the neuronal degeneration is localized. If this degeneration is largely in the cerebrum and the peripheral nerves, a Korsakoff's syndrome results. If the degenerative changes occur in the long peripheral nerves of the alcoholic, the result is known as "alcoholic neuritis." If the greatest deficiency is in niacin and the degeneration is marked in the cerebrum, less in the spinal cord and least in the peripheral nerves, the vitamin deficiency encephalopathy assumes the form of pellagra. If the brain stem is the site of the degenerative process, the syndrome is that of Wernicke's disease. Frequently these syndromes are not sharply defined but merge one into another, the pattern depending upon the vitamin in which the deficiency is greatest and upon the sites and extent of the degeneration. For example, symptoms of Korsakoff's psychosis and Wernicke's disease or of Wernicke's disease and pellagra may be associated. In fact, in nutritional encephalopathy it is possible in the same individual to see delirium tremens, Korsakoff's psychosis, niacin deficiency encephalopathy, and the Wernicke syndrome.

The nutritional encephalopathy is probably caused by the fact that in the absence of ample quantities of thiamine and nicotinic acid there is an impaired oxidation of pyruvic acid during the breakdown of glucose.

The histopathology of Korsakoff's psychosis consists of diffuse parenchymatous changes. Among these changes are axonal alterations, a deposition of excessive amounts of normal lipochrome pigment in the nerve cells, glia, microglia, and around the blood vessels in the prefrontal and motor cortex, and acute chromatolytic changes in the larger nerve cells in these areas, especially in the Betz cells.

Symptoms

The most conspicuous symptoms have already been indicated. Superficially, consciousness may appear clear and the seriousness of the mental disorder may not be apparent. On questioning the patient, however, one is often surprised to discover the extent of mental impairment. Although possessing a relatively good grasp of what is in sight, he is disoriented as to that which is beyond immediate observation and dependent on memory. At first the memory loss is most marked for events occurring since the onset of the disease, but later the memory for remote events is lost also. The amnesia is anterograde, and frequently the patient cannot recall what has just been said to him. He usually presents a superficial cheerfulness and often evades inquiries by jocularities. In his confabulation the patient relates fictitious memories which superficially conceal the actual amnesia. The pseudo-reminiscences which usually vary from day to day can often be suggested and guided by leading questions, with the result that the patient will narrate whatever fictitious reminiscence is proposed. Presumably the patient's confabulations serve as a defense against anxiety by concealing from himself his defective functioning. The patient characteristically presents a jovial mood and often misidentifies people about him. Disorientation, especially as to time, usually exists. The polyneuropathy, which is sometimes absent, is most marked in the legs, with pain, tenderness over the nerve trunks, absent knee jerks, and, in severe cases, foot drop and wrist drop. The disease is relatively more frequent in women.

Course and Prognosis

Many cases clear up after six or eight weeks, with approximate restoration to mental health. If the process is not fully reversible, the disease continues for several months, with a gradual improvement but without complete return of memory. In some cases there is a permanent impairment of efficiency and a certain degree of intellectual, emotional, and esthetic deterioration. The neuropathy usually improves rather rapidly and often completely disappears. A Korsakoff-like amnesia with confabulations serving to fill in the losses of memory may occur in uremia, after brain trauma, in general paresis, and in other organic and toxic diseases of the brain—conditions in which the pathogenesis does not seem related to dietary deficiency. If irreversible changes have not already occurred, the active symptoms may rapidly disappear. Insight is not usually regained.

Treatment

The first step in treatment is the discontinuance of the use of alcohol. To correct the deficiency of vitamin B_1, 20 to 50 gm. of thiamine chloride may be given daily for a few days, to be followed by 20 gm. of powdered brewers' yeast in iced milk three times a day. Milk, fruit, eggs, meat, and other foods rich in vitamin B complex should be liberally provided. It is probably advisable to administer ascorbic acid also. If irreversible structural changes have already taken place, the symptoms are not affected by vitamins. As in other mental disorders associated with chronic alcoholism, daily doses of insulin are often advisable. When acute neuropathy exists, rest in bed is desirable. Care should be exercised to prevent permanent foot drop. As soon as pain and tenderness in the legs have disappeared, massage and electricity are of value. The patient should then be encouraged to move his feet.

ACUTE HALLUCINOSIS

Since excessive indulgence in alcohol is the occasion of the symptom complex to be considered, it has usually been classified as an alcoholic psychosis. The present tendency is to look upon it as a psychogenic reaction liberated by alcoholic excess rather than as a purely toxic expression. It seems reasonably safe to state that the clinical characteristics are determined by personality factors. Some cases lead one to believe that the disorder is a schizophrenic reaction released by alcohol. However, recent clinical studies have disclosed that the majority of individuals with this syndrome are cyclothymic or extroverted individuals, with a family and developmental history quite unlike that of the schizophrenic. Cases diagnosed as chronic alcoholic hallucinosis ultimately become obvious paranoid schizophrenic reactions.

From the histories of cases of prolonged inebriation with onset shortly after withdrawal of alcohol or restriction of intake, it appears likely that this acute condition represents a type of an alcoholic abstinence syndrome, perhaps occurring in individuals with a constitutional predominance for auditory imagery. Pure alcoholic hallucinosis occurs much less commonly than does delirium tremens or hallucinatory states with both visual and auditory hallucinations.

Symptoms

As in the case of delirium tremens, acute alcoholic hallucinosis develops only after the prolonged and excessive use of alcohol, although usually it is precipitated by increased indulgence. Descriptively the reaction may be summarized as one of auditory hallucinosis occurring in a clear sensorium accompanied affectively by marked fear. In the majority of cases, the hallucinations are usually accusatory, or threatening, or both. The voices are particularly apt to accuse the patient of homosexual practices and to call him indecent names. In women, as in men, the hallucinations are frequently accusatory and of sexual content. The voices, however, accuse the patient of heterosexual offenses rather than of homosexual ones as in men. The hallucinated voices often refer to the patient in the third person and threaten him with such expressions as, "Now shoot him;" "Let's cut him up tonight." The patient may hear the firing of pistols or other sounds suggesting a threat of attack. Not infrequently, in the case of the operator of some mechanical equipment, the hallucinations appear at first to come from his machine and to be synchronous with the rhythmical sound of its operation. In a few the vocal hallucinations are benign and may or may not affect the behavior of the patient. Olfactory hallucinations are not infrequently associated. Illusions of sight are not uncommon. Visual hallucinations may be intermingled to a slight extent but are rarely present in a typical case.

The patient's ideational content and his behavior are determined by the acceptance of his hallucinations as reality. Ideas of reference and misinterpretations are common. A delusional system is rapidly acquired, while additions and elaborations are quickly introduced. The patient may appeal to the police for protection or arm himself in self-defense.

In contrast to its disturbance in delirium tremens, consciousness remains clear in alcoholic hallucinosis and the patient continues to be oriented, projecting his hallucinations into a real environment. In another respect, too, acute hallucinosis differs from delirium tremens: After recovery there is no amnesia for events occurring during its course.

The disturbance in mood is usually pronounced, being characteristically one of fear and apprehension. Terror-stricken by the threats of his imaginary pursuers, or reduced to despair by the accusing voices and his panic state, the patient may attempt to end his own life. The fear may at times be accompanied by anger or depression. Not infrequently

there is an element of irritability, while during the temporary cessation of the hallucinations the characteristic alcoholic humor may be manifested.

Course

Recovery from alcoholic hallucinosis usually occurs in five days to a month. Recurrences are common if the patient again indulges excessively in alcohol. Unlike delirium tremens, alcoholic hallucinosis is never followed by the Korsakoff syndrome. Occasionally the hallucinatory episode continues beyond the usual period and merges into a manifest schizophrenia.

Psychological Factors

Mention has already been made of the fact that acute hallucinosis is not always an uncolored alcoholic psychosis. There seems reason to believe that if a certain type of personality takes large quantities of alcohol over a considerable period of time, a psychogenic reaction of an acute schizophrenic nature may be liberated. The frequent history of unsuccessful heterosexual adjustment in the patient with alcoholic hallucinosis and the homosexual character of the hallucinations suggest that in some cases, at least, unrecognized homosexual tendencies may be the psychopathogenic factor which has both prompted the use of alcohol and determined the nature of the hallucinations. As to the psychogenic determination of the mood in alcoholic hallucinosis, one may speculatively suggest that the unconscious sense of threat to the personality in the biologically destructive and socially prohibited homosexual impulse is greater than the feeling of guilt which this repressed impulse sometimes arouses; hence the mood is usually one of fear rather than of depression. From the standpoint of self-respect, too, fear is psychologically preferable to shame. If the sense of guilt is relatively strong, then the patient exhibits the depression occasionally seen in the disease.

Treatment

The treatment consists in placing the

patient under such supervision that he may neither commit an indiscreet act nor do harm to himself. All alcohol must, of course, be withdrawn. The continuous bath assists in calming fear and anxiety. Chlorpromazine or related tranquilizing agents are useful for this purpose. The administration of food is not so difficult as in delirium tremens, but it should be given regularly and in abundance. It is well to give large amounts of orange juice, also vitamin B complex.

ALCOHOLIC PARANOIA

Clinically it is convenient to describe alcoholic paranoia, although its recognition as a true alcoholic psychosis is scarcely warrantable. Here, too, there may be a common factor—the repressed homosexual impulse—beneath both the alcoholism and the psychosis. Usually the patient has never established a wholesome, mature heterosexual relationship. In the prepsychotic life of the patient, we often find the same incomplete developments, fixations, traits of personality, and psychopathological processes as in other paranoid psychoses. In alcoholic paranoia, the use of alcohol, prompted by these tendencies, weakens repression and causes the vicious psychopathological circle of homosexual conflict, alcoholic indulgence, and paranoid delusion to continue without interruption. Psychologically the conditions were favorable for the development of a psychosis before the use of alcohol became excessive. In some cases one might almost say that a latent psychosis already existed and that the alcohol did no more than hasten its appearance. The previous personality pattern has been characterized by stubbornness, suspiciousness, resentment, projection, and other defensive mechanisms. The history of the future patient usually shows that he has accepted discipline poorly and that he has preferred the society of men.

Symptoms

This clinical manifestation is typically characterized by delusions of jealousy and infidelity. At first the patient is irritable, fault-finding, and distrustful. To these unpleasant defensive characteristics are later added accusations of marital infidelity, as evidence of which are cited the most insignificant and absurd arguments. With his jealousy motivated by an unrecognized sense of guilt and fear based on the odious trends and impulses of his own personality, the suspicious husband devises numerous schemes to entrap his wife and her supposed paramour.

A noncommissioned officer in the Army, whose enlistment had perhaps been prompted by an unrecognized homosexual interest, argued that he could not be the father of the child to which his wife had given birth inasmuch as it was born 279 instead of 280 days following marital relations with her. As evidence that the family physician was the father of the child, he cited the fact that on one occasion the doctor had not submitted his bill promptly. On several occasions, he threatened the life of the physician and finally actually attempted to shoot him.

Because of their incompletely developed and poorly integrated personalities, these patients are peculiarly inadequate for the sustained demands for social adaptation which marriage brings. By imputing to the wife, too, the interest which they fundamentally feel for other men, they secure an alleviation of anxiety. The ideas which follow are psychologically protective but adjustively disruptive. At times, with the increased use of intoxicants, impotence, produced by the toxic action of the alcohol on the central nervous system, increases the patient's sense of insecurity and incompetence, the prevention of any recognition of which requires a further development of ideas of infidelity.

Prognosis

The prognosis in the alcoholic paranoid state is not good. With the decrease in demands for adjustment that follows removal to a hospital, the patient may improve and no longer entertain his delusional ideas. At other times, having observed that the expression of his ideas has resulted in a deprivation of his liberty, he may dissimulate and maintain that he now recognizes he was in error and that he no longer doubts the fidelity of his wife. At any rate, after the return to the old situation, the former delusions and threatening behavior usually soon reappear.

WERNICKE'S SYNDROME

This encephalopathy, resulting from a deficiency in vitamin B, may be associated with alcoholic addiction or with other conditions in which this deficiency exists. It will be discussed in Chapter 18, Chronic Brain Syndrome Associated with Other Disturbances of Metabolism, Growth, or Nutrition.

ALCOHOLIC DETERIORATION

A considerable number of persons who consume large amounts of alcohol over a prolonged period ultimately suffer a certain disintegration of personality, the change ranging from an impairment of emotional stability and control to a noticeable dementia. The principal organic damage that alcohol inflicts upon the human nervous system is caused by avitaminosis rather than by primary toxic injury itself. From the standpoint of anatomical pathology there is, in the more severe cases, a progressive, chronic parenchymatous nervous degeneration, sometimes affecting a considerable part of the neuraxis. As previously indicated, so-called alcoholic dementia is caused by progressive atrophy of the cortex of the frontal lobes. The reaction seems to result from the toxic effects of ethanol rather than from malnutrition (avitaminosis).

Symptoms

One of the earliest mental symptoms of the abuse of alcohol is an increased tendency to act impulsively in accordance with primitive instinctive forces and the momentary affectivity. Because of various factors, particularly through a sense of rejection and frustration, the alcoholic patient develops resentment, hostility and feelings of guilt. Although, at least for a considerable period, a capacity for ethical sentiments remains, yet these are not sustained or applied, with the result that ethical purposes and strivings suffer, will is weakened, perseverance of endeavor is lost, and the patient becomes untruthful and unreliable. His tendency to deceive and to gloss over whatever is discreditable in behavior or character is but a part of a fundamental inability to face the facts of reality and of his own situation. He blames others for his failure and represents himself as abused and as the victim of circumstances for which he is in no way responsible, while at the same time he exaggerates his own achievements.

Affection is lost and ambition disappears. The confirmed alcoholic becomes careless as to his personal appearance and neglectful of his family. With an increasing egocentricity, his former sense of social or other responsibility disappears, or rather is avoided by the process of evasively treating it facetiously and superficially. Usually the patient's mood is one of unwarranted euphoria and carefree good humor, but a word of implied reproval may evoke a violent and profane outburst of irritability. A word of commiseration calls forth a ready tear, but, with a hearty slap on the back, his tears promptly give way to a cheerful laugh. With his friends, the alcoholic may be a congenial and welcome companion who enters enthusiastically into their pleasures, but at home he may be brutal, surly, and without shame. In nearly every instance, the patient's sex life is poorly adjusted, this failure in some instances serving as a cause of the alcoholism and in others representing a result. Not infrequently, this maladjustment operates to continue the vicious circle. A defensive attitude is assumed toward those who are not alcoholic in their habits, and the patient is touchy, irritable, and critical in the presence of those who he believes do not approve his excesses. There is an increasing poverty of ideas, with a growing incapacity for sustained attention and for more delicate discriminations. After a time, memory becomes impaired, and the insidious dementia finally becomes extreme. One patient, a physician, whose practice had been ruined by his habits, had abused his children and accused his wife of neglect and infidelity; he was unable to remember how long he had been in the hospital or give the name of his ward physician who had seen him daily for months. Psychometric examinations performed on alcoholic patients indicate that impairment of the mental functioning of various abilities precedes any clinical evidence of brain lesion.

Course and Outcome

If the use of alcohol is discontinued as soon as any early character changes are noted, there may be a nearly complete restoration to former mental health which, however, must always remain precarious, since the alcoholic was never well adjusted to life. Moreover, the alcoholic, in spite of his protests to the contrary, rarely wants to get well because alcohol provides the easiest way of escape from the difficulties which his inadequately integrated personality has precipitated. Deterioration of personality is permanent, and any actual dementia is, of course, quite irremediable.

Treatment

Unfortunately, alcoholism has long been regarded as simply a moral problem, with the result that the complex contributing factors have not received the scientific attention they have merited, and attention to therapy has not been commensurate with the extent of the social problem. "Even mental disease, one of the most persistently misunderstood and mismanaged of our social problems, is accorded better treatment than inebriety. The schizophrenic, the paretic, the manic depressive, provided, of course, that they make themselves sufficiently obnoxious to be legally adjudged 'insane,' are hospitalized and given treatment in a state-supported institution. But the inebriate, who, in addition, may well be a schizophrenic, or manic depressive, and who certainly makes himself even more obnoxious, is sternly admonished to mend his ways and is sentenced to the workhouse, there to seek insight into his behavior."*

Alcoholism should be looked upon as a psychic illness rooted in a personality disorder or immaturity. The tension-producing factors which have led to the alcoholism may be of a wide variety. Sometimes there has been a close mother attachment with resulting personality fixations and immaturities, again there may be latent or frank sexual maladjustments. Pathogenic intrafamily relationships are not rare. As in the psychoneuroses, with which alcoholism has much in common, the patient is usually unaware of the particular personality problems from which he has sought relief through the escape and anxiety-relieving mechanisms which alcohol facilitates. Theoretically, therefore, the object of treatment should be directed toward preventing the patient from desiring alcohol rather than toward restraining him from it. He must recognize, however, that he should never drink again. No addictive alcoholic can ever become a moderate, social drinker. All too rarely, even in the early days of his habit, will the patient co-operate in any adequate dynamic study of his personality or adjustment, or aid in the adoption of emotional compensations or socialized psychological substitutes that will relieve his anxiety and other tensions.

The patient should be approached with the attitude that his disorder is one of personality rather than of morality. The emphasis should not be on the alcoholism but on the individual in whom it occurs. Psychiatric treatment should have a basic routine program of active physical exercise, constructive occupational work, agreeable social relaxation, and psychotherapy. The patient's mental life and experiences should be reviewed for the purpose of discovering the main factors which have caused him to become dependent on alcohol. One must, therefore, obtain a thorough understanding of the

* Hewitt, C. C.: A Personality Study of Alcohol Addiction. Quart. J. Stud. on Alcohol, 4:368–386, 1943.

patient as a person and of his particular life situation. A psychoanalytically oriented approach, based on a careful understanding of psychodynamics, is the one that offers the greatest promise of success. Orthodox psychoanalytical techniques are usually not practicable with the addictive drinker, partly because of his instability and low tolerance to stress. Because of these characteristics, he usually resumes drinking whenever painful, unconscious material begins to come to the surface. A constructive analysis of his personality difficulties must be accompanied by a prolonged re-educational effort.

The alcoholic is usually a dependent personality and therefore needs continuous support over a long period of time, frequently for years. Frequently, too, he is a hostile, anxious, guilt-ridden person. Primitive or restraining measures that increase the patient's sense of being wronged and stir aggressive and resentful feelings should be avoided. The therapist should not condone his patient's alcoholic habits, yet he should not be critical. His attitude should be objective and impersonal. It should be remembered that the patient's rationalized reasons for his alcoholism are not the real reasons. It is often necessary to carry out the treatment in an institution, although in one where the patient can lead as normal a life as possible. In those instances in which there is a demonstrated dependent relationship upon a protecting person, often the mother, wife, or lover, who provides the alcohol and gives in to the insatiable demands of the alcoholic, this individual must also receive treatment in order to break the pathological bond that perpetuates the habit. Better results are secured in special institutions for alcoholics where planned psychotherapy is used. Psychotherapy is of course possible only in the habitué whose intellectual equipment is still sound. If dementia has occurred, he must usually be committed to an institution where he can no longer secure intoxicants and where both the patient and society may be protected from the results of his intellectual and moral defects.

Group psychotherapy of alcoholics is being employed with greater frequency and promises to become an increasingly useful method of treatment. The experience of being with other similarly afflicted people seems to make the alcoholic accept more readily treatment in the group environment. The interpretations offered by other members make the attainment of insight easier and less frightening. Individual psychoanalysis seems to be useful only in carefully selected cases. Its objectivity and depth of searching are apparently more than most alcoholics can tolerate.

ALCOHOLICS ANONYMOUS. In recent years an organization, Alcoholics Anonymous, established in 1935 in Akron, Ohio, and conducted by former alcoholics, has produced many temporary and even prolonged cures of alcoholic addiction. The organization now has over 100,000 members. Although it was organized without psychiatric guidance, and although its movement is largely limited to a social-religious program, it has been of great value in re-orienting many addicts in a socially-efficient way of life. Despite the fact that this program is very heavily weighted with an unrealistic optimism, it has constructively utilized many principles of group psychotherapy.

As a rule, members of Alcoholics Anonymous are above the average in intelligence, education, and social status, and their attitude toward the addict is tolerant and constructive. The organization offers the confirmed addict an opportunity to escape from his former psychosocial isolation, from the feeling that no one really understands or cares about him and that he can trust no one. In his group, the addict has a sense of belonging, of being understood and accepted, and of sharing common convictions. By means of his allegiance to the group, the member develops a religious fervor, and when he answers a call to aid another alcoholic at the cost of inconvenience and self-denial, his religious devotion is constructively internalized. An inspirational and mass-suggestion approach is an important feature.

By arousing a deep desire to help others and by creating a sense of responsibility for doing so, the organization contributes to the addict's cure. The opportunity to talk about himself in the group meetings affords the addict an opportunity for narcissistic satisfaction, for self-expression, and for therapeutic catharsis. The program of Alcoholics Anonymous ignores the cause of the alcoholic's addiction and focuses directly on the drinking itself. The permanency of the organization remains to be determined, but thus far it has escaped the dangers of sentimentalism and of misguided enthusiasm.

Unfortunately, certain individuals addicted to alcohol are unwilling to join this organization. The reasons for their lack of motivation for this group affiliation remain unclear. Some do so as a denial of the addiction, others appear to have competing loyalties, are perpetuating a defense of self-sufficiency against dependent strivings which would arouse shame, or are prone to develop intolerable anxiety in group situations.

DISULFIRAM OR ANTABUSE THERAPY. In 1948 two Danish investigators, Jens Hald and Erik Jacobsen, in search of a vermifuge, tried disulfiram (tetraethylthiuram disulfide). They observed that persons who had ingested this substance previous to the consumption of alcohol showed symptoms which differed quantitatively and qualitatively from those present in the common picture of alcoholic intoxication. The discomfort after alcohol consumption in persons taking this drug was so great that these investigators decided to use it as a remedy for alcoholism. It is believed that the discomfort is caused by intereference with the excretion of acetaldehyde, an intermediary product in the oxidation of alcohol.

When a patient who has taken 0.5 to 1 gm. of disulfiram within the preceding 12 hours partakes of alcohol, he experiences within 5 to 15 minutes a feeling of heat in the face soon followed by an intense vasodilation in the face

and neck, the skin of which may assume a purple-red color. At the same time, the conjunctiva is injected, and the patient suffers from tachycardia. These symptoms are soon followed by headache, dyspnea, dizziness, chest pain, nausea, palpitation, and vomiting. There is an initial rise of blood pressure followed by a fall, perhaps to 80 mm. of Hg. The discomfort following the imbibition of alcohol so long as disulfiram is in the blood is so great that the patient does not care to drink. The dose of disulfiram should be individualized, but usually 0.125 to 0.50 gm. once a day, preferably in the morning, is sufficient. Rarely 1.0 gm. is required. Initial treatment with a drug possessing such serious toxic potentialities should be under constant medical supervision. Cardiovascular complications, including myocardial infarction, may occur. Although it was originally believed that persons suffering from marked disease of the liver, coronary disease, arteriosclerosis with hypertension, or diabetes should not receive disulfiram, experience with a large series of patients suggests that the only important contraindication is cardiac decompensation. There have been several reports of psychoses occurring during the use of the drug.

Formerly the administration of disulfiram was not begun until after an abstinence from alcohol for one week, but in recent years disulfiram has been given even when the patient is intoxicated. In such instances, the initial dose is one-half or less of the usual one (7.5 mg. per kilogram of body weight) and is given with an antihistaminic drug, such as 25 mg. of Promethazine, and 5 gm. of sodium chloride in one-half glass of water.

A new agent, citrated calcium carbimide, is now under study. This drug shows effects similar to those of disulfiram; however, there are effects immediately after ingestion, though there is little duration of action after the final dose. Citrated calcium carbimide may offer a useful substitute for disulfiram in certain patients.

Disulfiram therapy must be considered

as a variation of the conditioned reflex aversion method. In contrast to other forms of conditioned reflex methods, the unpleasant effects not only are present each time the patient takes a small but adequate dose of disulfiram and drinks alcohol, but they actually increase with continued ingestion of the drug. If continued, it probably helps to overcome the craving for alcohol. For the treatment to be successful, however, it is necessary for the patient to have a real desire to be helped, to be willing to take the drug with consistency, and to co-operate in psychotherapy. Daily uninterrupted administration of disulfiram makes it physiologically impossible to continue to use alcohol as a defense mechanism. To remove this protection, however, without at the same time eliminating its need by psychotherapy can scarcely lead to a cure of the patient. As long as the basic difficulties which led to the alcoholism are not resolved, the desire for alcohol persists and along with it, an unwillingness to take the medication. During psychotherapy the psychiatrist will aim to discover both the internal, anxiety-producing factors and any social and family conditions that led to the alcoholism. With the aid of a social worker, in some instances various stressful social conditions and unhealthy habits may be uncovered and corrected.

BIBLIOGRAPHY

Adams, R. D., and Foley, J. M.: Neurological Disorder Associated with Liver Disease. (In Metabolic and Toxic Diseases of the Nervous System. Res.) Publ. A. Res. Nerv. Ment. Dis., 32:198–237, 1952.

Davidson, E. A., and Solomon, P.: The differentiation of delirium tremens from impending hepatic coma. J. Ment. Sc., 104:326–333, 1958.

Himwich, H. E.: The physiology of alcohol. J.A.M.A., 163:545–549, 1957.

Idem: ed.: Alcoholism: Basic Aspects and Treatment. Washington, Am. Assoc. for Advancement of Science, 1957.

Isbell, H., Fraser, H. F., Wikler, A., Belleville, R. E., and Eisenman, A. W.: An experimental study of the etiology of "rum fits" and delirium tremens. Quart. J. Stud. on Alcohol, 16:1–33, 1955.

Levy, R. I.: The psychodynamic functions of alcohol. Quart. J. Stud. on Alcohol, 19:649–659, 1958.

Martensen-Larsen, O.: Five years' experience with disulfiram in the treatment of alcoholics. Quart. J. Stud. on Alcohol, 14:406–418, 1953.

Myerson, D. J.: An active therapeutic method of interrupting the dependency relationship of certain male alcoholics. Quart. J. Stud. on Alcohol, 14:419–426, 1943.

Panmill, F. C., and Smith, J. A.: The chronic alcoholic. J.A.M.A., 171:2299–2303, 1959.

Pfeffer, A. Z., et al.: A treatment program for the alcoholic in industry. J.A.M.A., 161:827–836, 1956.

Ritchie, O. W.: A sociohistorical survey of Alcoholics Anonymous. Quart. J. Stud. on Alcohol, 9:119–156, 1948.

Schultz, J. D.: et al.: Chlorpromazine in the management of acute alcoholic states. Quart. J. Stud. on Alcohol, 16:245–250, 1955.

Sutton, T.: Tracts on Delirium Tremens, on Peritonitis, and on Some Other Internal Inflammatory Affections and on the Gout. London, Thomas Underwood, 1813.

Thompson, G. N., Ed.: Alcoholism. Springfield, Charles C Thomas, 1956.

Usdin, G. L., and Robinson, K. E.: Psychosis occurring during Antabuse administration. Arch. Neurol. & Psychiat., 66:38–43, 1951.

Victor, M., and Hope, J. M.: The phenomenon of auditory hallucinations in chronic alcoholism. J. Nerv. & Ment. Dis., 126:451–481, 1958.

Victor, M., Herman, K., and White, E. E.: A psychological study of the Wernicke-Korsakoff syndrome. Quart. J. Stud. on Alcohol, 20:467–479, 1959.

Williams, W.*: The society of Alcoholics Anonymous. Am. J. Psychiat., 106:370–375, 1949.

Zwerling, I., and Rosenbaum, M.: Alcoholic Addiction and Personality. In Arieti, S., Ed.: American Handbook of Psychiatry. New York, Basic Books, Inc., 1959, pp. 623–644.

* Co-founder with Robert H. Smith, M.D. (deceased) of Alcoholics Anonymous.

Chapter Eleven

MENTAL DISORDERS CAUSED BY OR ASSOCIATED WITH HEAD TRAUMA

With the mounting occurrence of accidents incident to industry and traffic and with the enactment of industrial compensation laws, there has been a marked increase in traumatic mental disorders and their medico-legal importance. For these reasons, the relationship of head trauma to the development of mental disorders often presents an important and difficult problem. Not infrequently the difficulty of this problem is increased by the fact that the clinical picture may become complicated by the addition of psychogenic symptoms to an organic syndrome. In order to arrive at an accurate diagnosis, it is often necessary not only to make detailed mental and neurological examinations but also to obtain a precise history of the patient's mental status prior to his injury. The opinion popularly entertained that injuries to the head are a frequent cause of mental disorders is an error. Undoubtedly severe trauma to any part of the body may occasionally serve as a contributing or precipitating agent in schizophrenia and manic-depressive psychosis in persons predisposed to these respective reactions. At times, too, trauma of the head, without recognizable injury to the brain, may activate an asymptomatic paretic process and lead to clinically active syphilitic meningo-encephalitis. Such psychoses, however, are not included among the traumatic mental disorders.

The mental disturbances associated with head trauma are divided into those caused by acute brain disorder and those caused by chronic brain disorder. This classification will be explained as these disorders are considered.

ACUTE DISORDERS CAUSED BY, OR ASSOCIATED WITH, HEAD TRAUMA

The acute (at times subacute) disorders following trauma of the head tend to fall into the following syndromes:
- (a) Concussion
- (b) Traumatic coma
- (c) Traumatic delirium
- (d) Korsakoff, or amnesic-confabulatory, syndrome

Concussion Syndrome

In concussion, there is a momentary

physiological interruption of cerebral processes because of head injury, but there are no histological changes or clinical signs. Recovery is rapid and complete. There is not only amnesia for the moment of injury but also for a period, usually seconds or moments, before the injury. Concussion follows the impact of a severe, functionally paralyzing force upon the head, especially of a force that causes abrupt acceleration or deceleration. In recent years it has been suggested that concussion may be the result of the cavitation phenomenon in the cellular fluids. Experiments show that an impulse applied to the skull by a severe mechanical blow or by an underwater explosion produces first a momentary positive pressure wave followed by a negative one. Although this negative wave is sustained for only an infinitesimal period of time, it apparently causes minute bubbles to form momentarily in the cellular fluids. This phenomenon of cavitation, with its molecular-disrupting action, produces a momentary generalized cortical electric discharge that renders the patient unconscious. This discharge is followed by a depression of function.

Recently brains of animals subjected to concussion and examined by fine techniques several days after the trauma have disclosed histological changes in nerve cells. These suggest that some of the remote symptoms following concussion may develop on the basis of nerve cell changes taking place some time after the concussion. The period of unconsciousness may be momentary or may continue for hours. Many patients vomit as they regain consciousness. There is apparently no relationship between the severity of the concussion as measured by the duration of unconsciousness and the severity of the psychiatric sequelae. In regaining consciousness, the patient may wake up suddenly or may pass through a state of clouded consciousness and confusion. He will subsequently have a loss of memory (post-traumatic amnesia) for this period, even though he seems alert and able to carry on a conversation. Usually recovery is complete in a short time, but occa-

sionally a chronic personality disorder may follow.

Contusing and lacerating injuries do not in themselves produce concussion, although they may be associated with it. On the other hand, a severe injury may be sustained without concussion. The diagnosis of uncomplicated concussion can be made only in retrospect. Only after the regaining of consciousness can one be sure that no organic sequelae will follow. Although cerebral concussion is an acute syndrome, there is frequently an aftermath of variable, even prolonged, duration. These postconcussion symptoms will be discussed on page 188.

Traumatic Coma

Severe concussion without injury, or more frequently, concussion accompanied by contusion (a mechanical disruption of tissue usually accompanied by minute capillary hemorrhages) or by laceration (a gross tearing of tissue) may produce prolonged coma. Coma is, of course, characterized by absence of response on stimulation. It may last for hours or for several days, the duration depending upon the degree and extent of the injury. In the absence of localizing signs of laceration or of pressure (as by subdural hemorrhage), coma for more than 24 hours usually means a major contusion. Following coma there is a period of stupor, restlessness, and clouding of consciousness, from which the patient may emerge into clear consciousness or at times pass into traumatic delirium. Coma is often interrupted by intervals of semistupor. Prolonged coma is frequently followed by a period of delirium succeeded by a longer period of amnesia or by the amnesic-confabulatory syndrome known as Korsakoff syndrome.

Traumatic Delirium

If delirium follows the suffering of head trauma, it usually begins during the gradual emergence of the patient from traumatic stupor or coma. The underlying cause may be concussion, contusion, laceration, hemorrhage, or increased intracranial pressure. In a majority of cases, delirium is mild and consists of haziness, irritability, dreamy fabrications, restlessness, and mild disorders of the sensorium. The patient does not grasp the finer points of situations and events of his surroundings. Although most of the time he may realize that he is in a hospital, he does not remember how he came to be there, may not recognize persons about him, and may not understand why he is detained. Other patients may be definitely bewildered. Not a few are apprehensive and fearful. In some cases the delirium is concerned with the patient's occupation. Many patients are resistive, noisy, irritable, unco-operative, and verbally abusive. Some patients are belligerent, demanding, and aggressive. If hallucinations occur, they are usually visual. In the more severe cases, there may be such confusional excitement and a tendency to wander about that restraint becomes necessary. Violent, impulsive outbursts making the patient dangerous to himself or others may occur. As their noisy delirium subsides, some patients remain talkative and show a perseveration of words. At times, after the stage of irritability, the emotional state may be characterized by a childish elation and happiness. As in delirium resulting from other causes, the course may be characterized by fluctuations between relative clearness and confusion. In some instances, the syndrome may be that of a twilight or dream state instead of delirium. With or without preceding delirium, various degrees of post-traumatic defect may follow major contusions with their diffuse degeneration of ganglion cells. Delirium continuing for more than a week suggests considerable damage. An estimate of the final residual defect should not be given for at least six months. Delirium or coma of more than a month's duration usually means serious tissue destruction. An estimate of the final deterioration and other results of tissue destruction should not be made until 12 to 18 months after the injury. The final mental defect will usually not be as serious as early symptoms suggest.

Korsakoff, or Amnesic-Confabulatory, Syndrome

A relatively frequent syndrome following head trauma is that first described by Korsakoff as associated with chronic alcoholism. The most striking feature of this syndrome is confabulation, although this is accompanied by disorientation and impairment of perception and recent memory. The fabrication of memory may be a mixture of truth and fiction or purely new fabrications. Suggestive questions may often elicit contradictory statements. The patient may superficially appear alert but on closer examination it will be found that perception is greatly deranged. Many patients with the Korsakoff syndrome show serenity and mild euphoria or even facetiousness but readily become irritable on questioning. The polyneuritis resulting from thiamine deficiency and seen in some instances of Korsakoff syndrome does not occur in the post-traumatic symptom complex. Since polyneuropathy is not present in the syndrome originally described by Korsakoff, the term "amnesic-confabulatory syndrome" is more appropriate. The symptoms are of shorter duration following trauma than in the alcoholic Korsakoff syndrome.

In practice it will be found that the acute and subacute symptoms of traumatic mental disorder do not usually occur in such distinct classificatory types as have been described. In severe cases one often observes mixed and transitional reaction types. Delirioid and Korsakoff symptoms are particularly apt to be associated.

Treatment of Acute Traumatic Mental Disorders

Except for the surgical procedures required in the case of definite injuries to the head, operative interference is to be avoided. The patient should be closely watched for any signs of increased intracranial pressure, and also, for the occurrence of any complication.

The initial objective is to quiet the patient. Rest in bed and as limited a use of sedatives as possible are important. Narcotics are contraindicated. In the acute stages, careful note should be made as to the state of awareness and the presence or absence of signs of injury to the cerebral substance. Vital signs should be recorded at intervals of two to four hours. Fluids and a soft or liquid diet may be administered if the patient is conscious and able to swallow. With the presence of coma, either feeding by a nasal tube or the administration of parenteral fluids is indicated. Daily dosage of penicillin is necessary to prevent pulmonary infection. Fluids and salt should be restricted but not to the point of leading to dehydration and acidosis. The fear of cerebral edema should not lead to their over-restriction. Patients with simple concussion require at least 24 hours of observation and may then return to their usual activities. The period of bed rest and convalescence of patients with more severe injuries is determined by the reactivity of the patient to the treatment. It is important that the severity of the injury not be overemphasized or the period of hospitalization unduly prolonged. There should be a gradual increase of activity with continuance of convalescence at home through the medium of graduated exercises. Active work should be deferred for two to three months following discharge from the hospital. Patients should be advised that alcohol tolerance is diminished following head injury.

Of utmost importance in the treatment of the acute traumatic mental state is the continued awareness of the possibility of severe complications. Such changes in the vital signs as slowing of the pulse and respiration, fluctuating states of consciousness, or the development of signs of focal disturbances of the brain, including paresis, suggest strongly the possibility of serious pathology. In particular, the possibility of subdural hemorrhage must be kept in mind.

Subdural Hematoma

Following injury to the head, subdural hematoma is said to occur in one to 10 per cent of individuals. In a series of 3,100 consecutive autopsies of psychotic patients, 8 per cent showed evidence of subdural hemorrhage. Subdural hematoma may be associated with any variety of psychotic reaction but occurs particularly in the senile, epileptic, alcoholic, and paretic individual. Such patients are especially prone to head injury.

Subdural hematoma consists of a collection of blood between the dura and arachnoid in the subdural space. The bleeding in this space is of venous origin and follows tearing of small veins reaching the subdural space. The fluid in the space may be admixed with cerebrospinal fluid if the arachnoid tears. Blood extravasated into this area fails to be absorbed and eventually is organized and encapsulated by the dura. Fibroblasts proliferate from the inner surface of the dura and invade the clot when in contact with the dura. Capillaries extend into the clot and gradually absorb the liquified fluid. If the clot is small, it may become completely organized, but if large, fibroblasts may form an encapsulating membrane by growing both along the inner surface of the clot and on the surface adjacent to the dura.

Subdural hematomas may occur either acutely following the head injury or at later periods. In either case the symptomatology may be brought to the attention of the psychiatric consultant. Headache is invariably present. Perhaps most important is the variable state of consciousness. Following recovery from the initial coma, the patient becomes irritable or confused. His mental status frequently changes from day to day or even from hour to hour. Focal signs of cerebral damage are not present in more than one-half of the cases. The most frequent signs are hemiplegia or central facial weakness. In chronic cases the symptoms are similar, but in addition, slight to severe intellectual impairment is usually noted. The initial trauma may not be remembered.

Cerebrospinal fluid is usually bloody

and under increased pressure. Roentgeno-logic examination of the skull may or may not show evidence of a linear fracture. The electroencephalograph is often help-ful in defining an abnormality on one or the other side of the brain. The diagnosis is firmly established only by placing a burr hole on both sides of the skull with discovery of the characteristic hematoma. Other complications that may follow head injury in the acute phase are extra-dural hemorrhage, intracerebral hemor-rhage, subdural hygroma, and cerebral thrombosis. When a subdural hemor-rhage or other traumatic vascular lesion is suspected, neurological and neurosur-gical consultations are immediately indi-cated.

CHRONIC DISORDERS CAUSED BY, OR ASSOCIATED WITH, HEAD TRAUMA

A definite classification of mental dis-turbances caused by, or associated with, head trauma into a group of acute dis-orders and a group of chronic disorders is somewhat arbitrary, but in general there are two groups of syndromes both in respect to their temporal relation to the trauma and in respect to clinical features. The chronic disorders may also be divided into two subgroups. One sub-group consists of those disorders pre-senting symptoms which are the direct result of the trauma, and the other, those in which the syndrome is only a second-ary result of the head trauma. The fol-lowing classification of the chronic trau-matic disorders is therefore suggested:

I. Caused primarily by head trauma:
   Post-traumatic personality disorders
   a. of adults
   b. of children
   Post-traumatic defect conditions
   a. traumatic encephalopathy of pugilists (punch drunk)
   b. traumatic convulsive disorder (traumatic epilepsy)
II. Caused secondarily by head trauma:
   Psychoneurosis with head trauma

Chronic Mental Disorders Caused Primarily by Head Trauma

Psychopathology which occurs follow-ing lesions of the brain is now regarded not only as an expression of changes that the patient's personality undergoes as the result of cerebral lesions but also as an expression of the efforts of the brain-damaged personality to adapt to these defects and to those demands that can no longer be met because of these de-fects. In his work on persons with brain injuries consequent to war wounds, Gold-stein emphasized that various types of symptoms must be evaluated and under-stood in this context if a rational therapy is to be applied in the treatment of indi-viduals with chronic disorders resulting from head injury.

Symptoms

The effort of such patients to find the new adjustment necessary because of the head injury results in three types of symp-toms: The first expresses the conflict that the individual faces; the second reflects the tendency to build up substitutive performances so as to adapt to the de-mands of the environment in the most effective manner under the circumstances of the defect consequent to the injury; and a third group of symptoms is the direct result of the impairment of the brain-functioning itself. In the third group, the defect may be ameliorated by training, and it is here in particular that the impairment of the "abstract attitude" described by Goldstein is to be found.

Among the symptoms exposing the pa-tient's defect is that now commonly known as the "catastrophic reaction." Confronted with a problem he cannot solve, the brain-injured individual be-comes suddenly anxious and agitated and may appear dazed. A change in his color may appear, he fumbles at the task, and may present other evidences of auto-nomic disturbances, such as irregular pulse and changes in respiratory rate. If he was initially in good spirits, he now be-comes evasive, sullen, irritable, and even aggressive. The "catastrophic reaction" develops simultaneously with the attempt to perform the task in which he fails, and not following the performance. Thus it does not represent the patient's response to the awareness that he has failed. As a consequence of such catastrophic reactions, a definite behavior pattern evolves in many of those with brain injury. Some, when confronted with tasks they cannot solve, lose consciousness. Others avoid exposing themselves to such situations by isolating themselves from individuals, or by avoiding tasks through apparent inability to understand directions. Some brain-injured individuals attempt to prevent up-surges of anxiety by continuous activity, which exposes the patient's inability to adopt a reflective attitude, to take himself for granted, or to place himself in the position of a detached spectator. The over-activity may be of the type commonly spoken of as "occupational delirium" and seen in patients with dementia. Certain patients appear to be unable to follow directions and carry out tasks. Essentially they avoid the task in the anxious expectation of precipitating the unpleasant catastrophic response. Others adapt themselves through an excessive orderliness. This may express itself in a meticulousness not only in relation to one's own property but also to that of others in the home.

The brain-injured person tends to suppress knowledge of his disability. Such denial, according to Goldstein, is more easily achieved in the patient with complete destruction of some function than in the individual with incomplete disturbance.

In addition to the efforts of the brain-injured person to avoid the catastrophic reaction by restricting his environment, his brain defect expresses itself through evidence of increase in the threshold of excitability, with the result that greater stimuli are required to bring forth responses. At the same time, the patient may appear unusually susceptible to exposure to various external stimuli because of his easy distractibility. Owing to his difficulty in discriminating between the object to which he is exposed and the background or setting in which the object is presented, the brain-injured patient suffers doubt and anxiety in his perceptions of common objects presented under ordinary circumstances. Thus his capacity for solving problems is impaired as a consequence of this perceptual weakness.

Goldstein has described what he terms the "abstract attitude." He defines this as the capacity to assume a mental set voluntarily; to shift from one aspect of a situation to another; to retain simultaneously several aspects of a situation; to break up and isolate the whole into its constituent parts; and to abstract common properties, plan ahead ideationally, and think or behave symbolically. The "concrete attitude," on the other hand, is a form of thinking fixed and unable to proceed beyond the stimulus of an immediate experience or object. To him the brain-injured person is impaired in his ability to assume the "abstract attitude" and has difficulty in moving easily from the "abstract" to the "concrete."

Post-traumatic Personality Disorders

Although these personality disturbances are primarily a result of injuries to the cranial contents, psychological factors usually participate to a varying degree. A decision as to the relative importance of the brain injury, of environmental factors, and of the previous personality pattern of the patient is not always easy. Sometimes the impression is gained that the patient has always had an immature attitude or, as a result of the accident, has reverted to such an attitude, accompanied by a reluctance to face former responsibilities. Again, the mental symptoms appear nearly all or entirely psychogenic and merge into a neurosis secondary to the trauma (accident neurosis).

Among the names applied to the personality syndrome caused directly by the head injury are "postconcussion syndrome," "post-traumatic general cerebral syndrome" (Foerster), "minor contusion syndrome" (Symonds), "traumatic constitution" (Meyer), "traumatic psychopathic constitution" (Ziehen), "traumatic encephalopathy," and others. In adults this primary post-traumatic personality syndrome may assume two forms: a milder and more frequent form known as postconcussion syndrome or postconcussional neurotic state, and a more serious disturbance to which the name post-traumatic personality disorder is applied in a narrower and more specific sense.

POSTCONCUSSION SYNDROME. Whether the injury that preceded this syndrome was mild or severe, the presenting symptom is anxiety. Other symptoms are headache, vertigo, fatigability, oversensitivity to strong sensory stimuli, insomnia, impairment of memory and of ability to concentrate, a narrowing of interests, a lessening of spontaneity, aggravation of symptoms by heat, excitement, or exertion and a reduced tolerance of alcohol. Headache and vertigo are aggravated by quick movement, by stooping, or by psychological tension. Many patients are emotionally labile, irritable, and easily moved to tears. Many complain of decreased sexual potency. Some become "head-conscious." This is perhaps to be expected, since the head is the most significant part of the body-image. Head injury, therefore, is more commonly experienced as a form of psychic trauma than injury to almost any other part of the body. If the injury occurred under conditions of discontent or dissatisfaction, psychogenic symptoms are particularly likely to follow.

Diagnosis and Prognosis. The chief problem in the diagnosis of the postconcussion syndrome is to determine when a postconcussional headache and other symptoms having an organic basis cease to be a result of organic causes and are carried on by psychological influences. The relative importance of psychogenic and physiogenic factors is often difficult to determine. If the headache is paroxysmal, throbbing, aggravated by postural alterations or physical exertion, it may be that it persists from an encephalopathic rather than from a neurotic state. The same is true if mental functions tend to be sluggish and if the emotional status is sanguine and not characterized by gloom, ready annoyance, and apprehension. If the symptoms are definite, constant, are not modified by suggestion, and the patient's interest is in rehabilitation and not in indemnification, they are probably not of psychogenic origin. The postconcussive or neurotic state is discussed elsewhere in this chapter. Most, but not all, patients with the postconcussion syndrome recover if complications of psychoneurotic symptoms are not too numerous or too severe. Recovery may be delayed for one or two years.

Treatment. In certain respects, the most important aspects of therapy are careful and adequate surgical and medical treatment at the time of injury, combined with subsequent discreet management in adjusting the patient to his symptoms and to the general situation with which he is confronted. Too early return to strenuous labor should be discouraged, yet too long a rest may lead to a secondary neurotic syndrome. Nearly every patient with concussion should have supportive and suggestive psychotherapy.

POST-TRAUMATIC PERSONALITY DISORDER OF ADULTS. In some instances, the most conspicuous sequel of head trauma is a change from the original personality make-up of the patient. The amiable, placid individual may become irascible, irritable, and impulsive. He may become quarrelsome and subject to outbursts of rage, aggression, and motor excitement. Family and other obligations and responsibilities are disregarded. Ambition and initiative are lost. The patient becomes petulant, resentful, self-centered, willful, and selfish. Some become morose and tend to develop paranoid reactions toward persons about them. Others lose all interest in activities and withdraw from social contacts. Not uncommonly, some degree of organic mental deterioration accompanies these changes in the psychological structure of the personality.

POST-TRAUMATIC PERSONALITY DISORDERS OF CHILDREN. In general, children withstand head injury better than adults. Not rarely, however, brain-damaged children may present serious behavior problems. Children without serious destruction of brain tissue may show much disorganization of behavior. The behavior disorders are similar to those seen following the epidemic encephalitis of the 1920's but they are more severe and of poorer prognosis. The previously normal child becomes disobedient, distractible, impulsive, aggressive, destructive, cruel, quarrelsome, and antisocial. Constant restlessness and overactivity are the rule. There may be some degree of intellectual deficit. The child is dominated by instinctive and emotional impulses and shows no regard for the welfare of others. Although there is little impairment of original intellectual capacity, the child does not concentrate, shows little interest in school work, and does poorly in the classroom, where he is intolerably disruptive. The usual methods of training and discipline are ineffectual, and eventually the most serious delinquents become institutionalized.

Although the emotional disorders seen in the brain-injured child probably have organic roots, they certainly have psychogenic ones. Because of his handicap, the child is in need of emotional support. Parental feelings and their attitude toward his handicaps may greatly influence his behavior. Some parents may manifest a smothering overprotectiveness and others may be unsympathetic and rejecting. An impatient attitude and unjustified blame by the teacher increase the child's anxiety and result both in more disturbed behavior and in less ability to learn. Environmental pathology becomes, therefore, the crucial determinant of the disturbances in behavior.

Post-traumatic Defect Conditions

Mental deterioration (dementia) following severe head trauma may or may not have been preceded by traumatic delirium. It not rarely happens that, as consciousness returns following delirium, an impairment of former mental capacity will become manifest. In milder forms, this may consist only of loss of initiative, mental slowing, loss of sense of responsibility, and impairment of ability to recognize abstract relationships. In somewhat more serious disturbances, memory is impaired, attention is reduced, reaction time is slowed, and defensive confabulations may be expressed. Judgment is impaired and finer affective feelings are blunted. Social values are not appreciated. Tasks that were formerly performed easily become difficult or impossible. The patient may consider himself normal, although it is apparent to his intimates that he has never been the same since his injury. The degree of dementia varies greatly according to the site of the lesion, the nature and extent of the injury, and its secondary results (atrophy, meningo-encephalic adhesions, distortion of ventricles). A permanent mental deterioration to a degree requiring institutional care is uncommon after contusion. If laceration has been extensive, the dementia may be great and associated with epileptiform seizures, paralyses, aphasia, deafness, and other neurological signs.

Difficulty sometimes arises in differentiating post-traumatic mental deterioration from psychoses of arteriosclerotic origin complicated by head injury. Careful inquiry should be made as to any symptoms of arteriosclerosis existing before the injury. The possibility that the confusion of arteriosclerosis or of a cerebral attack may have led to the injury should be kept in mind.

Severe, chronic dementia is hopeless, yet caution should guide the therapist in expressing a prognosis in acute or subacute cases, since with time many patients show a surprising improvement.

Traumatic Encephalopathy of Pugilists (Punch Drunk)

A chronic post-traumatic personality disorder first described by Martland is that to which he gave the name "punch drunk." This syndrome occurs among pugilists who have sustained repeated severe blows on the head over a period of at least a few years. The more skillful the fighter, the greater is the probability that he will either escape the causative injuries or remain relatively free from them for a considerable period of time. The disorder probably results from successive and accumulative petechial hemorrhages and foci of necrosis deep in the cerebrum. The patient shows an insidious impairment of skill, a slowing of muscular action, a little uncertainty in equilibrium, slight confusion, and deterioration in attention, concentration, and memory. Speech becomes thick and hesitating. The patient "continuously simulates a person who is just a little drunk." Most patients are voluble and euphoric. Confusion and defects of memory become more marked, and intellectual impairment continues to a disabling degree. The tremor, propulsive gait, and mask-like facies of the parkinsonian syndrome may appear. The symptoms progress for approximately a year, then become stationary. The degree of deterioration depends upon the extent and degree of brain injury.

Traumatic Epilepsy

One of the sequelae of brain injury may be epilepsy. There is so wide a variation in statistics as to the incidence of epileptic seizures following head injury— 4.5 per cent (Sargant) to 34 per cent (Denny-Brown)—that they are probably of little value. Study of 279 American personnel who sustained wounds of the brain in World War II showed that 36 per cent developed seizures within two years after injury, and 41.6 per cent within three years after receipt of penetrating brain wounds. The incidence is greatest in patients who suffer a penetration of the dura. Penfield showed that the most frequent epileptogenic lesions in post-traumatic convulsive state are cerebrodural or cerebral cicatrix and focal atrophy. Epilepsy is therefore more common after penetrating than after closed injuries and is not the result of generalized damage to the brain. Seizures do not develop after a simple concussion.

A lesion causing the convulsive state does so as a result of irritation of adjacent areas of the brain. The pattern of the attack and the march of motor phenomena during the seizure may betray the epileptogenic point of origin. Electroencephalography may be of much value in localization of the lesion. In the typical focal or jacksonian seizure, consciousness is not lost. Clonic twitches develop in one part of the body and spread consecutively to other parts of the same side. In a large percentage of cases, however, consciousness is disturbed in the manner of either the petit mal or grand mal seizure. There may also be the same paroxysmal periods of depression, exaltation, or fugues. Mental deterioration may be slight or extreme.

Chronic Mental Disorder Secondary to Head Trauma: Psychoneurosis

Although Chapter 28 will be devoted to a description of the psychoneuroses, those associated with head trauma have features sufficiently significant to justify special mention of them in a discussion of mental disorders following head injury. It is not generally considered that traumatic neuroses are the direct result of anatomical or physiological changes produced by the trauma, yet a subjectively disturbing postconcussion syndrome or other post-traumatic symptoms may facilitate or become the nucleus for neurotic attitudes. This is especially true if the trauma occurred at a time, or in a setting, in which anxiety-producing factors existed. There may, for example, have been economic insecurity, occupational dissatisfactions, family tensions, or inability to secure work. The circumstances under which the trauma was sustained—compensable accidents, in contrast to accidental falls in the home or injuries in sports—may have a significant etiological relation. There is also a contributing element in the fact that the head, particularly the brain, is an organ on which the patient sets particular value. If, therefore, the injury is followed by dizziness and headache, or if other physical symptoms are associated with it, a sense of insecurity and an associated anxiety may readily develop. Not rarely, complicating situational stresses arising from, or relating to, the injury tend not only to create but also to perpetuate the neurotic symptoms. Feelings of discontent or of grievance predispose to their development. Fear, suggestion, and wishful thinking may all be important psychological factors in the production of symptoms.

Diagnosis

The onset of psychoneurosis associated with head trauma occurs not at the time of injury but at a variable period after it. Frequently there is a history that the patient recovered from the organic symptoms produced by the trauma and was about to return to his usual employment, or even resumed work for a brief period, when a return of headache, dizziness, and other symptoms rendered employment impossible. This period between the time of the injury and the appearance of neurotic disability is often described as one of "incubation and contemplation." The patient who has had a resentful, dissatisfied attitude toward his work and was protected from resuming former responsibilities by reason of the acute physical symptoms that followed the head trauma is prone to the development of a neurosis. With the loss of the protecting physical disability, other means of avoiding a return to a distasteful situation must be sought. This means is readily provided by a return of headache, vertigo, impairment of memory, fatigability, irritability, and other symptoms. Likewise, both the man who is fundamentally covetous and indolent, or who was harassed by debts or other financial obligations before his injury, and the apprehensive, suggestible man fearful of losing compensation by return to work may develop similar psychoneurotic symptoms to assure a continuation of compensation. The sympathy and solicitude of friends, lack of occupation and interest, suggestive examinations, misdirected treatment, continued compensation, and other subconscious motivations tend to fix the symptoms. Various factors, such as fears related to the injury, head-consciousness,

and accentuation and elaboration of preexisting conflicts concerning occupational and financial problems, contribute to the development of anxiety, which is often a conspicuous symptom. Other symptoms are physical and mental fatigability, depression, apprehension, neurasthenic and hypochondriacal reactions, and a volubility and elaboration in expression of complaints. Symptoms tend to be vague, numerous, and inconstant.

Undoubtedly the organic concussion syndrome, with disturbance of consciousness, subsequent dizziness, and the feeling of insecurity connected with it, facilitates the production and suggests the nature of neurotic symptoms. As organic symptoms continue, they often tend, therefore, to acquire an overlay of psychoneurotic ones. Frequently, indeed, the post-traumatic concussion syndrome becomes the basis for psychological elaborations of a hysterical type. As a result, psychogenic symptoms may coincide or may be interwoven with organic sequelae of head injuries. With this tendency of neurotic attitudes to crystallize around the nucleus of head injuries, the differentiation between organic and psychogenic symptoms is not always easy; every combination of organic and psychiatric symptoms may, in fact, exist. The relative significance of these two groups may be a matter of personal opinion.

Treatment

Since the pretraumatic personality and the setting and circumstances of the accident are often more significant than the severity of the injury in producing post-traumatic mental disability, apprehension should not be manifested either by the physician or the patient's relatives. Prolonged rest in bed after head injury suggests that the injury is serious, engenders anxiety, and predisposes to the development of the post-traumatic syndrome. The stay in a hospital should not be prolonged, and the patient should return to his work as soon as practicable. Planned activity even before return to regular employment is desirable. Reference has already been made to the fact that occupational and home worries and concern for compensation favor the persistence of symptoms. Gain from the injury in any way deters recovery. A speedy settlement of any compensation question is advisable. Since the association between head injury and psychiatric factors is close, the "pre-neurotic interval" between the injury and the development of the neurosis is one in which preventive psychotherapy is advisable.

Rehabilitation of the brain-injured should commence immediately after the patient has become conscious. Such patients are often highly fearful and suggestible. Explanation as to the nature of the injury and reassurance as to outcome should be given. Efforts should be made to avoid inquiry concerning symptoms that are not spontaneously presented. As soon as the patient is able, he should move about, and a carefully-planned program of progressive activity should be established. Such a program should not overtax his capacities intellectually, emotionally, or physically. Those with chronic defects require more than a regimen of occupational therapy, games, and exercises, even though such activities assist in restoring self-confidence and an awareness of capacity for performance. Treatment is most effectively managed in hospitals with well-established departments for rehabilitation, including occupational, recreational, and vocational therapies. Many advances have been made in the methods used in the re-education of those with chronic brain damage, particularly of those who manifest, in addition to disturbances of the abstract attitude, specific defects in the field of language, motor disabilities, and perception, as Goldstein has indicated. Such patients require a careful psychological evaluation and then re-training by skilled persons. There is a continuing need for the insight of the psychiatrist and his assistants in dealing with the emotional problems of patients. However, in addition to this type of therapy, the utilization of the psychologist trained in the pedagogy of the brain-injured, also of the social worker if there are particular family needs, must be considered. The outcome varies according to the severity of the lesion and the pretraumatic personality of the individual. In some cases, intellectual tests may fail to reveal serious disturbances, yet when the patient has returned to work his impairment in judgment and capacity for work may be demonstrated. Here the well-established rehabilitation center, with the opportunity for testing performance in a workshop, is most useful in determining the eventual capacity of the individual for an occupation and the proper type of vocation for the future. In those rare cases of dementia with severe personality change, the prognosis is grave. No final assessment of the degree of damage should be made in less than 12 to 18 months after the injury.

BIBLIOGRAPHY

Adler, A.: Mental symptoms following head injury. Arch. Neurol. & Psychiat., 53:34–43, 1945.

Allen, A. M., Moore, M., and Daly, B. B.: Subdural hemorrhage in patients with mental disease. New England J. Med., 223:324–329, 1950.

Association for Research in Nervous and Mental Diseases, Vol. XXIV: Trauma of the Central Nervous System. Baltimore, Williams & Wilkins Co., 1945.

Courville, C. B.: Commotio Cerebri: Cerebral Concussion and the Postconcussion Syndrome in their Medical and Legal Aspects. Los Angeles, San Lucus Press, 1953.

Critchley, M.: Medical aspects of boxing. Brit. M.J., 1:357–364, 1957.

Denny-Brown, D.: The sequelae of war head injuries. New England J. Med., 227:771–780 and 813–821, 1942.

Idem. Disability arising from closed head injuries. J.A.M.A., 127:429–436, 1945.

Eisenberg, L.: Psychiatric implications of brain damage in children. Psychiatric Quart., 31:72–92, 1957.

Friedman, A. P., and Brenner, C.: Amnestic-confabulatory syndrome (Korsakoff psychosis) following head injury. Am. J. Psychiat., 102:61–66, 1945.

Goldstein, K.: After-effects of Brain Injuries in War. New York, Grune & Stratton, 1942.

Guttmann, E.: Psychiatric aspects of head injury. J. Ment. Sc., 90:328–350, 1944.

Idem. Late effects of closed head injuries. J. Ment. Sc., 92:1, 1946.

Ingram, T. T. S.: A characteristic form of overactivity behavior in brain-damaged children. J. Ment. Sc., 102:550–558, 1956.

Kozol, H. L.: Pretraumatic personality and psychiatric sequelae of head injury. I. Arch. Neurol. & Psychiat., *53*:358–364, 1945. II. Arch. Neurol. & Psychiat., *56*:245–275, 1946.

McConnell, A. A.: The cephalic post-traumatic syndrome. J. Ment. Sc., *102*:330–335, 1956.

Martland, H. S.: Punch drunk. J.A.M.A., *91*: 1103–04, 1928.

Rowbotham, G. F.: The long-term results of injuries of the head. J. Ment. Sc., *95*:336–354, 1949.

Ruesch, J.: Intellectual impairment in head injuries. Am. J. Psychiat., *100*:480–496, 1944.

Idem, and Bowman, K. M.: Prolonged post-traumatic syndromes following head injury. Am. J. Psychiat., *102*:145–163, 1945.

Siegal, L. J.: Craniocerebral postconcussive personality states. Psychiatric Quart. Supplement, *24*: 65–72, 1950.

Strauss, A. A., and Lehtinen, L. E.: Psychopathology and Education of the Brain-injured Child. New York, Grune & Stratton, 1947.

Tobias, J. S., Lowenthal, M., and Maringer, S.: Evaluation and management of the brain-damaged patient. J.A.M.A., *165*:2035–2041, 1957.

Chapter Twelve

ACUTE BRAIN SYNDROMES ASSOCIATED WITH METABOLIC DISTURBANCES

Although chronic brain syndromes are more frequently associated with diseases of metabolism, endocrine disturbances, and vitamin deficiencies than are acute ones, reversible syndromes may also occur at times with these disorders.

Although their relations are complex and imperfectly understood, and although the psychological and physical interrelations of *endocrine derangements* are poorly correlated, it is apparent that mutually influencing reactions occur among the central nervous system, mental functioning, and the endocrines. It is reasonable to assume that interactions between emotional and metabolic processes may produce endocrine disturbances, and these, in turn, may affect cerebral functions and mental reactions. The psychological consequences of a given hormonal action are not uniform. A certain hormonal change may or may not have a psychological effect. If it does produce an effect, it is not necessarily the same in all cases but will depend upon the previous personality organization of the individual and upon all the other influences acting upon the personality.

It is not clear, however, whether endocrine abnormalities will in themselves produce a psychosis. Some endocrine disturbances produce changes in brain function by influencing brain metabolism, but this is no indication that such changes are related to disturbances in behavior. This is well illustrated when thyroid function is considered. Although psychotic and other types of reaction occur in association with hyperthyroidism, it has been shown by recent work that the cerebral metabolic rate is not elevated from normal in this condition. On the other hand, in myxedema there is a reduction of oxygen consumption by the brain and a retardation in expression at the psychological level.

In the evaluation and management of the personality disorders associated with metabolic and endocrine disturbance, the degree of stress consequent to the metabolic shift and the rate of change of bodily functions secondary to that shift must be weighed against the constitutional and experiential development of the specific individual. The time in development at which such changes take place is highly significant.

Preceding the onset of personality disorder, there exist chemical, metabolic, physiological, and sometimes anatomical changes in contrast to what is now known of the functional psychoses and neuroses. Such changes are perceived, and must be adapted to, by the specific individual in his own environment. When endocrine disorder produces gross changes in the body, creating psychological and social stresses which vary from one person and culture to another, the adaptation is particularly difficult because the body-image is disturbed. Thus the patient may see himself as deformed, inadequate, or sexually misidentified and, in turn, suffer ridicule or attack. He then develops feelings of shame and inadequacy. His responses may be anxiety, hostility, guilt or social withdrawal, or both. In those instances in which the metabolic change induces largely subjective perceptions, there is likely to result only a shift in the affective life and the level of the drive. It is clear that the symbolic significance of change induced by the metabolic shift depends on the ego attitude toward the body and its functions, derived during psychosocial development. Thus young women exposed to the masculinization resulting from an adrenal tumor develop anxieties as to their sexual role and functions, associated with activation of sexual fantasies and doubting, an attitude which would not be observed in the young child who has suffered since birth with the symptom complex due to adrenal hyperplasia.

Hyperthyroidism

In the mental disorders associated with hyperthyroidism—an association in which there is a striking interaction between emotional and metabolic processes—it has long been noted that a special type of personality seems usually to have existed before the clinical signs of Graves' disease were apparent. This disease arises largely in sensitive, impressionable persons who react keenly to life, have a marked feeling of insecurity, and an unusual sense of responsibility. The general hypermotivity, emotional excitability, alertness to every sound and impression, the tendency to walk, talk, and eat rapidly, and the mild anxiety, apprehensiveness, and irritability commonly observed in Graves' disease and characterized by the laity as "nervousness," represent in many ways but an exaggeration of a previously-existing pattern of response to ordinary life problems. In other words, these persons have been anxious individuals with psychiatric problems giving rise to tension. In them it is frequently impossible to tell where anxiety stops and hyperthyroidism begins.

Psychiatric studies have shown that, usually long before the onset of the clinical symptoms of hyperthyroidism, patients who succumb to this illness have suffered emotional and psychological maladjustment. The majority of those who have examined groups of patients indicate that the basic need of such patients is for the satisfaction of an exaggerated dependency relationship. With chronic frustration, their response is aggressive and leads to the welling up of death wishes toward the hoped-for gratifying party. As a means of adapting to such wishes, the patients may respond by an over-depressed relationship to the significant person or turn away from this person and attempt a striving at self-sufficiency which is often premature. Women with the illness have many conflicts and fears in relation to childbirth; yet at the same time they manifest a strong desire for children. The dependency needs are satisfied while the child is small, but when the time comes for the child to seek its own independence, the mother responds often with anxiety and anger or with the reaction formation of anxious over-concern. These psychological defenses are not specific for the hyperthyroid patient and may be seen in many other conditions. Nevertheless, the strivings of individuals with this type of personality structure relate well to those observations that show that the psychiatric problem frequently precipitating the hyperthyroid activity is that of the loss of a key person in the patient's life.

Although the usual mental symptoms associated with hyperthyroidism are those of tension, overactivity, and emotional instability already mentioned, in about 20 per cent of acutely thyrotoxic patients a psychotic reaction appears. In extreme cases a fairly typical manic excitement may develop as if in accordance with the increased tempo of all organic processes. In other instances there may be an acute hallucinatory delirium accompanied by great restlessness and insomnia. Other patients present depressed, anxious, agitated reactions. Paranoid states with systematized delusions may occur. In general the symptoms manifested are exaggerations and caricatures of the previous personality. It will usually be found that persons with recurrent hyperthyroidism after thyroidectomy are still struggling with serious and unresolved personality difficulties.

The treatment of hyperthyroidism is often a joint task for the psychiatrist and the internist. The internist directs his efforts to the restoration of the metabolic rate to normal limits. The function of the psychiatrist is to aid patients who are disturbed emotionally in accepting the need for therapy through bringing insight to their denial of symptoms. Continued psychotherapy is indicated for those hyperthyroid patients who present clear evidence of psychological maladjustment prior to the onset. Here psychotherapy is an important adjunct in bringing about a permanent euthyroid state with reduction in emotional and psychological symptomatology.

Hypocalcemia

The most common cause of hypocalcemia is the removal or damage to the parathyroid glands during thyroidectomy. Psychological symptoms are observed in such patients in addition to the characteristic clinical signs of paresthesia, cramps, carpopedal spasms, tetany, or laryngeal stridor. The most common symptoms are those of depression, memory loss, disturbance of deep reflexes, and emotional lability. Such symptoms may persist for years, yet are often quickly relieved by correction of the hypocalcemia with the administration of calcium salts orally and with vitamin D; the dosage is carefully controlled by regular determination of the serum calcium. Parathyroid hormone has not been effective for such control.

Cushing's Syndrome

In his original descriptions in 1932 of what has come to be known as Cushing's Syndrome, Harvey Cushing called attention to the frequent co-existence of mental symptoms. It is now recognized that these occur in not less than a fifth of those with the syndrome. Originally thought to be associated with a basophil adenoma of the pituitary gland, Cushing's syndrome now is regarded generally as the result of adrenocortical hyperfunction with either neoplastic or hyperplastic expression in the adrenal glands.

The diversity of the associated personality disturbances is such as to indicate that they represent the defensive adaptations of the individual to the endocrine imbalance and, also, to a considerable extent, the disfiguring alteration in the patient's appearance. Thus, as the illness progresses, the patient's appearance may change from that of an attractive young woman to that of an obese and bearded lady whose activities are restricted by weakness and easy fatigability.

A reactive depression is the most frequently encountered response. In relatively few patients is it associated with psychomotor retardation. Other patients, without depression, are anxious, and have crying spells, or are agitated or stubborn in their behavior. Irritability, paranoid ideation, and rarely a florid schizophrenic response are sometimes seen. Less than a fourth of those with associated personality disturbance suffer serious personality decompensation with psychosis. Obviously this syndrome presents symptoms similar to those induced by the administration of cortisone, other adrenal steroids, and corticotropin and discussed in an earlier chapter.

DIAGNOSIS. This is made with observation of the complaints of marked weakness and easy fatigability and an often painful adiposity, which may develop rapidly in a characteristic distribution of fat in the areas of the face and neck (moon face) and trunk. The combination of supraclavicular fat pads and dorsal kyphosis due to osteoporosis sometimes gives a lumped posture. There may be depressed purple streaks over the abdomen, thighs, and upper arms, with increased susceptibility to bruising. There is a diminished carbohydrate tolerance due to increased gluconeogenesis from protein, sometimes with diabetes. Hypertension and peripheral edema may occur. Women, the most frequently affected, are usually amenorrheic and show masculinization, with deepening of the voice, hirsutism, growth of the clitoris, and acne. Men are often impotent. The definitive diagnosis is established by laboratory evidence of increased excretion of 17-hydroxycorticoids in the urine. Also helpful are the findings of an eosinophil count below 50 per ml., lymphopenia, neutrophilia, polycythemia, and glycosuria and evidence by x-ray of osteoporosis.

TREATMENT. Abolishment of the adrenal hyperfunction by subtotal resection of the adrenal gland or removal of an adrenal tumor usually relieves both the personality and physiological disturbances. However, the return to health is not immediate and requires time. Those who develop hypoadrenalism after surgery and in whom substitution therapy proves inadequate often have persistence of the personality disorder. Others, particularly young women, who have suffered severe disfigurement due to hirsutism, bony deformities, and the scars of acne also are apt to have a stubborn perpetuation of symptoms.

Adrenogenital Syndrome

The virilizing effects of excessive secretion of adrenal androgens, whether due to bilateral hyperplasia at birth or an adrenal tumor (often carcinomatous) occurring later in life, have serious consequences for personality development. The condition is frequently associated with psychosis.

When the syndrome develops in women after puberty with the physical deformity resulting from overgrowth of sexual hair, deepening of the voice, absence of breasts, enlargement of the clitoris, and amenorrhorea, it leads to marked anxiety. Female patients particularly are pre-occupied with their masculinized appearance, develop doubts as to their gender and sexual role, often become depressed and withdrawn socially, and are obsessed with thoughts of homosexuality or guilt relative to masturbation.

DIAGNOSIS. This is established definitively by demonstration of increased secretion of adrenal androgens and 17-ketosteroids. Other forms of precocious sexual development and hermaphroditism may be distinguished by special differential analyses of steroid secretions.

TREATMENT. Small doses of cortisone suppress the virilizing activity of the adrenals. If this treatment is given in early life, the female patient develops normally and at puberty matures and menstruates regularly. Removal of a tumor or partial adrenalectomy is the treatment of choice for those late in life.

Hypoglycemia

It is now recognized that spontaneous —in distinction from therapeutically induced—hypoglycemic states may occasionally exist. At times the clinical picture of such hypoglycemic attacks may be dominated by mental symptoms, usually transitory in nature. There is no single psychic syndrome characteristic of the condition. Among the many mental phenomena that may be prominent are the following: apathy, irritability, restlessness, anxiety, negativism, somnambulism, confusion, disorientation, fugue states, delirium, syncope, stupor, or coma. Thinking may be confused and retarded and speech may be disturbed. Grasp may be impaired and emotions unstable. Hallucinations and delusions may be present. The patient may complain of weakness, fatigability, and hunger. He perspires and may suffer from tremor, unsteadiness of gait, diplopia, and convulsions. There is no recollection of the attack. There is a tendency for the symptoms to appear after exertion or when the patient is hungry. Complete relief from the symptoms follows the administration of sugar. Hypoglycemia should always be suspected as the cause of any mental symptoms appearing in a diabetic who is receiving insulin.

DIAGNOSIS. The diagnosis of spontaneous hypoglycemia is made on evidence of depression of the blood sugar level. Since the periods of the condition are transient, it is often difficult to establish its presence by simple study of the fasting blood sugar. A definitive diagnosis is evident if the blood sugar determination occurring during an attack falls below 50 or 60 mg. per 100 ml. If the attack is convulsive in nature, the blood sugar may be elevated following the seizure. Glucose tolerance tests have limited value but may suggest the diagnosis if the blood sugar level falls to 50 mg. per 100 ml. three to five hours after the stimulating dose of glucose. When hypoglycemia is not demonstrated by these means, a 24 or 48 hour fast should be instituted and blood sugar determinations made at periods of 12, 18, and 24 hours. With the onset of symptoms and their prompt alleviation by the use of intravenous glucose, the diagnosis is established. Electroencephalographic changes occur in association with such attacks and show local or widespread dysrhythmias which again are relieved on ingestion or intravenous application of glucose.

ETIOLOGY. Once the diagnosis of hypoglycemia is established, its etiology must be determined. Although the majority of such patients will be found to suffer from hyperinsulinism caused by islet cell tumors of the pancreas, the functional cases with an associated neurosis are of particular interest to the psychiatrist. It has not been determined whether this type of condition may occur as a somatic manifestation of a psychoneurosis or whether the majority of these cases fall into the group of induced hypoglycemic states symbolic of a sadomasochistic neurotic conflict. A number of such induced hypoglycemic cases have been observed, usually in women and most frequently in nurses who have had experience with the utilization of insulin. The diagnosis was established on one occasion by tagging the insulin used by the patient with radioactive phosphorus and then detecting the excretion of the radioactive material in the urine the following day. In some instances the patient suffered from diabetes and had numerous unexplained attacks of hypoglycemia, though denying the use of insulin.

The following case history illustrates such a problem and its management:

The patient, a 44-year-old married nurse, with a history of episodic attacks of hunger, weakness, sleepiness, sweating, vertigo, and occasionally unconsciousness, was referred for study. The attacks were always aborted by eating. They were so severe that six months previously the patient had to give up a fast. Another physician had diagnosed an islet cell pancreatic tumor and advised surgery. The patient refused operation, stating that she had gained weight and was not suffering any pain. She consulted other physicians in an attempt to obtain a different diagnosis. She expressed her fear to these physicians that if operated upon she would become diabetic and require insulin.

A careful medical examination failed to reveal any evidence of tumor. The patient sustained a fast without the development of hypoglycemia. In view of previous experiences with patients who had induced hypoglycemia, the patient's room was searched while she was having a diagnostic test and several bottles of insulin and a syringe were found. At this point a psychiatric examination was requested.

In consultation the patient reported that her mother, who died two years previously, had been a diabetic and had been nursed in her terminal illness by the daughter. The patient had lived a restricted life and had entered nursing to relieve herself of her loneliness. Some four years previously she had undergone a hysterectomy performed by the physician who had advised her that she had an islet cell tumor.

Following the initial psychiatric interview, the patient stated that she proposed to sign out of the hospital. Since it was considered that her condition was dangerous in the sense that she was exposing herself to a potentially major surgical procedure, the psychiatric consultant concluded that it was advisable to suggest the possibility of induced hypoglycemia to the patient. This was done by informing her of the conclusions reached by the medical service on the basis of finding the bottle of insulin and the previous experience of the hospital with others with similar conditions. The patient was gently told that, if this was the case, she must have some underlying emotional problems which had led her to the desperate expedient of the self-administration of insulin and that she might therefore wish to solve the major conflicts which had driven her to such action. The suggestion was met by immediate denial. When seen the following day, the patient asked assurance that any information given by her would be considered inviolate. When this was given, she broke down, cried, and gave the following information.

She stated that her drive for the self-administration of insulin began about four months previously during the period of a fast when she felt weak and unable to continue her work. Believing that she might obtain a dispensation from a religious fast from the physician who had removed her uterus some years earlier, with whom she worked and toward whom she had a strong positive attachment, she asked if he would assist her in securing a dispensation for medical reasons. He replied that he would do so if he found her to be suffering from hypoglycemia. Shortly before blood was to be drawn for the determination of its sugar content, the nurse, without the knowledge of the physician, took her first injection of insulin. Naturally, hypoglycemia was found. The physician therefore gave her the desired recommendation that dispensation be granted from the obligation of fasting before communion.

The nurse then revealed that she had developed a feeling of depression after her hysterectomy. She feared that she had not healed properly and wondered whether she would develop a cancer. Her father had died of cancer and had suffered from fears relating to mental disease. He was given insulin to relieve his depression. The patient herself had given insulin in mental hospitals and recalled her anxiety on being shown the brain of a patient who had died during insulin shock therapy. Throughout her life she had felt hungry, had been an extremely heavy eater, and had felt weak when she fasted. The patient had always devoted herself to the care of her mother and an aunt and had spent months at home each year nursing them for their various ailments. The mother had written her that she should provide nursing services not only for herself and the aunt but also for her brothers, if she really loved her family. She always seemed fearful of losing the love of her relatives. Perhaps it is not surprising that upon the death of her parents she expressed the sentiment that her brothers "beat her out" of her patrimony.

The nurse declared that she had devoted the same amount of attention to the care of her physician's patients as she had to her own family. She admitted that her response to his rejection of her request for a medical dispensation had been one of anger and resentment. On the other hand, she felt so anxious concerning the possibility of losing his respect and good will and so guilty in relation to the church that she felt obliged to continue the self-administration of insulin when faced with another medical examination. Following these revelations, which were responded to with sympathetic interpretation of her emotional reactions and their origin, the patient returned home to her profession and made a satisfactory adaptation, with no recurrence of the hypoglycemic attacks.

Acute Vitamin Deficiency Syndrome

Chronic mental syndromes are not exceedingly rare in cases of chronic avitaminosis, particularly in thiamine deficiency, but acute mental syndromes are quite uncommon. Jolliffe, however, called attention to what he called "acute nicotinic acid deficiency encephalopathy." This syndrome is characterized by delirium, sucking and grasping reflexes, cogwheel rigidities, and irregular jerking movements of the extremities. This readily disappears after treatment with niacin.

Exhaustion Delirium

At times acute, confusional, delirioid reactions accompany marked states of exhaustion. Since such reactions are not associated with infection, they may best be considered in a discussion of acute syndromes resulting from disturbances of metabolism. Exhaustion delirium is not common but it may occur occasionally, associated with hemorrhage, unusual and extremely prostrating physical exertion, starvation, prolonged insomnia under conditions of stress or emotional tension, and debilitating effects of a chronic wasting disease such as carcinoma. This acute hallucinatory confusion ("confusion mentale") was described by Chaslin under the term "primary mental confusion" and by Meynert under the designation "amentia," a term still applied to this syndrome by English and German but not by American psychiatrists, who occasionally employ the word as synonymous with feeblemindedness.

The onset is usually with insomnia, some clouding of consciousness, mild confusion, difficulty in collecting one's thoughts, perplexity, perhaps of a distressed type, vague fears, restlessness, illusions, fleeting hallucinations, and changing delusions. The patient's mood varies with his thought content. The environment appears obscure and distorted. As the condition increases in severity, the patient becomes more bewildered; his perceptions are more impaired; he misidentifies persons and objects and becomes disoriented. Sometimes speech is of a question and answer form. Frequently the patient may seem to be groping in a mental fog, as if attempting to differentiate his confused, dreamlike world from that of reality and gain a point of contact with his previous normal life. Sometimes he may be comparatively clear for a period, only to return to his previous confusion.

This confusional, toxic–exhaustive state may continue for several weeks, but recovery finally takes place. After his recovery, the patient may be able to give considerable retrospective interpretation of his delusions and hallucinatory experiences.

Postoperative Neuroses and Psychoses

Since metabolic changes (acidosis, acetonuria, glycosuria, hypoglycemia, and hepatic insufficiency) may in some instances act as contributory agents to many postoperative mental disturbances, these should be included among acute brain syndromes resulting from metabolic and endocrine disorders. It is probable, however, that other factors, both somatic and psychogenic, are of equal or greater importance. Postoperative anxiety and other neurotic states are, too, more frequent than postoperative psychoses. Their source is to be sought in emotional factors.

Physical agents, other than metabolic changes, causing disturbances may include the anesthetic and sedative drugs. Other factors may be toxic and infectious complications and also nutritional disturbances with associated dehydration, ketosis, or avitaminosis. Among psychological factors are fear and apprehension preceding the operation. The fear of mutilation, of loss of part of one's body, and of possible death is important. The strangeness of the setting, the sights and sounds in the operating room, and all the other preoperative procedures, including anesthesia with the fear of losing consciousness, contribute to the tension and apprehension. The importance to the patient of the particular organ operated upon will affect the possibility of a postoperative psychosis and will influence the character and content of any psychotic ideas. Psychotic reactions are most frequent following operations upon the eyes and the genitals. There is usually a postoperative interval of three to ten days before the onset of the psychosis.

The most frequent type of postoperative syndrome is delirium with its confusion, disorientation, hallucinations, paranoid delusions, fear, apprehension, and restlessness. Similar disturbances may follow amputations of limbs and other external appendages. In these instances, the clinical picture is complicated by the patient's reaction to the "phantom phenomenon" (described in Chapter 28). A not uncommon postoperative mental syndrome is that which occasionally follows the removal of a cataract. The patient becomes suspicious and confused and manifests fear and panic-like excitement, particularly at night. The loss of familiar landmarks adds to the sense of insecurity. It is now thought that those psychotic reactions which occur due to the covering of the eyes after cataract removal are induced by deprivation of visual perception as described in Chapter 6.

Manic states, depressions, and schizophrenic reactions determined by long-standing personality factors may be released by emotional, toxic, or other agents incident to the operation.

Surgery may be accompanied by trauma not only to the body but also to the personality. Psychological factors such as those mentioned may also act in the production of anxiety and occasionally of hysterical syndromes. In addition to these factors, ill-considered remarks by the surgeon or his assistants, technical bedside discussions, or the demonstration of charts or roentgenograms that create apprehension on the part of the patient may produce alarm in the insecure personality. Genital evisceration in the woman highly desirous of bearing children may prove so frustrating that a permanent neurosis results. Although scarcely pertinent to the present topic, it should be borne in mind that many a failure of surgery to relieve a disabling symptom occurs because an attempt has been made to remove surgically the somatic expression of an emotional illness. All too often such attempts merely lead to their repetition.

BIBLIOGRAPHY

Blackburn, C. R.: Effects of hypocalcemia on the central nervous system. Rocky Mountain M. J., *54*:441–444, 1957.

Bleuler, M.: Endokrinologische Psychiatrie. Stuttgart, Georg Thieme Verlag, 1954.

Bursten, B.: Psychosis associated with thyrotoxicosis. Arch. Gen. Psych., *4*:267–273, 1961.

Harn, G. C., et al.: Dynamic Aspects of the Personality Features and Reactions Characteristic of Patients with Graves' Disease. In Proceedings of Association for Research in Nervous and Mental Diseases, Vol. XXIX. Baltimore, Williams & Wilkins Co., 1950.

Himwich, H. E.: Brain Metabolism and Cerebral Disorders. Baltimore, Williams & Wilkins Co., 1951.

Kepler, E. J., and Moersch, F. P.: The psychiatric manifestations of hypoglycemia. Am. J. Psychiat., *94*:89–109, 1937.

Kleinschmidt, H. J., Waxenberg, S. E., and Cuker, R.: Psychophysiology and psychiatric management of thyrotoxicosis. J. Mt. Sinai Hosp., *23*:131–153, 1956.

Kolb, L. C.: The Painful Phantom. Springfield, Illinois, Charles C Thomas, 1954.

Lidz, T.: Emotional factors in the etiology and therapy of hyperthyroidism. J. Mt. Sinai Hosp., *20*:27–40, 1953.

Mandelbrote, B. M., and Wittkower, E. D.: Emotional factors in Graves' disease. Psychosom. Med., *17*:109–123, 1955.

Rome, H. P., and Robinson, D. B.: Psychiatric Conditions Associated with Metabolic, Endocrine and Nutritional Disorders. In Arieti, S. (Ed.): American Handbook of Psychiatry. New York, Basic Books, Inc., 1260–1288, 1959.

Rynearson, E. H.: Hyperinsulinism among malingerers. M. Clin. North America, *31*:477–480, 1947.

Sokoloff, L., Wechsler, R. L., Mangold, R., Balls, K., and Kety, S. S.: Cerebral blood flow and oxygen consumption in hyperthyroidism before and after treatment. J. Clin. Investigation, *32*:202–208, 1953.

Tethowan, W. H., and Cobb, S.: Neuropsychiatric aspects of Cushing's syndrome. Arch. Neurol. & Psychiat., *67*:283–309, 1952.

Titchener, J. L., and Levine, M.: Surgery as a Human Experience. New York, Oxford University Press, 1960.

Ziskind, E., Jones, H., Filante, W., and Goldberg, J.: Observations on mental symptoms in eye patched patients: hypnogogic symptoms in sensory deprivation. Am. J. Psychiat. *116*: 893–900, 1960.

Chapter Thirteen

CHRONIC BRAIN DISORDERS

The mental syndromes discussed in Chapters 8 to 12 inclusive are, for the most part, the result of temporary, reversible, diffuse impairment of brain tissue function. The present and several succeeding chapters are concerned with chronic organic syndromes resulting from relatively permanent, more or less irreversible, impairment of cerebral tissue function. Usually some impairment of "intellectual" functions, such as memory, comprehension, and judgment, as well as affect, persists permanently.

SYPHILITIC MENINGO-ENCEPHALITIS

The chronic brain syndrome associated with syphilitic meningo-encephalitis, formerly known as general paresis, general paralysis of the insane, or dementia paralytica, is a disorder produced by a progressive syphilitic meningo-encephalitis leading to a degeneration of brain parenchyma with an infiltration of interstitial elements. Clinically, general paresis is characterized by a comprehensive but variable syndrome of neurological and mental disturbances associated with fairly constant serological changes.

History
Although Haslam of Bethlehem Hos-pital, in a monograph entitled "Observations on Insanity," described in 1798 the associated mental and physical symptoms that occur in general paresis, yet the credit for its recognition as a clinical and pathological entity belongs to the French psychiatrist, A. L. J. Bayle, who published his thesis in 1822 at the age of 23. An opinion that paresis was caused by syphilis was first expressed in 1857 by Esmarch and Jessen. At first this theory received little credence. Finally it became accepted that syphilis was a cause in some cases, although many psychiatrists continued to believe that other causes might be operative. The latter opinion was maintained by only a few after Alzheimer and Nissl in 1904 demonstrated the histopathology of the disease. Later the development of the Wassermann reaction indicated the existence of syphilis in practically all cases of paresis. Any remaining doubt that syphilis is the sole determining cause was dispelled in 1913 when Joseph W. Moore at the Central Islip (New York) State Hospital, demonstrated the *Treponema pallidum* in the brains of paretics. This finding was confirmed by Hideyo Noguchi of the Rockefeller Institute. It is now possible to demonstrate treponemata in fresh paretic brains taken at necropsy and studied by darkfield illumination. They may also be discovered in brain

tissue obtained by puncture in living paretics.

The disappointment arising from the failure of the brain lesions to respond to arsphenamine as did the signs and symptoms of syphilis elsewhere in the body stimulated research into other forms of treatment. In 1917 Wagner-Jauregg of Vienna found that artificial fever induced by inoculation with malaria resulted in an arrest of the paretic process and an improvement of the patient. Within the next few years, other methods of producing artificial fever, some of them equally effective, were developed. In 1919 the discovery of tryparsamide, a pentavalent arsenical, by Jacobs and Heidelberger at the Rockefeller Institute added a valuable chemotherapeutic agent. In 1943 penicillin was found to be an active spirocheticidal agent and has since then proved to be an effective means of treating both general syphilis and neurosyphilis. Thanks to these discoveries and to the more widespread use of lumbar puncture as an early diagnostic measure, paresis, instead of being an invariably fatal disease, can now be prevented in a vast majority of cases if treatment of syphilis is early and active. If paresis arises because of the absence or inadequacy of treatment, it can nevertheless be arrested in 70 to 80 per cent of the cases, and if early treatment is instituted, 50 per cent of the affected patients can be restored to their former station in society.

Frequency and Pathogenesis

Prior to 1920, 8 to 10 per cent of the patients committed to public hospitals in the United States were suffering from general paresis, whereas at the present time about 2 per cent of the patients admitted for the first time are suffering from this disease. This decline in admissions is probably a result of both a decrease in syphilis and earlier and more adequate treatment.

The *Treponema pallidum* is one of the few microorganisms which can penetrate the blood-brain barrier with ease. It is now believed that during the period of generalized spirochetemia this invasion of the neuroaxis occurs in most, if not all, patients infected with syphilis. In the majority of cases, this original invasion never produces symptoms, physical signs, or changes in the cerebrospinal fluid; the organisms which have penetrated the nervous system are spontaneously eliminated by obscure immune processes not yet understood. The reason for the development of paresis in some luetic individuals while others remain free from the disease is not known, but perhaps the incidence is determined by the virulence of the infection and by immune factors in the host. There probably is not a special neurotropic strain of treponemata.

Abnormalities of the spinal fluid found to persist for more than two years after infection suggest that the central nervous system may be seriously involved. Even though the patient then shows no clinical signs or symptoms of neurosyphilis, he is extremely likely to do so later and is particularly prone to develop paresis. It is therefore exceedingly important that examinations of the spinal fluid be continued during the first three years following infection and, if found positive, that treatment continue until it is negative. A normal spinal fluid three years after the primary lesion, whether therapy has been given or not, is nearly always assurance against future parenchymatous neurosyphilis. With adequate treatment of syphilis in its early stage followed by prolonged observation, general paresis can be prevented in almost 100 per cent of the cases.

Paresis occurs four times more frequently in men than in women. The cause for this strikingly higher incidence in men is uncertain, since the probable ratio of primary syphilis infection among men as compared with women is not greater than 2 to 1 (Merritt and Moore). Parenchymatous neurosyphilis is also much less frequent among Negroes than among white subjects in spite of the greater incidence of syphilis among the former. Not a few persons develop syphilitic meningo-encephalitis without previous knowledge of their luetic infection.

Pathology

The basic pathology of paresis is a chronic syphilitic meningo-encephalitis in which two pathological components—inflammation and degeneration—are at work. The process with its progressive degeneration of nerve cells begins largely in the frontal region, but as the disease progresses, any part of the cortex, cerebellum, or bulb may become involved. The pia mater is typically thickened, edematous, and infiltrated, often presenting a cloudy, frosted appearance. Frequently it is firmly attached to the surface of the brain, so that on attempting to remove it, portions of the brain substance are torn away, with the result that the cortex may present a flaking appearance. The thickening of the meninges is largely a result of infiltration with lymphocytes and plasma cells and proliferation of the endothelial cells. Because of diffuse atrophy of the cerebral cortex, the sulci are widened and the convolutions are less distinct than in the normal brain. The atrophy is greatest in the frontal lobes and progressively decreases toward the posterior poles of the hemispheres. There is an increase in both the subarachnoid and the ventricular cerebrospinal fluid. The ventricular ependyma is thickened, and often, particularly on the floor of the fourth ventricle, presents a frosted or granular appearance known as granular ependymitis.

Microscopically the perivascular lymph spaces of the vessels are crowded with proliferated endothelial cells, occasional mast cells, and, most important of all, lymphocytes and plasma cells. The pia mater is similarly infiltrated with lymphocytes and plasma cells. A sprouting of the capillaries produces increased vascularity, while the "cuffing" of these capillaries by the perivascular infiltration mentioned gives rise to one of the important histopathological features of paresis, although it is not confined to general paralysis but occurs also in epidemic encephalitis and in trypanosomiasis. The ganglion cells are cloudy and suffer degeneration, and many disappear, particularly in the middle layer of the frontal cortex. It has not yet been determined whether the degenerative changes are caused by the action of the spirochetes themselves or by their toxic products. The usual cortical architecture, with lamination and column formation of the neuron cells, is disorganized. The glia is proliferated. Scattered about through the cortex are numerous cylindrical-appearing cells known as rod cells or "stäbchenzellen," first described by Franz Nissl: "An extraordinary long cell, whose cell body does not appear plainly or adheres to both poles in the form of a single thread."

Another constant finding in the brain of the paretic subject is the presence of iron pigment in the walls of the blood vessels and in the cortical microglia. Many pathologists consider that the presence in the rod cells of a substance giving a Prussian blue reaction is to be considered as characteristic and pathognomonic of general paresis. Spirochetes are found in about 80 per cent of the untreated cases.

The degree of the brain changes is believed to be dependent upon the multiplication of the parasites and, perhaps, upon the production of a toxin. Probably of significance is the increased permeability in the barrier between the blood vessels and the cerebrospinal fluid, as determined by the passage of bromides, which may allow the toxins of syphilis more easily and freely to secure entrance into the brain tissue.

Incubation Period

General paresis develops from five to thirty or more years after the primary infection with syphilis. In one-half of the cases, the incubation period is from 10 to 20 years; in one-fourth the period is under 10 years, and in one-fourth it is over 20 years. The peak in the curve of incidence occurs between the ages of 35 and 45. Invasion of the nervous system by *Treponema pallidum* is first manifested by a rising cell count in the cerebrospinal fluid. Three to six months later the protein becomes elevated, and this is then followed by the development of positive Wassermann and colloidal reactions. If the nervous system has not been invaded by the end of the second year of the disease, it is unlikely that it will ever be involved.

It is established that there is a preclinical period during which the only evidence of the condition consists of spinal fluid findings characteristic of the disease. During this period the patient may be said to be suffering from *asymptomatic paresis*, the forerunner of clinical paresis. The difference between the asymptomatic phase and the symptomatic one is only a matter of degree. For this reason, every patient having a positive Wassermann reaction of the blood serum should also have an examination of the cerebrospinal fluid, even if there are no signs or symptoms of central nervous system involvement. Also, a spinal fluid examination should be made on every patient with early syphilis within 12 to 24 months after completion of treatment.

Trauma as Etiologic Factor

The question as to whether trauma may play a precipitating role in the production of general paralysis in a person already suffering from syphilis is one that occasionally confronts industrial accident and other boards exercising similar judicial functions. Medical evidence and judicial precedent indicate that there is a connection between head trauma and the development or acceleration of the paretic process. The limits usually set for this causal relationship are six weeks to three months as a minimum and two or three years as a maximum. There is, however, divergence of opinion as to the severity of injury necessary for a relationship between the injury and the development of the disease.

To justify the opinion that trauma precipitated or aggravated the general paralysis, it must be shown that the trauma involved the head and was of sufficient intensity to injure the brain by concussion, or more likely by contusion. It is not probable, in such a case, that the injury initiated the paretic process but that the trauma activated an asymptomatic paresis and caused clinical symptoms to appear. It cannot be stated whether or not, in the absence of trauma, a person in such a preclinical stage would have developed general paresis. At times the trauma does not activate a pathological process but perhaps aggravates one that already existed, although its symptoms had thus far not been recognized.

Probably most psychiatrists feel that the role of trauma in the precipitation or aggravation of the symptoms of general paresis has been inadequately established on a scientific basis. Since there is basis for controversy in individual cases, the therapist should be conservative in expressing any conclusions as to relationship. By far the most frequent relation between trauma and general paresis is that the injury was sustained in an accident that resulted from the impairment of judgment, apperception, or co-ordination produced by the unrecognized existence of the disease. Such accidents serve to call attention to the menace in industry of the early paretic, the existence or nature of whose symptoms has escaped recognition.

Symptoms and Signs

The description of syphilitic meningoencephalitis may conveniently be considered under the following headings: (*a*) personality disturbance, (*b*) physical and neurological signs, and (*c*) serological changes.

PERSONALITY DISTURBANCE. Changes in personality and disturbed mentation commonly are the first noted signs of the illness. The clinical findings often fail to reflect the extent of the pathological process. Frequently the mental symptoms develop so insidiously that the patient's family has not recognized that a deteriorating change in personality has been taking place. The physician often has difficulty in determining the exact time when symptoms first existed. The early symptoms may consist largely of an extension and exaggeration of previous personality traits. Other early symptoms may be irritability, fatigue, difficulty in concentration, depression, periods of confusion, disturbed sleep, and headache. The early paretic individual is often opinionated and perhaps quarrelsome. Frequently he becomes neglectful of his dress, unkempt in appearance, inconsiderate of others, and forgetful of social amenities and proprieties and manifests an insidious breakdown of higher ethical and cultural sentiments and standards. The moderate user of alcohol may become dissipated; sexual activities may become excessive. The man whose previous life has been quite exemplary may not only suddenly show some surprising defect of character but feel no concern for his dereliction.

Early in the disease there is often an impairment in professional skill or in craftsmanship. Unaccustomed slips and failures in the discharge of ordinary duties occur. The consequences of errors are not foreseen. The patient may conceive ambitious schemes of an extremely impracticable and extravagant nature. The businessman may no longer show his former capacity for successful management and, because of failing judgment, may dissipate the resources upon which the livelihood of his family depends. There is often a contented indifference—an apathy and unconcern that at first may be mistaken for laziness. Frequently there is a tendency to drowsiness. The patient becomes incapable of submitting his impressions and conclusions to a critical examination, nor does he recognize the insidious deterioration that is going on in the intellectual, feeling, and social aspects of his personality. The man previously regarded as possessing an acute and well-trained mind and sound judgment surprises his acquaintances by his failure to grasp the finer shades of meaning or by some puerile, inept remark. Associations are characterized by their slowness, superficiality, and poverty.

A change of mood is common in the early stages, the frequent mood being apathy or depression. Sometimes the early stages are characterized by anxiety. In some cases, euphoria and expansiveness exist from the beginning, but more often these mood trends appear somewhat later. Momentary periods of confusion or an inability to grasp a situation and to act promptly and correctly leads to automobile accidents in early paretic patients whose mental disorder has not yet been detected. One paretic subject whose disorder had not yet been recognized left his home dressed only in night clothes, coat, and hat to attend the funeral of a friend. Occasionally, particularly in the early stages of the disease, there may be a tendency to a Korsakoff type of confabulation, the content of which is characterized by the narration of fantastic experiences.

Delusions occur at some period of the disease in a majority of the patients. It has usually been emphasized that the delusions are gradiose, yet not more than 50 per cent of the subjects express delusions of this nature. Expansive delusions may reach the height of absurdity. The patient may declare, for example, that he owns a railroad freight train, each car of which is loaded with million-dollar treasury notes. Ideas of boundless benevolence may be expressed, including fantastic schemes for the welfare of all mankind. However, delusions often are depressive, self-accusatory, nihilistic, or persecutory. Hallucinations occasionally occur but are not of diagnostic significance. In the very early stage of the paretic process, individuals who, before the development of the psychosis, showed a definite tendency to schizoid or cyclothymic manifestations, frequently exhibit, at the onset of the mental disturbance, features suggestive of schizophrenia or manic–depressive psychosis.

The dementia of general paresis, even at a comparatively early stage, tends to be of a diffuse type involving memory, judgment, emotional life, and conative expressions. Intelligence tests show a mental deterioration with defective reasoning and an impairment of social ability, memory, and learning. Unlike the dementia of senility, it is not at first limited largely to memory. As the disease advances, the dementia becomes progressive. Affectivity and emotional response suffer improverishment, inadequacies of perception prevent contact with the environment, memory fails, associations become slow and limited, apperception is destroyed, spontaneous activities cease, and finally, the mental processes, devoid of conscious participation, are reduced to those at the reflex and vegetative level.

PHYSICAL AND NEUROLOGICAL SIGNS. As numerous and varied as are the mental symptoms that may exist in paresis, the physical and neurological symptoms are equally so. During the stage of onset, the patient may become easily fatigued and may lose weight. Numerous somatic complaints referred to the various bodily systems are frequent in the early course of the disease. The diagnosis in many paretic patients has been neurasthenia. Many patients complain of headache, caused probably by the thickening of the meninges and by an increase in pressure of the cerebrospinal fluid. Because of the loss of tone in the facial muscles, the lines of expression become smoothed out. This relaxation of the facial muscles, together with the blunting of emotional response, gives the facies a vacant, fatuous appearance. There seems reason to believe that this loss of expression, the tremors, and the spasticity to be mentioned later may well be a result of changes in the basal ganglia and substantia nigra.

Disturbances, varying greatly in degree, occur almost certainly at some period in the eye, or in its innervation or reflexes. Papilledema, syphilitic retinitis, or primary optic atrophy may occur. Bruetsch reports that complete optic atrophy occurs in 2 per cent of the cases and that incipient and intermediate stages of atrophy occur in 62.5 per cent. Probably optic atrophy is the end result of direct infection and inflammation of the optic nerve and chiasm, causing destruction and disappearance of nerve fibers, disappearance of myelin sheaths and connective tissue, and glial overgrowth. More frequent than optic atrophy are the disturbances of the pupils, which may be unequal in size, irregular in outline, much contracted, or widely dilated. Reaction to light is often sluggish or lost, as may also be the convergence reaction. The pupil first described by Argyll Robertson in 1869 will be found in over half of the paretic patients. This is a miotic pupil which contracts when the eyes converge and accommodates for near vision but does not contract when strong light is suddenly thrown on the eye. Occasionally there may be some degree of ptosis of one lid or weakness of one of the external muscles of the eye, especially the external rectus. It is to be distinguished from Adie's myotonic pupillary response, which also is seen to be associated with absent deep reflexes. The myotonic pupil is never miotic but is dilated, sometimes oval, and after a period in the dark it slowly contracts with exposure to light.

A progressive weakness and inco-ordination of all voluntary muscles occurs. There is tremor of the facial muscles, first observed in the lips when the patient attempts to speak or show his teeth. As enunciation becomes more difficult, there is an overactivity of all the facial muscles when speech is attempted. The tremor of the tongue is coarse and is best demonstrated when the latter is protruded. This muscle weakness and inco-ordination lead to the disturbance of speech, which, when associated with the blandly inane facial expression already noted, constitutes a syndrome so characteristic that the experienced psychiatrist can often make a diagnosis as the patient speaks. At first this speech defect is often manifested in the form of a hesitation, drawl, or slurring. Later there is omission, reduplication, or transposition of syllables. The speech disturbances are often best demonstrated by asking the patient to repeat polysyllabic words or phrases containing labial or dental types of consonants (as "electrical artillery brigade"). Omission of syllables, slurring, a terminal clipping of words, and even a forgetting of some of them will often be demonstrated if the patient is requested to repeat the words three or four times. As the disease progresses, the speech may become quite unintelligible. Transient, incomplete aphasic attacks may occur, at times rather early in the disease.

Deterioration in handwriting is often an early clinical symptom. Because of loss in delicate muscular co-ordination, it is often tremulous. There may also be reduplication or elision of letters in syllables. Characters show irregularity in spacing or size, a diminutiveness of which is particularly common. As progression of the disease continues, the patient usually becomes unable to write at all from dictation, and if he attempts to form characters, he produces only an unintelligible scrawl.

Muscular inco-ordination gives rise also to many other symptoms. Among early ones is a tremulous inco-ordination of finer movements of the hand. Later the patient is unable to button his clothing or even to dress himself. Station and gait then become uncertain, all movements are clumsy, and finally, because of his weakness and ataxia, the patient is confined to his bed. The muscles of deglutition do not escape involvement, with the result that difficulty in swallowing may occur.

Disturbances of the deep tendon reflexes are the rule. More frequently these are exaggerated, when ankle clonus and spasticity are usually present, but if, as not infrequently happens, a tabetic process co-exists, the knee jerks are absent. Disturbances of the rectal and vesical sphincters are common in the terminal stages. The bladder may become greatly distended, resulting in a dribbling of urine caused by an overflow of retention. Rupture of such a bladder may occur upon receipt of slight trauma. Trophic changes may occur in the bones, causing them to be easily fractured.

It is not uncommon for the paretic subject suddenly to develop a marked rise in temperature without evidence of infection or of additional somatic disease. These apparently causeless fevers are probably a result of disturbances of the heat-regulating centers.

About three-fourths of all these patients suffer from convulsions at some time during the course of the disease. Occasionally a convulsion, particularly of an abortive type, may be the first symptom to attract attention to the illness, although more frequently convulsions do not occur until the disease is well developed. The occurrence of a convulsion in a person of early middle age who has never previously suffered from a seizure should always suggest the possibility of general paresis. The seizures may show numerous variations in type but are most frequently of an epileptiform nature. Convulsions in syphilitic meningo-encephalitis must be considered of serious significance, as not a few patients die during or soon after a seizure. The cause of these convulsions is not known, but they are perhaps a result of sudden deprivation of oxygen at some area by reason of vascular disturbances.

Another form of episodic attack is apoplectiform in type. These attacks are sudden in onset, are accompanied by disturbances of consciousness, and are followed by hemiplegia or more localized paralyses. These paralyses are usually temporary in nature, often clearing up without residuals in a few days. Less frequently a hemorrhage occurs, leaving a permanent paralysis.

SEROLOGY. Serological changes supply important diagnostic evidence as to the existence of general paresis. The spinal fluid syndrome provides the best guide to the activity of a syphilitic infection of the central nervous system and to the effect of treatment. In nearly all cases of untreated paresis, the Wassermann reaction on the blood serum is positive. Of much greater importance, since they indicate not only the presence of neurosyphilis but also its parenchymatous nature, are certain changes in the cerebrospinal fluid. In general paresis, the patient usually suffers less headache and discomfort following the withdrawal of 10 ml. of the fluid than does the person with intact nervous system. The normal limits of pressure of the cerebrospinal fluid when the patient is prone are generally considered to be from 70 to 160 mm. of water. In general paresis this pressure may be increased, and in approximately 8 per cent of the cases it will exceed 200 mm. of water.

Spinal fluid Wassermann reaction. The important tests in the examination of the cerebrospinal fluid for the existence of general paresis are the Wasserman reaction, protein tests, the cell count, and a colloidal test, preferably the gold test. In untreated syphilitic meningo-encephalitis, the Wassermann reaction in the cerebrospinal fluid is positive with 0.2 ml. of the fluid in 90 per cent of the cases and is always positive with 1 ml. A positive Wassermann reaction does not, of course, signify that the neurosyphilis is of the paretic type, nor does it necessarily indicate that the process is active. Under ordinary conditions, the protein content of the spinal fluid is chiefly albumin and globulin in the ratio of 4 to 1. An increase of protein to 50 to 150 mg. per 100 ml. (normal, 25 mg.) with a disproportionate increase of globulin is the rule in paresis, although these increases are merely indicative of a disorder —not necessarily syphilitic—within the nervous system. The total protein and the amount of globulin are greater in general paresis than in any other type of neurosyphilis except acute meningitis. The more active the paretic process, the larger the amount of these substances. The normal cell count of the spinal fluid varies from one to five small lymphocytes per cubic millimeter. In paresis, the number of cells in the spinal fluid may remain normal or may reach one hundred, the average being twenty-five to fifty. An excess of this number indicates that a syphilitic meningitis also exists. The cell count affords the most valuable information as to the activity of the infection. It is also the first abnormality to return to normal as a result of treatment.

Colloidal gold test. Given a positive Wassermann reaction of the spinal fluid and other evidence of neurosyphilis, one of the most valuable tests in determining its type is the colloidal gold test described by Lange in 1912. This test depends on the precipitation and varying degrees of decolorization of a solution of gold chloride by a series of dilutions of the cerebrospinal fluid. The precipitation is considered to be caused by globulin, the curve of precipitation depending on the relative amounts of globulin and albumin present in the arachnoid fluid. Since, of the various forms of neurosyphilis, paresis shows the largest amount of globulin in the cerebrospinal fluid, the greatest precipitation of gold chloride occurs in the form which gives a first-zone curve. The precipitation is complete in the first three to six tubes that contain the greatest amount of cerebrospinal fluid, and becomes progressively less complete with the greatest dilutions. Degrees of precipitation show as changes from the normal salmon-red color of the solution and range through a slight change to deeper red, to lavender, violet, red-blue, and the colorless solution representing complete precipitation of the gold. For convenience, these shades of color are graded by numbers, the colorless fluid of total precipitation being represented by 5, red-blue 4, violet 3, lavender 2, deeper red 1, and the transparency of a brilliant salmon color with no precipitation by 0. Changes which are graded as 1 or 2 are not usually of pathological significance, but a grade of 3 or higher always indicates an abnormal fluid. An intense paretic reaction might be as follows: 5555554432; one less marked reaction might be: 55432111000.

In multiple sclerosis, Schilder's disease, and other types of neurosyphilis, the decolorization curve with colloidal gold may follow that of general paresis. The collodial gold reaction is no longer thought to be diagnostic of any particular disease of the central nervous system but is simply an indication of an abnormality of the protein content of the fluid. It does not reflect the activity of the disease. This, as previously stated, is best indicated by the cell count.

Clinical Types

Because of the conspicuousness of certain presenting symptoms, different clinical types of syphilitic meningo encephalitis are usually described. Such a division into forms is artificial and possesses the merit of descriptive convenience only. Some cases, too, do not fit into such a classification, and in others the symptoms may shift during the course of the disease.

SIMPLE DEMENTING TYPE. In this form, the chief symptom is an insidious, progressive dementia with few, if any, delusions and no psychomotor disturbance except the declining activity indicative of the failing interest and capacity. Following closely upon the gradual loss of ambition and of mental alertness, there appears the flabby, vacuous facies, presenting a syndrome that can scarcely be mistaken. This type of paretic subject often gains weight during the early stages of his disease, maintaining the additional flesh until his disorder is far advanced. Remissions are rather uncommon in the simple dementing form. Someone has said that the paretic patient lives apathetically in the present, whereas the patient suffering from senile dementia lives in the past.

The following brief abstract indicates the general clinical picture often occurring in the simple dementing form.

A woman of 26 was brought to the hospital because she had become lost when she attempted to return home from a neighboring grocery store. About seven months before the patient's admission, her husband noticed that she was becoming careless of her personal appearance and neglectful of her household duties. She often forgot to prepare the family meals, or, in an apparent preoccupation, would burn the food. She seemed to have little appreciation of time and would not realize when to get up or go to bed. The patient would sit idly about the house, staring uncomprehendingly into space.

At the hospital the patient entered the admission office with an unsteady gait. There, by way of greeting, the physician inquired, "How are you today?" to which she replied in a monotonous, tremulous tone, "N-yes-s, I was-s op-er-a-ted on for 'pen-pendici-ci-tis." She never made any spontaneous remarks and when, a few days after her admission, she was asked if she were sad or happy, she stared vacantly at the physician and, with a fatuous smile, answered, "Yeah." The patient sat about the ward for hours, taking no interest in its activities. Sometimes she would hold a book in her lap, aimlessly turning the pages, never reading but often pointing out pictures like a small child and showing satisfaction when she found a new one to demonstrate. Neurological examination showed dilated pupils that reacted but slightly to light and on convergence. There was a tremor of lips and facial muscles on attempting to speak. The protruded tongue showed a coarse tremor. All deep tendon reflexes were hyperactive. The Wassermann reaction was strongly positive in both blood serum and cerebrospinal fluid. There were 24 cells per ml. of spinal fluid; the Pandy reaction was two plus, as was also the Ross-Jones reaction. The colloidal gold curve was 5555543210.

EXPANSIVE TYPE. The expansive form, while no longer emphasized as distinctly characteristic, is nevertheless regarded as one of the most important of the clinical types. In the early stages, the patient is self-satisfied and has a superficial good humor, but becomes easily irritated. If handled with good-natured and tactful suggestion, he is quite amenable, but if interfered with, his resentment may lead to violence. Although his grandiose ideas may be most absurd, the paretic patient sees nothing incredible in them.

The following report illustrates the defective judgment and grandiose ideas of the expansive type:

M., aged 41, a roofing salesman, was transferred to a state hospital from the jail to which he had been sentenced for violation of the motor vehicle laws. The prodromal symptoms of the patient's oncoming disease were apparently slight. The informant, his sister, who had seen him but infrequently, stated that she had not noticed any change in him except that for a year he had seemed somewhat "worried." While driving his car, he disregarded the collector at a toll bridge and drove across the structure at high speed. When overtaken by a police officer, the patient was found to have no license to drive an automobile, the permit having been revoked several years previously. Three days later, while awaiting trial for this offense, he was again arrested for driving an automobile without a license. He was given a short sentence in jail, where a physician soon recognized the patient's disorder and had him committed to the hospital.

On arrival at the admission office of the hospital, he told the office attendant that he was going to give her a million dollars because she was "a nice lady." As he was being questioned for the usual admission data, he began to boast of his wealth, claiming that he had three automobiles, thousands of dollars in the bank, a "diamond watch," and much other valuable jewelry. His son, he said, was lieutenant governor of the state, was soon to be governor, and later would be president of the United States. After having expressed various absurdly grandiose plans, he added, "I have another plan, too. I'm going to the wardens of the prisons in this state and all the other states and I'm going to buy the prisoners. I'll have an agreement with the warden to take their prisoners and put them to work on farms, and I'll charge each prisoner $300 for doing it and for getting him out of jail. I made $105,000 with prisoners just last week, and when I get going, I'm going to make plenty of money." The neurological signs were all consistent with those of syphilitic meningo-encephalitis, and the serology was in all respects typical of the disease.

As a subgroup of the expansive type may be mentioned an excited or galloping form. Included in this subgroup are those who show great motor excitement, often with confusion. Some of these patients run a rapid course, quickly exhaust themselves, and die within a few weeks after the appearance of the excitement.

DEPRESSED TYPE. The depressed forms are those characterized by melancholia and frequently by hypochondriasis or by nihilistic delusions. Some of these patients have ideas of persecution and many have ideas of unworthiness and attempt suicide. In spite of the depression, there is often a certain element of apathy, and observation usually detects some dementia.

B. J., a woman of 37, was admitted to the hospital in September, 1949. The date of her infection is uncertain. In 1939 at the out-patient department of a municipal hospital she was discovered to have a positive Wassermann but failed to secure treatment. Six months before her commitment, she became depressed, declared she had tuberculosis and refused food because, she said, her stomach was too small to contain any food. On one occasion, she drank iodine, and attempted suicide, but failed through lack of resolution.

On arrival at a public hospital, her facies was noted to be ironed out, her hair unkempt, her clothing loosely arranged and soiled; her posture was stooped and her movements were slow. The Wassermann reaction was positive in both blood and cerebrospinal fluid. The latter contained 97 cells per cu. mm. and an excess of albumin, showed the presence of globulin, and the colloidal gold curve reading was 554432100. It was often impossible to secure any replies to questions, and those obtained were given with considerable delay and incompleteness. She left her tray of food untouched because her stomach was not "working any more." She looked fixedly toward the floor; she declared that her condition was hopeless and that her blood was "all gone." She said, "Look at what a mess I have made around here. The only way I can be happy is down there," pointing downward. When a specimen of blood was taken for the Wassermann test, she appeared to enjoy it, adding that she "ought to suffer." Later she became assaultive, often attacking the nurses, all of whom, she said, God had told her to kill.

CIRCULAR TYPE. Interesting, but not particularly common, are the circular forms of paresis presenting alternations of mood that in their course and clinical manifestations resemble manic–depressive psychosis. It has been suggested that the organic disease is superimposed on a cyclothymic personality.

J. T. was admitted when 53 years of age. The informant, who either did not know or was unwilling to divulge much concerning the patient's earlier life, stated that for three months he had been irritable, childish, and forgetful, and would go to sleep when callers were present. He went to a city in a neighboring state to look for work, but he was arrested for carrying a concealed weapon when he visited the city police department and exhibited a revolver. After a short term in jail, he was committed to an institution for mental diseases, from which he was transferred to a state hospital. In the admission office he was friendly, talkative, and exalted. With a marked pressure of speech, he insisted on telling about his various activities as a detective for numerous police departments, for the United States Government, and as a crusader against the anarchists. He owned, he said, the largest arsenal in the world, used exclusively for the purpose of entertaining his distinguished friends. On the ward he was superior and patronizing in his manner. When not otherwise engaged, he was busy writing letters to the officials of various organizations and to women of his acquaintance, particularly to the nurses connected with the hospital from which he had been transferred. He declared his life to them and proposed marriage to two of them. The neurological and serological findings were typical of paresis.

In less than two months from the date of his admission, the patient had so improved that he was given freedom of the hospital grounds and placed in charge of the laboratory animals. For a month he appeared practically well; then he gradually grew depressed, slept poorly, and lost much weight. He was pre-occupied with ideas about his body and expressed depressive, nihilistic, and persecutory delusions. "Something has gone wrong with me. My gizzard has been cut. I can only breathe that gas you are putting in me. I am the worst person in the world. I wish you would take me out and kill me." One day he was found with a table cover tied about his neck. Gradually he gained weight and strength, but 18 months after the depression began he was still melancholy.

LISSAUER'S TYPE. This is a form with atypical clinical and pathological features. It was named after the pathologist by whom, in collaboration with Storch, it was first described. Pathologically this form, in addition to the usual lesions of syphilitic meningo-encephalitis, is characterized by unilateral localized atrophies, macroscopically apparent, and located particularly in the precentral, postcentral, occipital, and rolandic areas, thus giving rise to the focal symptoms to be mentioned later. A specific feature of these lesions is their laminar distribution. Microscopically these atrophic areas are characterized by extreme pathological changes in the cortex which cause these foci to present a moth-eaten appearance known as status spongiosus. In these areas, all parenchymatous components of the cortex at the focus involved may be destroyed, the only tissue remaining being fibrous glia. Demyelination of infracortical white matter may be extensive. The cause of status spongiosus is unknown, but it may be of local vascular origin. Clinically, in addition to the symptoms associated with the usual forms of paresis, there are localizing signs and symptoms determined by the foci of maximum atrophy, such as aphasic speech disorders, epileptiform attacks confined to one side of the body, unilateral facial paralysis, hemiplegia, hemianopia, hemianesthesia, apraxia, unilateral asteognosis, cortical deafness, and similar disorders.

TABO–PARESIS. Patients with neurosyphilis show evidence not only of the parenchymatous involvement of the brain seen in general paresis, but also symptoms and signs of involvement of the posterior columns met with in tabes dorsalis. The co-existence of both of these diseases is known as tabo–paresis. The symptoms of tabes usually precede those of paresis.

The tabo–paretic patient manifests not only the mental symptoms of general paresis, but also the ataxia and other physical evidence of tabes. Frequently there is a history of difficulty in walking in the dark, of "shooting" pains in the legs. The knee jerks are absent. A Romberg's sign is present, and there is a loss of sense of position in the lower extremities. Primary optic atrophy may occur. The colloidal gold curve may be of the second zone type.

JUVENILE PARESIS. This form, which occurs in the child or adolescent suffering from congenital syphilis, was first described by Clouston in 1877. Infection is transmitted from the mother to the offspring by the transplacental route after the fifth month of pregnancy. It is estimated that rather less than 1 per cent of the cases of congenital syphilis develop general paresis. The age of the juvenile paretic subject at the time of the onset of symptoms corresponds approximately to the length of the incubation period in adult paresis. The child will generally, therefore, be from 5 to 20 years of age at the time of onset of symptoms. In about one-third of the cases, there is retardation of physical development. Many, perhaps 40 per cent, are found always to have been feebleminded. In those who have been markedly feeble-minded, the onset is usually so vague that it is impossible to set a time of onset. In the moderately feeble-minded, and in those who have a period of normal development before the onset, there is an insidious but definite failure of previously-learned accomplishments, followed by a progressive dementia.

The child's history may reveal that he had attended school and had acquired knowledge with fair success until 8 to 14 years of age, when insidious dementia began to develop. Many patients show confusion and restless, purposeless behavior. Because of the impairment of intelligence and the appearance of convulsions, not a few of the cases are diagnosed as epilepsy or idiocy with epilepsy. Delusions and euphoria are much less frequent in the juvenile than in the adult form of paresis. Trophic and other neurological disturbances are often conspicuous. Optic atrophy is not uncommon. Remissions of the type seen in paresis resulting from acquired syphilis are uncommon. The average duration of the disease is four to five years. In the final stages, the child is mute, untidy, and emaciated, and lives at merely a vegetative level. Treatment is less effective than in adult forms.

The following is a fairly illustrative case of juvenile paresis.

J. C. was admitted to a hospital in 1929 when 17 years of age. The first pregnancy following his parents' marriage terminated at seven months, the child dying almost immediately. The patient was the next child in order of birth. His early development was said to have been normal. He attended school from 6 to 13 years of age and is said to have been promoted each year. The first symptoms appeared in October, 1925, when, as his father explained, the boy "became draggy and droopy" and "didn't want to serve his paper route as before." In December, 1925, the teacher reported that he was failing in school. In the spring of 1926, the patient "began to talk funny and was thick-tongued." At practically the same time, the parents noticed a weakness of the left leg and arm. His difficulty in walking increased, his speech became almost unintelligible, and he occasionally soiled himself.

On admission to the hospital, the patient was found to be of rather small stature but fairly well nourished. He walked somewhat in the manner of a mechanical doll, with his elbows pressed close to his ribs, his forearms extended straight before him, and his fingers separated. His steps were short and shuffling, with his feet widely separated as if to maintain his balance. His pupils were widely dilated (the right more than the left), were irregular, and did not react to light, but showed a little contraction on convergence. Both nerve heads were found to be somewhat atrophic. His tendon reflexes were exaggerated, there was a bilateral Babinski reaction, and he showed tremor of the fingers. Co-ordination in fine movements was defective. Attempts to secure the finger-to-nose tests were unsuccessful, as the patient could not be made to comprehend the instructions. The Wassermann reaction was positive on both blood and spinal fluid. The latter contained 19 cells and an excess of globulin and showed a colloidal gold curve of 5555422210.

Mentally the patient's manner suggested that of a high-grade idiot. His facial expression was smoothed-out, and he frequently exhibited a silly grin. He co-operated in the eager, ineffective manner of a mentally defective and responded to all questions with "Huh?" He could not utter a single intelligible word but obeyed simple requests, such as "Shut your eyes," "Close your mouth." The Wassermann reaction on the father's blood was found to be positive.

Because of the active effort now made to ascertain if pregnant women are infected with syphilis and the efficacy of treatment with penicillin, cases of congenital syphilis are relatively rare. Juvenile paresis is therefore now an uncommon disease.

Psychological Considerations

Although the major etiologic factor causing the clinical picture of general paresis is the brain destruction consequent to the spirochetal invasion of the nervous system, in the early stages of the illness the adaptive efforts and psychological defenses largely contribute to the variable clinical picture. The organic damage to the central nervous system produced by the paretic process may permit less restrained expression of previous personality maladjustments and often releases tendencies which had formerly been successfully repressed. In the early stages, therefore, important symptoms may, to a considerable extent, be determined by the individual's previous personality features, its organization, motives, problems, and experiences.

It seems obvious that neither the spirochete nor the destruction of brain tissue can explain the grandiosity of one case, the stupor in another, or the paranoid delusional system in a third. Some symptoms may be the expression of attempts on the part of the personality to cope with threats to its integrity. The patient's delusions, for example, may well be looked upon as psychologically reparative and defensive processes on the part of a personality, the integrity of which is threatened with disorganization because of the destructive assault upon its organic aspect. Finally, the defect and other symptoms caused by the progressive organic disease of the brain come to overlie and more or less conceal the underlying deviation in personality. Since, because of his age, a desire for wealth or social distinction has not come to be a matter of such concern to him as to the adult, the juvenile paretic patient's ideas are rarely expansive.

The paretic subject is not aware of the insidious dissolution going on in his personality. Kinnier Wilson tells of a psychiatrist who suffered from paresis, yet never realized that he was succumbing to the disease on the histology of which he was an acknowledged expert.

Course and Prognosis

If not treated, syphilitic meningo-encephalitis leads inevitably to dementia and death, and if not arrested within a reasonable period, it produces a permanent but varying degree of dementia and economic dependence. In the absence of treatment, death usually occurs from two to five years after the first appearance of symptoms. The course may be interrupted, however, by spontaneous remissions in slightly over 10 per cent of the untreated cases. The clinical improvement that may occur in these remissions may seem almost miraculous and often leads the patient's relatives to the erroneous conclusion that improvement will be permanent. Remissions are more frequent in those cases in which the onset has been comparatively sudden and stormy. The duration of the remissions is quite variable, extending from one or two months to five or six years. The average life expectancy in the untreated patient is four years. The prognosis in the treated patient depends upon the promptness and thoroughness of treatment. Active treatment with adequate doses of penicillin during the asymptomatic stage should prevent the development of clinical symptoms in at least 85 per cent of the cases. If treatment is begun in the early clinical stages, 60 or more per cent of the patients will improve sufficiently to permit them to return to work. It is generally believed that a spinal fluid that is negative after three years from the date of infection will not become positive. In hospitals where patients are admitted in all stages of the disease, the number recovering rarely exceeds 30 per cent, the death rate is 20 to 30 per cent, and further progress is arrested in 30 to 50 per cent of patients.

Symptoms which may be described as organic are caused by the changes produced in the central nervous system by the spirochete; some changes are of an inflammatory nature, while others are degenerative. If the spirochetes can be destroyed by treatment, it is probable that the inflammation caused by them will subside, and the symptoms attributable to inflammatory lesions will disappear, but those caused by degenerative changes will persist. The prognosis depends, therefore, upon the relative extent to which degenerative changes have occurred before the activity of the paretic process is arrested by treatment. Frequently the relative extent to which these two processes exist cannot be ascertained until treatment has been undertaken. The results of structural injury already suffered cannot be remedied.

Diagnosis

The data presented by mental, neurological, and serological examinations provide evidence of a syndrome that can scarcely be mistaken. If the neurological signs alone are considered, cerebral arteriosclerosis may at times be confused with dementia paralytica. The mental symptoms in the early stages of paresis may suggest neurasthenia or one of the phases of manic–depressive psychosis. Dementia, slurring speech, tremors, epileptiform seizures, and even pupillary disturbances may occur in chronic alcoholism, but the serological changes of dementia paralytica are, of course, absent. Paresis has been confused with Alzheimer's disease, Pick's disease, multiple sclerosis, senile dementia, cerebral tumor, or other diseases producing cerebral damage, particularly to the frontal lobes.

The spinal fluid findings constitute the most important differential criterion. In order of diagnostic value and activity of process, these are: (a) increased cell count, (b) increased concentration of protein, (c) positive serological reaction for syphilis, and (d) abnormal reaction in the colloidal gold test. The results of these four tests, interpreted as a whole, give reasonably accurate information as to the presence or absence of neurosyphilis and as to its type and activity. A normal number of cells and normal amount of protein indicate that the process is inactive, even though Wassermann and colloidal reactions are positive.

Treatment

Penicillin is the treatment of choice in the treatment of syphilitic meningoencephalitis. A course of penicillin, repeated if necessary, is effective in a large proportion of both symptomatic and asymptomatic forms of the disease. The patient should receive a course of penicillin intramuscularly totaling 12,000,000 to 15,000,000 units. Different types of penicillin are used by different clinics. Many physicians use 600,000 units daily of procaine penicillin G, given intramuscularly for 20 days.

The results of the spinal fluid tests serve as a guide for both the activity of the paretic process and the effect of treatment. The spinal fluid should be examined four to six months after the completion of treatment. The first change in the cerebrospinal fluid following penicillin therapy is a reduction in the number of cells, which usually reach normal limits within six months. This is followed by a drop in total protein level. If the increased cell count has reverted to normal or near normal, the amount of protein has decreased, and the patient seems improved, no further treatment is needed. The complement–fixation reaction and results of the colloidal test may not revert to normal for several months or years and cannot be used to gauge adequate treatment. If the cell count and protein value remain high, a second course of treatment is mandatory. The second course should be the same as, or more intensive than, the first one. When the response is favorable, the spinal fluid should be examined at intervals of four to six months for the first year after treatment, then yearly until the spinal fluid is no longer abnormal. Less reliance is placed upon clinical features than upon spinal fluid changes as a guide to further treatment.

In greatly overactive patients, also in those with prominent affective components, it is often well that the administration of penicillin be preceded by a course of electroshock treatments.

FEVER THERAPY. If two courses of penicillin fail to effect good results, a few physicians use fever therapy, but it is rarely employed. However, malaria, or another antibiotic such as chlortetracycline, is sometimes administered to the patient.

EMPLOYMENT OF RECOVERED PARETIC. Frequently the question arises as to when the paretic who has become free of clinical symptoms through treatment may resume activities involving the safety of others. It should be advised that he not operate an automobile until his cerebrospinal fluid is negative in every respect. Should his occupation involve still greater responsibility, such as that of locomotive engineer, he should probably never resume it.

TREATMENT OF JUVENILE PARESIS. The treatment of juvenile syphilitic meningo-encephalitis is less satisfactory than the usual adult form of the disease. It is generally considered, however, that the most complete and most persistent remissions are secured by penicillin. Spinal puncture should be done in all cases of congenital syphilis, followed by treatment in the manner described if the cerebrospinal fluid suggests involvement of the central nervous system.

TREATMENT OF ASYMPTOMATIC PARESIS. Attention has been called to the fact that every case of symptomatic general paresis is preceded by an asymptomatic stage when examination of the spinal fluid reveals the paretic formula but clinical manifestations are still absent. It is therefore axiomatic that no patient suffering from systemic syphilis should, regardless of serological tests on his blood, be discharged from treatment until the cerebrospinal fluid has been examined and found to be normal. Even without treatment, the treponemata may be eliminated from the central nervous system within the first five years of infection. Examinations of the cerebro-spinal fluid should, however, be made annually for five years. Should the spinal fluid at any time show the paretic formula, the patient should, even though there be no clinical signs or symptoms of paresis, at once receive penicillin therapy. With adequate treatment, the prognosis of asymptomatic paresis is excellent.

BIBLIOGRAPHY

Bruetsch, W. L.: Penicillin in Neurosyphilis. New York, Grune & Stratton, 1949.

Dattner, B., Thomas, E. W., and de Mello, L.: Treatment of neurosyphilis. J.A.M.A. *141:*1260, 1949.

Hahn, R. D., et al.: Penicillin treatment of general paresis. A. M. A. Arch. Neur. & Psych., *81:*557–590, 1959.

Merritt, H. H., and Solomon, H. C.: Relation of trauma to syphilis of the nervous system. Ann. Surg., *117:*623, 1943.

Moore, M., and Solomon, H. C.: Contributions of Haslam, Bayle, and Esmarch and Jessen to the history of neurosyphilis. Arch. Neurol. & Psychiat., 32:804, 1934.

Robertson, G. M.: Discovery of general paralysis. J. Ment. Sc., 69:1, 1923.

Smith, R. H. F.: Permeability of the blood-brain barrier to penicillin in cases of parenchymatous neurosyphilis. J. Ment. Sc., 97:340–361, 1951.

Chapter Fourteen

MENTAL DISTURBANCES WITH OTHER FORMS OF SYPHILIS OF THE CENTRAL NERVOUS SYSTEM

Syphilitic meningo-encephalitis is a form of neurosyphilis in which the important pathological lesions are confined largely to the cerebral cortex, the inflammatory and degenerative processes being mainly limited to the parenchyma. Frequently, however, the lesions of neurosyphilis are predominantly interstitial, the parenchyma escaping the syphilitic process. Except for the comparatively rare cases of discrete gummata, this interstitial involvement is meningovascular in distribution. By common consent, the meningovascular forms of brain syphilis, in distinction from the meningo-encephalitic forms of brain syphilis, are spoken of as cerebral syphilis, and any psychotic reactions that are associated with them are referred to as psychoses with cerebral syphilis. This distinction from parenchymatous brain syphilis is important, not merely from the standpoint of pathology, but because the symptoms, course, and prognosis of meningovascular brain syphilis are typically quite different from those of the meningo-encephalitic form. In many cases, both meninges and blood vessels are diffusely involved, although again the pathological changes may be largely confined to one or the other of these mesoblastic structures. The mesoblastic forms of syphilis of the central nervous system tend to produce distinguishable groups of symptoms, yet no clear distinction can be drawn. For ease of description, the symptoms of the more characteristic pathological processes will be presented as if the lines of distinction were more clearly drawn than often obtains. It should be remembered, however, that although syphilis of the central nervous system is classified pathologically into meningeal, vascular, and parenchymatous according to the element most seriously involved, these classifications are not mutually exclusive, and many cases show a mixture of two or all three types.

Syphilitic Meningitis

It is customary to divide syphilitic meningitis into three types, depending on the site of selective involvement.

ACUTE SYPHILITIC HYDROCEPHALUS. This is a relatively rare form of neurosyphilis and is not characterized by selective involvement. Signs and symptoms include headache, nausea, vomiting, choked disc, stiffness of the neck, and Kernig sign. The symptomatology is caused by an excessive formation of cerebrospinal fluid and an impairment of the absorption of the fluid resulting from the inflammatory reaction.

BASILAR MENINGITIS. In this form, the inflammatory process is concentrated around the base of the brain. Basilar meningitis, which is one of the commonest forms of neurosyphilis, usually develops from one to three years after the primary infection. Thickening and infiltration of the pia mater occur in the cerebellopontine angle and in the interpeduncular space. With the infiltration of the former region, the sixth, seventh, and eighth nerves are affected, and as exudative processes occur in the latter space, the second and third nerves are involved.

Headache and perhaps dizziness appear; the patient shows mental hebetude, impairment of memory for recent events, sleepiness, difficulty of comprehension, perhaps clouding of consciousness, confusion, and delirium, and occasionally stupor. The degree of disturbance of consciousness and of impairment of the more strictly intellectual functions varies roughly with the extent to which intracranial pressure is increased, as well as the degree to which the cortex is involved. The mental symptoms, however, if present, are usually so clearly of an organic type, are associated with obvious neurological signs, and yield so quickly to treatment that comparatively few patients reach the mental hospital. Signs

resulting from involvement of the optic nerve and of the nerves controlling the extrinsic muscles of the eye appear early and are perhaps fluctuating and inconstant at first. Ptosis, diplopia, strabismus, pupillary disturbance, papilledema, and choked disc therefore are present. Loss of corneal reflex, facial anesthesia, peripheral facial palsy, deafness, or signs of involvement of other cranial nerves may occur. Even in the absence of treatment, the mental symptoms may disappear, only shortly to reappear.

VERTICAL MENINGITIS. This type of cerebral syphilis usually occurs later than the more focal forms of syphilitic meningitis and involves the meninges of the convexity rather than of the base of the brain. Severe paroxysmal headache, often worse at night, is common. Dizziness is frequent. Sometimes the mental symptoms are so indefinite and combined with such an ineffectiveness of personality that the patient is thought to be neurasthenic. More frequently there occur irritability, loss of ability for sustained effort, progressive hebetude, slow thinking, inertia, amnesia, and other signs of intellectual impairment. There is often much irregularity in the impairment of intellectual functions, some being retained much better than others. The nucleus of the personality is less impaired than in syphilitic meningo-encephalitis. Retarded speech, brief attacks of aphasia, and other speech difficulties occur. Generalized or jacksonian convulsions may appear, and hemiplegia is not uncommon. Confusion, delirium, and stupor may be present in relatively acute cases. Paranoid reactions may exist, but here, as in the other forms of nonparenchymatous forms of brain syphilis, there is less disturbance of behavior, judgment, and social reactions, and there are fewer delusional trends, than in paresis.

Syphilitic meningitis is accompanied by a positive Wassermann reaction in both blood serum and cerebrospinal fluid, cells are markedly increased, there is an excess of albumin, and globulin is present. Typically, the precipitation of colloidal gold is greatest in the second zone, giving what is called the "luetic curve" (0123443210).

Vascular Neurosyphilis

This type of cerebral syphilis may give rise to symptoms within a few months after infection or as late as 10 or 12 years after the primary lesion, the majority of cases appearing in the first three to five years of the disease. Vascular involvement in the early stages of syphilis is usually an accompaniment of syphilitic meningitis and consists of thrombosis secondary to the inflammatory reaction around the vessel. Vascular symptoms during later stages are caused by thickening of the intima and adventitia, with such damage to the walls that thrombosis, obliteration, miliary aneurysm, or hemorrhage may occur, leading to atrophy, softening, and degeneration of brain substance.

SYMPTOMS. Among the early symptoms is intermittent headache, often worse at night, and aggravated by mental or physical effort. Dizziness is another troublesome symptom, as is insomnia. Periods of intense sleepiness or of stupor may occur. The patient becomes irritable and emotionally unstable and shows loss of interest in, and lack of capacity for, work, an increasing apathy, and impairment of memory. With or without the prodromal symptoms mentioned, the majority of cases of vascular cerebral syphilis develop symptoms or neurological signs of a focal nature. Since these vascular accidents are usually thrombotic, the signs are ordinarily of slow onset and are quite variable in their intensity and permanency. Consciousness is often not lost, and there is a surprising tendency to recovery from serious neurological disturbances. Hemiplegias are common, the particular syndrome depending on the site of the lesion—cortical, capsular, pontine, et cetera. Aphasias, usually transient, are frequent. After these apopletic attacks, the patient is frequently left with a certain impairment of effectiveness and of intellectual capacity. Subarachnoid hemorrhages may also occur as a result of syphilis of the meningeal vessels.

The Wassermann reaction of the blood serum is, of course, usually positive. This reaction is frequently positive in large amounts of cerebrospinal fluid but may be entirely negative, a fact that should be borne in mind. Protein is usually increased, and cells may or may not be increased. The colloidal gold reaction in vascular neurosyphilis is quite uncertain, since, while it often gives a curve of the luetic type, it may not be distinctive or may even be negative. It will thus be seen that the serology in the vascular form of cerebral syphilis may be conclusive but that the absence of positive findings may not exclude its existence.

The following abstract will illustrate a case of mental disorder resulting from interstitial brain syphilis, the lesion of which was probably vascular in nature.

J. L. was admitted to a public mental hospital at 48 years of age. Four years previously he had contracted syphilis. Five months before he had suffered a "clot back of the eyes." For a short period he was nearly blind but soon recovered. About this time a change in personality occurred. He lost interest in his home, drank heavily, began to gamble, and was discharged from the position he had satisfactorily held for 22 years. Some months later he suffered an apoplectic stroke with hemiplegia of the right side. He was described as semiconscious for three or four weeks, following which he had difficulty in talking. Following another stroke four months later, the patient became sullen, irritable, suspicious, and threatening, and at times abused his wife. Just prior to his hospital admission he threatened his daughter with a knife and drove his family from the house. The following day he refused to eat, declaring that his food was poisoned.

On arrival at the hospital, the patient was found to be fully oriented and well in touch with his environment. His memory was fair but his fund of information was impaired and his capacity for apperception was faulty. Neurologically he showed a slight ptosis of both upper lids and slight external strabismus of the left eye; the pupils were unequal but reacted to light and convergence. His speech was characterized by dysarthria; the right arm and leg were moderately spastic and presented exaggerated tendon reflexes; the right foot showed ankle clonus. The Wassermann reaction on the blood serum was positive but was negative on the cerebrospinal fluid; the latter contained 2 cells per cu. mm., and gave a "suspicious" Pandy reaction and the following gold curve: 1122110000. Under treatment the serology became entirely negative. Four years later he was still in the institution, where he was well behaved, had freedom of the grounds, and worked in the hospital industrial shop. His higher intellectual functions were obviously much impaired, however, and he was quite incapable of supporting himself or adjusting independently in the community.

TREATMENT. The treatment of meningeal and vascular forms of neurosyphilis is the same as that of the meningo-encephalitic form, i.e., with penicillin. Treatment with this antibiotic is usually followed by excellent results unless vascular or meningeal inflammation has already caused permanent damage to the nervous tissue. Routine laboratory examinations of both blood and cerebrospinal fluid should be made every six months.

BIBLIOGRAPHY

Dattner, B.: Penicillin in Neurosyphilis. New York, Grune & Stratton, 1949.

Merritt, H. H.: The early clinical and laboratory manifestations of syphilis of the central nervous system. New England J. Med., 223:446–450, 1940.

Idem, Adams, R. D., and Solomon, H. C.: Neurosyphilis. New York, Oxford University Press, 1946.

Chapter Fifteen

BRAIN SYNDROMES ASSOCIATED WITH CHRONIC ARTERIOSCLEROSIS

*"It is not a divinity but the mystery of arteriosclerosis that shapes the earthly endings of most lives."**

The designation "Psychoses with Cerebral Arteriosclerosis" is, strictly speaking, a misnomer. The term *arteriosclerosis* may still be used in a generic sense applied to a group of vascular diseases characterized morphologically by hardening of the vessel wall. It does, however, place undue emphasis upon the hardening aspect of the changes that occur with age in the walls of blood vessels. It is now known that the hardening per se is a relatively benign process that produces little if any interference with the flow of blood. On the other hand, the process known to the pathologist as atherosclerosis is vastly more serious since it is characterized by the *narrowing* or *obliteration of the lumen*. It is an occlusive disease that affects the nutrient vessels of the brain, heart, or kidney, and by progressively choking off the flow of blood leads to functional alteration and even to disability or death. When, therefore, the term arteriosclerosis is used in this chapter, it should be borne in mind

that the real nature of the pathological vascular process is an atherosclerosis with its distinctive morphological feature of stainable lipid within the atheromatous lesions.

From the physiological standpoint, the narrowing of the lumen of the blood vessels leads to reduction in cerebral blood flow and to progressive hypoxia. Thus there follow disturbances in cellular metabolism and eventual death of cells. Although it is true that some individuals with cerebral arteriosclerosis associated with markedly diminished general cerebral blood flow appear to show good personality and cerebral function and to withstand well sudden additional lowering of that flow, it must be kept in mind that the presently used techniques of measuring flow do not determine levels in localized subcortical areas but rather present quantitative changes only in the circulation of the brain as a whole.

The part played by age in the genesis of atherosclerosis has been discussed at great length by pathologists. Although it is now generally agreed that arteriosclero-

* The "little strokes," New England J. Med., 246:155, 1952.

sis (atherosclerosis) is not a necessary result of age, it is indirectly related to the aging process in the sense that it is a cumulative and slowly progressive disease that becomes increasingly manifest with the passage of time. It is therefore natural that, with the progressive lengthening of the life span during the present century, there has been a great increase in the number of persons suffering from arteriosclerosis. There is perhaps no better evidence of this fact than the striking increase in the number of admissions to public mental hospitals of persons suffering from mental disorders incident to this disease. Persons suffering from brain syndromes associated with cerebral arteriosclerosis constitute approximately 22 per cent of first admissions to New York State psychiatric hospitals.

With the progressive diminution in caliber of the relatively narrow vessels of the brain, the flow of blood is slowly throttled and the nutrition of the parenchyma affected. Ganglion cells gradually deteriorate and areas of atrophy develop around the constricted arterioles. Hemorrhage or thrombosis and embolism with infarction may occur. Thrombosis is much more frequent and probably accounts for 85 per cent of vascular accidents.

Symptoms

The age of onset of the arteriosclerotic psychoses varies widely, but in general it is between 50 and 65. Prodromal symptoms in the form of fatigue, headache, dizziness, diminution of capacity for prolonged concentration, drowsiness in the afternoon or evening, and an insidious impairment of physical and mental abilities are common. Frequently latent character features are revealed or previous trends become pathologically exaggerated. Any apparent change in character in a person over 50 should suggest the possibility of cerebral arteriosclerosis if syphilitic meningo-encephalitis is excluded. There is much evidence that states of vasoconstriction do occur in the brain and that they are of functional significance. In somewhat more than half

of the cases, a sudden attack of confusion is the first obvious mental symptom. Episodes of confusion or of excitement or, particularly, of their combined association, constitute a frequent symptom of the arteriosclerotic syndrome. There are clouding of consciousness, incoherence, and restlessness, sometimes extreme. In other cases the onset is insidious and represents what has been descriptively characterized as "a slow dying at the top." Among such symptoms are easy mental fatigability, a lessening of initiative, an impairment of attention, emotional instability with outbursts of weeping or laughter, and perhaps a tendency to depression. Some patients are irritable, aggressive, meddlesome, quarrelsome, obstinate, jealous, and paranoid. Finer sentiments, such as affection, may be destroyed. Some patients become garrulous. Memory is impaired to varying degrees. At first it may consist merely of difficulty in recollecting names, but later it may become general. The facies may become increasingly immobile and inanimate. Nocturnal attacks of bewilderment, of delirious, anxious states or of violence may occur. Frequently the arteriosclerotic patient becomes neglectful of his personal appearance, his clothing may not be clean, and he may fail to bathe. Delusions may be expressed and are particularly apt to be of a persecutory nature, although ideas of ruin and hypochondriacal delusions are not uncommon. The patient may be distressed by ideas of jealousy concerning his wife or other members of his family. His ideational content, like other expressions of his psychosis, is influenced largely by former types of mental mechanisms and other patterns of personality expression. Occasionally a patient is noted who expresses ideas of grandeur representing a compensation for failing sexual capacity. As in senile dementia, defective judgment and decreased inhibition may result in sexual indiscretions or offenses.

Characterological changes representing alterations in adaptive mechanisms and personality defenses may occur. Defenses against feelings of dependency may, for example, be replaced by acceptance of these needs. Hostile impulses that were previously suppressed may be released. Premorbid defensive drives, such as for perfectionism, may be relaxed.

Among persons with more advanced cerebrovascular disease are those subject to "the little strokes" (Alvarez). Such individuals may become intermittently psychotic or subject to periods of delirium. In the case of sclerosis of the large cerebral vessels, the first gross symptom may be an apoplectic stroke, aphasic attack, or other focal disturbance, although other evidence of vascular disease usually appears first. Vertical headaches that are worse in the morning, giddiness, short periods of confusion, and fleeting loss of power in arm or leg, or momentary aphasias or apraxias usually give warning of subsequent more serious focal lesions. Station becomes insecure, its base wide, the gait uncertain, and the steps short and spastic. Pupillary inequalities are not uncommon, although recent studies have shown that there is no close relationship between retinal atherosclerosis and sclerosis of the small arteries supplying the brain. Coarse tremors may appear, and the patient may finally experience much difficulty in feeding himself. Cardiovascular disease in the form of cardiac hypertrophy, coronary sclerosis, or chronic valvular disease is common. Numerous paralytic lesions appear—evidence of focal destruction of nervous tissue by occlusion or by rupture of a vessel of considerable size. Upper motor neuron paralyses and various aphasias and apraxias are most frequent. Paraphasia, or confusion of words, may occur. Deterioration and dementia are hastened by these focal lesions, especially by those that result in serious speech disturbances. Certain intellectual functions may be much impaired while others remain comparatively intact. Epileptiform attacks, either jacksonian or general, may take place, caused, some believe, by temporary anemia or edema.

Sands has called attention to the fact that patients with cerebral arteriosclerosis are peculiarly apt, on the occasion of a mild infection, to suffer from episodes characterized by confusion, disorientation, misidentification of persons, anxiety, fear reaction, suspiciousness, and delusional trends.

Contrary to the dementing senile patient, the arteriosclerotic patient, at least in the early stages of his deterioration, recognizes that there is a decline in the quickness and accuracy of his mental functions. He often feels keenly his difficulty in finding a word, his weakness of memory, and the diminution of physical and mental capacity.

The following abstract of a patient's clinical record illustrates some of the more frequent symptoms resulting from the physiological disturbances of brain function through arteriosclerotic changes.

W. B., aged 66, a bookkeeper by occupation, was brought to a mental hospital from the Ab. Hospital to which he had been admitted one month previously. The family physician reported that the patient had had elevated blood pressure for 10 years. Three weeks before admission to the general hospital he suddenly suffered from an attack of vertigo and severe headache lasting for about 20 minutes. He then resumed his daily task although he felt weak and tired. On the following day, "for no reason that he can explain, as he claims he was not dizzy," his brother reported, "he just lost his balance and fell downstairs." He was then referred to the hospital for study and diagnosis.

The patient's brother added that 18 months previous to this episode the patient first showed a change in behavior. He talked much less and "would often sit and look at absolutely nothing for long periods. For the past year he had been saying rather peculiar things. He became silly, flighty, and confused." While in the general hospital to which he had been admitted, he was constantly worrying over loss of his money, although there was no basis for such a belief. The brother described the patient's behavior in the general hospital as follows: "He was very confused. He would not remain in bed, and instead of getting out of the side of the bed, he would crawl over its foot to get out."

Upon arrival at the mental hospital, his systolic blood pressure was found to be 240 and the diastolic fluctuated from 100 to 140. He said he had come from the B. General Hospital and had never heard of the Ab. Hospital. When asked the dates when he became ill, he maintained that he had not been ill. He gave his age, his birth year, and the current year correctly, but when asked the present date he replied, "The New York Giants won the first game, Brooklyn won the second game, and the third game was going home when I went." A month after admission he conversed freely and usually rationally with other patients and showed concern about the condition of the feeble ones. He continued, however, to manifest difficulty in concentration, in apperception, and in memory for recent events. He was then fully oriented as to time and place and recognized that his memory was impaired. He remarked to his physician, "I don't know. If I have to keep on this way, maybe the good Lord ought to take me." Four months after admission he was described as having periods of memory loss. Although the United States was then intently pre-occupied with World War II, he took no interest in the world situation and important events. At times he showed difficulty in choosing the proper word and occasionally became quite irritated at himself for having this difficulty. Although he had completed three years of college, he was unable to answer simple mathematical questions and failed in an attempt to subtract from 100 by using 7 as the subtrahend and the successive differences as the minuend. Under the simple routine of hospital life and freedom from responsibility, the patient improved still further. Five and a half years after admission he was described as discussing his business affairs intelligently and as showing an interest in hospital activities and as being well informed on current events. Three years later there developed periods of 24 hours' duration during which he became excited, screamed at anyone who approached him, and often became quite threatening, although he never did violence to them. At such times he was somewhat confused.

Prognosis

The prognosis is naturally unfavorable, but the course is not always uninterruptedly progressive. It frequently happens that a patient, particularly if he has cardiac and general vascular disease also, will enter an institution in a greatly confused, perhaps excited, state, so that he appears to be quite demented. After rest and several days or a few weeks of the simple regimen of hospital life, the patient may become clearly conscious and apparently recover from the acute symptoms. There is constant danger, however, that an apoplectic stroke or another confused episode may occur at any time. Many patients, nevertheless, retain considerable, although impaired, capacity for several years before dementia or physical helplessness removes them from the scene of activity. In many cases death is hastened by general arteriosclerosis associated with cardiorenal disease.

Diagnosis

The mental disorder from which the differentiation of arteriosclerotic psychosis is most frequently required is senile dementia. Since the two forms of deterioration are often associated and the manifestations of both are about equally prominent, differentiation may be difficult or impossible. Arteriosclerotic psychosis occurs somewhat more frequently in men than in women, while senile dementia occurs more frequently in women. Arteriosclerosis usually arises earlier in life than senile atrophy. Usually there is less intellectual impairment in arteriosclerosis. Headache, dizziness, or apoplectic phenomena occur in about half of the cases of arteriosclerotic psychosis. Fainting attacks, convulsive seizures, or attacks of cardiac dysfunction likewise suggest an arteriosclerotic origin. Sudden attacks of confusion often occur in arteriosclerotic psychoses. In younger persons the clinical picture may be strongly suggestive of syphilitic meningo-encephalitis, but laboratory tests quickly provide differentiating data. When depression and anxiety are present, the differentiation from a depressed phase of manic-depressive psychosis or from involutional melancholia may not be easy. Although in all three disorders the presenting picture may be an affective one, yet in arteriosclerotic disease there will usually be evidence of an underlying organic impairment of mental capacity or of signs of beginning vascular disease. Fluctuations in the sensorium and other episodic manifestations are often significant of involvement of the cerebral vessels. It should be remembered that acute confusional states resulting from toxic and biochemical factors are not uncommon among the aged, associated, at times, with dehydration.

Treatment

Since our knowledge concerning the causes of cerebral arteriosclerosis is so limited, little can be done to prevent its development. The milder psychoses with cerebral arteriosclerosis may be cared for at home; the severe ones require institutional treatment. In either case a carefully regulated mode of life is a fundamental requirement in treatment. Although neither heavy manual labor nor mental tasks involving burdensome responsibilities or emotional stress should be permitted, an agreeable occupation of simple type should be continued as long as possible, due attention being paid to recreation and physical rest. It should be borne in mind that suicide is not rare in arteriosclerotic depressions. The arteriosclerotic patient will be wise to refrain from alcohol. Any inadequacies of nutrition should be improved, and attention should be directed to any associated cardiorenal or other pathologic condition. The value of low cholesterol, low fat diets, estrogens, heparin, choline, or inositol as a means of influencing the presumed disturbed lipid metabolism remains controversial. Hydrotherapy in mild forms, carefully supervised, may be employed, but measures that are too long or too vigorous may be harmful.

Chlorpromazine has been helpful with some patients in reducing nocturnal insomnia and restlessness, confusion, excitement, and aggressive, destructive behavior, but care must be taken in the case of the arteriosclerotic patient because of the possibility of a hypotensive reaction following administration of the drug. For this reason, oral administration is preferred, commencing with small doses (10 mg. three times daily) and gradually increasing the amount. The use of other sedatives often may be discontinued. The dosage needed and tolerated is highly variable. Psychotherapy should not be forgotten in the anxious patient. Barbiturates will sometimes aggravate the confusion associated with cerebral arteriosclerosis and hypertensive encephalopathy. Reese and Kant report that the dizziness, headache, insomnia, confusion, and delirious confusion occurring in these disorders is often relieved by the administration of aminophylline in doses of 4 grains each four times a day. Nicotinic acid or its amide is often used to improve the cerebral circulation. The use of anticoagulants to prevent cerebral thrombosis is now widely practiced.

BIBLIOGRAPHY

Allen, E. B.: Psychiatric aspects of cerebral arteriosclerosis. New England J. Med., *245*: 677–684, 1951.

Idem: The management of cerebral anteriosclerosis: psychiatric aspects. Bull. New York Acad. Med., *31*:366–375, 1955.

Alman, R. W., and Fazekas, J. F.: Disparity between low cerebral blood flow and clinical signs of cerebral ischemia. Neurology *7*:555–558, 1957.

Freyhan, F. A., Woodford, R. B., and Kety, S. S.: Cerebral blood flow and metabolism in psychoses of senility. J. Nerv. & Ment. Dis., *113*:449–456, 1951.

Malzberg, B.: The expectation of psychoses with cerebral arteriosclerosis in New York State. Psychiatric Quart., *19*:122–138, 1945.

Pollack, B.: The addition of chlorpromazine to the treatment program for emotional and behavior disorders in the aging. Geriatrics, *11*: 253–259, 1956.

Raskin, N., and Ehrenberg, R.: Senescence, senility, and Alzheimer's disease. Am. J. Psychiat., *113*:133–137, 1956.

Rothschild, D.: Neuropathologic changes in arteriosclerotic psychoses and their psychiatric significance. Arch. Neurol. & Psychiat., *48*: 417–436, 1942.

Idem: The note of the premorbid personality in arteriosclerotic psychoses. Am. J. Psychiat., *100*:501–505, 1944.

Idem: The clinical differentiation of senile and arteriosclerotic psychoses. Am. J. Psychiat., *98*:324–333, 1941.

Simon, A., et al.: Lipoproteins in general and cerebral arteriosclerosis. Am. J. Psychiat., *108*: 663–668, 1952.

Wright, I. S., and Luckey, H. E., Eds.: Cerebral Vascular Diseases. New York, Grune & Stratton, 1955.

Chapter Sixteen

BRAIN SYNDROMES ASSOCIATED WITH CONVULSIVE DISORDERS (EPILEPSY)

"As for this disease called divine, surely it too has its nature and causes whence it originates, just like other diseases, and is curable by means comparable to their cure."

Hippocrates

The term *epilepsy,* derived from the Greek word meaning to seize or fall upon, has long been applied to a group of explosive reactions formerly believed to constitute a disease *sui generis.* The name has persisted, although it is now generally agreed that epilepsy is not a disease entity but is a symptom complex characterized by periodic, transient episodes of alteration in the state of consciousness which may be associated with convulsive movements or disturbances in feeling or behavior, or both. The following may be regarded as a reasonable clinical definition of epilepsy: "Episodic, recurrent, limited periods of altered consciousness with or without involuntary movements, not the result of bodily disorders such as failure of circulation, low blood sugar, emotional disturbance, or use of soporific drugs or intoxicants."*

ETIOLOGY, TYPES, AND SYMPTOMS

Physiologically, epilepsy may be regarded as a disturbance in the electro-physiochemical activity of the discharging cells of the brain, a disturbance that may be produced by a variety of irritative stimuli impinging upon them from within or from without. This physiological disturbance may be expressed in the form of: (*a*) a change in electric potential as recorded in the electroencephalograms, (*b*)

* J.A.M.A., *164*:1706, 1957.

varied disorders of consciousness, (c) disordered functioning of the autonomic nervous system, and (d) convulsive movements or psychic disturbances. The nature of the disturbance of the internal milieu which, in so-called idiopathic epilepsy, alters the activity of the cortical neurons or of basal gray matter and precipitates an abnormal discharge of electrical energy in the brain is unknown, but there is much to suggest that biochemical changes which increase the excitability of neurons may be the pathophysiological abnormality. Epilepsy, therefore, is probably neurogenic rather than psychogenic, although psychogenic factors may precipitate a seizure in a person who has a tendency to them.

Precipitating Factors

Although it appears that, in the majority of patients, the attacks are not precipitated by obvious external stimulation, in some they are always induced by a specific type of physical or perceptual stimulation. The arousal of anxiety either through some immediate interpersonal conflict or through fantasy of such a conflict often acts as a precipitating factor. In patients whose attacks originate in such a manner, psychiatric management may be helpful. In other cases specific sensory stimuli act as the precipitants.

Sudden sounds, occasionally listening to music, flickering lights (as when driving through an avenue of trees in sunlight, watching sunlight on water, or by rapidly moving the hands before the eyes) may induce seizures. Seizures induced by flickering lights are now designated as *photogenic epilepsy*. In some instances, only complex visual stimuli prove excitatory. Prolonged reading has initiated an attack, which commences with "clicking" or movement of the jaws. Some patients are able to terminate such an attack if they discontinue reading with the initiation of the jaw "clicking."

In female epileptic patients, the occurrence of a seizure in association with the menstrual period is common, but it is not known in what way the premenstrual hormonal interplay acts to precipitate attacks. The final metabolic derangement that results in a seizure is probably not the same in all patients or even the same at all times in any one patient. If the equilibrium of the internal milieu is in delicate balance, an attack may be precipitated by a minor physiological disturbance, such as that produced by hyperventilation.

Electroencephalography

Although the occurrence of an abnormal discharge of energy in the cerebral cortex coincident with epileptic attacks has only relatively recently been proved by electrical methods, Hughlings Jackson (1834-1911), the father of clinical neurology, conceived the idea nearly 75 years ago that such a discharge must be the basis of epilepsy. In 1929 Hans Berger of Jena discovered that by perfecting technical methods of amplification he could record through the intact skull the changes in electric potential already known to accompany cortical activity. The electroencephalogram (EEG) indicates alterations in electrical, and thus physiological, activity within the brain. Further study showed that normally about 10 electrical impulses originate in the brain every second, and that when these currents are recorded in the electroencephalogram they show a pattern of voltage and frequency (height and rate of the waves) more or less characteristic of the individual.

It was then found that in epilepsy there are paroxysmal bursts of abnormal cortical activity with resulting changes in the rhythmic pattern of the EEG, indicating abnormalities in both rate and voltage of these currents. For this reason Lennox introduced the term "paroxysmal cerebral dysrhythmia" as applicable to epilepsy. Although abnormalities are to be observed in the electroencephalogram in many conditions other than epilepsy, yet in this disorder these abnormalities tend to assume certain patterns. Further, these patterns are distinctive for certain types of seizures. The electroencephalogram reveals the presence of these dysrhythmic discharges but fails to reveal their pathogenesis. When the focal discharging lesion is in the parietal, occipital, or frontal lobes, the symptomatology is largely neurological; if the disorder is in one or both temporal lobes, the symptomatology is largely psychiatric or that of psychomotor epilepsy.

It is generally estimated that 5 to 10 per cent of normal persons exhibit abnormalities of their electroencephalograms similar to those seen in epileptics. It is believed that such persons are predisposed to epilepsy, although the disturbance in cortical electrodynamics as represented by the EEG is not so serious as to result in seizures unless the cerebrum suffers some pathological alteration. It has also been found that about 85 per cent of persons with a history of epilepsy show abnormalities of electroencephalographic rhythm during a 15-minute recording in the interval between convulsions as compared to 10 per cent in the average population. When such abnormalities of the EEG exist in the interparoxysmal period, they tend to be of the same general type as those observed in the form of seizure from which the patient usually suffers. These types will be described later. There are, however, undoubted epileptics in whom abnormal tracings have never been obtained even by repeated examinations.

It will thus be seen that the electroencephalogram has its limitations. Although the finding of seizure discharges creates a presumption that clinical seizures have occurred or will occur, a negative report (no seizure discharges) does not rule out epilepsy. This is because (*a*) seizure discharges can be present in the depths of the brain and not appear in standard recordings from the surface of the head and (*b*) discharges may occur so infrequently that there is almost no likelihood of one occurring during the relatively short period of recording required in a routine examination. In the waking state, but more especially during sleep, seizure discharges occur, as evidenced by the electroencephalogram, that are not immediately associated with clinical symptoms. Eighty per cent of patients with a history of convulsive epileptic seizures have non-convulsive seizure discharges while asleep. When not asleep, only 35 per cent of this group have subclinical seizure discharges.

To be of value, it is essential that the making of an encephalogram be carried out with meticulous care by a thoroughly-trained technician. The requirements in this respect are far more exacting than for other diagnostic procedures in common use. Artifacts resulting from technical errors or mechanical defects may easily arise. Even greater technical knowledge and experience is required in the interpretation of the encephalogram. The individual who interprets the record must have all the information available regarding the patient if the test is to be really useful and dependable. With the possible exception of a minority of cases of idiopathic epilepsy, it is rarely if ever possible to make a conclusive diagnosis on the basis of an EEG alone. In about 48 per cent of persons with a history of seizures, a routine EEG is of great value in diagnosis and in about 42 per cent it is of little or no value.

Idiopathic and Symptomatic Epilepsy

In many instances clinical seizures develop in persons with pre-existing cerebral dysrhythmia but in whom no visible or otherwise demonstrable alteration of cerebral tissue can be discovered. For this reason seizures of unknown origin have long been known as *idiopathic epilepsy*. It is now generally acknowledged, however, that epilepsy is not a disease in itself but rather a symptom of some underlying cerebral disorder. Perhaps in the so-called idiopathic, or better, cryptogenic, epilepsy there is some metabolic disorder of the brain cells as a result of which they are apt to discharge in an explosive way. This may happen at any time and without apparent cause. About 77 per cent of all epileptics fall among those in whom no cause of the condition can be found. Cases in this group tend to manifest themselves early in life. In other instances tumors, trauma, inflammation, or other discoverable lesions precipitate seizures in a person who may or may not have had a pre-existing cerebral dysrhythmia. Those seizures in which a cerebral lesion either brought out a subclinical dysrhythmia or produced seizures in the absence of pre-existing dysrhythmia are known as *symptomatic or acquired epilepsy*. A growing recognition of the multiplicity of etiological and contributing factors continues to displace the traditional idiopathic versus symptomatic point of view.

Frequency of Epilepsy

It is generally estimated that the incidence of epilepsy in the United States is 1 in 200 of the population. This means that there are over 700,000 epileptics in this country. Because of the development of new drugs in recent years for the treatment of the disorder, fewer patients than formerly require institutional care. For the most part these epileptics are chronic, mentally deteriorated patients. The incidence in males is slightly greater than in females, probably because of the greater frequency of head trauma in the male both at birth and in adult life.

Age of Onset

Idiopathic epilepsy may develop at any age but a majority of the cases appear between the ages of 10 and 20. Not a few occur before 10 years of age, but the first appearance of a seizure after 20 requires study by all known methods before the conclusion is reached that it is idiopathic. Infantile convulsions appearing without obvious cause should be regarded with apprehension. It is reported that infantile convulsions associated with fever or other physical disturbance increase the chances of epilepsy five times.

Inheritance

The exact degree to which heredity influences the development of seizures is a controversial subject. The work of Lennox and his associates strongly suggests that it is of considerable influence, while Alstrom, a Swedish epileptologist, although believing epilepsy to be a symptom and not a disease *sui generis*, concludes that it is rarely gene-determined. After a careful study of 897 families in which one or more members suffer from the disorder, he concluded that the incidence of epilepsy among close relatives of epileptics does not significantly exceed that of the general population. Lennox, Gibbs, and Gibbs, on the other hand, found from an electroencephalographic examination of parents of epileptics that these parents had abnormal brain waves much more frequently than did control persons. In the opinion of these authors, the "presence of abnormal brain waves in the parents of epileptics is presumably evidence that the cerebral dysrhythmias associated with epilepsy are inheritable and that parents who show such cortical dysrhythmias are 'carriers' of the disorder." These authors found that 60 per cent of the near relatives of non-institutional epileptics had dysrhythmia and 2.4 per cent of them had a history of seizures. Of their controls, 10 per cent showed dysrhythmia. Of course none had seizures.

It has been found that among identical twins idiopathic epilepsy occurs eight times more frequently in both individuals than it does in both of fraternal twins. It is estimated that epilepsy occurs about five times more frequently among near relatives of idiopathic epileptics than it does in the general population. The existence of a predisposition to the disease in the child of an epileptic is often demonstrable in the form of cerebral dysrhythmia. There is also a striking likeness of brain-wave abnormalities in epileptics with the same heredity. A person afflicted with epilepsy who marries a non-epileptic may, however, expect only one child in 50 resulting from the union to suffer from convulsions.

Not infrequently the psychiatrist is asked concerning the advisability of marriage for the epileptic or the probability that his children may inherit the disease. Lennox points out the following factors as tending to minimize the chances of the disease in the child of an epileptic; a family history devoid of epilepsy or migraine for the spouse as well as the patient; a minimal abnormality of their electroencephalograms; some acquired condition that is at least partially responsible for seizures; late onset of the illness, and a normal mental endowment. In his opinion the genetic factor in epilepsy is probably no greater than it is in many other common diseases.

Types of Seizures and Their Symptoms

Three major types of clinical seizures are usually described: grand mal, petit mal, and psychomotor seizure or psychic equivalent. Heredity is of importance in determining the pattern of seizure. The seizures of all types are irregular and unpredictable. There are many variants of epilepsy which, because they depart so far from the "usual" forms of seizures, are apt to escape recognition. Loss of consciousness with or without convulsive spasm is the criterion of epilepsy. It is probably not sufficiently appreciated that in many attacks consciousness is not lost but is merely disturbed. The patient may be aware of all that is going on around him, may hear and understand what is being said, but is for the time being unable to collect his thoughts or reply to a question. Not rarely the occurrence of a major epileptic fit suddenly renders clear the meaning of obscure minor events that may have existed for years. These may have been myoclonic, local muscle spasms, defects of attention, "absences," dreamy states, or brief periods of mental inhibition when mental processes seemed to be arrested and the mind a blank. The form that epilepsy takes depends not so much on the pathological features of the lesion as on its site and the violence of the neuronal discharges in the neighborhood of the lesion and the extent of their spread to the rest of the brain.

GRAND MAL. The grand mal seizure with its intense spontaneous neuronal activity is the most dramatic of the epileptic manifestations. Seizures of this type tend to be accompanied by an increase in speed and voltage of brain waves which are recorded in the electroencephalogram as sharp spikes, often at the rate of 25 per second.

Aura. From a moment to several seconds before the loss of consciousness, about half of the patients with a grand mal type of attack have an *aura*, or warning, that a seizure is immediately imminent. The aura is not really a premonition but the first manifestation of the neuronal discharge. The form of the aura depends primarily upon the site of the epileptogenic focus. Lesions of the precentral region generally give rise initially to motor phenomena and of the postcentral region to sensory phenomena. The aura may consist of numbness, tingling, uncomfortable sensations, of a feeling of distress in the epigastrium, perhaps passing up toward the head, or of a hallucination of the special senses, such as flashes of light, certain noises, or olfactory hallucinations. The aura is usually affectively unpleasant. Sometimes the aura is motor in nature and consists of a twitching or stiffness in a certain group of muscles preceding the loss of consciousness.

Tonic phase. The loss of consciousness is sudden and complete. The patient falls at once, and as there is rarely any opportunity to protect himself, he may sustain serious injuries. As he falls, the entire voluntary musculature goes into a continuous contraction, remaining in this *tonic* phase from 10 to 20 seconds. The muscles of the chest often contract at the same time as do those of the larynx; air is thereby forcibly expelled and results in the peculiar sound known as the epileptic cry. At first the face is pale, but as the muscles rigidly contract, the superficial veins become engorged. At the same time the chest becomes fixed and the aeration of the blood ceases, thus adding to the cyanosis of the face. During this tonic phase and for a variable period afterward, the pupils are dilated and do not react to light and the corneal reflex is absent. The Babinski reflex is present and the tendon reflexes are absent or decreased. During the general muscular contraction, the bladder is often emptied and occasionally the rectum.

Clonic phase. The tonic stage is followed by intermittent or *clonic* muscular contractions, at first rapid but gradually growing less frequent. If at this time the tongue happens to fall between the teeth during a relaxation, it may be bitten when a clonic contraction follows. As respiration returns, the saliva, which could not be swallowed, may become intermixed with air and thus appears in a foam, perhaps tinged with blood.

Coma. In the *postconvulsive coma,* the pupils are rigid, tendon reflexes are absent, respiration is stertorous, the face is congested and covered with perspiration, and the lips are cyanosed. If an arm or leg be lifted and then released, it drops heavily as in a state of flaccid paralysis. If left undisturbed, the patient may sleep for an hour or two, complaining of headache, fatigue, and perhaps of a painful tongue on awaking. As the patient emerges from the coma, he is often bewildered and may perform semi-automatic acts, move aimlessly about, exhibit chewing movements, fumble at his clothing, or attempt to remove it. Sometimes clouded states persisting for a few days may develop after several successive convulsions. They are more frequent in men than in women.

Some patients have convulsions during sleep as well as in their waking hours, while in some patients the convulsions are always nocturnal. Many have their seizure just as they are falling asleep. It should be remembered that occasionally an epileptic who is subject to nocturnal seizures is suffocated by burying his face in a pillow during a convulsion.

Status epilepticus. Sometimes a patient may pass from one seizure into another without intervening recovery of consciousness. This condition, known as status epilepticus, always involves danger to life. It is sometimes precipitated by abrupt withdrawal of medication, particularly if the patient has been receiving phenobarbital. It may follow alcoholism or excessive fatigue, but frequently no precipitating factor is evident. It is not rare after cerebral operations on epileptics. If preventive measures are not taken, the temperature may rise to dangerous heights. The patient may become profoundly exhausted, lapse into coma, and die from cardiac dilation or pulmonary edema.

PETIT MAL. Abortive seizures of various degrees and types occur, in all of which there is usually some disturbance of consciousness. The most frequent of the minor forms is that of petit mal, which is characterized by a transient interruption of the stream of consciousness. The electroencephalogram of petit mal consists of a slow, round wave followed by a quick, sharp spike. Groups of these alternately slow and fast waves occur three times a second. It is the most distinctive of any of the epileptic brain-wave records. The details of these minor attacks differ widely among individual patients, but the most frequent form consists of a loss of consciousness lasting from 5 to 30 seconds. They begin and end abruptly and are without warning or sequel.

The patient does not fall. He may become pale, with his posture fixed, his eyes staring and expressionless; his attention cannot be secured; he may suspend his occupation and, through loss of muscle tone, drop whatever article may be in his hand. Usually there is a little rhythmic twitching of eyelids, eyebrow or head. After a few seconds, consciousness abruptly returns and the patient resumes his activities. Most patients recognize that an attack has occurred, but some remain unaware of this "absence."

The onset of petit mal is usually between 4 and 8 years of age. After 18 years of age it tends to disappear or to be replaced by other types of seizure. Petit mal attacks usually occur much more frequently than grand mal seizures. From one or two to a few hundred attacks may occur in a day. The two forms frequently co-exist. Two of every three children with petit mal subsequently develop grand mal.

Many children with petit mal are often socially and emotionally maladjusted.

R. FRONTAL

R. TEMPORAL

R. PARIETAL

R. OCCIPITAL

L. FRONTAL

L. TEMPORAL

L. PARIETAL

L. OCCIPITAL

1 SEC.   50 uV.

R. & L. EAR REFERENCE

Figure 1. Normal adult record characterized by 11 c.p.s. alpha rhythm, which is most prominent in the occipital areas.

R. FRONTAL - R. MOTOR

R. MOTOR - R. PARIETAL

R. PARIETAL - R. OCCIP.

L. FRONTAL - L. MOTOR

L. MOTOR - L. PARIETAL

L. PARIETAL - L. OCCIP.

50 μ V.

1 Sec.

Figure 2. One of a number of types of tracings found between attacks in patients with grand mal epilepsy. The record shows a burst of irregular, slow waves and atypical spike and wave discharges from all areas.

Figure 3. Spike discharges from the left anterior temporal lobe seen between attacks in a patient subject to psychomotor seizures of temporal lobe origin.

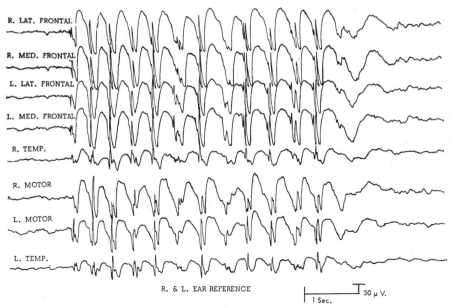

Figure 4. A short, clinical, petit mal attack accompanied by continuous 3 per second spike and wave discharges. Both the attack and the electrical discharges begin and end abruptly. (Records by courtesy of Dr. E. Goldensohn.)

This maladjustment often appears to be explained on the basis of an impaired parent-child relationship which affects the child's personality formation. The impaired relationship apparently grows out of a conscious or unconscious parental rejection. The lack of basic security occasioned by the impaired parent-child relationship tends to extend and pervade all relationships. Sometimes the child, believing that all adults are like his parents and that all experiences will be frustrating, develops a pattern of antagonism and rebellion.

Usually included in the petit mal form are myoclonic twitches in which single contractions of the flexor muscles of the arms occur without loss of consciousness, also akinetic attacks in which there is a sudden falling with muscular hypotonia. Like the classical petit mal, the latter two forms show a wave-and-spike rhythm of electrical discharge. Formerly the term pyknolepsy was given to what was believed to be a special type of seizure allied to petit mal. It is now considered to be a true petit mal. The name should therefore be dropped.

PSYCHOMOTOR EPILEPSY. Of greatest importance to the psychiatrist is psychomotor epilepsy, since it is characterized by trance-like attacks and confusional episodes which often lead to its misdiagnosis as schizophrenia or psychoneurosis. It is much more common in adults than in children, although in minor forms of the condition the attacks are very similar to those of petit mal. They differ from petit mal, however, in various ways. The attacks last longer, from one-half to two minutes, and are frequently associated with movements of the muscles concerned with mastication, swallowing, or speech, so that the patient may smack his lips, chew, or make incoherent verbalizations. Also, the clouding of consciousness is greater than in petit mal, with amnesia persisting for one-half to several minutes after the attack. In other instances, either brief episodes of automatic thought formations of a delusional nature and auditory or visual hallucinations may take place. In the case of the former, the patient may report only an amorphous repetitive and ill-defined thought, a crystallized thought percept, an internally-located voice usually in the head but sometimes in the abdomen or elsewhere or placed in the external environment. The visual hallucinations also may be apprehended either internally or externally. Finally, the electroencephalographic record is not similar to that of petit mal and its focus is the anterior pole of the temporal lobe.

Some patients describe brief affective states of fear, vague alarm, terror, rage, and occasionally of well-being or pleasure. The patient's behavior is appropriate to his mood. Other episodic but sustained moods may be in the form of extreme irritability, depression, ill humor, or bad temper. Sometimes the psychomotor seizure takes the form of a clouded state characterized by confusion, bewilderment, excitement with hallucinations, outbursts of violence, or occasionally ecstatic moods with religious exaltation. Clinically the clouded state suggests a delirium with liberation of aggressive, and occasionally, self-destructive impulses. Acts of violence may be committed in these automatisms and may be of a strikingly brutal nature, the patient pursuing his crime to a most revolting extreme.

These furors are characterized by their suddenness, absence of premeditation and of precaution, and amnesia for them. The extraordinary degree of discrimination and judgment displayed in the psychomotor attack often gives the patient's acts a misleading appearance of deliberation. It may be difficult to accept the fact that the author of the crime was not responsible for his acts. Usually these psychomotor seizures continue for only a few minutes, but they may go on for hours or even days. Sometimes the seizure may assume the form of a fugue. Occasionally the patient may report feelings of loneliness, strangeness, or typical "déjà vu" phenomena as if he had undergone the same experience in the dim past. Psychomotor seizures may occur in pure form, but in many cases grand mal seizures may also be present. Their frequency increases with age.

Probably to be included among the psychomotor epilepsies is the syndrome known as *epilepsia cursiva* ("running fit"). This is an episodic alteration of awareness associated with running. Consciousness may be clouded to a variable degree. Sometimes the running fit occurs immediately after a grand mal seizure. There may or may not be an aura. The duration of the running is brief. Frequently one finds a history of conflicts with members of the family that seem to have acted as precipitating factors.

The distinguishing feature of the electroencephalogram in the psychomotor seizure is the presence of spike seizure discharges at the rate of four to eight a second. It is believed that the focus of electroencephalographic activity is the anterior part of the temporal lobe. There is an increasing tendency to use the term *temporal lobe epilepsy* as a synonym for the psychomotor type, or to refer to the seizures characterized by hallucinations, memory disturbances, and automatisms as "temporal lobe" in preference to "psychomotor." Penfield and his co-workers, by stimulation of the cortex of the temporal lobe in patients with temporal lobe epilepsy, produced complex hallucinations, vivid memories, and dreams that were often identical with the content of the seizures.

A 10-year-old girl was brought to the clinic by her mother after she had suffered a number of episodes of loss of consciousness. These were described by the mother in the following way.

She awakened with a headache, seemed listless, and then was noticed by her mother to develop a twitching movement of the left side of her mouth and eyes. Her arms assumed an "odd," stiff position and became unresponsive. This condition persisted 5 minutes, to be followed by another similar episode 10 minutes later in which she urinated and defecated. These attacks were followed by five others preceded by an aura of "fear"—as the child stated, being "scared." The patient had total amnesia for the attacks.

Physically, no abnormalities were noted. An electroencephalogram showed a right occipito-temporal focus of high voltage, 31/second activity aggravated by hyperventilation. Other studies were negative. Psychiatric and psychological examinations at this time showed no pathology. She was treated with phenobarbital and Dilantin in increasing doses, with reduction in the occurrence of attacks and in their intensity.

For years she reported only daily brief episodes of "scary feelings." It was necessary to increase the dosage of the anticonvulsant medication, and mebaral was prescribed as well. At age 14 she was admitted to the hospital with an acute delirious state due to barbiturate overdosage. Following this hospital admission, her mother noticed a character change in that she became resentful and hostile, expressed the attitude that she was disliked, and seemed depressed. Then "slow spike waves" were observed over the left temporal region during periods of sleep.

At this time she commenced to have episodes of loss of consciousness, occurring without warning and with subsequent amnesia, in which she suddenly rushed away from her place of work, walking rapidly and aimlessly through the streets, impulsively removing her stockings and placing them in her purse or suddenly staring blankly, smacking her lips, giggling foolishly, and then mumbling incoherently. High-dosage combinations of various anticonvulsants failed to control these seizures. Due to her progressive social disability and withdrawal, in spite of medical therapy, a craniotomy with resection of the right temporal lobe was performed when she was 20 years old. Following the operation she was free of seizures and resumed her work on treatment with Dilantin alone.

Narcolepsy

The term *narcolepsy* was introduced in 1880 by Gélineau to describe a "rare neurosis characterized by an invincible need for sleep, ordinarily of short duration, occurring at longer or shorter intervals of time, often several times a day, forcing the subject to fall to the ground or to lie down in order to avoid falling." It has often been described as a variant of epilepsy. Probably, however, this is not the case, and it should be considered as a special clinical type in a group of sleep disorders. In many cases a history of previous epidemic encephalitis has been obtained. In some instances narcolepsy may be a sequel or a continuing form of that disease.

Narcolepsy is characterized by a sudden, irresistible desire to sleep. Regardless of the situation in which he may be placed or of the activity in which he may be engaged, the patient falls fast asleep. The sleep is apparently natural; the patient may be awakened, but the period of sleep usually lasts from seconds to 30 minutes. After he has awakened the patient usually states that he feels refreshed. Nocturnal sleep is not modified. The condition is most frequent in young male patients. Sexual impotence, obesity, and lymphocytosis are often associated symptoms. It is generally believed that some anatomical pathologic condition, the result of localized encephalitis, trauma, or neoplasm, exists in the gray matter surrounding the third ventricle at the level of the ocular nuclei or in the hypothalamus. Lesions of the hypophysis may be secondary.

Cases supposed to be psychogenic have

been reported. Psychometric studies in certain groups of patients with the narcoleptic syndrome have shown a common background of emotional conflict. The individuals felt themselves to be caught in a life pattern which they resented but felt obligated to conform to it. Frustrated in their efforts to achieve an autonomy in another pattern of their own choosing because of their dependent emotional attachments, those affected develop the narcoleptic complex which relieves the anxiety of open conflict.

Many consider narcolepsy as a syndrome that may occur in several pathological states. It is probably not a disease *sui generis*. Electroencephalographic records do not show the cerebral dysrhythmia of epilepsy. When the individual is alert, the electroencephalogram appears normal. On the other hand, a large proportion of patients with the syndrome demonstrate the electrical patterns of drowsiness, the earliest stage of sleep, and maintain such patterns for prolonged periods during examination. For this reason, some regard narcolepsy as a reversible dysfunction of the reticular-activating system and not as a paroxysmal convulsive disorder.

Narcolepsy does not respond to bromides, phenobarbital, or other sedatives, but is controlled by dextro amphetamine sulfate (10 to 50 mg. twice daily) or racemic amphetamine sulfate 10 to 50 mg. twice daily). If taken after midday, such drugs may produce insomnia.

DIFFERENTIATION FROM HYPERSOMNIA. Since this disorder may have psychogenic determinants or may be confused with hypersomnia as a symptom of an emotional disturbance, careful psychiatric evaluation is indicated in all suspected cases. Psychogenic hypersomnia differs in that the patterns of drowsiness or sleepiness last for several hours rather than for 15 to 30 minutes and are often associated with a history of disturbed nocturnal sleep, obesity, and the personality characteristics of passivity, with anxiety aroused by any situation threatening expression of criticism or anger to others. Such situations, particularly when the emotional outburst might be directed toward the person to whom they hold a strong dependent relationship, is the usual precipitant of the hypersomniac period. In hypersomnia, in contrast to narcolepsy, the amphetamines are unlikely to be useful, but their use may enhance the possibility of working out psychotherapeutically the psychodynamic conflict. Psychotherapy is reported to be helpful in certain instances.

Cataplexy

Apparently related to narcolepsy are the paroxysmal attacks known as cataplexy in which, under the influence of emotional excitement, there is paralysis of voluntary movements, a postural collapse of the whole body. The patient suddenly loses power and tone of all skeletal muscles, his knees give way, and he sinks helplessly to the ground. Many patients are unable to speak during the episode, although consciousness is fully preserved during its existence. Laughing, in particular, appears to provoke an attack, although anger, anxiety, or annoyance may act similarly. Narcolepsy and cataplexy are probably allied reactions, since cases of a transitional nature, including narcoleptic attacks provoked by emotion, are observed. Some writers consider cataplexy as a symptom of narcolepsy. The attacks of narcolepsy and cataplexy constitute what is often spoken of as the narcoleptic–cataplectic syndrome.

Epileptic Personality

Reference is often made to a so-called epileptic personality. The idea, however, of an "epileptic personality" as a precursor and an essential background of epilepsy has been discarded. Undoubtedly, some epileptic children are overly-aggressive, irritable, restless, overactive, moody, stubborn, oversensitive, and shy, and may manifest such conduct disorders as lying, stealing, fighting, sex misbehavior, cruelty, and destructiveness. By no means do all epileptic children show these characteristics. If they exist they are probably a result of bad home environment and of the frustrations, social rejection, state of insecurity, constant anxieties, and other emotional difficulties arising from the child's handicap.

Psychiatrists whose contacts with adult epileptics are limited to institutionalized patients usually assert that the epileptic patient has a rigid, unpleasant, irritable, self-centered personality given to rage on frustration. On the other hand, physicians who see no epileptics except those met in the office and clinics report that their patients do not exhibit more undesirable traits than do persons free from the disease. Undoubtedly, however, the patient who feels that he is handicapped through his disorder, who is constantly struggling for a place in his community, who fears exposure and is convinced that he is destined to be an abnormal member of the family has periods of irritability and depression. The sense of resentment that he often feels may produce unhappiness, add to his problem of adjustment, and perhaps create anti-social tendencies. Discouragement and hopelessness may lead to contraction of interests and mental slowness. The religiosity shown by some epileptics may have its origin in a search for security, solace, and self-esteem.

Epileptic Deterioration

In a certain number of epileptics, the range of interests narrows as the convulsive reaction continues. A psychic slowness develops, attention, intellectual processes, and emotional responses become increasingly dull, and comprehension and memory become impaired. The patient suffers from a poverty of ideas, shows a tendency to stress the trivial as much as the important, to become circumstantial in his ideational expression, to disregard the interests of others, to become selfish, affectively self-satisfied, boastful, lazy, and careless in appearance; his facies are characterized by expressionless vacuity. His speech comes to be slow and monotonous, with but little variation as to accent or tone, and his vocabulary becomes limited.

The degree to which dementia progresses, if it occurs, varies greatly. In extreme cases this dementia is great, the patient existing at a purely vegetative level, having no interest in, and no intelligible communications with, his social environment. Dementia is a much more frequent outcome in those who develop epilepsy in early childhood than in those in whom it appears in later years. Deterioration occurs less frequently if the patient was mentally normal at birth and if his seizures are of the petit mal or of infrequent grand mal types. It is more frequent in institutional patients than in the non-institutional ones. Of the latter, about one-third show some degree of mental impairment, although in only about 10 per cent is it so gross as to be immediately evident.

It is possible that deterioration may, in fact, be the result of the repeated anoxia and increased intracranial pressure that accompany repeated convulsions. In part it may be the result of the prolonged toxic effect of drugs; in considerable part it may be a response to the problems and situations which the very nature of the disease creates. The social and intellectual ostracism from which the epileptic often suffers, the deprivation of normal educational advantages, his feelings of inferiority, and his discouragement and hopelessness lead to a contraction of interests and to an impoverishment of personality.

The following case is fairly illustrative of the type of epileptic that enters institutions for mental disorders:

T. C. was admitted to a state hospital at the age of 31. He was described by his family as having a rather bad temper, being somewhat stubborn and inclined to boast. At 17 he began to suffer from mild seizures with loss of consciousness but without generalized convulsive movements. Not until age 27 did seizures occur more than two or three times a year. At that time they began to occur once or twice a month. At 29 the seizures became more severe, with marked convulsive movements and longer periods of unconsciousness. Because of a seizure at his place of employment, he lost his position in an ice factory. Unable to find other employment, the patient became somewhat depressed, worried, irritable, and "hard to get along with." His seizures became more frequent and severe.

One day following a period of moody pre-occupation, during which he seemed unaware of his wife's presence, he said to her, "Catherine, I've done good today. I've made my fortune." He then added, "Call the doctor and the priest, I'm afraid I am going to die." That night he walked about all night, talking constantly about becoming rich, quoted passages from the salesmanship instructions issued by a concern for which he had recently attempted to canvass, and paid little heed to his environment.

The following night he became so uncontrollable that, at his family's request, he was taken to the police station, and on the following day, he was committed to the state hospital. He was brought to the institution in straps, and in the admission office he shouted in a loud tone, "I drank a lot. I don't need that fellow. I thought an awful lot of that fellow. I think an awful lot of my mother. I told them plenty. I said, 'No! No!'" At intervals he struggled violently to escape from the two officers who were holding him. When asked any questions he would shout, "None of your business."

On examination at the hospital, he was noted to be a tall, ungainly individual, his large ears standing out prominently nearly at right angles to his skull. The conformation of his facies suggested that he was a biological variant. He remained clouded for about six weeks, at times apparently hallucinated, sometimes pre-occupied, mute, and having to be tube-fed, again talking in a loud, angry tone. When not in the continuous bath, he was usually to be found in his room, frequently with his prayer beads hanging from his mouth, often nude, and when approached would spontaneously make such remarks as: "I'm—I'm trying to solve the problem. I'm trying to find the solution. Irish! Irish! Captain I, an eye for an eye, and a tooth for a tooth. I've tried to save my soul."

After this prolonged clouded state, the patient remained clear for two months, occasionally suffering from a convulsion. Four months after admission he again became cloudy. At times he was stuporous, at times excited, and on several occasions attempted suicide. Nine months after admission he was paroled to his family, and for seven months he remained well except for occasional light convulsions. At the end of that period, while attending church, he suddenly arose during the services and began to pray loudly. He held a crucifix high above his head, and when led from the building, seemed much confused. The patient was then returned to the hospital, where the clinical course was much like that of the first residence.

DIAGNOSIS

If the attack is witnessed by the physician or by a trained observer, the diagnosis of the typical grand mal, with its unconsciousness and sequence of tonic cramp, cyanosis, clonic convulsive movements separated by intervals of gradually increasing length, stertorous breathing, perhaps automatic activity, stupor, and hebetude, is comparatively easy. In the case of petit mal or of an atypical and incompletely developed seizure, the diagnosis may be difficult. One should inquire for a history of migraine and of fainting attacks, and ascertain if any disturbances of consciousness have been accompanied by biting of the tongue, relaxation of the sphincters, or injury to self. If observed by the physician, the discovery of fixed, dilated pupils, of loss of the corneal reflex, and the presence of a Babinski reflex may confirm suspicion as to the epileptic nature of the paroxysm. The diagnosis of epilepsy is, however, not always easy. Attacks of loss of consciousness, of muscle-twitching, of feelings of faintness or of unreality will usually suggest epilepsy, but often a diagnosis must be based on retrospective facts found by careful questioning of the patient and observers.

The electroencephalogram is of assistance in establishing a diagnosis, but the evidence supplied by it must be supplemented by clinical observation. It must be remembered that about 5 per cent of the persons who never suffer from seizures of any kind show minor dysrhythmia in the EEG, and occasionally the EEG in such normal persons may be characteristic of the records made in epileptics between attacks. This is particularly true in the relatives of epileptics. In rare instances an epileptic with definite clinical seizures may in intervals between convulsions show an entirely normal EEG. It is estimated that the chances are nine in ten that any disturbances of consciousness occurring in a person with a positive EEG are epileptic. Activation of the abnormal electrical potentials may be induced occasionally by hyperventilation, or by small doses of metrazol intravenously. It is of interest that mescaline and diethyl lysergic acid diethylamide (d LSD 25) are incapable of activating the attacks or the typical electroencephalographic abnormality in those who have temporal-lobe seizures.

Hysterical patients with attacks resembling epilepsy usually have normal electroencephalograms. The seizures of the hysteric occur in the presence of others, and there is often some fairly obvious gain or domination to be secured by the paroxysm. The hysterical person rarely injures himself in a seizure. It is important to remember the make-up of this type of individual with his tendency to histrionic poses and simulation of symptoms. Although there may be a history of emotional disturbance just prior to an epileptic convulsion, yet any dramatic staging of a seizure points strongly toward hysteria. The hysterical seizure is usually grotesque in its manifestations, lacks the characteristic "march" of phases seen in epilepsy, and is not accompanied by ocular signs indicated in the previous paragraph, by sphincter incontinence, Babinski sign, or so deep a loss of consciousness. In hysteria there is never any biting of the tongue as in epilepsy. There may be difficulty in the differential diagnosis of temporal-lobe epilepsy and hysterical amnesic periods with automatism. The presence of psychogenic factors and the absence of the psychomotor type of electroencephalogram will point to the latter. It is often said that no epileptic attack is "motivated" and that no motivated act is epileptic.

The diagnosis of syncope from epilepsy is not always easy. The loss of consciousness in epilepsy is primarily caused by paroxymal discharges within the brain, while in syncope it results primarily from a fall in blood pressure. In syncope a cause—postural, emotional or physical—seems apparent. In syncope there is a fairly long warning. The patient often comments "I feel faint," and adopts some protective action, such as sitting. Pallor and hot or cold sweating are apparent. Consciousness usually returns without any confusion or sequel except sweating. The epileptic's loss of consciousness is usually followed by drowsiness and frequently associated with headache. In a Stokes-Adams attack, syncope and a convulsion may be closely linked. Here a rapid fall of blood pressure caused by cardiac arrest produces convulsions through cerebral anemia.

COURSE AND PROGNOSIS

Today the average epileptic enjoys an incomparably brighter prognosis than he did 20 years ago. Credit belongs mainly to the widespread availability of the electroencephalograph for diagnosis, to an ever-expanding group of non-sedative drugs that in many cases suppress epileptic phenomena, and to an increasing education of the public concerning the disorder with a resulting lessening of the rejection and social stigma from which the epileptic suffers.

The institutional physician may acquire altogether too pessimistic a view as to the prognosis of epilepsy. Most epileptics are intelligent and normal persons apart from their attacks and are quite able to earn a living. In a large percentage of the patients seen by the private physician, deterioration does not occur at all; if it does, it is but slight. This does not mean that essential epilepsy is not a serious symptom complex, one in which the prognosis must always be guarded. The prognosis is least favorable if the onset is in childhood. The prognosis as to recovery is worse in petit mal than in grand mal, but, contrary to general opinion, the mental life does not suffer so much in petit mal.

To a considerable extent, the prognosis is dependent upon the promptness of diagnosis and treatment. Both rate and extent of deterioration vary greatly but tend to be influenced by the age of onset, the frequency of seizures, and the effort made to maintain wholesome, constructive, satisfying, unselfish interests and constant employment. The emotional handicap produced through faulty attitudes such as shame or overprotectiveness on the part of the patient's family may operate against recovery. In its more malignant forms, the deterioration may proceed until the patient lives at an essentially vegetative level. A few epileptics become psychotic and require care in a hospital for mental diseases. However, with the use of anticonvulsant drugs now available, complete control or total abolition of grand mal seizures can be secured in 80 per cent of the patients.

TREATMENT

General Management

The medical profession is beginning to modify its fatalistic attitude toward the epileptic syndrome. In a minority of cases, epilepsy leads to a devastating impoverishment of personality, but much more frequently it is not incompatible with the functioning of the patient as a normal citizen. The social handicap remains, however, out of all proportion to the seriousness of the disease.

One of the fundamentals of treatment is the maintenance of optimum physical health. Physical and mental activities should be encouraged, especially those that afford a combination of muscular exercise, intellectual interest, and pleasure. It should be remembered that conscious or unconscious parental rejection may seriously warp the developing personality of the child. He should not be the object of oversolicitous fear and overprotection. Petit mal attacks, even if frequent, should not prevent attendance at school, nor should infrequent major attacks. The epileptic patient should be employed, but at a job wherein his own safety or that of others would not be jeopardized should he suffer a seizure. If possible, safety should not be purchased at the cost of active participation in life. Although it is usually necessary to raise the seizure threshold through medication, psychiatric treatment should not be omitted. Emphasis should be placed upon the relief of emotional or other psychic stress and upon the promotion of a normal life within the limits of the patient's psychobiological equipment. He should be given an opportunity to preserve his self-respect, develop his abilities, and maintain social usefulness. Many epileptics tend to daydream and

to indulge in idle dissipations that increase the frequency of their seizures and hasten deterioration. The epileptic should be encouraged to plan his own work, studies, and activities. Sustained work is often a difficult habit for him to establish but one of great importance.

There has often been an unnecessary restriction of the epileptic's diet. Ordinarily he should eat the same food as other members of the family, but attacks may be precipitated by hypoglycemia. The patient should therefore not go too long without food. The ingestion of an abnormal amount of fluid at one time may precipitate an attack. Food should be moderate in amount, and alcohol should be avoided.

Drug Therapy

The aim in treatment is to give medicine which will counteract the explosive tendency of the brain cells. For over 60 years bromides, first suggested in 1857 by Sir Charles Locock, constituted the principal form of medication. They have now been largely displaced by newer drugs.

Phenobarbital, or phenylethylbarbituric acid, first recommended by Hauptmann in 1912, is one of the drugs most widely used for raising the convulsive threshold of the epileptic. In persons 12 or more years of age, one may begin with a dose of 0.1 gm. once a day. In adults this may, if necessary, be increased to 0.3 to 0.4 gm., administered in divided doses. In children under five, 0.05 gm. may be used. If the seizures are nocturnal, it may be given at bedtime. If they are diurnal, it may be taken in the morning. Should seizures be frequent and severe, the patient may receive the drug three times a day. Even ordinary doses may produce drowsiness at the beginning of its use, but this effect usually disappears in a few weeks. Toxic doses may produce apathy, slow mental reactions, ataxia, slow speech, and muscular weakness. A sudden discontinuation of its use usually leads to an increase in the number of seizures and even to status epilepticus. Phenobarbital, nevertheless, is usually the most effective drug in alleviating grand mal seizures and least frequently produces toxic symptoms. It is of little value in petit mal, which should usually be treated by Tridione. Methylethylphenylbarbituric acid (Mephobarbital or Mebaral) acts similarly to phenobarbital but is more effective with certain individuals. For adults the dosage is 0.3 to 0.6 gms. daily.

In 1937 Merritt and Putnam introduced sodium diphenylhydantoin sodium, generally known as Dilantin, an anticonvulsant that has proved of great value. Not being a hypnotic, it does not cause drowsiness, as is so often the case with phenobarbital. The usual dose is 0.1 gm. capsule three times a day. The maximum amount that adults tolerate is approximately 0.6 gm. daily. If necessary for the control of seizures, this may be increased somewhat. In psychomotor seizures, it is the most efficacious of the antiepileptic drugs and in grand mal may be effective in some cases in which phenobarbital has failed. There is apparently a synergy between phenobarbital and Dilantin sodium that makes the combination more effective than when either drug is used alone. In toxic amounts, Dilantin causes gastric distress, a symptom that usually ceases after one or two weeks of treatment. Less frequently it causes dizziness, ataxia, tremors, nystagmus, diplopia, drowsiness, and hyperplasia of the gums. Its sudden, complete discontinuance may induce status epilepticus.

Another anticonvulsant which is now rather extensively used is Mesantoin. The usual doses are 0.1 gm. three times a day for children and 0.2 gm. for adults. Since it may be toxic, blood counts should be made once a month. Combined with Dilantin or phenobarbital, it may be effective in cases resistant to other drugs. Its combination with Tridione is to be avoided.

Trimethadione, introduced in 1945 under the trade name Tridione, has been found to produce gratifying results in the treatment of petit mal but may aggravate other types. The starting dose of trimethadione is 0.3 gm. three times a day for adolescents and adults. Gradual increases in dosage are carried out until a therapeutic effect is obtained, the optimal dosage being usually between 1.5 and 2.7 gm. daily. In children under two years of age, 0.15 gm. two or three times is the initial dosage, with increments of 0.15 gm. Toxic symptoms in the form of skin eruptions, "glare phenomenon," a photophobia in which objects appear to shimmer and blurring of vision, drowsiness, dizziness, and headache may occur. Toxic action on the blood-forming elements of the bone marrow followed by death has been reported. For this reason, the blood should be examined once a month for agranulocytosis. For some persons, paramethadione dimethylethyloxazolidine dione (Paradione) is more effective than Tridione. N-methyl-*alpha*-phenylsuccinimide (Milontin) may also be used for petit mal, though it is less effective than the diones. For adults, the dose is 0.9 to 3.0 gm. daily, and for children, 0.6 to 1.8 gm. daily.

Another drug which has been increasingly employed in therapeutically-resistant convulsive disorders since 1949 is Phenurone (phenacetylcarbamide). This may be used in both grand mal and psychomotor seizures, but seems to be more effective in the latter type. It may be given in 500 mg. doses three times a day. After the first week of treatment, an additional 500 mg. may be taken on rising. One-half the adult dose is recommended for children from 5 to 10 years of age. It seems to be especially useful in combating drowsiness and lethargy in patients who are affected in this manner by phenobarbital and other drugs. Patients receiving Phenurone should be watched carefully for the possible development of serious damage to the hematopoietic system and to the liver.

Primidone (Mysoline) is safer than phenurone and is reported to be of much value in the treatment both of psychomotor epilepsy and grand mal. Dosage range is from two to eight 250-mg. tablets a day.

All types of seizure patients show some improvement under anticonvulsant therapy, and those with focal and grand mal seizures respond best. Phenobarbital and Dilantin usually give the best results in seizures of those types.

Because of the danger of status epilepticus, anticonvulsive drugs should not be withheld abruptly. The occurrence of status epilepticus constitutes a medical emergency and is best handled in a hospital. Prolonged status epilepticus may lead to irreversible cerebral changes and even death. The patient must be placed under heavy sedation and kept in that condition for 24 hours. This is best accomplished with a solution of amobarbital sodium, 1.0 gm. in 20 ml. for injection, given slowly intravenously at the rate of 1 or 2 ml. per minute until the seizure stops and deep sleep results. Sleep is maintained with a continuous intravenous drip of 0.5 gm. amobarbital sodium (Amytal) in 500 ml. of isotonic saline solution. The patient should be turned every half hour to prevent hypostatic and aspiration pneumonia. Mild Trendelenburg position is maintained, and mechanical aspiration of secretions is often necessary. Oxygen is given through a nasal catheter when indicated. Additional sedation may be obtained without depressing respiration with the use of paraldehyde suppositories, each containing 4.5 ml. of paraldehyde, repeated every four hours. A parenteral preparation of diphenylhydantoin sodium (Dilantin) is now commercially available and may be injected either intramuscularly or intravenously. This has been found valuable in status epilepticus in a dosage not to exceed 500 mg.

In the case of seizures secondary to meningocerebral cicatrix formation resulting from trauma or infection, relief has at times been secured by surgical removal (Penfield) of the cicatrix. Surgery is being increasingly employed in the treatment of seizures of focal nature.

Because of the physical hazards involved, the epileptic should be safeguarded from obvious environmental and occupational risks.

It is agreed that an epileptic whose disorder is not well controlled should not be permitted to operate a motor vehicle. In many states a known epileptic is forbidden by law to operate one. In recent years there has been a tendency to be more permissive in the case of persons with well-controlled epilepsy. In 1949 the Wisconsin legislature, with the support of the state medical society, enacted legislation to allow the person with controlled epilepsy to drive a motor vehicle subject to the following provisions.* When the epileptic can present medical certification that he has been completely free of attacks for two years, he can obtain a driver's license, renewable every six months, upon application to the motor vehicle division. Medical forms are sent to him to be filled out by his physician attesting to the fact that his condition has been completely controlled for over two years. This license is automatically renewable every six months upon application and medical certification that the patient's condition has remained under complete control during the previous six months.

It is reported that, during the period 1949–1957, 553 licenses to operate a motor vehicle were granted, 96 licenses were denied after review by the medical review board, and but one accident occurred during the period because of an epileptic seizure by a driver.

BIBLIOGRAPHY

Bandler, B., et al.: Role of sexuality in epilepsy. Psychosom. Med., 20:227–234, 1958.
Barrow, R. L., and Fabing, H. D.: Epilepsy and the Law. New York, Paul B. Hoeber, Inc., 1956.
Berger, H.: Ueber das Elektrenkephalogramm des Menschen. Arch. f. Psychiat., 87:527–570, 1929.
Bradley, C.: Behavior disturbances in epileptic children. J.A.MA., 146:436–441, 1951.
Bridge, E. M.: Epilepsy and Convulsive Disorders in Children. New York, McGraw-Hill Book Company, 1949.
Daly, D. D., and Yoss, R. E.: Electroencephalogram in narcolepsy. Electroenceph. Clin. Neurophysiol., 9:109–120, 1957.

* J.A.M.A., 164:1705–6, 1957.

Davidson, D. T., Jr., and Lombroso, C.: Epilepsy. New England J. Med., *251*:853–858, 897–903, 1954.

DeJong, R. N.: "Psychomotor" or "temporal lobe" epilepsy. Neurology, 7:1–14, 1957.

Falconer, M. A., et al.: Treatment of temporal lobe epilepsy by temporal lobectomy. Lancet, *1*:827–835, 1955.

Fox, J. T.: Social aspects of epilepsy. Lancet, *1*:775, 1947.

Gélineau, J. B. E.: De la narcolepsie. Gaz. d. hôp., *53*:626–628, 1880.

Gibbs, F. A.: Ictal and non-ictal psychiatric disorders in temporal lobe epilepsy. J. Nerv. & Ment. Dis., *113*:522–528, 1951.

Idem, and Gibbs, E. I.: Atlas of Electroencephalography. Cambridge, Mass., Addison-Wesley Press, Inc., 1950–1952.

Glaser, G. H., and Dixon, M. S.: Psychomotor seizures in childhood. Neurology, *6*:646–655, 1956.

Goldstein, N. P., and Giffin, M. E.: Psychogenic hypersomnia. Am. J. Psychiat., *115*:922–928, 1957.

Hill, Denis, et al.: Personality changes following temporal lobectomy for epilepsy. J. Ment. Sc., *103*:18–26, 1957.

Karagulla, S., and Robertson, E. E.: Psychical phenomena in temporal lobe epilepsy and the psychoses. Brit. Med. J., *1*:748–752, 1955.

Langworthy, O. R., and Betz, B. J.: Narcolepsy as a type of response to emotional conflicts. Psychosom. Med., 6:211–226, 1944.

Lennox, W. G.: The genetics of epilepsy. Am. J. Psychiat., *103*:457–462, 1947.

Idem: Tridione in the treatment of epilepsy J.A.M.A., *134*:138–143, 1947.

Idem: Psychiatry, psychology and seizures. Am. J. Orthopsychiat., *19*:432–446, 1949.

Idem: The heredity of epilepsy as told by relatives and twins. J.A.M.A., *146*:529–536, 1951.

Livingston, S.: The Diagnosis and Treatment of Convulsive Disorders in Children. Springfield, Illinois, Charles C Thomas, 1954.

Penfield, W., and Erickson, T. A.: Epilepsy and Cerebral Localization. Springfield, Illinois, Charles C Thomas, 1941.

Idem, and Jasper, H. H.: Epilepsy and the Functional Anatomy of the Human Brain. Boston, Little, Brown & Co., 1954.

Robertson, E. G.: Photogenic epilepsy: self-precipitated attacks. Brain, *77*:232–251, 1954.

Schwarz, B. E., Bickford, R. G., Mulder, D. W., and Rome, H. P.: Mescaline and LSD-25 in activation of temporal lobe epilepsy. Neurology, *6*:275–280, 1956.

Taylor, J.: Selected Writings of John Hughlings Jackson. London, Hodder and Stoughton, 1931–1932.

Yahr, M. D., and Merritt, H. H.: Current status of the drug therapy of epileptic seizures. J.A.M.A., *161*:333–338, 1956.

Chapter Seventeen

SENILE PSYCHOSES

"He who is of a calm and happy nature will hardly feel the pressure of age."

Plato

In 1900, 1 in 25 living persons was over the age of 65; in 1950 this ratio had changed to 1 in 13. The total population of the United States doubled between those years, but the number of persons of 65 years or over almost quadrupled and is said to be increasing at the rate of 1000 per day. This has naturally been reflected in the number of aged people who develop mental disorders. In the past 30 years, the number of first admissions to New York state hospitals of persons aged 60 or more has increased from 19.1 per cent to 40 per cent of all admissions.

A gradual wearing down of energy, a decline in responsiveness, a waning of initiative and of creative imagination, a narrowing of interests, an increase in egocentricity, and a certain warping of personality must be looked upon as a normal involutional process operating with the passage of time. With advancing age, there is a progressive loss of physical and mental resources, a loss that tends to arouse feelings of helplessness. These feelings serve to create anxiety that the individual tries to overcome by mechanisms that he has long employed in making his adjustments. As one grows older, therefore, he "grows more like himself." The stress of increasing physical and mental limitations, loneliness resulting from the loss of friends and relatives, and perhaps rejection by children produce an anxiety that may evoke various protective mechanisms. Among them may be a turning to and perhaps embellishment of the past, a paranoid projection or a self-assertiveness to the point of being domineering. Other elderly persons, through feelings of insecurity or inadequacy, become ill-natured and contentious or regress to a dependent state. Both biological and sociopsychological factors contribute therefore to the personality changes of old age.

From these mild, senescent mental changes, there is a sliding scale to the extreme impoverishment of mental resources that characterizes senile dementia. The dividing line may be a matter of individual opinion. Often the senile dementia patient is one who has not felt secure and whose pattern of living has long been constricted. The person of cheerful disposition who maintains contact with the outside world, has been well adjusted in previous years, and has built up emotional and intellectual resources may well escape the dementia of senility. The person who develops senile dementia has often been characterized by rigid and static habits. Persons who have always had difficulty in adjusting to the demands of life are prone to react to the inevitable retirement from business and professional posts of honor, to deaths of friends and relatives, and the loosening of family and social ties that accompany old age by the development of mental symptoms.

The more immature and maladjusted, too, have been the adaptations of earlier life, the smaller is the stress required in old age to produce disorganized or disturbed behavior. That social activities and a wholesome variety of mental occupation may retard mental senility has long been recognized. In one of his famous dialogues, Cicero said, "Old men retain their intellects well enough if they keep their minds active and fully employed." It will therefore be seen that, although of great importance, organic disease of the brain is often not the only factor in the development of senile psychoses. It is increasingly recognized that frequently they result from the interaction of organic and psychological factors.

Pathology

It is generally accepted that the anatomical changes associated with senile dementia are a result of deficiencies in cerebral blood flow, with a concomitant decrease in brain metabolism and available oxygen. In many cases arteriosclerotic changes apparently equal in extent to those observed in senile dementia are found in elderly persons who manifest little or no dementia. It would appear, therefore, that not all the factors producing senile dementia are known. Perhaps there are predisposing constitutional ones. As already indicated, psychological factors may also contribute to personality breakdown of the aged.

The gross pathology of the brain in senile dementia is typically characterized by cerebral atrophy, but frequently this is not easily demonstrated. If atrophy is apparent, it will be greatest in the frontal lobes where wide sulci and narrowed gyri may give the brain a wrinkled appearance. In extreme cases, the ventricles are widened and the ependyma presents granular excrescences. On section, the gray matter may be less atrophied than the white. One of the most significant histopathological changes, if demonstrable, is the reduction in the number of cells. Occasionally, however, more severe neuropathological disturbances are found in brains of senile dementia patients who are not psychotic than are found in the brains of those suffering from unquestioned senile dementia. On the other hand, psychotic senile patients may show only mild histological changes in the brain. In other words, there is not always a correlation between the degree of histological changes and the degree of intellectual impairment.

Mental Symptoms

The transition from usual old age to senile dementia is ordinarily gradual, and any decision as to when the imaginary line is passed must often be an arbitrary one. A dislike of change, a reduction in ambition and activity, a tendency to become constricted and self-centered in interests, an increased difficulty in comprehension, an increase in time and effort necessary for the performance of familiar duties, an increasing difficulty in adapting to new circumstances, a lessened sympathy for new ideas and views, and a tendency to reminiscence and repetition are scarcely signs of senile dementia, yet they pass imperceptibly into mental destitution and personality regression. Many elderly people have little capacity to express warm and spontaneous feelings toward others.

During relatively early stages and before mental impairment is advanced, periods of reactive depression following some specific event are common. Physical illness or severe emotional disturbance may quicken mental deterioration. Rarely are the symptoms of waning mental capacity sufficiently marked to warrant the diagnosis of senile dementia until after 60 years of age. The decreased impressionability, impaired registration, and declining interest in environment and in present affairs predispose to the loss of memory for recent events that often serves as the earliest clinical criterion for the diagnosis. Limitation of ideas and impairment of capacity for abstract thought usually appear early, as may also an indifference to the ceremonies and courtesies of social life. The patient resents what he considers as interference by younger persons and may complain that he is neglected. Some show a hostile but anxious and fearful dependence. Natural affections become blunted and may turn to hatred.

A certain tendency to isolation occurs. This tendency to self-isolation and to hostility toward some living person is most frequent if some close member of the family has been lost. Altruistic sentiments are usually lost early, while egoistic, selfish ones are intensified and, like the instinctive ones, may be crudely manifested. Irritability, either as an expression of egocentric trends or a defensive reaction to the impairment of memory, is common. Exaggerated sexual activities or sexual indecencies may be exhibited, in which case they usually represent not merely a weakening of inhibitions but a defensive effort at psychological compensation for the waning of a fundamental function. Some senile dementia patients become careless in habits of toilet and dress; pride of appearance is forgotten. At times there is a tendency to be distrustful, prying, and suspicious. Hoarding and delusions of theft, of poisoning, of poverty, or of not being wanted are common.

Exaggerations and caricatures of the previous personality betray its earlier tendencies. Anxiety, irritability, timidity, and other personality changes frequently seen in senility are not attributable solely to changes in the brain. Many of them are caused by the fact that the individual has been shoved into a position that frustrates his wishes and deprives him of his usefulness and of his status as an autonomous person. A failure to find the satisfactions necessary to replace those the elderly person had when he felt needed, important, and productive tends to lead to regressive changes.

Although frequently occurring to some degree, these regressions of personality are less constant and less progressive than the impairment of the more strictly psychic functions. Accompanying, or even preceding the amnesia, is a tendency to reminiscence, the theme being characteristically personal. As memory for recent life sinks further away from recollection, the limits of recall are forced back further and further until the patient, with the loss of his ability to assimilate new ideas and experiences, comes to live in the distant past, often in the period of his childhood. The patient may speak of parents or grandparents as still living, and persons are often misidentified. Any recollection for the simplest events of recent life may be lost. This retention of memory for remote events and loss for recent ones seems reasonable in view of the theory that the hypothetical neuronal circuit patterns responsible for memories become more strongly established with time. The longer, then, the pattern has been established, the more strongly does memory resist degenerative states such as those of senility.

Orientation becomes defective, and in his confusion the patient may wander away and become lost. Judgment becomes impaired; the personal hazards of traffic or other situations are not recognized. Frequently the patient forgets where he has placed articles and accuses other persons of having stolen them. He may leave the gas jet burning and is careless with matches and fire. He may become the victim of unscrupulous persons, particularly if their technique involves an appeal to the patient's vanity, either in matters of competence or of sex.

Many are restless at night and either wander about the house or engage in some aimless, perhaps destructive, activity in a confused manner. This nocturnal delirium is due apparently to the limitations of vision in darkness. Those with senile states become disoriented within an hour when placed in darkened rooms due to failure to retain their spatial location; they then become anxious and more confused.

Through the day, on the other hand, the patient may sleep much of the time. Hoarding of articles of no value is common, quantities of worthless objects being carried in the patient's pockets or jealously guarded in some cherished hiding place. Hallucinations may occur; in some cases absurd delusions are conspicuous.

Physical Symptoms

Physically, the patient usually exhibits conspicuous signs of senility. The skin is often thin, atrophic, and wrinkled. In advanced forms the special senses lose in acuity, weight is lost, the muscles are wasted, the gait becomes unsteady and shuffling, the voice harsh and the speech slow. The handwriting becomes tremulous, while tremors of head and hands are common. Co-existing sclerosis of the cerebral arteries frequently gives rise to headache, dizziness, and the episodic and focal disturbances incident to vascular accidents.

Clinical Types

Different clinical types, such as simple deterioration, delirious and confused, depressed and agitated, paranoid and presenile types are described, but there is frequently so much overlapping that the assignment to any particular group is an arbitrary matter.

SIMPLE DETERIORATION. This is the most frequent form of senile psychosis; it is characterized largely by progressive memory defect, at first for recent events but later for remote ones, a narrowing of interests, loss of initiative, sluggishness of thought, apathy, irritability, and nocturnal restlessness. Contact with the environment becomes less and less, and a vegetative, mildly stuporous state may finally develop.

DELIRIUM AND CONFUSION. The nature of the delirious and confused type is indicated by its name. The onset of this delirioid and confused reaction is comparatively acute and may accompany a variety of physical illnesses. Among them are alkalosis, anoxia, hypoglycemia, and urinary infection. An incautious use of bromides, morphine, barbiturates, or other drugs may precipitate an attack. The reaction may be associated with dehydration occurring in fever or following a surgical operation (such as prostatectomy) requiring general anesthesia. Less frequently it may be caused by vitamin deficiency. In milder cases the patient is perplexed, disoriented, and perhaps inaccessible. Insomnia is marked, and hallucinations are frequent. In more severe cases, the patient is restless, resistive, and noisy and may exhaust himself. Strictly speaking, such a reversible process is not a part of senile dementia but represents a reaction to which the elderly person is particularly prone. Some senile subjects, however, present a chronic confusional state. Such a person may present a bewildered expression, move about in a vague and aimless fashion, and be only dimly aware of his whereabouts.

DEPRESSION AND AGITATION. The depressed and agitated type presents not merely the memory loss and intellectual impoverishment of senile dementia but also a marked egocentricity, persistent agitation, and melancholic, hypochondriacal, and nihilistic delusions.

PARANOIA. The paranoid type is distinguished by the conspicuousness of delusions, most frequently of a persecutory nature. Sometimes helplessness is used as an effective means of securing and wielding power. Many paranoid senile individuals are irritable, quarrelsome, hostile and demanding. Complaints of bad treatment are nearly always expressed. This type of behavior usually occurs in persons whose life personality pattern has been characterized by dissatisfaction, projection, and other defensive mechanisms. As its physical substratum suffers the degenerative changes of senility, the personality is no longer able to cope with its problems, its former defensive and compensatory mechanisms are exaggerated, and delusional beliefs falsify reality to protect the personality and maintain its self-esteem. Memory loss may be absent or comparatively insignificant for a long time. As memory defect appears, delusional extension and further defensive emotional reaction may take place in an attempt to repair the additional psychobiological defect. Similarly, as judgment fails the delusions become more absurd, partly because beliefs are no longer subject to any critical scrutiny, and partly because the damaged personality requires more fantastic beliefs for its support. Hallucinations and illusions occur more frequently than in any other type of senile psychosis. Consciousness is not disturbed, and orientation usually remains unimpaired. Of the various types of senile psychosis already mentioned, the paranoid form stands out most clearly as a special type. Transitions and admixtures of the various types described are common.

PRESBYOPHRENIA. The presbyophrenic type is characterized largely by a defect of retention with confabulation. It is doubtful if it should be accorded a special classification. Probably it should be regarded as a somewhat precocious form of senile dementia exhibiting certain clinical symptoms. It occurs rather more frequently in women than in men. Usually it will be found that the premorbid personality was characterized by cheerfulness, energetic activity, a certain vivaciousness, and a good adjustability. The previous personality is fairly well retained, and the patient continues to manifest a warm emotional response but with a tendency to be suggestible and to vacillate between friendliness and irritability. Most presbyophrenic patients are talkative, apparently alert individuals who, however, when addressed, are found to be quite out of touch with their environment. Impressibility and retention are defective, and memory is greatly impaired. Without the slightest realization of his memory fault, the patient supplies the deficiencies with confabulations, often accepting with good humor and amplifying as facts the fabrications that are suggested to him. His absurd contradictions and repetitions pass unnoticed by him.

Many presbyophrenic patients are constantly busy with a restless, unproductive, even destructive, activity. With a certain amiable eagerness, as if occupied with his usual vocation, the patient intently disarranges or destroys his bed. The fabrication and memory disturbances are suggestive of the Korsakoff syndrome, but the age of the patient, the gradual onset, complacent loquacity, progressive deterioration, and absence of neuritic symptoms serve to differentiate presbyophrenia from Korsakoff's psychosis.

The following case history abstract is illustrative of simple senile dementia with an admixture of paranoid features—a not uncommon association.

H. S. was admitted to a public hospital for mental disorders when 72 years of age. When 6 years old she sustained a fracture of the hip. Four years later an operation was performed in an effort to correct the deformity and disability. It was necessary to strap her to the bed for 6 months following the operation. The functional results of this operation were disappointing, and the patient was always self-conscious concerning the considerable degree of disability that persisted. She always felt that people did not wish to mingle with her because of this infirmity and did not seem comfortable in the presence of others. It is quite possible that the few paranoid features accompanying the patient's senile dementia may have had their origin in this defensive characteristic.

Five years before the patient's admission her adopted son with whom she resided noted that she was becoming forgetful, especially concerning her usual household duties and recent incidents. She hoarded articles and sometimes said that someone had stolen them. She remembered events of her childhood quite well and at times was somewhat boresome in her accounts of early experiences. Her adopted son noted that she became increasingly neglectful of her personal appearance. For many months prior to her admission she would not bathe unless reminded to do so. Recently she often went to bed without removing either clothing or shoes. At times she put on her clothing "inside out." For four years prior to admission she seemed to find it difficult to prepare meals at accustomed times.

On many occasions she completed the preparation of the midday meal at 8 a.m. and insisted that the family should eat at that time. In preparing coffee she often put sugar instead of coffee in the coffee pot but failed to recognize her error. In a few instances she wished to pay bills that she had already paid. She was restless at night but often slept during the day. The patient became increasingly confused in surroundings with which she had formerly been quite familiar. Often, when crossing the street, she paid no attention to approaching automobiles. At times she wandered away from home.

There were periods during which she constantly packed and unpacked her clothing. During recent months she had often failed to recognize friends. She became increasingly suspicious, said that neighbors were talking about her, spoke of them in extremely derogatory terms, maintained that her son lied to her and had tried to poison her, and that her neighbors had threatened to kill her. She claimed that her son and an elderly woman who had been employed to give her protective care had been secretly married. She complained that everyone was trying to control her activities and threatened to commit suicide if not permitted to do as she wished.

When the patient was brought to the mental hospital, she rose to meet the admitting physician, shook his hand, asked him where he was and if there was anything she could do for him. She knew her name but could not give her address or other identifying data. She claimed that her son, who had really been extremely devoted to her, had ejected her in order to secure possession of her house, which was located "down the hill." At the time of this writing she has been in the hospital for 18 months. Affectless and placid, she sits in a rocking chair all day, paying little or no heed to her environment. Her existence is now but little above a vegetative level.

Prognosis and Course

The prognosis of advanced senile dementia is manifestly hopeless. No well-defined remissions are to be expected, although in the depressed and excited types subsidence may occur. The course is progressive; the patient gradually becomes more demented, although life may continue for 10 years or even longer before death supervenes. Not a few mental disorders in the aged are, however, precipitated by situational problems such as isolation, exhaustion, and toxic and nutritional factors. Many of these are quite amenable to appropriate management.

Diagnosis

In well-developed, simple senile dementia, the age of the patient, the progressive egocentricity, and the characteristic memory loss, particularly for recent events, makes the diagnosis easy. In the paranoid form, the memory loss and evidences of dementia may be comparatively slight. Since these senile paranoids have usually had a life pattern of a defensive, paranoid type, the matter of deciding when this exaggerated pattern

crosses the psychotic line may be one of arbitrary decision to be determined largely by social criteria and by the interpretation and values accorded to reality. In such paranoid personalities, their progression to a psychotic degree may, in both arteriosclerotic and senile disease of the brain, follow from the threat to the integrity of the personality contained in the degenerative, structural changes taking place in the organ which constitutes the important physical substratum of the personality. When arteriosclerotic changes in the brain, rather than the histological ones of senility, are the basis for such paranoid psychoses, the patient usually suffers from easy mental fatigability, dizziness, or slight confusion, suggestive of changes in the smaller vessels of the cerebrum. Some depressed and agitated types of symptoms suggest involutional melancholia. The differentiation must be made largely by the age of the patient and particularly by the presence or absence of deterioration. Differentiation from arteriosclerotic psychoses is discussed in Chapter 15. A restricted diet in the aged may lead to avitaminosis suggestive of senile psychosis. Toxic psychoses are frequently mistaken for senile dementia. It should be remembered that, in the aged, mental disturbance may be caused by uremia, anemia, decompensated heart disease, or pulmonary disease rather than by senile dementia. The differentiation of presbyophrenia from Korsakoff's disease has already been mentioned.

Treatment

The discussion in the early part of the chapter has already suggested the importance of prophylactic factors in the prevention of the senile psychoses. It is therefore highly desirable that the aged person maintain a feeling of emotional security and a sense of dignity. One will accordingly attempt to see that the old person's needs for affection, for a feeling of belonging, for achievement, and for recognition and approval are met.

The milder form of senile dementia

should be cared for in the home. It is there that the patient's roots are deeply imbedded. Unless circumstances are such that either the safety of the patient or that of the family is endangered, it is well to attempt to care for him in the usual and familiar environment. The patient is ordinarily happier there than in the unaccustomed and rather rigid routine of an institution, where the habits of a lifetime have to be reconstructed. It is true, however, that the patient's inability to recognize his failing physical and mental vigor may present a serious problem to his family. In not a few cases, too, hospital care becomes necessary because of nocturnal restlessness, disturbing response to paranoid delusions, marked irritability, assaultiveness, sexual play with children, exhibitionism, or ill-considered plans for marriage. Impaired judgment in business affairs may make the appointment of a legal guardian necessary. Care must often be exercised to prevent the confused patient from setting fire to clothing or furniture, to prevent wandering from home or falling with resulting fracture of the neck of the femur. It is particularly important to maintain the visual orientation of the senile patient at night. This may be done by providing adequate night lighting, available if he awakens. During the day, the presence of familiar objects also supports his orientation.

Because of the danger of suicide, patients suffering from depressed or agitated types of senility should receive hospital care. Mild hypnotics may be required at night. Chlorpromazine is often useful in the treatment of agitation, restlessness, irritability, confusion, and delirium. The dosages and problems of treatment are similar to those described in Chapter 15, Brain Syndromes Associated with Cerebral Arteriosclerosis. If appetite has been poor or diet restricted, it is advisable to prescribe ascorbic acid, thiamine chloride, niacin, and glutamic acid. Preparations are now available in which is supplied the latter agent in its utilizable form, monosodium L-glutamate. Vitamins are frequently of value in confused and delirious senile states. In the depressive forms, electroshock therapy can often be used safely and with great success.

BIBLIOGRAPHY

Busse, E. W., Barnes, R. H., et al.: Studies of the processes of aging. Am. J. Psychiat., *111*: 896–901, 1955.

Cameron, D. E.: Studies in senile nocturnal delirium. Psychiat. Quart. 15:47–53, 1941.

Clow, H. E.: Psychiatric factors in the rehabilitation of the aging. Ment. Hyg., 34:592–599, 1950.

Doty, E. J.: The incidence and treatment of delirious reactions in later life. Geriatrics, 1:21–26, 1946.

East, W. N.: Crime, senescence and senility. J. Ment. Sc., 90:835–850, 1944.

Ebaugh, F. G.: Age introduces stress into the family. Geriatrics, 11:146–150, 1956.

First National Conference on Aging: Man and his Years. Raleigh, N. C., Health Publications Institute, Inc., 1951.

Gibson, A. C.: Psychosis occurring in the senium. J. Mental Sci., 107:921–925, 1961.

Hoch, P. H., and Zubin, J. (Eds.): Psychopathology of Aging. Proc. Fiftieth Ann. Meet. Am. Psychopathological Assoc. New York, Grune and Stratton, Inc., 1961.

Kay, D. W. K., and Roth, M.: Physical accompaniments of mental disorder in old age. Lancet, 2:740–745, 1955.

Kolb, L.: Mental hospitalization of the aged: is it being overdone? Am. J. Psychiat., 112:627–636, 1956.

Lansing, A. I., Ed.: Cowdry's Problems of Aging, 3rd ed. Baltimore, Williams & Wilkins Co., 1952.

Lemkau, P. V.: The mental hygiene of aging. Public Health Reports, 67:237–241, 1952.

Litin, E. M.: Mental reaction to trauma and hospitalization in the aged. J.A.M.A., *162*: 1522–1524, 1956.

McFarland, R. A.: The psychological aspects of aging. Bull. New York Acad. Med., 32:14–32, 1956.

Newton, R. D.: The identity of Alzheimer's disease and senile dementia and their relationship to senility. J. Ment. Sc., 94:225–249, 1948.

Pollack, B.: The addition of chlorpromazine to the treatment program for emotional and behavior disorders in the aging. Geriatrics, 11: 253–259, 1956.

Proceedings of Association for Research in Nervous and Mental Disease: The Neurologic and Psychiatric Aspects of the Disorder of Aging. Vol. XXXV. Baltimore, Williams & Wilkins Co., 1956.

Rothschild, D.: The clinical differentiation of senile and arteriosclerotic psychoses. Am. J. Psychiat., 98:324–333, 1941.

Stieglitz, E. J., Ed.: The Care of the Aging and the Aged, 2nd ed. Philadelphia, W. B. Saunders Company, 1949.

Titchener, J., Zwerling, I., Gottschalk, L., and Levine, M.: Psychological reactions of the aged in surgery. Archiv. Neurol. & Psychiat., 79:63–73, 1958.

Wilson, D. C.: The pathology of senility. Am. J. Psychiat., *111*:902–906, 1955.

Chapter Eighteen

CHRONIC BRAIN SYNDROMES ASSOCIATED WITH DISTURBANCE OF METABOLISM, GROWTH OR NUTRITION

ALZHEIMER'S DISEASE

In 1906 Alois Alzheimer (1864–1915) described the case of a woman who had died at age 51 following a rather rapidly progressing dementia and whose brain tissue showed the development of tangled, threadlike structures occupying much or all of the body of many cortical ganglion cells. These agglomerated neurofibrils are stained black and silver. This degenerative change may involve even one-fourth of the ganglion cells. It is now known that they are not limited to this disease but may be observed in senile dementia and even in the brains of the normal senium. There are accompanying diffuse gliosis and an abnormal amount of fatty pigment in the nerve cells. Another histopathological change that practically always exists is the presence of senile plaques with their amorphous and homogeneous core. Plaques are most frequent in the frontal cortex and in the cornu Ammonis. In Alzheimer's disease the cortical degeneration is diffuse and involves the outer layers of the cortex, especially those of the frontal and temporal lobes. The cerebral atrophy can be demonstrated by pneumoencephalography. Changes in the basal ganglia are regularly found. Air encephalograms show a dilation of the ventricular system and increased cortical markings.

The onset of Alzheimer's disease is usually between 50 and 60 years of age, although earlier appearances have been reported. The disease begins insidiously, with a reduction of spontaneity, progressive intellectual deterioration, and alterations in behavior. There is no characteristic pattern in either the intellectual impairment or the behavioral disturbances. Disorientation, memory impairment, defects in calculation and general information, emotional lability, and decrease in concreteness in thinking are present in varying degrees and combinations. Pronunciation is difficult, spoken language is comprehended poorly, and errors are made in reading and writing. The patient makes mistakes in the routine details of his everyday life, words are forgotten, and speech disorders are common. A not infrequent disturbance is a perseveration of speech in the form of logoclonia. In advanced stages of the disease, speech becomes an incoherent jargon without sentence formation. Prolonged periods of restless over-activity, anxiety, and depression may occur. Agnosia, apraxia, and temporary hemiplegic or paraplegic weakness may exist. Syncopal and epileptic attacks are common. A Parkinson-like difficulty in gait is often seen. Facial paresis and hypertonicity of muscles are frequent, and in late stages there may be contractures of the extremities. At this stage the patient becomes extremely demented, is entirely out of touch with his environment, and becomes reduced to a mere vegetative existence. The usual duration of the disease is five to ten years, but the course may be characterized by remissions.

Little is known concerning the factors contributing to this form of presenile dementia. The clinical differentiation from Pick's disease is often difficult and at times impossible. Certain symptom differences are mentioned in the discussion of the latter disease in Chapter 20. The following is a rather typical clinical history of a patient suffering from this disorder.

W. M. was admitted to the hospital at the age of 52. The patient's early life, including medical history, does not appear to have been significant. The onset of his mental disorder was so insidious that his wife was able to give only an approximate date. About five or six years before his admission, he began to show less affection toward his family. His wife added that at about the same time "he grew lazy and his interests gradually dulled. He had a habit of just sitting around the house. For years he has not mentioned the payment of the interest on his mortgage or his taxes." About three years before admission his wife noticed that he could not tell time correctly and that he would make errors in writing a check. "He would set out for the store to buy feed for his cows and forget to do so. One time he wanted to walk to his father's place, thinking that it was just down the road, whereas it was a matter of 60 miles. He grew confused, and on one occasion he stopped the car in the middle of an intersection. He would put on his trousers backward and his overalls inside out. Sometimes, when a dish of food was put on the table for the whole family, he would eat the entire amount himself."

The pre-admission history is obviously that of an insidiously developing and progressive dementia. On admission the patient appeared to be older than he actually was. He was completely disoriented for time and place. He did not know whether his home was in Pennsylvania or New Jersey. On the day of admission he said he was 34 years of age; on the following day he gave his age as 25 and a few weeks later, as 80. He was careless and untidy in dress and wandered about the ward in a confused and bewildered manner, often mistaking the nurse for his wife.

On admission, general hyperreflexia was noted, but there were no other neurological abnormalities. Prior to his death his extremities showed spasticity. The patient became incontinent of urine; he gradually grew weaker and even more demented. In August, 1945, nearly two and one-half years after admission, he suffered a rather typical epileptic seizure. About September 1, 1945, he became comatose and died nine days later.

At autopsy the brain weighed 1250 gm. A coronal section through the frontal lobes showed pronounced cortical atrophy, with enlargement of the sulci. The island of Reil was also atrophic. On microscopic examination, a marked cortical atrophy was found; there was also a decrease in the amount of subcortical white matter. In some convolutions the white matter was reduced to a narrow band. The subcortex showed moderate general demyelination. Sections through the plane of the substantia nigra showed this to be depigmented. A section further caudad showed the posterior horns of the ventricles to be considerably enlarged at the expense of the white matter. Stained sections showed a focal and general loss of ganglion cells, the presence of ghost cells, severe degenerative changes in the cells that remained, and a uniform gliosis. Special silver stains demonstrated numerous senile plaques, also neurofibrillary degeneration of many ganglion cells. These showed thickening and agglutination of the neurofibrils, their displacement to the periphery of the cells, and their bizarre arrangement within the cells.

VITAMIN DEFICIENCY SYNDROMES

In recent years it has become recognized that there is a common factor operative in various mental and neurological phenomena which had been previously regarded as unrelated entities. This common factor is a vitamin deficiency, particularly a deficiency of vitamin B. The localization of the pathological process produced in different parts of the nervous system by the deficiency determines the neurological signs and releases the mental symptoms. The nature of the symptom or syndrome depends upon the particular member of the B complex in which the deficiency is relatively greatest and upon the part of the nervous system predominantly affected by the deficiency. If the deficiency of nicotinic acid is greatest, the clinical picture produced is that of pellagra. If, as is not rare, a peripheral' "neuritis" is also associated or if a Korsakoff syndrome is observed, a deficiency of thiamine exists also. If, because of chronic alcoholism, the patient suffers from thiamine deficiency, he may suffer from a painful thiamine neuropathy, or "alcoholic neuritis." If at the same time there is nerve cell degeneration in the cerebral cortex resulting from deficiency of another member (or members) of the B complex (probably niacin), the patient will present an alcoholic Korsakoff syndrome.

Wernicke Syndrome

In 1881 Wernicke described a syndrome consisting of ophthalmoplegia, memory loss, confabulation, apathy, progressive dementia, ataxia, clouding of consciousness, and even coma. It is now known that it is invariably associated with thiamine deficiency and that usually there is a deficiency of niacin also. Because of the thiamine avitaminosis, there is an impaired oxidation of pyruvic acid, which is formed during the breakdown of glucose. As a result, pyruvic acid accumulates in the blood.

Wernicke's "encephalitis" mainly affects chronic alcoholics but has also been described in pernicious anemia, hyperemesis gravidarum, and gastric cancer, and in prisoners of war. Delirium usually precedes its development. The Wernicke syndrome, formerly observed occasionally in pernicious vomiting of pregnancy or after abdominal or pelvic operations when solutions of glucose were administered in considerable amounts, is now seen much less frequently, apparently because thiamine is given with the glucose as a usual procedure. This syndrome has almost disappeared since 1942. This disappearance is ascribed to the fact that enrichment of bread and flour began in that year.

The pathological changes are mainly in the brain stem and involve the mammillary bodies and the regions adjacent to the aqueduct and to the third and fourth ventricles. The lesions are characterized by various degrees of necrosis of both nerve cells and nerve fibers, together with reactive changes of microglia and astrocytes, alteration of small blood vessels, and, in some instances, petechial hemorrhages.

The ocular disturbances takes the form of horizontal and vertical nystagmus and various degrees of paralysis of conjugate gaze and of the external recti.

H. B., aged 62, a chronic alcoholic who had been arrested many times for drunkenness, was taken to a general hospital October 1, 1951, because of confusion and difficulty in walking. There was a history that following a long alcoholic debauch he had been taken into custody by the Salvation Army. For several days the supervision of this organization made it impossible for him to secure alcohol. He then remained at its hotel for several days more, performing light duties until his physical disabilities made employment impossible. Soon after entering the general hospital he became confused, restless, demanding, and was noisy at night. He was then transferred to a psychiatric hospital where the confusion soon subsided. On neurological examination, he showed marked bilateral ptosis, his pupils reacted very slightly to light, and he was totally unable to follow a light in any direction. His speech was thick and slurred; there was a great defect in co-ordination of his extremities; all tendon reflexes, except the biceps, were absent. The calves of both legs were tender, and he was unable to walk unaided. A diagnosis of Wernicke's syndrome plus peripheral neuritis was made. He was at once placed on large doses of thiamine. He soon began to improve, but the evidence of ophthalmoplegia did not completely disappear for seven months.

If the thiamine deficiency produces peripheral neuropathy, cardiac hypertrophy, myocardial weakness, and edema, the clinical manifestation is that of beriberi, a form of deficiency without mental accompaniment. Beriberi may, however, be associated with Wernicke's encephalopathy. An uncomplicated thiamine deficiency without any associated neurological phenomena may produce a neurasthenic syndrome characterized by feelings of weakness, easy fatigue, emotional instability, irritability, moodiness, quarrelsomeness, forgetfulness, apathy, mild depression, and vague fears. These symptoms soon disappear after the intake of thiamine is increased.

In nutritional encephalopathy, there is almost never a single vitamin deficiency. In the same individual one may see delirium tremens (the cause of delirium tremens is uncertain, but it is probably a result of a disturbance of cerebral metabolism incident to vitamin deficiency), Korsakoff's psychosis, nicotinic acid encephalopathy (pellagra), and the Wernicke syndrome. There may also be a neuropathy in the form of an "alcoholic neuritis."

Psychoses with Pellagra

Pellagra was first described in 1735 by a Spanish physician, Gasper Casal, under the name *mal de la rosa*. He attributed the disease to a poor diet, but not until 1915 was its dietary origin conclusively demonstrated by Goldberger. In 1937 it was discovered that nicotinic acid (niacin) is the pellagra-preventive vitamin. The principal deficiency, therefore, is in nicotinic acid, although it appears that the disease may also result from a deficiency in the amino acid, tryptophan. Usually there are also other associated deficiencies, particularly of thiamine and riboflavin. Often, too, there is a deficiency of ascorbic acid. Many of the neurological symptoms in pellagra are presumably a result of the associated thiamine deficiency.

Pellagra occurs most frequently in communities where the prevailing low economic status leads to extensive nutritional deficiencies. Isolated cases occur among chronic alcoholics whose food has consisted largely of alcohol and has therefore been deficient in vitamin B complex. It is not rare in aged, destitute people who, living alone and in deprivation, suffer from vitamin deficiency. Sporadic cases may also occur in persons suffering from intestinal lesions that interfere with the absorption of food.

It should not be forgotten that pellagra may develop in persons who are already psychotic. This was formerly common in institutions for mental diseases. With more abundant and better balanced diets, such institutional cases are no longer common.

Morbid Anatomy

There is but little experimental evidence indicating that uncomplicated niacin deficiency results in injury to the nervous system. In well-developed cases, neuronal and capillary changes are found distributed throughout the neuraxis, usually most marked in the cerebrum. In the frontal lobes and in the hippocampus, the ganglion cells lose their Nissl substance and may eventually disappear. There may be proliferation of glia cells and of capillary endothelium. The similarity of these changes to those of Meyer's "central neuritis" and to those of Wernicke's syndrome has long been noted. There now seems reason to believe that the same factor is common to all these conditions, that the histopathological changes in all of them are caused by thiamine deficiency or by a polyavitaminosis of the vitamin B complex, since it is known that single vitamin deficiencies rarely if ever occur. Until the pathological changes become somewhat advanced, they are reversible.

Symptoms

The early mental symptoms of pellagra are often regarded as psychoneurotic and consist of vague headache, irritability, difficulty in concentration, forgetfulness, restlessness, apprehension, and a feeling of inability for mental or physical effort. These early symptoms are followed by those of an organic syndrome and consist of memory defects, confusion, disorientation, intermittent delirium, Korsakoff's syndrome, and dementia. Some patients show a manic excitement, while others may be depressed, anxious, apprehensive, or paranoid. Although organically released, the particular type of such reactions will be determined by the patient's previous personality pattern. Later in the disease there may be evidence of irreversible neurological impairment resulting from advanced encephalopathy of the deficiency. This may be in the form of stupor, convulsions, incontinence, muscular rigidity, irregular involuntary movements, hypertonia, defective sensation, and muscle paralysis.

Mild mental symptoms are usually the first evidence of pellagra, but after some months these are followed by stomatitis and by glossitis; the tongue is red and painful and the papillae are atrophic. Digestive disturbances with achlorhydria and diarrhea are common. An early erythema of the skin is followed by coarse scaling and a deep red-brown pigmentation. The dermatitis occurs characteristically on the extensor surfaces of the extremities and on the vulva and inner surfaces of the thighs.

Prognosis

If treatment is begun early before irreversible neuronal changes have taken place, the prognosis is good, but in neglected cases, permanent impairment of memory and persistent dementia result.

Treatment

Mild, ambulatory cases of pellagra are relieved by 100-mg. doses of niacin or niacinamide given three to six times a day. In extremely severe cases the patient should receive 1200 to 1500 mg. a day for several days. Sodium nicotinate may be given intravenously or intramuscularly in 100-mg. doses. Parenteral liver extract given intramuscularly in doses of 20 cc. three to five times daily is indicated in severe cases. Since a thiamine deficiency usually co-exists, this vitamin should also be given. The patient should receive

from 40 to 200 gm. of powdered brewers' yeast daily, best tolerated in iced milk. The diet should be liberal and include a quart of milk daily, wheat germ, lean meat, liver, and such vegetables as lettuce, spinach, asparagus, fresh peas, cabbage, and tomatoes. Diets high in carbohydrate and fat are contraindicated. The patient should receive and retain a well-balanced diet of approximately 4000 calories daily.

MENTAL SYNDROMES ASSOCIATED WITH PERNICIOUS ANEMIA

Although Addison in his original descriptions of pernicious anemia in 1849 and 1855 spoke of the occasional "wandering of the mind," the mental disorders associated with the disease have received less attention than have the associated neurological disturbances incident to the accompanying degeneration in the spinal cord, first recognized by Lichtheim in 1886. Mental symptoms, however, are not at all rare in the disease. They are probably secondary to disturbances in cerebral metabolism. It is estimated that 35 per cent of the patients with pernicious anemia manifest minor mental symptoms. If the patient is observed for delirioid reactions, mental changes will be noted more frequently than has usually been reported. Symptoms of a degree sufficient to be called psychotic have been reported by various clinics as occurring in from 4 to 15 per cent of the patients suffering from the disease. With the effective and early treatment now available, these symptoms are encountered less frequently. Mental symptoms may be present alone or in association with cord disturbances.

Morbid Anatomy

Degenerative foci in the white matter of the brain similar to the degenerative plaques in the cord were first demonstrated by Barrett, although they are not always present. Areas of degeneration occur also in the gray matter, the pyramidal cells undergoing disintegration, with the presence of rod cells and other changes, particularly an increase in glia, increase in lipoid products in cells, swelling and proliferation of intimal cells in cerebral blood vessels, and miliary hemorrhages. Ferraro and his associates have pointed out that the pathological changes, both in their location and in their nature, are suggestive of those found in Wernicke's encephalopathy.

Symptoms

The time of onset of mental symptoms in relation to the course of pernicious anemia is variable. Although any associated psychosis was formerly thought to be a terminal condition, it is now recognized that mental symptoms may also occur early, even before the typical blood picture of pernicious anemia is established. Except sometimes in the case of confusion, there is no relationship between the degree of anemia and the intensity of the mental symptoms. Although there is no mental syndrome characteristic of pernicious anemia, the mental picture tends to fall into one of the following groups: acute delirioid state, paranoid condition, affective reaction, and organic deterioration. Probably the organic changes release a psychosis, the type of which is predetermined by previous psychogenic factors and psychological mechanisms. Characteristics of the respective groups are as follows.

ACUTE DELIRIOID STATE. The acute confusional, delirioid state is the most frequent form of psychosis. It is characterized by fluctuations in degree of consciousness, by illusions, and by transitory and terrifying hallucinations. The patient may show drowsiness, with incomplete awakening, impaired ability to maintain attention, and decreased ability to utilize abstract concepts. As in delirium resulting from other causes, the content of thought, and hallucinations, and frustrating dreams is more dependent upon the previous life experience and psychological development of the pa-

tient than upon the nature of the underlying physical cause. The delirious states may continue for several weeks or even longer. Because of the occasional failure to recognize the source of these states in pernicious anemia, it is well in the case of a toxic–infectious type of reaction of undetermined origin in a person over 40 years of age to look for glossitis, a disturbance in vibratory sense, and other signs of cord sclerosis and to make a careful blood examination.

PARANOID STATE. Patients with mild paranoid reactions present an irritable, complaining, discontented attitude, with a tendency to be verbally abusive to persons charged with their care. Others become suspicious, state that their food has been poisoned, or develop other ideas of persecution based on affective and other psychological factors. As a result of these delusions, the patient may become restless, noisy, and abusive. Not rarely the patient's delusions center around members of his family. In one of the authors' cases, the patient developed delusions of persecution concerning his daughters, with the result that he excluded them from the list of beneficiaries named in his will.

AFFECTIVE REACTIONS. These are usually in the form of depression, agitation, and apprehension. In rare cases the patient may end his life.

ORGANIC DETERIORATION. In patients with the organic deterioration syndrome, there is a gradual disintegration of intellectual functions, with impairment of memory and judgment and, at times, periods of confusion.

There is a tendency for mental symptoms to improve with liberal doses of liver extract or with vitamin B_{12}. Both should be administered parenterally. During the first week of treatment, 30 micrograms of vitamin B_{12} or its equivalent as liver injection USP should be given intramuscularly each day. Thereafter the same dose is given twice weekly. After two months, if the response is satisfactory, a single injection every other week is sufficient.

PORPHYRIA

This condition, first described in 1911 by Günther, is a constitutional metabolic disorder resulting in the production of abnormal types of porphyria which appear in the urine. Three types of porphyria are usually described: congenital, acute intermittent, and mixed. The congenital type is seen only in childhood, and the mixed has mostly dermatological symptoms. The acute intermittent type is the one with which mental symptoms are most frequently associated.

This last type is commonly familial and thought to be inherited through a Mendelian dominant trait. Congenital porphyria, on the other hand, appears to be transmitted as a Mendelian recessive. Biochemically, it has been suggested that inhibited synthesis of purines with consequent overproduction of porphyrins and their precursors takes place as a consequence of poisoning of the succinate glycine cycle. In this cycle, α-amino levulinic acid is the common precursor of both porphyrins and purines. Inhibition of the oxidative de-amination of this acid may block purine synthesis and lead to overproduction of the porphyrins. This biochemical explanation remains to be confirmed. Dean recently has stated that in the acute intermittent type the urinary porphobilinogen and α-amino levulinic acid levels continue at high levels for years in contrast to the mixed or variegate form. On the other hand, coproporphyrin and protoporphyrin excretion in the stool are raised only during the acute attack, in contrast to the condition in the mixed form.

Pathologically the changes in the nervous system consist of patchy areas of demyelinization with or without the destruction of axis cylinders, particularly in the spinal nerves. Retrograde degeneration of the motor cells occurs in the central nervous system and the sympathetic ganglia. These findings are inconstant and nonspecific. In rapidly fatal cases no changes may be evident in the central nervous system. The liver may show fatty degeneration, cirrhosis, or cell injury. In the hematopoietic type the bone marrow is hyperplastic and normoblastic. Splenomegaly and hemolytic anemia exist. The teeth may be reddish brown, as are the bones, as a result of uroporphyrin deposit.

Symptoms and Signs

Porphyria occurs much more frequently in women than in men. The disease may be suspected in a patient who presents a combination of abdominal, neurological, psychiatric, and at times dermatological symptoms. The acute attack often starts with colicky abdominal pain, sometimes associated with nausea, vomiting, and constipation. The gastrointestinal symptoms often suggest appendicitis, with the result that laparotomy is performed. The patient continues to complain bitterly of abdominal pain and becomes anxious, irritable, argumentative, and perhaps obviously psychotic. As the disease progresses, the patient loses much weight and may become quite cachectic.

Psychiatric manifestations are varied and may be the most prominent presenting symptoms. They are probably due to a direct, possibly reversible, metabolic effect of the disease. They usually precede the neurologic symptoms. Agitation, depression, and disturbances of memory and of the sensorium, with delirious and psychotic-like hallucinatory and delusional experiences, are among the most common symptoms.

The neurological manifestations are greatly varied. Perhaps the most frequent are motor weaknesses, which may be irregularly distributed but are most frequent in the extremities and less so in the muscles of the trunk and abdomen and in the muscles innervated by the cranial nerves. Of the latter, the facial and oculomotor muscles are most often involved. The motor weaknesses may be accompanied by severe pain and paresthesias, but there is usually little or no objective sensory disturbance. The paralysis is flaccid, and tendon reflexes are usually absent or depressed. Convulsions may occur. Cases of both receptive and expressive aphasia have been reported. Bulbar involvement with dysphonia, dysphagia, tachycardia, and respiratory and vasomotor dysfunction may occur.

The following case report illustrates the acute intermittent form.

A woman registered for examination at a medical clinic at the age of 40 with a history of five attacks of pain in the right upper quadrant of the abdomen during the previous eight months. The attacks of pain were described as continuing from a half hour to two hours. Results of the general physical examination were essentially normal. A cholecystogram made at this time was reported as disclosing nothing abnormal. A brief note by the medical consultant suggested the existence of an emotional disturbance associated with an unsatisfactory marital relationship. The diagnosis of porphyria was not made at this time.

A history of brief attacks of pain in the right upper quadrant of the abdomen recurring periodically over a period of 11 years was obtained. The present attack began 10 days before the patient's visit to the clinic. This attack was more severe than usual, was accompanied by fever, and persisted much longer. The severity of the pain was such that for the first time the patient allowed her physicians to administer narcotic agents by hypodermic injection. These consisted of one tablet of scopolamine and morphine administered nine days before admission and 100 mg. of meperidine hydrochloride (Demerol) on the following days, when she was placed in a hospital elsewhere. No further sedatives were administered. Penicillin was given and plans were made to remove her gall bladder after the fever had subsided. The patient and her family, because of their religious beliefs, were opposed to this or any surgical procedure. Four days before her clinic visit her family noticed that she wrote unusual letters and displayed peculiar, incessant to-and-fro movements of her hands and arms to the extent that she had no rest. She withdrew from contact with others. The day before her admission to the clinic she refused to accept food or fluids.

At the time of her registration, the patient held herself in a rigid position, with her right arm stiffly raised in a cataleptic pose. Her hands were clenched tightly, and her eyes were closed, and she muttered incoherently. When she was spoken to, she closed her eyes more tightly and repeated in a rhythmic way, "Are they laughing at her?" She resisted attempts to change her position by strong muscular contractions wherever she was touched. When she was left alone, she opened her eyes; occasional jerky, sucking movements of her mouth were observed. Results of the neurological examination were essentially negative. With great difficulty she was examined by a surgeon, who found no evidence of an acute abdominal lesion.

The patient's history was obtained from the husband. She was the eighth of 11 children. The father was alcoholic until 15 years before his death at 85 (four years prior to the time of this report). The parents' attitude toward surgical treatment had always been, "What God put there was meant to stay." The patient had repeatedly refused cholecystectomy. She had been in good health except for the repeated attacks of pain in the right upper abdominal quadrant previously mentioned. Information about the patient's relatives indicated that in general they had lived to advanced age and had been free of abdominal complaints and mental symptoms.

During her first seven days in the hospital, repeated physical examinations failed to disclose abnormalities except for the behavior disturbance. The patient's temperature remained persistently elevated between 99.6° and 102.8° F. Oliguria was present. The specific gravity of the urine was 1.030. Grade 4 albuminuria was noted. The value for urea nitrogen was 68 mg. per 100 ml. of blood. After the subcutaneous administration of fluids, the output of urine increased and there occurred a decrease in the content of albumin in the urine and a rapid decrease in the level of the blood urea nitrogen. On the third hospital day, qualitative study of the urinary porphyrins showed no uroporphyrins, but the presence of coproporphyrin. On the fourth and fifth hospital days, the patient was mute. On the sixth day she was either crying out incoherently or whispering and muttering unintelligibly. On this day the diagnosis of porphyria was established by the detection of porphobilinogen in the urine. (Quantitative porphyrin test, 24 units; uroporphyrin, none; porphobilinogen, 2.6 Ehrlich units; coproporphyrin, 333 micrograms.)

The patient's rectal temperature reached 105° F. on the seventh hospital day. She remained withdrawn, mute, and uncommunicative until the twelfth hospital day, when she began to talk irrelevantly. Visual and auditory hallucinations occurred on the fourteenth hospital day. She sang and talked incoherently and screamed for long periods. She soiled and smeared herself with feces. She spoke of being crucified, of sinning so terribly that she would never be forgiven, and of committing sexual misdemeanors. On the nineteenth hospital day, results of qualitative tests for urinary porphyrins were reported negative. The behavior disturbance remained unchanged.

Electroshock treatment was initiated on the twentieth hospital day. Immediately after this treatment, the patient inquired as to where she was and what she was doing. She declared she wished "to get better." Following the second electroshock treatment, the patient spoke to the ward personnel and began to eat without assistance. She declared that she had burning sensations (paresthesias) and complained of pains in the distal portions of her extremities.

Her verbal production still indicated suspicion and misinterpretation of her environment.

Six electroshock treatments were administered between the twentieth and thirtieth hospital days. After the fourth treatment the patient's temperature again became normal. She was oriented and was able to recall recent and past events except for the period of acute illness, although she did not recall her fright and some of the hallucinations which occurred in this period. At this time there was slight increase in the sensitivity of her feet to touch and pinprick. She was returned to her home thirty-three days after admission.

Diagnosis

The diagnosis depends upon the finding in the urine of uroporphyrin or porphobilinogen in excess, or both. Porphobilinogen is found only in patients showing combined abdominal and nervous manifestations. With the excretion of large amounts of uroporphyrin, the urine attracts attention because of its characteristic red, port-wine color. Spectroscopic examination readily permits identification of the uroporphyrin. It is important to stress the fact that the presence of reddish urine is by no means a general rule. Frequently a fresh urine specimen is nearly normal in color, while in other instances it is light yellow or dark amber. When porphyria is suspected, it is unwise to discard a sample of urine merely because it fails to show the characteristic port-wine color. Such specimens should be kept in the light; they will then darken, and appropriate laboratory tests for uroporphyrin may be performed. Porphobilinogen may be detected in fresh urine by means of the Ehrlich aldehyde test. Excessive coproporphyrin may be found in such urines. Recently α-amino levulinic acid has been found also.

The triad of variable abdomen pain, gradually increasing paralysis of the arms and legs, and toxic–organic mental symptoms should suggest the possibility of this rather uncommon and not rarely misdiagnosed disease.

Prognosis

The outlook for life is relatively good in the erythropoietic and in the dermatological or photosensitive types; in the intermittent acute variety the mortality is relatively high, particularly in those with symptoms referable to the bulbar nervous system.

Treatment

Chlorpromazine is the most helpful remedy thus far available in the treatment of acute porphyria. It does not affect established paralyses, may not prevent fatalities from bulbar or respiratory paralyses, and does not appear to influence porphyrin metabolism directly. At the outset it may be necessary to give as much as 100 mg. four to six times in 24 hours intramuscularly; however, it is usually possible to reduce this dose quite rapidly and often to discontinue it entirely. There are some cases in which a small maintenance dose is necessary. Electric shock therapy has been tried in several patients with psychotic symptomatology, and the response has been variable. Conflicting reports have been expressed concerning the effectiveness of cortisone and of corticotropin (ACTH). Alcohol, barbiturates, and other toxic agents should be avoided. It is important also that emotional stresses be avoided insofar as possible. These are often decisive in precipitating attacks.

HEPATOLENTICULAR DEGENERATION

This rare condition, described by S. A. K. Wilson in 1912, is associated, almost invariably in its later course with evidence of personality disorder. In some instances, emotional lability or even gross behavioral deviations are the most prominent early symptoms. It has been, and is, most likely to be confused with schizophrenia, paranoid, hypomanic, and depression reactions, and hysteria.

Characterized by degenerative changes in both brain and liver, it is associated in over half of those affected with it with a characteristic greenish yellow ring seen on the undersurface of the cornea near its margin (the Kayser-Fleischer ring). Hepatolenticular degeneration appears to be inherited as a recessive character and represents a primary metabolic defect.

Symptoms

The illness may occur in a rapidly progressive form, which commences most commonly in childhood and early adolescence to terminate by death after a few months or several years. Emotional lability of the pseudo-bulbar type (forced crying and laughing), thought of as childishness, and behavioral disorder occur with the development of dysarthria and dysphagia, slowing of voluntary movements, rigidity, and dystonic movements. The acute type is often associated with fever.

Those cases developing in later adolescence or early adulthood more frequently run a more prolonged course, without fever, and are characterized by tremulousness, titubation, later contractures, and sometimes convulsive seizures, with eventual evidence of general cerebral insufficiency. These are the patients whose personality disturbances resemble the schizophrenic, hypomanic, and hysterical reactions. The tremor is characteristic, most often involving the distal portion of the extremities. It becomes progressively more violent. When the arms are extended, it appears as though the patient were waving his hands (wing beating).

There is usually little evidence of hepatitis, although occasionally jaundice may precede the illness. The liver is seldom enlarged.

Diagnosis

In addition to the various clinical symptoms, the presence of the Kayser-Fleischer corneal ring, there exists an increased urinary excretion of copper and amino acids and a diminution in serum ceruloplasmin. Minor symptoms of nausea and anorexia may precede or accompany the neuropsychiatric disturbance. More recently it has been found in x-ray studies that many patients with Wilson's disease have osteomalacia with pseudo-fractures and marginal bone fragmentation resembling the changes in the Fanconi syndrome.

Pathology

There is gross degeneration of the lenticular nuclei, particularly in the putamen and caudate nuclei. Histologically, neuronal degeneration with loss or pathological changes are found not only in the cells of the basal ganglia but also in those of the cerebral cortex and cerebellum. There are generally nodular cirrhosis of the liver and splenomegaly. Excessive deposition of copper is found in the brain, liver, Descemet's membrane of the cornea, and other organs. It appears that an excessive absorption of copper takes place from the intestinal tract. It has been suggested that the excessive copper is toxic due to a blocking effect on coenzyme A or a related enzyme which leads to disturbed pyruvate metabolism.

Treatment

Weekly intramuscular injections of 2,3-dimercaptopropanol (BAL or British anti-lewisite) in doses of 1.0 to 1.5 ml. of 10 per cent solution in peanut oil should be given indefinitely. A chelating agent (Versene) and penicillamine should be given in doses of 1 to 4 gm. daily, with BAL. In order to reduce the absorption of copper in the diet, 20 mg. of enteric-coated capsules of potassium sulfide should be given with each meal, in association with a diet low in copper-containing foods.

MYXEDEMA

Although Ord, in 1877, first proposed the term "myxedema," Gull, four years earlier, had presented a paper entitled, "On a cretinoid state supervening in adult life in women." Accompanying mental changes were noted in the early descriptions of the disease. Among the most frequent mental symptoms are slowness and difficulty in apprehension, thought, and action. These retardations, together with indecision and listlessness, may suggest depression. Memory may be impaired, the defect being more marked in respect to recent events. Speech is frequently slow, and changes in articulation may occur. Recently these clinical findings have been interpreted as the result of impairment of the level of awareness leading to defects in attention, concentration, endurance, and conceptual use without sensory activation. In cases showing such manifestations, there is associated an electroencephalographic abnormality with diminution in mean frequency and voltage, resulting from impaired cerebral metabolism. The serial subtraction test is said to expose the defect in awareness most effectively. Associated with their hebetude, many patients show an unusual fretfulness, irritability, and a paranoid trend. The clinical picture is determined largely by individual emotional and personality factors. There may, therefore, be paranoid characteristics, delusions of persecution, and hallucinations. Mild degrees of thyroid insufficiency are not infrequently seen in middle-aged persons who complain of fatigue, pains, and headache and are pessimistic.

Treatment with thyroid extract not only relieves the above symptoms but corrects the electroencephalographic disturbance in those without permanent cerebral damage. Treatment with the extract should be initiated with caution, is best carried out in a hospital under careful observation, and should be commenced with low dosages of 15 mg. daily. The sudden changes in metabolism are particularly dangerous for those with cardiovascular disorders.

ACROMEGALOID PERSONALITY

Manfred Bleuler (son of Eugen Bleuler) of the Zurich Psychiatric Clinic, Burghöltzli, has called attention to the fact that, while acromegaly does not in itself lead to a psychosis, it is quite regularly accompanied by an alteration of personality. This change consists mainly of a lack of initiative and spontaneity and a change in mood. Some patients show

brief periods of moodiness without apparent cause, sometimes manifesting cheerfulness, self-satisfaction, and elation, with passivity and indifference. Again, the mood may at times be anxious, resentful, tense, and unpleasant. In advanced acromegaly, even without increased intracranial pressure, there are slow reactions and a slowness in stream of the thought. There is no intellectual impairment except that referable to apathy and slowness of thought and action. The patient's social attitude is usually characterized by egocentricity, lack of consideration for and interest in other people, impatience, irritability, and over-sensitivity during social contacts. Bleuler does not mean that this type of personality is specific to acromegaly, but he speculatively raises the question whether the endocrine disturbance of acromegaly and the emotional and other psychological disturbances may not, as in other fields of psychosomatic medicine, be merely different aspects of a single life process. To support this hypothesis, Bleuler calls attention to the fact that it is now conceded that psychogenetic factors are of importance in many forms of hyperthyroid disorders, in Cushing's disease, and in other endocrine derangements.

BIBLIOGRAPHY

Alzheimer, A.: Ueber eine eigenartige Erkrankung der Hirnrinde. Centralbl. f. Nervenh. u. Psychiat., *18*:177–179, 1907.

Asher, R.: Myxoedematous madness. Brit. M. J., *2*:555–562, 1949.

Association for Research in Nervous and Mental Disease. Vol. XXII. The Role of Nutritional Deficiency in Nervous and Mental Disease. Baltimore, Williams & Wilkins Co., 1943.

Bailey, F. W.: Histopathology of polioencephalitis hemorrhagica superior (Wernicke's disease). Arch. Neurol. & Psychiat., *56*:609–630, 1946.

Bleuler, Manfred: The psychopathology of acromegaly. J. Nerv. & Ment. Dis., *113*:497–511, 1951.

Browning, T. B., Atkins, R. W., and Weiner, H.: Cerebral metabolic disturbances in hypothyroidism. Arch. Int. Med., *93*:938–950, 1954.

Brunsting, L. A., Mason, H. L., and Aldrich,

R. A.: Adult form of chronic porphyria with cutaneous manifestations. J.A.M.A., 146:1207–1212, 1951.

Cleghorn, R. A.: Endocrine Influence on Personality and Behavior. In The Biology of Mental Health and Disease. New York, Paul B. Hoeber, Inc., 1952.

Dean, G., and Barnes, H. D.: Porphyria in Sweden and South Africa. South African Med. J., 33:246–253, 1959.

Ferraro, A., Arieti, S., and English, W. H.: Cerebral changes in the course of pernicious anemia and their relationship to psychic symptoms. J. Neuropath. & Exper. Neurol., 4:217–239, 1945.

Freeman, J. G., and Kolb, L. C.: Acute intermittent porphyria: Associated psychiatric symptoms treated by electroshock. Proc. Staff Meet. Mayo Clin., 26:401–406, 1951.

Harris, S.: Clinical Pellagra. St. Louis, C. V. Mosby Co., 1941.

Hieros, R.: Changes in the nervous system in acute porphyria. Brain, 80:176–192, 1957.

Himwich, H. E.: Brain Metabolism and Cerebral Disorders. Baltimore, Williams & Wilkins Co., 1951.

Holmes, J. M.: Cerebral manifestations of vitamin-B_{12} deficiency. Brit. M. J., 2:1394–1398, 1956.

Korsakoff, S. S.: Eine psychische Störung, combiniert mit multipler Neuritis. Allg. Ztschr. f. Psychiat., 46:475–485, 1890.

Melby, J. C., Street, J. P., and Watson, C. J.: Chlorpromazine in the treatment of porphyria. J.A.M.A., 162:174–178, 1956.

Money, J.: Psychologic studies in hypothyroidism. Arch. Neurol. & Psychiat., 76:296–309, 1956.

Newton, R. D.: The identity of Alzheimer's disease and senile dementia and their relationship to senility. J. Ment. Sc., 94:225–249, 1948.

Samson, D. C., et al.: Cerebral metabolic disturbance and delirium in pernicious anemia. Arch. Int. Med., 90:4–14, 1952.

Scheinberg, I. H., and Sternlieb, I.: Long-term management of hepatolenticular degeneration (Wilson's Disease). Am. J. Med., 29:316–333, 1960.

Spillane, J. D.: Nutritional Disorders of the Nervous System. Baltimore, Williams & Wilkins Co., 1947.

Stengel, E.: A study on the symptomatology and differential diagnosis of Alzheimer's disease and Pick's disease. J. Ment. Sc., 89:1–20, 1943.

Visher, J. S., and Aldrich, C. K.: Acute intermittent porphyria. Psychosom. Med., 16:163–168, 1954.

Walshe, J. M.: Changing concepts of the pathogenesis of Wilson's Disease. Ann. Intern. Med., 51:1110–1115, 1959.

Wernicke, C.: Lehrbuch der Gehirnkrankheiten, Vol. II, p. 289. Berlin, T. Fischer, 1881.

Chapter Nineteen

CHRONIC BRAIN SYNDROME ASSOCIATED WITH INTRACRANIAL NEOPLASM

Brain tumors with accompanying mental disorder are more frequent than indicated by the diagnostic statistics provided from hospitals. Summaries of the total incidence of intracranial tumors found at autopsy in patients in mental hospitals in the United States give a figure of 3.7 per cent against that of 2.35 per cent for patients without diagnosed psychiatric disorder in general hospitals. Meningiomas are found much more frequently in autopsies performed on patients in mental hospitals than in the general hospitals. The number of brain tumors discovered at necropsy is much larger than the number diagnosed correctly antemortem. Probably in only a minority of early cases of brain tumor are the mental symptoms so pronounced as to form a conspicuous part of the clinical picture of the neoplasm, although there are few cases that remain entirely free of manifestations of mental disorder. There is need to recognize that the initial symptoms of tumor may be masked by preexisting or concomitant mental and emotional disturbances. There is a great statistical disparity as to both the frequency and the nature of mental symptoms in brain tumor. Clouding of consciousness and disturbance of memory occur most frequently. There is, however, no symptomatic picture which may be considered characteristic of a brain tumor.

Symptoms

The genesis, pathological structure, neurological signs, and electroencephalographic records of brain tumor will not be discussed. Generally speaking, the symptoms and signs of brain tumor fall into three groups: (*a*) signs of increased intracranial pressure; progressive impairment of consciousness and energy with headache, vomiting, and papilledema; (*b*) focal neurological symptoms and signs determined by the location of the tumor, (*c*) psychiatric symptoms which tend to fall into two types. Symptoms of the first type, which often appear early, perhaps before those caused by increased intracranial pressure or the site of the tumor, are psychogenically determined by the characteristics of the patient's pre-morbid personality structure and his particular stresses, conflicts, and defenses. In some cases the first and, perhaps for a time, the only symptoms may be psychiatric and consist of accentuations of personality tendencies. Some patients show a loss of inhibitions with blunting of social or moral sense, egotistic tendencies, shamelessness, and even gross sexual or other misbehavior. Psychiatric symptoms of the second group stem from cerebral damage incident to the tumor and to increased intracranial pressure.

Among early symptoms may be absentmindedness, later becoming an obvious memory defect, especially for recent events, easy fatigability, a raising of the threshold of consciousness, disturbances of sensorium, difficulty of grasp, impairment of calculation and of reasoning abilities, defective attention, hebetude, drowsiness, confusion, and disorientation. Psychomotor retardation is not uncommon. Fluctuations of consciousness may occur. Sometimes the patient may confabulate as in Korsakoff's psychosis. Loss of libido is common.

Temporal lobe tumors frequently are mistaken for schizophrenic disorders. Often they present paroxysmal motor, affective, and perceptual disturbances. These may be crude and disagreeable olfactory or gustatory hallucinatory experiences. The disturbances are characteristically repetitive, and although the patient is absorbed in, and may suffer anxiety with, the experience, he is usually capable of perceiving the existence of both the present environment and the hallucination. Either then or later he is able to distinguish the experience as ego alien—outside his usual personification of self-functioning. "Déjà vu" phenomena occur in such tumors, but more frequently patients describe emotional reactions and transitory experiences of strangeness, loneliness, or dreamy states. Also noticed are episodic and short-lived affective states consisting of feelings of dread, terror, or overwhelming fear. Some patients have reported either unexpected angry affect or feelings of well being.

Motor automatisms may take place in which the patient may carry out sudden aggressive or assaultive actions or other complex performances for which he has no memory.

Frontal lobe tumors are particularly prone to produce symptoms affecting the functioning of personality over time. Slow-growing meningiomes compressing the frontal lobe are among the most frequently undiagnosed tumors of the brain that produce symptoms of a psychiatric nature. Tumors in this area produce insidious and subtle changes in personality functioning.

A flattening of affect coupled with a growing apathy concerning personal and business affairs is frequent. Other emotional disturbances are instability, irritability, depression, and anxiety. Euphoria and facetiousness ("witzelsucht" of Oppenheim) are probably a little more frequent in tumors of the frontal lobe but are not specific for any one location in the brain. It well may be that this lightness of spirit and tendency to be witty is merely a defense reaction against the threat to the integrity of the organism by the destructive growth.

Occipital lobe tumors are associated more frequently with unformed simple visual hallucinating experiences which consist of flashes of light or of colored lights. Moving objects may be hallucinated. Complex visual and auditory hallucinations are more frequent in tumors of the temporal lobe. Olfactory hallucinations in the form of disagreeable odors may occur in the case of tumors on the undersurface of the hemispheres.

It is generally agreed that tumors of the corpus callosum are accompanied by intellectual impairment, difficulty in concentration and in thinking, and failure to respond to stimuli, particularly to auditory stimuli.

The conspicuousness of the symptoms and, to some extent, their nature are determined by the rate of growth of the tumor. In the case of slowly growing meningiomas, there may be simply a slowly developing mental deterioration. In rapidly developing gliomas (spongioblastomas), there may be an active delirium suggesting a toxic state, with confusion, disorientation, and perhaps stupor. In those that develop unusually rapidly, both the mental and neurological signs may suggest an inflammatory lesion.

Diagnosis

If increased intracranial pressure appears suddenly and develops rapidly, mental symptoms are usually produced and may be severe. If pressure increases slowly, there may be no mental symptoms. Many tumors, because of their site and the particular structures they injure, produce neurological signs of great localizing value. Mental symptoms by themselves have, however, little or no value in localizing a tumor of the brain. It is stated that mental symptoms are nearly twice as frequent in case of supratentorial tumors as in infratentorial growths. In case the brain tumor causes convulsions, difficulty may arise in evaluating the mental symptoms, with the result that they may be attributed to idiopathic epilepsy. Convulsions occur in about 8 per cent of the cases and may be either of grand mal or petit mal type. Seizures are rare in cerebellar tumors and most frequent in those of the parietal and temporal lobes.

Difficulty in diagnosis may also arise if the patient suffered from cerebral arteriosclerosis prior to the appearance of the mental symptoms. If the patient suffers from sensory or motor aphasia or from apraxia by reason of the location of the tumors, the resulting inability of the patient to communicate his ideas adequately may make it difficult to determine the presence or extent of mental symptoms. In the terminal phase the patient may be stuporous and lose control of both rectal and vesical sphincters.

The electroencephalogram is an invaluable aid in detecting those tumors present in "silent areas" or not productive of increased intracranial pressure early in their course. The use of the electroencephalogram has been recommended as a routine procedure for patients admitted to mental hospitals. However, its serial application is necessary in many instances to insure detection of tumors. Metrazol for activation of the electroencephalogram is valuable, particularly for the diagnosis of temporal lobe tumors.

BIBLIOGRAPHY

Association for Research in Nervous and Mental Disease. Vol. XVI: Tumors of the Nervous System. Baltimore, Williams & Wilkins Co., 1937.

Bailey, P.: Intracranial Tumors, 2nd ed. Springfield, Illinois, Charles C Thomas, 1948.

Idem: Buchanan, D. N., and Bucy, P. C.: Intracranial Tumors of Infancy and Childhood. Chicago, The University of Chicago Press, 1939.

Mulder, D. W., Bickford, R. G., and Dodge, H. W., Jr.: Hallucinatory epilepsy: complex hallucinations as focal seizures. Am. J. Psychiat., 113:1100–1102, 1957.

Idem: and Daly, D.: Psychiatric symptoms associated with lesions of the temporal lobe. J.A.M.A., 150:173–176, 1952.

Patton, R. B., and Sheppard, J. A.: Intracranial tumors found at autopsy in mental patients. Am. J. Psych., 113:319–324, 1956.

Soniat, T. L. L.: Psychiatric symptoms associated with intracranial neoplasms. Am. J. Psychiat., 108:19–22, 1951.

Strauss, I., and Keschner, M.: Mental symptoms in cases of tumor of the frontal lobe. Arch. Neurol. & Psychiat., 33:986–1007, 1935.

Waggoner, R. W., and Bagchi, B. K.: Initial masking of organic brain changes by psychic symptoms. Am. J. Psychiat., 110:904–910, 1954.

Chapter Twenty

CHRONIC BRAIN SYNDROMES ASSOCIATED WITH DISEASES OF UNKNOWN OR UNCERTAIN CAUSE

DEMYELINATING DISEASES

Although demyelinization within the nervous system occurs as the consequence of vascular lesions, infectious illnesses, and nutritional and toxic disturbances, this type of pathological lesion is not the primary phenomenon in these disorders. Multiple sclerosis and the various forms of diffuse sclerosis (encephalitis periaxialis diffusa of Schilder, encephalitis periaxialis concentrica of Balo, and the several forms of progressive cerebral sclerosis) form the group of primary demyelinizing disorders. The etiology of these structural disturbances of the nervous system is unknown. Their importance to the clinical psychiatrist springs from the concomitant personality disturbance noticed in the course of the illness, or the behavioral abnormalities often confused with other disturbances of personality. Their differentiation is important for therapeutic and prognostic reasons.

Multiple Sclerosis

Despite the fact that multiple sclerosis is definitely a structural disease of the nervous system, in a considerable percentage of patients personality problems are present at the onset or during the course of the disease. Both in multiple sclerosis and in Parkinson's syndrome enough concomitant psychiatric symptoms may be present to mask the organic picture, with the result that a psychiatric instead of a neurological diagnosis is made. Psychotic symptoms that require commitment are, however, rare.

There is no characteristic syndrome determined by the organic pathology of the disease. The general nature of the symptoms tends to be dependent upon the personality make-up of the individual patient. Not rarely, therefore, we see paranoid, depressive, hypomanic, or expansive reactions. Previous personality patterns of these types may, through the damage sustained by the personality at

267

the organic level, become exaggerated. As a compensating psychological reaction to the disorganizing, destructive effect of the disease, one often observes a pathological complacency, cheerfulness, and even euphoria. These symptoms occur so frequently that they have often been erroneously regarded as a particular feature of the disease process itself.

Sometimes the patient's reaction to his disability is marked by an irritability or emotional instability that seriously disturbs interpersonal relationships. Impaired control over the expression of laughter and of crying resulting from bilateral upper motor neuron defects is often a significant feature. The emotional instability is associated with the clinical impression of intellectual impairment. If the explosive and forced laughing or crying occurs, the patient does not feel any affect such as the emotional signs suggest. A few patients manifest serious behavior disorders. These are occasionally observed in patients who are impotent but nevertheless have an increase in sex urge. Emotional lability and intellectual impairment are often found in patients with marked neurological disability.

Examination of cerebrospinal fluid will reveal some abnormality in cell count, total protein, or colloidal reaction in a majority of the cases. The electroencephalogram is abnormal in half of the patients, although there is no pattern specifically diagnostic.

Diffuse Sclerosis

The most common type is that known as Schilder's disease, which occurs as a rapidly progressive disorder productive of various mental symptoms, convulsions, loss of vision, and motor or sensory defects. Fatal cases show extensive demyelinization of the cerebral hemispheres. The signs and symptoms are inconstant from patient to patient and depend upon those areas of the cortical hemispheres involved. Headache, vomiting, and vertigo are common. Memory defects, apathy or irritability, personality changes, or confusion with disorientation and dementia may occur. The neurological signs are extensive. Cortical blindness is common. Hemianopsia, optic atrophy, and choked discs have been observed. All varieties of motor and sensory disturbances, with the associated defects in neurological examinations, may occur. Occasionally these conditions are confused with brain tumors caused by the increase in intracranial pressure. Early in the course of these illnesses they have been confused with hysterical or schizophrenic reactions. The spinal fluid shows no consistent changes. In the majority of instances, these illnesses are clinically progressive and terminate fatally following the development of dementia and quadriplegia with decerebrate rigidity. Remissions occasionally occur. Treatment consists presently in providing symptomatic care and nursing.

PARALYSIS AGITANS

In his "Essays on Shaking Palsy," published in 1817, James Parkinson, himself a victim, described the disease of late middle life now known as paralysis agitans. With its degenerative lesions of the extrapyramidal system, particularly of the corpus striatum and substantia nigra, the neurological symptoms are the conspicuous features of the clinical picture. The chronic progressive muscular rigidity, the immobile facies, the posture of flexion of neck, trunk, and extremities, the poverty of movement, and the slow, rhythmic tremor affecting the extremities to varying degrees constitute a striking syndrome. In many cases there are no mental symptoms. Most patients present a good-natured complaisance, but some, in reaction to their disability, are irritable, peevish, and dissatisfied. The fact that the patient finds himself in a continuously contracting environment in which he becomes more and more dependent on other members of the family creates many emotional problems.'

Drugs of the solanaceous group have been used for over 80 years in the treatment of this disease. Recently several synthetic antispasmodic drugs have been introduced, of which trihexyphenidyl (Artane) is now most widely employed. The initial dose is 1 mg. on the first day, increased to 1 to 2 mg. daily up to a total of 4 to 8 mg. divided into three or four doses. Elderly patients usually can take only 1 to 2 mg. daily. Toxic effects of these drugs are dryness of the mouth, excessive mydrioses, gastrointestinal upsets, and rarely a delirious reaction.

In cases of severe muscle rigidity, contracture, and spasm, the powerful muscle-relaxant action of benztropine methanesulfonate (Cogentin) may prove helpful. It is longer acting than other antispasmodics and can be taken in doses of 0.5 to 1 or 2 mg. in older patients and 1 to 4 mg. in younger patients, usually once a day on retiring.

Procyclidine hydrochloride (Kemadrin hydrochloride) is one of the newest of the synthetic antispasmodic drugs. It combines antirigidity action with a strong cerebral-stimulating action that is helpful in patients with somnolence and depression. The initial dose is usually 2.5 mg. three times daily, gradually increasing to 5 mg. three times daily.

Another anti-parkinsonian drug which has been increasingly employed is orphenadrine hydrochloride (Disipal). The average dose is 50 mg. three times a day. It is a harmless preparation with minimal side reactions. Its chief drawback is the tendency for the good effects to wear off in the course of months.

Since changes may be produced in the basal ganglia by infections (viral, spirochetal), by toxins (carbon monoxide, manganese) and by trauma, a symptomatic parkinsonism may be produced by various pathological agents.

HUNTINGTON'S CHOREA

Huntington's chorea is a degenerative disease of the central nervous system resulting from a dominant mutation. The first distinctive description of the disease was given in 1872 by Dr. George Huntington, whose father and grandfather had practiced medicine at East Hampton, Long Island, for a period conjointly covering 78 years and had observed families among the adult members of which an incurable chorea had existed for generations. No person, not descended from a progenitor so tainted, has ever been known to develop the disease. It is inherited as a pure mendelian characteristic. It behaves as a dominant with the result that from one-fourth to one-half of the offspring of a sufferer will develop the disease. Kennedy quotes over 1000 cases in the United States as having been traced to three individuals who emigrated from an English village in 1630. Its organic basis was demonstrated by Alzheimer. The essential pathology consists of a slow degeneration of the cells of the caudate nucleus, of the putamen, and of the cerebral cortex.

Symptoms

The onset of Huntington's chorea is insidious and, generally speaking, occurs between the ages of 30 and 45 years. Frequently a change of character antedates or accompanies the appearance of the choreiform symptoms. The patient may be irritable, obstinate, and moody and lack initiative. In other cases the picture may be one of fatuous euphoria. Esthetic and ethical senses are blunted. Many patients become fault-finding, spiteful, irascible, and even destructive and assaultive. There is an increasing lack of spontaneity in activity, of concern as to the disease, and of solicitude as to obligations of conscience, affection, or ideals. Suspiciousness, jealousy, and paranoid trends, even to the extent of well-developed delusions of persecution appear. Some patients experience hallucinations. With the increasing emotional deterioration, there is a coincident impairment of attention, memory, and judgment. Interest in life becomes progressively narrower. There is also a poverty of ideas and a disorderliness of thought. The dementia may become extreme.

The choreiform movements usually appear first in the upper extremity, neck, and face. These involuntary movements are clumsy, irregular, jerky, stretching ones. In the early stages it appears as if the patient were merely inattentive or careless in his movements, which gradually increase in intensity and inco-ordination. The contractions of the facial muscles result in grimaces while those of the tongue, lips, and respiratory muscles lead to a hesitating, explosive, poorly articulated type of speech which, in advanced cases, is difficult to understand. The choreiform movements result in a shuffling, dancing type of gait associated with irregular movements of the trunk. The movements usually cease during sleep. As the disease progresses, there is interference with swallowing, walking becomes impossible, and the patient may become bedridden. The tendon reflexes are increased. Suicide is not uncommon.

R. A. was admitted to a mental hospital at the age of 56. The familial incidence of Huntington's chorea was striking. A maternal grandmother, a maternal uncle and his daughter, the patient's mother and four of the patient's siblings exhibited definite symptoms of Huntington's chorea. Two members of the family committed suicide after they had developed the disease. Prior to her illness the patient was apparently an attractive, well-adjusted person. She was a Girl Scout leader and took part in community affairs. Shortly before she was 35 years of age she began to show an insidious change of personality. She discontinued her church, Girl Scout, card club and other activities; she lost interest in her family and at times wandered away from home, returning at night but giving no information as to where she had been. In this same period she began to drop articles and to show twitching of her hands.

The patient became neglectful of her personal appearance, refused to comb her hair, bathe, or change her clothes. She refused to launder soiled garments and would hide them in closets or corners. The choreiform movements increased in extent, and she occasionally fell. At times she showed temporary alertness and interest in anticipation of a visit from her daughter, but after one or two days she drifted back into her former seclusiveness and deteriorated habits.

On many occasions she threatened and even attacked her husband, sometimes with a knife, and on one occasion inflicted a four-inch scalp wound. She became profane and her favorite term in addressing her husband was, "You G - d - fool." She was subject to tantrums in which she would threaten to jump from a window. She came to be known to the children in the neighborhood as "the old witch on the third floor." Finally, the choreiform movements became so extreme that it was difficult for her to go up and down stairs and she often fell.

On arrival at the hospital, her facial expression was vacant and she showed such uncoordinated and choreiform movements of her legs that she had difficulty in walking without assistance. There were gross choreiform movements of the head and all extremities. Her constant grimacing, blinking of her eyes, and twitching of her fingers were quite striking. The co-ordination of her hands was so poor and the movements of her head were so extreme that she had difficulty in eating. Her speech was explosive and difficult to understand. Although somewhat irritable, demanding, and distrustful, she adjusted to the hospital environment without serious difficulty.

Treatment

There is no effective treatment. The average duration of life is 15 years.

PICK'S DISEASE

This uncommon chronic brain syndrome, first described by Pick of Prague in 1892, is characterized pathologically by atrophy and gliosis in the associative areas. The motor, sensory, and projection areas are relatively unchanged. Several reports of multiple cases in one family suggest that the disease may be a heredodegenerative disorder, but it does not show any simple mendelian pattern. The involvement is of cortical areas which are relatively younger genetically, areas which are concerned with higher associative functions. The mechanisms of speech and of thinking are therefore especially impaired. It has been suggested that the disease is a premature and localized neuronic aging, a senile process limited to a genetically young area. The frontal lobe may look as if a constricting band had been applied to it. The clinical symptomatology is the result of a combination of the diffuse and focal processes. The majority of cases have been in persons between the ages of 45 and 60 years, the youngest being 31.

Local areas of the brain, particularly the frontal and temporal lobes, may be severely atrophied, and the total weight of the brain may be reduced to less than 1000 gm. (the average normal male Caucasian brain weighs 1340 gm.). The whole depth of the cortex may be involved. Microscopically the lesions are found to be degenerative and not inflammatory. Usually there is distortion in the arrangement of the cyto-architectural layers of the atrophic convolutions. Chromatolysis of the nerve cells is marked, there is a progressive disappearance of the chromatic substance, the nucleus becomes pale and is displaced to the periphery, and the granulations are lost. Ballooned cells, not found in Alzheimer's disease, are regularly seen in Pick's disease. The loss of ganglion cells become marked, and many of those remaining are swollen and show argentophilic granules. There is hypertrophy of the neuroglia, and the microglia presents a swollen appearance, with relatively numerous fatty granules. Senile plaques and Alzheimer fibrillary changes frequently found in senile dementia and Alzheimer's disease are rarely found. The white matter atrophies early. Changes in the basal ganglia are regularly found in Alzheimer's disease but are rare in Pick's disease.

The affliction occurs twice as frequently in women as in men. Among the earliest symptoms are lack of spontaneity, loss of memory, difficulty in thinking and concentration, and a blunting of emotions. The patient becomes taciturn, indifferent, and bewildered and is unable to deal with new situations. The memory for the execution of normal, concrete tasks is relatively well preserved, but the capacity for abstract behavior is more seriously impaired. Dementia is usually well established within a year. Some patients show a euphoric contentment, while others are irritable, depressed, and suspicious. Common focal symptoms include apraxia, alexia, agraphia, or aphasia until such time as their characteristics are obscured by general dementia. The patient may have difficulty in naming objects, although he may remember their use and properties. A rather important characteristic of these aphasias is that they are of gradual rather than of sudden onset and the spontaneous logorrhea often found in aphasia due to vascular disease is not present. Echolalia and stereotyped reactions are not infrequent. The pupils, other reflexes, and spinal fluid are not disturbed.

As the disease progresses, the patient becomes asthenic, is confined to bed, and scarcely moves. Dementia becomes extreme, sphincter incontinence develops, the capacity for speech practically disappears, and cachexia becomes marked. The patient usually dies in from four to six years of some intercurrent infection.

Diagnosis

Clinical differentiation of the disease from Alzheimer's disease is extremely difficult. Many clinicians believe that this differentiation can be made only on postmortem examination of the brain. The age period, slowly progressive course, and intellectual impairment are similar in both diseases. Convulsions, facial paresis, and muscular rigidity common in Alzheimer's disease are rare in Pick's disease. Aphasic disturbances with perseveration and logoclonia are frequent in Alzheimer's disease but rare in Pick's. Motor impulsiveness and aggression are more common in Alzheimer's. Indifference is common in Pick's disease and anxiety in Alzheimer's disease. Defects of memory seem to occur earlier in Alzheimer's disease, and in late stages memory may be practically obliterated, whereas some retention of it continues in Pick's disease. Delusions, hallucinations, and confabulations, rather frequent in the former disease, are not common in Pick's disease. Hyperactivity is common in 'Alzheimer's disease; in Pick's disease the patient tends to be underactive. Many believe that deterioration of emotional factors, and especially of habit, progresses more rapidly in Pick's than in Alzheimer's disease. In the former, neurological signs are more frequently focal than in the latter. Finally, Pick's disease occurs much less frequently than does Alzheimer's.

Cerebral arteriosclerosis can usually be differentiated by the antecedent history of headache, dizziness, apoplectic phenomena, and other evidences of vascular disease.

LUPUS ERYTHEMATOSUS

To a psychiatrist practicing in the general hospital, lupus erythematosus disseminata is now frequently encountered as a condition with various reaction formations, or with delirious and psychotic manifestations. This condition, once considered rare, is now frequently diagnosed on the medical services because of the increasing awareness of the symptomatology and a better knowledge of the tissue and cellular pathology, including the existence of the now well known "LE cells."

Lupus erythematosus disseminata is one of the group of conditions now known as diseases of the collagen tissues. In lupus the primary damage is to the subendothelial connective tissue of capillaries, small arteries, and veins, and the endocardium and synovial membranes. Approximately 85 per cent of all clinically-recognized cases occur in women. The onset of the illness usually takes place in childhood but is most commonly recognized during adolescence and early adult life. The pathological changes are found in the ground substance and collagen which serves as a matrix and binding substance for the capillaries and small blood vessels in various parts of the body. Gross thickening is found in the endocardial and pericardial tissues, while the small arteries and arterioles of various organs, including the brain, show a fibroid degeneration and necrosis in the connective tissue matrix of the vessel wall. In certain of the affected areas of connective tissue, the intercellular ground substance shows deep metachromatic staining or the presence of eosinophilic masses, thought to be a result of the swelling and fibroid degeneration of collagen fibers. Certain deep purplish staining material found in some of the affected areas has been identified histochemically as desoxyribonucleic acid.

This is apparently the abnormal chromatin material found in the so-called "LE cells" of the blood and bone marrow on dry smears.

In one series of cases, 50 per cent presented delirious or psychosis-like phenomena at some time during the course of their illness. Another small group developed neurosis-like symptoms, while a considerable number had neurological signs at one time or another. The early symptoms of the condition are easy fatigability, malaise, and fever. The so-called butterfly rash that occurs across the bridge of the nose and on the cheeks, often considered a traditional lesion of the disease, is not present or necessary for the diagnosis of systemic lupus erythematosus. Commonly the initial signs are those of migratory reactions of joint and fibrous tissue simulating rheumatic fever or rheumatoid arthritis. Examination sometimes discloses anemia, lymphadenopathy, and edema, or signs indicating pathology involving the pleura, lungs, heart, pericardium, or gastrointestinal tract. The differentiation of the illness from rheumatic fever or rheumatoid arthritis is suggested on finding hematuria. The "LE cell" is found in stained blood of bone marrow smears, particularly those made from clotted blood or the buffy layer of heparinized blood. They consist of phagocytes containing masses of chromatin material which stain deep purple with Wright's or Giemsa stain. Usually there are leukopenia, elevation of sedimentation of the erythrocytes, and occasionally intermittently or falsely positive serological reactions for syphilis.

At the onset of the illness, anxiety is often evident, and the patients may manifest personality changes which are frequently considered to be reflective of the personality structure. Phobic, depressive, and schizophrenic pictures have been seen as well as delirioid reaction. The psychiatric disorders have been thought by many to be related to the use of steroid therapy in the course of this illness. The psychotic reactions are usually apparent some 12 days after the institution of steroid therapy, with a maximum of 30 days and a minimum of two. It must be concluded, however, that the steroid therapy per se is not related to the occurrence of the disturbance of mental functioning. In one group of patients, a large number recovered from the initial delirioid psychotic reaction only to have an active recurrence of lupus at a later time. The majority, when placed on an equivalent dose of ACTH or cortisone, did not again present the mental aberration. Exacerbation of the lupus erythematosus itself, rather than the usage of the steroids, appeared to increase the possibility of the occurrence of psychiatric disturbances.

Although remissions may occur, and cortisone and ACTH have proved effective in inducing prompt improvement, most sufferers ultimately die from renal insufficiency and intercurrent pneumococcal or streptococcal infection. The majority who present psychotic disturbances have characteristic lesions in the cerebral hemisphere at autopsy.

The behavior disturbances associated with this illness often require protective hospitalization and careful nursing. Cortisone and ACTH should be administered. The former is usually given in dosages of 0.025 gm. every six hours intramuscularly. Cortisone may be administered orally, 0.15 to 0.30 gm. in four divided doses during the day. Following seven to ten days on this dosage, the agents may be gradually reduced each succeeding two or three days until a maintenance level is reached, below which evidences of clinical activity are observed to recur. The majority of the patients require a small maintenance dosage for indefinite periods. The careful collaboration of a psychiatrist and the internist is often indicated in the treatment of disseminated lupus erythematosus.

J. M.: Five months before her admission to a general hospital, this 18-year-old girl noticed fatigability, sore throat, and fever associated with pain on movements of the ankles, fingers, and joints. These symptoms improved. About four weeks before admission she suffered nausea, loss of appetite, and intermittent vomiting. Eleven days before admission she developed double vision on lateral gaze, at first intermittent, but later constant. A few days later her vision was blurred. On admission her temperature was 98.8° F., pulse 82, respiration rate 14. She had lost 22 pounds in weight.

At this time her behavior and mental status were not unusual. She appeared thin, showed some unsteadiness in standing, and had double vision on lateral gaze, but otherwise there seemed to be no conspicuous physical disturbances. Her urine contained albumin; there was evidence of liver dysfunction with a positive cephalin flocculation test. Electroencephalogram was abnormal with disorganization and slowing in the temporal areas and periods of low voltage, 4 to 7 per second activity. At this time the sedimentation rate equalled 82 mm. per hour. Bilateral papilloedema developed. A medical consultant suggested that the patient either had rheumatoid arthritis or possibly disseminated lupus erythematosus. An internal carotid arteriogram was normal. Treatment was commenced with cortisone. The spinal fluid contained 460 mg. of protein per 100 ml. The patient's symptoms increased, particularly those referred to the joint pains. When she finally received 100 mg. of cortisone daily two months after admission, her symptoms subsided quickly. She was then discharged to her home on cortisone, 75 mg. daily.

She remained well at home until three months later, when she became very elated and overactive. She spoke of her body and brain shrinking; she said that she was becoming a baby again and would shortly die. Her return to the hospital was precipitated by a series of convulsions. She then seemed quiet and rather suspicious, but occasionally she called out for help in a loud voice. She failed to recognize certain physicians who had treated her before. The cortisone dosage was reduced from 125 to 75 mg. and her symptoms remitted.

Later the patient recounted that the psychotic disturbance occurred when she had the impression that she "was getting much better on the cortisone. I was getting stronger. About 8 p.m. when I was watching television I suddenly got the feeling that I was going to change into a baby. Previously I had talked to my relatives about this, but they didn't pay any attention to it. I felt that I was going to be bald, that all my hair was inside of my head, and that they couldn't operate to let the hair out. I felt that I was cramped up and couldn't move." (At this point she assumed the fetal position.) "I felt that I was going to die like a girl that I knew while in the hospital. I was in a dream." She declared that she felt that, when blood was being drawn from her arm, the purpose was to drain every drop of blood from her. "I felt that all the people in the ward were German spies. One of them had an Irish accent, but I felt it was a German accent. They were trying to electrocute me. When my mother came to visit me, I tried to push her off the bed so that she would not be electrocuted, but she didn't understand this. I felt that all the nurses were traitors—German spies." She seemed to interpret the slightest remark or facial expression as something of significance to her; she was frightened when the doctors approached her. Her sensorium was clear.

Some five days later the psychotic picture disappeared. A blood smear showed "LE cells." The encephalogram performed at the time of the behavior disturbance revealed an increase in the abnormality. The patient was discharged on 75 mg. of cortisone daily.

Because of increased weakness, joint pains, and general debility, she was readmitted to the hospital several months later. At this time no psychotic disturbance was evident, although she was carefully followed by a psychiatrist. She was from time to time pre-occupied by a fear of death and freely called for psychiatric help when most anxious. No recurrence of psychiatric symptoms took place on elevation of the daily dose of cortisone to 87 mg. Following another period at home, she returned to the hospital two months later with hemiparesthesia and expired shortly thereafter. Necropsy disclosed the typical pathology of lupus erythematosus.

BIBLIOGRAPHY

Bowman, L.: Diffuse Sclerosis: Encephalitis Periaxialis Diffusa. Bristol, John Wright & Sons, Ltd., 1934.

Braceland, F. J., and Griffin, M. E.: Mental changes associated with multiple sclerosis. Assn. Res. Nerv. & Ment. Dis., 28:450, 1950. Baltimore, Williams & Wilkins Co., 1951.

Dunlap, C. B.: Pathologic changes in Huntington's chorea. Arch. Neurol. & Psychiat., 18:867–943, 1927.

Greenfield, J. B., et al.: The pathology of parkinsonism. J. Nerv. & Ment. Dis., 122:200–201, 1955.

Huntington, G.: On chorea. Med. and Surg. Reporter, 26:317, 1872.

Malamud, N., and Saver, G.: Neuropathologic findings in disseminated lupus erythematosus. Arch. Neurol. & Psychiat., 71:723–731, 1954.

Idem, and Waggoner, R. W.: Genealogic and clinicopathologic study of Pick's disease. Arch. Neurol. & Psychiat., 50:288–303, 1943.

McCaughey, W. T. E.: The pathologic spectrum of Huntington's chorea. J. Nerv. & Ment. Dis., 133:91–103, 1961.

McClary, A. R., Meyer, E., and Weitzman, E. L.: Observations on the role of the mechanism of depression in some patients with lupus erythematosus. Psychosom. Med., 17:311–323, 1955.

Neumann, M. R.: Pick's disease. J. Neuropath. & Exper. Neurol., 8:255–282, 1949.

O'Connor, J. F.: Psychoses associated with systemic lupus erythematosus. Ann. Int. Med., 51:526–536, 1959.

Parkinson, J.: An essay on the shaking palsy. London, Sherwood, Neely & Jones, 1817.

Pick, A.: Ueber die Beziehungen der senilen Hirnatrophie zur Aphasia. Prag. Med. Wchnschr., 17:165, 1892.

Idem: Ueber einen Symptomenkomplex der Dementia senilis bedingt durch umschriebene Hirnatrophie. Monatschr. f. Psychiat. u. Neurol., 19:97, 1907.

Polatin, P., Hoch, P. H., and Horwitz, W. A.: Presenile psychosis. Am. J. Psychiat., 105:96–101, 1948.

Pratt, R. T. C.: An investigation of the psychiatric aspects of disseminated sclerosis. J. Neurol., Neurosurg. & Psychiat., 14:326–335, 1951.

Raskin, N., and Ehrenberg, R.: Senescence, senility, and Alzheimer's disease. Am. J. Psychiat., 113:133–137, 1956.

Ross, A. T., and Reitan, R. N.: Intellectual and affective functions in multiple sclerosis. Arch. Neurol. & Psychiat., 73:633–677, 1955.

Sjogren, T., et al.: Morbus Alzheimer and morbus Pick: A genetic, clinical and pathoanatomical study. Acta Psychiatrica et Neurologica, Supplement 83. Copenhagen, Ejnar Munksgaard, 1952.

Stengel, E.: A study on the symptomatology and differential diagnosis of Alzheimer's disease and Pick's disease. J. Ment. Sc., 89:1–20, 1943.

Stern, M., and Robbins, E. S.: Psychoses in systemic lupus erythematosus. Arch. Gen. Psych., 3:205–212, 1960.

Chapter Twenty-one

MENTAL DEFICIENCY

Definition

There exists a large group of individuals whose personality limitations rest essentially upon failure to develop sufficient intellectual capacity to cope with the demands of their environment and thus to establish an independent social existence. This lack of intellectual capacity derives from an innately imposed limitation in cerebral development, is the result of disease or injury to the brain suffered to, during, or in the immediate period after birth, or is the consequence of impaired maturation due to insufficient environmental stimulation from familial and cultural sources.

There is now little agreement as to the terminology and proper classification of these personality disorders. The general classification "Mental Deficiency" is retained by the American Psychiatric Association, while the American Association on Mental Deficiency recommends that of "Mental Retardation." By "Mental Retardation" the latter Association refers to "sub-average general intellectual functioning which originates during the developmental period and is associated with impairment of one or more of the following: (1) maturation, (2) learning, and (3) social adjustment."* "Mental

* A Manual on Terminology and Classification in Mental Retardation. Monograph Supplement. Am. J. Mental Deficiency, 642:1–111, 1959.

Deficiency" is commonly used now to refer to that group of cases due to disease or injury and more properly the province of action of the physician and psychiatrist. In considering general intellectual functioning, the upper age limit for the developmental period is arbitrarily set at 16 years.

In the early years of developmental impairment, the rate of maturation or the acquisition of various sensory–motor activities most frequently provides the evidence for the diagnosis of mental deficiency. Thus delays or failures in the sequential evolution of motility, language, control of evacuation of the bladder and bowel, and ability to interact with other children provide the clues. Inability to acquire and retain knowledge as the result of experience is an indication of a deficiency in *learning ability* and is best observed during the child's school years. If the mental defect is mild, the child may show little evidence of it until he enters school. Social adaptation becomes important as an indicator of mental retardation, particularly at the adult level, but is reflected earlier in the individual's capacities to relate to parents, teachers, and peers.

In terms of intellectual functioning, the mentally deficient have difficulty in retention and recall and thus in the acquisition of information. These lacks, in turn, limit their capacity for analysis and synthesis of information and for other than relatively simple efforts at problem solving. Under circumstances in which their intellectual capacities are overtaxed, whether these involve clear-cut intellectual tasks or a complex including emotional and social factors, these individuals appear inept and deficient in planning and judgment. When untaxed beyond their capacities, provided their emotional development has been healthy, they perform well in accustomed social and vocational settings.

Incidence and Prevalence

From various estimates it is known now that in the United States 3 per cent of the children born annually will never achieve the intellect of a 12-year-old, 0.3 per cent will fall below the level of the 7-year-old, and 0.1 per cent will be so impaired in their intellectual capacity that they will remain throughout their lives as completely helpless individuals incapable even of caring for their simplest biological needs.

In the United States, in individuals up to 18 years of age there are about 1,500,000 who are mentally retarded. Many are fairly well adjusted in their communities, but many more require training. About 150,000 are in special institutions for the mentally handicapped. There is considerable variation in the prevalence of mental deficiency from place to place and from one type of population to another. In areas where there is a high degree of illiteracy and isolation of culture, it is difficult to evaluate mental deficiency, since most tests presuppose certain common levels of education and culture. It is estimated that one bed per 1,000 population should be provided in public institutions for the mentally defective.

Eugenicists frequently point out that civilization tends to preserve the unfit and that therefore a general decline of physique and intelligence is to be feared. Penrose, an outstanding English investigator of mental deficiency, is of the opinion that the number of defective and subnormal individuals is not steadily increasing. He concludes that propagation of the unfit is not a danger to the community because such persons tend to propagate less efficiently. In his opinion, decisions about segregation or other disposition of high-grade defectives should be based solely on medical, psychological, and social grounds; he maintains that the equilibrium with respect to biological fitness and intelligence level will be retained. Probably the only areas where the average intelligence is falling are certain small rural communities in which there has been imbreeding of poor mental stock and a rapid emigration of better stock. The incidence of mental defect, particularly at the moron level, is distinctly higher in rural than in urban areas.

Determination of Intellectual Defect

In order to determine whether a child who is suspected of being mentally retarded really is, and in order to outline constructive treatment, one should study the many factors which led not only to his intellectual defect but to his unique personality pattern. If one or both of the child's parents are known to be defective, it may be found that heredity has been an important factor. It should be kept in mind, however, that intellectually defective parents contribute not only defective genes but usually a home atmosphere deficient in intellectual, social, and personality-forming influences which promote the potentiality of mental growth.

In many defectives there is some evidence either of a general biological inferiority or of the sequelae of former traumatic or inflammatory processes in the central nervous system. Other evidences of a biological inferiority are anomalies of the skull, such as microcephaly, oxycephaly or tower-shaped skull, hydrocephalus, the spherical skull of the mongol, and asymmetry of the skull. Low fronto-temporal hair line, asymmetries of the face, malformations of the external ear, anomalies of the eye and its appendages, uncomeliness of the nose, thickness of the lips, receding or protruding mandible, imperfectly formed or irregularly erupted teeth, and malformation of the palate are much more frequent in mentally defective individuals than among persons of average intelligence.

In most mentally retarded children there will be a history of delay in the development of physiological, psychological, or social functions. In the infant, early indications of deficit are shown in apathy, difficulties in sucking, and later, in commencing to use his motor apparatus at the customary stage of maturation, weakness or absence of the sucking, Moro, and grasping reflexes in the newborn, crying in response to painful stimuli, closure of the eyelids, and contraction of the pupils. By the second month, the healthy child may smile, and crying is now accompanied by tears. The head and eyes turn toward sounds. At the fourth month, the child usually begins to hold up his head; two months later he should be able to sit for several minutes. At this time, he should begin to crawl, may grasp for objects, holds up his arms to be taken, and begins to distinguish people. At the tenth month, he should stand, and at one year he should take a few steps, say "Mama" and "Papa," and recognize toys. At eighteen months, he should be walking well. Delay in the acquisition of these motor skills suggests impaired cerebral development.

There exists an important relation between intelligence and the capacity for development of correct and distinct speech. The degree of intelligence is closely indicated by the age of acquisition of speech; by the character of articulation, i.e., as to whether the articulation is clear, slovenly, slurring, or jerking; by lalling, or the substitution of one consonant for another; and finally, by the extent of vocabulary, since this measures rather well the stock of ideas. Usually the normal child should be speaking a few words at one year and should articulate clearly between the ages of three and four.

A more valuable indication of the presence or absence of defect than either the history of school progress or an examination in school work is the practical knowledge and general information possessed by the individual. Here we find that the ability for breadth and accuracy of observation, and the capacity for comparison, planning, and discrimination essential for the successful solution of the practical problems connected with occupation and the business life, are inadequate in the mental defective. His range of knowledge, too, concerning common objects and events in his environment is limited. The defectives often vary in their ability to apply their intelligence to concrete life situations.

In considering the field of social history and behavior, it should be kept in mind that social incompetency does not necessarily mean social delinquency. Such chronic social problems as pauperism, slumdom, and recidivism are associated not so much with mental defect as with a population of borderline intelligence. The extent to which criminality is a result of mental defect is usually overestimated. Studies by English psychiatrists show that the percentage of criminals who are definitely feeble-minded is about 3.5. Probably the percentage in United States is about the same. The percentage of criminals of borderline intelligence is doubtless higher. Although acquisitive crimes occur most frequently both among the feeble-minded and those of normal intelligence, it is estimated that serious sexual offenses are nearly ten times as common among defectives as among ordinary criminals.

Individual psychological as well as social factors contribute to delinquency among the feeble-minded. In the borderline defective, especially, it will be found that the precipitating factors of his delinquencies are emotional ones. Some behavior disorders may represent a rebellion against, or a flight from, a difficult environment. If the feeble-minded child is rejected by his home, feelings of hatred and resentment may be stimulated and transferred to all parental surrogates. Again, aggressive and destructive behavior may represent a compensation for an underlying sense of inadequacy. Some defective individuals, through their wish to gain recognition, are easily led into delinquency by stronger, dominant personalities. Because the defective person obtains thrills and satisfactions so quickly, he is apt to follow those who show evidence of bold and vicious behavior.

Although many who are not feebleminded may rate low in economic efficiency, yet because the feeble-minded cannot successfully compete with those of higher intelligence, the degree of economic efficiency possesses a certain practical value in determining intellectual endowment.

Psychometric Tests

From what has been said it will be realized that in ascertaining an individual's intellectual capacity one should make a comprehensive study of his personality in many fields. Despite the fact that psychometric tests reveal little information concerning his personality characteristics or emotional maturity, they do yield important information concerning the patient's native intellectual endowment.

Not until 1905 was there any standard psychological criterion for the determination of intellectual capacity. At that time Binet, a French psychologist, and Simon, a psychiatrist, the former's associate on a commission appointed to study the matter of instruction of defective children, developed a plan for ascertaining mental age irrespective of chronological age. They drew up a set of graded problems constituting a progressive scale arranged in steps of increasing difficulty. These problems constituted tests of imagination, attention, comprehension, suggestibility, logical memory, language functions, common information, and ability to discriminate concepts, detect absurdities, and solve problems. These tests, first introduced into the United States in 1910 by Henry Herbert Goddard of the Training School for Feeble-Minded Children at Vineland, New Jersey, were devised after studying the abilities of children of all ages up to 16 years, after which age it was found that there was little increase in native intelligence as distinguished from knowledge.

The Binet scale was restandardized in the United States in 1916 by Lewis M. Terman of Stanford University, who developed the idea of the intelligence quotient. This Stanford test was last revised in 1937, when some of the previous shortcomings were eliminated, new problems were introduced, and the scale was extended both for the higher and the lower mental ages. Most intelligence tests, particularly the revised Stanford-Binet, are now based on the assumption that full maturation of intelligence is reached at 15 years of age.

In the application of a test, the patient is given a standardized series of graded groups of tests (such as the Stanford-Binet), each successively more difficult than the preceding. The tests are grouped according to the age at which they are usually passed. Each succeeding group should be solved by a child one year older than he who solved the preceding one. One group of the series, for example, should be successfully solved by a child of six, and the next most difficult group in the series by a child of seven. The mental age of the person examined is the average of the series of tests which he can successfully pass, the lowest age group used in determining the average being that one in which all the problems were successfully solved, and the highest one being that in which at least one problem was solved.

INTELLIGENCE QUOTIENT. When this mental age is compared with the person's actual chronological age if he is 15 or younger, or with 15 if he is older, a measure of his retardation is secured. (The age of 15 is used for comparison since, as already stated, there is probably no further development of native intelligence after that age.) This measure of intellectual development is usually expressed in terms of what is known as the intelligence quotient. The intelligence quotient, or I.Q., is obtained by dividing the mental age of the patient by his chronological age (or by 15 if he is more than 15 years of age) and multiplying the quotient by 100 for the sake of eliminating decimals.

It should be remembered that, since intelligence tests are expressed in terms of numerical findings, their apparent definiteness is apt to be misleading. It should be remembered, too, that an adult who is, say, 10 years old mentally but 40 years old chronologically is a very different person from a child of 10. He may not be able to do any more with his intellect than a 10-year-old child, but he has had 30 more years of experience in living, and his emotional experiences, conditionings, and maturity may be very different. Routine intelligence tests are inadequate, too, to represent capacity for making a variety of social adjustments or, with proper training, for full or part adjustment to selected occupational or communal responsibilities.

VERBAL AND PERFORMANCE TESTS. Intelligence tests fall roughly into two classes, one largely verbal, the other performance. The degree of deviation from the average as revealed by a verbal intelligence test is not necessarily the same as that revealed by a nonverbal test. Neither tells one the nature of intelligence any more than an ammeter tells one the nature of electricity. Performance tests consist of various kinds of puzzles which do not have to be solved in language terms and are therefore particularly applicable in illiterates and those not adequately familiar with the language in which the test is given. In the past, the criteria employed in determining cognitive endowment have too often been confined to measurements of verbal intelligence. The performance tests indicate how well concrete material is handled and do better justice to the child whose powers of verbal expression may be poor. Among the best known performance tests are the Arthur scale, the Pintner-Patterson scale, and the Cornell-Coxe performance ability scale.

A verbal and performance test which is frequently used is the Wechsler-Bellevue Intelligence Scale developed by David Wechsler as a means of measuring the intellectual capacity of adults. This test obviates the necessity for resorting to tests devised primarily for the classification of children. In addition to the advantages of item selection and standardization on an adult population with allowance for changes with age, it permits direct comparison in equated terms of verbal ability and performance ability. The verbal division includes tests of information, comprehension, digit span, arithmetic, and similarities; the performance division includes picture arrangement, picture completion, object assembly, block designs, and a digit symbol test. A vocabulary test is also included in the scale. It is more reliable than the Stanford-Binet test in estimating average intelligence in adults.

LIMITATIONS OF TESTS. The question naturally arises as to whether in applying intelligence tests one is measuring native endowment solely or whether to some extent the subject's kind of experience and the results of it are being measured also. Although such tests as the Stanford-Binet, dealing with composite aspects of intelligence, are largely tests of innate endowment, they undoubtedly measure in part the use the subject has made of his experiences. The results of these tests will therefore be modified somewhat by the home environment and social status of the subject. Moreover, it is important to remember that in the main they measure ability to manage ideas rather than the ability to handle or manipulate concrete objects or to get along with other people. They are useful as guides to educational policy and, to some extent, to the complexity of the social and occupational situations to which adjustments may be expected. If the subject's score gives him a mental age of less than 10 years, it is not to be expected that he will be both self-supporting and capable of an unsupervised adjustment in an urban community. Although we can scarcely identify the various attributes and qualities that enter into what we call intelligence, yet there appears to be a number of more or less distinct components in mental ability, each of which can be measured by appropriate tests. Aptitude tests have been devised to discover evidence as to one's fitness for certain types of professions or occupations, but any conclusions based on them must be accepted with great discretion.

Not infrequently in medicolegal matters the question arises as to the responsibility of an alleged feeble-minded person. In general it may be said that no limitation of responsibility should be recognized if the offender has a mental age exceeding 10 years.

The various intelligence tests fall, also, in two groups insofar as technique of application is concerned. Some, like the Stanford test, must be given to one person at a time. Others, like the Army Alpha or the Kuhlman-Anderson, can be administered to groups.

SIGNIFICANCE OF I.Q. Of the individual tests, the Stanford-Binet, Standard Revision, has been most extensively used, but it has the disadvantage that it was based on results obtained by the examination of a group of individuals who were of more than average intelligence. As a result, its standard intelligence quotient of 100, although supposed to represent the general average intelligence, is too high. An intelligence quotient of 87 on this scale more nearly represents the general average at age 15, the age at which the Stanford test assumes that full intellectual development has been obtained. A child found on the Stanford-Binet scale to have an I.Q. of 30 and a mental age of five cannot be expected successfully to complete school work more difficult than that of kindergarten grade. An I.Q. of 45 and a mental age of seven will permit one to complete the second grade of school. An I.Q. of 50 and a mental age of eight are required for the completion of the third grade; an I.Q. of 65 and a mental age of 10 are necessary for the completion of fourth grade. An I.Q. of 80 and a mental age of 12 should enable one to complete the fifth or sixth grade. Persons with an I.Q. between 80 and 90 can sometimes complete grade school. Those with an I.Q. between 90 and 110 can often complete high school; those between 110 and 120 can complete college, and those above 120 can successfully pursue specialized graduate or professional training.

Degree of Defect

The diagnostic and statistical manual of the American Psychiatric Association classifies the degrees of intelligence defect as mild, moderate, or severe. An impairment of mild degree is such as would be expected in a person having an I.Q. of approximately 70 to 85. Moderate is used for a degree of functional impairment that will require such special training and guidance as would be expected in a person having an I.Q. of 50 to 70. Severe refers to a degree of defect such that the individual requires custodial or complete protective care. Usually this will apply to I.Q.'s below 50. The degree of defect should not be determined solely by psychological test scores but should take into consideration cultural, physical, and emotional determinants as well as school, vocational, and social effectiveness. Usually a person having an I.Q. between 70 and 90 may be said *to be of borderline intelligence.*

Since general intelligence tests are valid only if they measure overall capacity to solve mental problems, in recognition of the limitations of all presently available tests, the American Association for Mental Deficiency has proposed a *behavioral classification* of deficit which consists of the two dimensions of *measured intelligence* and *adaptive behavior.* Thus the measured intelligence dimension is scaled into five levels in terms of Standard Deviation units* which describe the distribution of test scores in the general population. The adaptive behavior dimension classifies four levels of behavior in the two areas of degree: to function and maintain oneself independently and to meet satisfactorily the culturally imposed demands of personal and social responsibility. This scale is given in the accompanying table.

Additional scales should be used to

---

* A statistical unit which expresses the dispersion from the mean of a range of measurements in a sample.

Adaptive Behavior Classification*

	PRE-SCHOOL AGE 0–5 MATURATION AND DEVELOPMENT	SCHOOL-AGE 6–21 TRAINING AND EDUCATION	ADULT 21 SOCIAL AND VOCATIONAL ADEQUACY
Level I	Gross retardation; minimal capacity for functioning in sensori-motor areas; needs nursing care.	Some motor development present; cannot profit from training in self-help; needs total care.	Some motor and speech development; totally incapable of self-maintenance; needs complete care and supervision.
Level II	Poor motor development; speech is minimal; generally unable to profit from training in self-help; little or no communication skills.	Can talk or learn to communicate; can be trained in elemental health habits; cannot learn functional academic skills; profits from systematic habit training. ("Trainable")	Can contribute partially to self-support under complete supervision; can develop self-protection skills to a minimal useful level in controlled environment.
Level III	Can talk or learn to communicate; poor social awareness; fair motor development; may profit from self-help; can be managed with moderate supervision.	Can learn functional academic skills to approximately 4th grade level by late teens if given special education. ("Educable")	Capable of self-maintenance in unskilled or semi-skilled occupations; needs supervision and guidance when under mild social or economic stress.
Level IV	Can develop social and communication skills; minimal retardation in sensori-motor areas; rarely distinguished from normal until later age.	Can learn academic skills to approximately 6th grade level by late teens. Cannot learn general high school subjects. Needs special education, particularly at secondary school age levels. ("Educable")	Capable of social and vocational adequacy with proper education and training. Frequently needs supervision and guidance under serious social or economic stress.

*Reprinted from Sloan, W., and Birch, J. W.: A rationale for degrees of retardation. Am. J. Ment. Def., 60:258-264, 1955-1956.

supplement the clinical judgments. For example, the Vineland Social Maturity Scale is useful at the preschool level and may be supplemented by items from the Gesell Developmental Schedules, the Cattell Infant Intelligence Scale, and the Kuhlmann Tests of Mental Development.

TERMINOLOGY. There is a tendency to discontinue the use of the descriptive terms idiot, imbecile, and moron. Since, however, they are still occasionally used, their definition, as adopted in 1934 by the American Association on Mental Deficiency, may be quoted: "An idiot is a mentally defective person usually having a mental age of less than three years, or if a child, an intelligence quotient less than 25. An imbecile is a mentally de-

fective person usually having a mental age of three years to seven years, inclusive. A moron is a mentally defective person usually having a mental age of eight years or upwards, or if a child, an I.Q. of 50 or more." As for the I.Q., the Association stated: "As a rule the upper limit for a diagnosis of mental deficiency should be an I.Q. of 69, but this limit should not be adhered to in cases where medical, social, and other factors clearly indicate that the patient is mentally defective."

APPARENT DEFECT. Several writers, notably Kanner, have called attention to a group of children who have often been neglected. This is composed of those who may be described as apparently feeble-minded or pseudo-feeble-minded. In many cases persons have been declared feeble-minded solely upon the basis of their intelligence quotient. Although usually the I.Q. correctly measures a person's intellectual capacity, at times conditions may mask a child's intellectual potentialities. Among such conditions are blindness, deafness, spasticity, specific reading or numerical disability, or emotional blocking, with consequent inhibition of intelligent behavior or of responses in psychometric tests.

The child with sensory defects often leads an isolated existence, full of frustrations and confusion and deprived of certain necessary types of stimulation and information, with the result that he may not demonstrate his real intellectual potential. Sometimes a learning difficulty actually caused by emotional retardation may be mistaken for an organic deficiency. Occasionally the awkwardness of the examiner stimulates a negativism that prevents an accurate assessment of intelligence. The authors are familiar with the case of a child whose admission to the public school system was refused because of his alleged imbecility as demonstrated by psychometric tests. The boy's parents, knowing that he was not feeble-minded, sent him to a private school where he soon demonstrated that he was of superior intelligence. At the usual age he entered a university, from which he graduated with honors.

Etiology

Mental deficiency, then, is a symptom associated with a large number of disease entities which affect the organism in its earliest stages of growth and development. It is not a clinical entity itself. The group of mentally retarded is by no means homogeneous; it is marked by wide dissimilarities in etiology, clinical phenomenology, and pathology linked only by the common criterion of subnormal intellect. To be excluded from the group are those instances of impairment of intellect which occur as the result of brain damage after adolescence and to which is applied the term dementia.

In the past it has been the custom often to classify the mental deficiencies in terms of the temporal relationship of the impairment factor to birth. From a clinical standpoint, it is convenient to divide them into those operating prior to birth, into those resulting from injuries at birth, and into those resulting from injuries or disease occurring after birth but before mental development has been fully attained.

The American Association on Mental Deficiency recently has recommended an etiologic classification of mental retardation with supplementary qualifications to indicate the existence of a genetic component, secondary cranial anomalies, impairment of special senses, and motor dysfunction. Since both classificatory systems are in use, a brief statement is provided of the etiologic factors recognized to function in the prenatal, neonatal, and postnatal periods. Later, specifically defined entities are described under the suggested etiologic headings of the American Association on Mental Deficiency.

CAUSES ACTING BEFORE BIRTH. It is often difficult to determine whether a mental defect was caused by factors inherent in the genes or whether toxic, infectious, endocrine, traumatic, nutritional, and other prenatal pathogenic factors operating on the germ cell or within the pregnant mother tended to weaken or distort developmental capacity of the brain. Among prenatal factors may be pertussis, mumps, and other viral infections, particularly the virus of rubella, which late in the first trimester of pregnancy may pass through the placenta and damage the brain. Anomalies of various organs often coexist with the defect.

Other causes may be toxoplasmosis, the Rh factor (usually if the fetus is Rh-positive and the mother Rh-negative), the influences responsible for the chromosomal disjunction mongolism, also damage to the fetus by therapeutic doses of roentgen rays. Fetal oxygen deficiency as a cause of brain damage and subsequent mental defect usually occurs during labor but may happen earlier also. The mental deficiency of cretinism may either be caused by thyroid deficiency at a very early prenatal age or may be co-ordinated with the hormonal defect rather than caused by it. Toxic, anoxic, and infectious states which, in the adult nervous system, may be reversible or completely recoverable can produce permanent neural changes in the fetal neural structures, leading to impairment of developmental potentiality. There are doubtless many possible causes for a failure of, or for accident to, neural evolution in intrauterine life, but they are inadequately understood. The extent to which feeblemindedness is caused by congenital syphilis is uncertain but probably does not exceed 1 per cent. It is now a much less frequent cause than formerly.

Probably from 50 to 65 per cent of the cases of feeble-mindedness arise from poorly understood causes existing prior to birth. It is now agreed that hereditary transmission of mental defect plays a much less important role than was previously believed.

Causes Acting At Birth. Birth trauma resulting in either mechanical injury to the brain or asphyxia with resulting anoxia may be a cause of mental defect. In recent years the surgical removal of subdural hematomas has prevented some degree of mental defect which would otherwise have followed birth injury. The most frequent immediate causes of cerebral hemorrhage at birth are prematurity and difficult labor. Asphyxia at birth is a common cause of mental defect. If the resulting anoxemia exists sufficiently long, it will produce permanent degeneration of the ganglion cells of the cerebral cortex, with resulting impairment of mental capacity. It is estimated that about 8 per cent of the mental defects result from causes acting at birth. Probably, however, 50 per cent of the children showing clinical evidence of brain injury are not mentally defective.

Causes Acting After Birth. The various forms of viral and bacterial encephalitis and of meningitis are the most frequent factors acting after birth in the production of feeble-mindedness. Although head trauma with brain damage in infancy or early childhood occasionally results in feeble-mindedness, this is much overemphasized by the laity. In institutionalized mental defectives, it will be found that the defect in about 1.5 per cent of the inmates is the result of postnatal cerebral trauma. Toxemia and vitamin deficiency in infancy and early childhood may, if long continued, produce irreversible changes in the cortex with varying degrees of mental retardation. Convulsive disorders often accompany mental defect resulting from organic disease of the brain.

In the congenitally blind and deaf, the reduced number of stimuli received from exteroceptors results in a certain degree of mental defect unless compensatory training is provided. It is generally agreed, too, that retardation in intellectual development may be caused by emotional factors without organic defect. Probably from 25 to 30 per cent of the cases of feeble-mindedness result from causes acting after birth.

ETIOLOGIC CLASSIFICATION

Due to Infection

Although there remains controversy as to whether maternal infections cause congenital brain damage without direct infections of the growing fetus, there is much evidence to show that in many conditions a direct fetal brain infection does take place. At times this infection may occur without clinical evidence of illness of the mother. There are five important entities in this group:

Cytomegalic inclusion body disease is a mild or subclinical virus infection in the mother which causes the fetal brain damage, hepatosplenomegaly, erythroblastosis, and jaundice. It is recognized by inclusion bodies in the urine, cerebrospinal fluid, and other tissues.

Congenital rubella, associated with illness of the mother in the first trimester of pregnancy, causes mental deficit and other congenital anomalies such as deafness, cataract and cardiac malformations.

Congenital syphilis is diagnosed on the basis of maternal infection with positive serologic tests for syphilis and the various signs of congenital syphilis in the child, including Hutchinson's teeth, interstitial keratitis, choroidoretinitis, and pupillary abnormalities. Juvenile parcsis, another form, is discussed in Chapter 13.

Toxoplasmosis is due to infection *in utero* from the mother with the protozoan-like organism, *Toxoplasma*. At birth, or shortly thereafter, the infant may show wasting, convulsions, spasticity, choroidoretinitis, hydrocephalus or microcephaly. The last group includes other infectious processes incurred by the fetus such as meningococcal meningitis and equine encephalitis.

Due to Intoxication

Bilirubin encephalopathy (kernicterus) may follow any condition which produces jaundice with a high level of serum bilirubin in the newborn. Since it may now be prevented by exchange transfusions, the potential danger of high levels of bilirubin in the first few days of birth is highly important. It is now widely accepted that a value of 20 mg. per 100 ml. of plasma bilirubin is indication for such transfusion. Oftentimes it is due to Rh incompatibility between the fetus and the mother, but it also may result from other blood incompatilities, including those between A, B, and O types.

In the absence of blood incompatibility, kernicterus is associated often with prematurity, and neonatal sepsis. The early stages of kernicterus are difficult to determine, but the condition may be assumed in the presence of drowsiness, poor feeding, unstable body temperature, a high-pitched cry, and alterations in the Moro reflex. Opisthotonus, loss of the Moro reflex, and ocular signs are indicative of marked damage. Mental defect, choreo-athetosis, and deafness are the common late sequelae.

Pathologic studies of the brain show yellow staining with bilirubin in the basal ganglia, cerebellar nuclei, hypocampus, and medulla, and, when severe, loss of cells, glioses, and demyelination are noticed.

Encephalopathies, caused by lead or carbon monoxide and those following the post-serum and post-vaccinal encephalitides are other more frequent causes of retardation due to intoxication. Lead poisoning has been discussed in Chapter 9.

Due to Trauma or Physical Agent

Difficulties of labor, such as those occurring with malposition or malpresentation of the child or disproportion between the head of the child and the pelvis of the mother, tend to the probability of damage to the infant's brain at birth. Common lesions with birth injury are meningeal tears and rupture of blood vessels and brain substance, often with intracerebral bleeding. Considerable hemorrhage leads later to brain softening and cyst formation, particularly after difficult forceps delivery. The falx cerebri or tentorium may be torn, resulting in subarachnoid or subdural hemorrhage. With time the structural evidence of acute injury at birth is supplanted in the process of repair with such non-specific tissue changes as glioses, cavitation, and areas of defective myelination.

The *diagnosis* of severe injury at birth may be immediately inferred with pallor of the infant, inability to make sucking movements, respiratory distress, high-pitched feeble cry, tense or depressed fontanel, nystagmus, and retinal hemorrhage. At later stages of growth, the brain-injured child may be over-active or under-active and show fluctuations of muscle tone, impaired associated movements, primitive reflex activity, difficulties in convergence, and trouble with posture.

The growing child finds himself at a disadvantage in learning *complex motor skills* such as walking, climbing, skating, and cycling, even though there may exist few or none of the classical neurological signs of damage to the motor system. *Perceptual processes* are impaired, and normal responses to stimuli are limited. The child with injury of the visual portion of the brain may discriminate with difficulty foreground from background or may show an inability to remember sounds, localize their source, and discriminate pitch; he also may present incapacity in perceiving and understanding spoken language. Some children have an inability to discriminate tactual stimuli.

The development of *social behavior* is deviate due to confusion and frustration, and although the most frequently encountered tendency is toward hyperactive aggressive behavior, other children may be passive and withdrawn or show ritualistic and compulsive activity. The symptomatic picture in an individual patient is highly specific, depending upon the locations, extent, and degree of the brain injuries. Thus there does not exist a universal clinical picture, and the clinician will make the diagnosis without the presence of the full range of sensory–motor or behavioral disturbances.

Mental deficiency of this type is caused as well by asphyxia at birth due to interference with the placental circulation, overdosage with anesthetic agents or drugs depressing respiration, or, much more rarely, by prenatal irradiation of the uterus.

Due to Disorders of Metabolism, Growth, or Nutrition

Perhaps in no other area has so much new understanding accrued from research in the past decade as in that concerned with the abnormalities of brain development due to the inherited specific metabolic defects. This group of conditions may be separated into those due to abnormalities in lipid, carbohydrate, and protein metabolism. The early recognition of many of these defects is highly important, since the institution of proper dietary measures may prevent or appreciably reduce the amount of brain damage and subsequent impairment of mental function.

CEREBRAL LIPOIDOSES. Of the lipoidoses, the infantile form of Tay-Sach's is the most common and is characterized by accumulation of lipid in nerve cells. The condition is transmitted by a single recessive gene. Thus, although both parents may appear healthy, if both are carriers, the probability exists of one out of four children suffering the disease. Marriages producing affected children represent an increased occurrence of consanguinity. The majority of cases are from Jewish families, but non-Jewish are also affected.

At birth the infant seems normal but within the first year the child's development is impeded. He becomes apathetic, appears to have muscular weakness, cannot hold his head steadily, and regresses in his ability to grasp objects. There is advancing visual deterioration, and ophthalmoscopic study of the retina shows a typical "cherry-red spot" in the macula. The course is progressive, with death ensuing in one to three years. In a late infantile form of the disease (Bielschowsky's disease) the onset is in the second or third years and it is more common in non-Jewish families.

Gaucher's Disease, due to deposition of kerasin in the reticulo-endothelial cells of the spleen, liver, and other organs, occasionally involves the cells of the cerebral cortex of infants. Here again the infant seems to grow well until the fourth or fifth month but then undergoes regression in development. He is found to have an enlarged liver and spleen as well as anemia, leukopenia, and thrombocytopenia. Death follows, again within a few years, Niemann-Pick's disease is a similar condition with, however, deposition of lipophosphotides in the reticuloendothelial system.

PHENYLKETONURIA. This is the most frequently encountered and most thoroughly understood of the specific metabolic disorders of protein. The condition was recognized in 1934 by Fölling, a Norwegian biochemist. Since the associated mental defect in this condition as with other disturbances of protein metabolism may be prevented by diagnosis shortly after birth, early recognition and treatment with proper diet, are highly important.

This form of familial mental deficiency is inherited as a simple recessive. Since each parent is a heterozygous carrier, a quarter of the children will have the illness, one-half will be carriers, and a quarter will be healthy non-carriers. For each pregnancy the chances are one in four of having a phenylketonuric child and three in four of bearing a normal child. Approximately one phenylketonuric occurs in 25,000 births; in institutions 1 per cent are estimated to have this condition.

Diagnosis. Clinically, retardation in motor and mental development is observed before the end of the first year, and it is thought that all damage to the nervous system takes place within the first two years of life. Although most untreated patients learn to walk, few speak; a quarter have grand mal convulsions, and electroencephalographic abnormalities are more common. The mental defect is severe, with the intelligence quotients usually below 50. One child has been reported with an I.Q. of 100. The children usually have fair hair and blue eyes, and there is frequently an associated dermatitis. Accompanying the marked mental deficiency and the metabolic error are neurological manifestations generally regarded as an extrapyramidal syndrome. The posture of the patient is usually that of general flexion, with bent head and body; both flexor and extensor muscles are rigid, the deep reflexes are active, and many patients show hyperkinetic or dyskinetic manifestations, such as tremor and athetosis. Encephalograms suggest that the extrapyramidal signs may be referred to cortical atrophy of the frontal lobe.

The urine has a penetrating, musty odor and contains abnormal amounts of phenylalanine and its derivatives, phenylpyruvate and phenylacetate, in the urine. Phenylpyruvic acid can be easily detected in the urine by adding a few drops of ferric chloride to an acidified specimen. An intense green color develops in the presence of phenylpyruvic acid. Other conditions and substances may lead to the report of a false positive test. For this reason the serum level should be examined as the amino acid phenylalanine is found in increased amounts in the blood, spinal fluid, and perspiration. At present the defect seems to be caused

by a blockage in the conversion of phenylalanine into tyrosine due to a deficiency of the enzyme phenylalanine hydroxylase, as shown by Jervis. Thus the unmetabolized amino acid accumulates in the body fluid and large amounts of its deaminated products—phenylpyruvic, phenyllactic and phenylacetic acids—are excreted with it in the urine. There is a marked failure of myelinization of the nervous system.

All infants should have their urine tested between the third and ninth weeks for this condition. Repeated urine tests should be done every two weeks on birth of siblings of a phenylketonuric until the tenth week if serum phenylalanine levels cannot be obtained. A few normal children may show elevations of serum phenylalanine during the first six weeks of life.

Treatment. Treatment with diet restricted in phenylalanine appears both to prevent and greatly limit cerebral damage. There is now available commercially an acid hydrolyzate of casein with phenylalanine removed but supplemented with additional amino acids, minerals, and choline. It may be given at the level of 2.0 to 2.5 gm. per kilogram of body weight, with additional fats and carbohydrates to meet caloric requirements. The casein hydrolyzate is supplied as Lofenalac, and the manufacturer provides full instructions for the diet. The phenylalanine levels of the blood serum should be maintained at the levels of 2 to 4 mg. per 100 ml. during the first year of life.

MAPLE SYRUP URINE DISEASE. Another of the specific inherited defects in amino acid metabolism described in 1954 by Menkes has been named due to the characteristic maple syrup-like odor of the urine. Within the first week of life, the infant appears spastic, loses the Moro reflex, and then undergoes progressive cerebral deterioration, with death in a few months. Studies of the urine show marked increase in excretion of the branched chain amino acids leucine, isoleucine, and valine as well as methionine, but cystine and other amino acids are abnormally low. Studies show that in this disease transamination of methionine and the branched amino acids occurs normally, with formation of keto acids, but that further degradation is blocked, with accumulation of these four keto and amino acids in the blood. There also appears to be a secondary disturbance of tryptophan metabolism. Therapeutic studies with diets low in these acids are encouraging but require further evaluation.

Several other amino acidurias have been discovered in a few mentally defective patients and are designated as *cystothioninuria* and *arginosuccinuria*. There are several conditions in which renal overflow of amino acids occur in which the body metabolism is normal but there exists a defective renal reabsorption, leading to overflow and loss. The familial *Hartnup disease* is a generalized amino aciduria associated with a pellagra-like rash, cerebellar ataxia, and often mental deficit. Other patients have been reported to have little mental deficit but personality disturbances and dermatitis later in life.

Congenital Galactosemia. Galactose diabetes, a specific metabolic defect of carbohydrate metabolism, is productive of profound disturbance in growth and development and leads to mental retardation unless recognized early and properly treated. It appears that galactosemia represents a single block in the formation of the enzyme, galactose-l-P-uridyl transference which leads to collection of galactose-l-phosphate in cells. The eventual effects of galactosemia relate to the amount and duration of galactose consumption and are reversible by removal of this substance from the diet.

The infant born with galactosemia seems to be normal for several days but shortly commences to show difficulty with feedings, vomits, and may develop diarrhea. If milk feeding is continued, there may occur noticed jaundice, enlargement of the abdomen because of ascites and hepatomegaly, nuclear cataracts, and the indications of mental defect in delay in standing, walking, and talking. Sugar is present in the urine, which is nonfermentable with heat.

The condition may be diagnosed just after birth by incubating erythrocytes of cord blood with galactose; in the galactosemic blood, galactose-l-phosphate accumulates in the cells. Galactose tolerance tests are abnormal, and the cephalin flocculation is elevated. If milk is eliminated from the diet and soy bean or casein hydrolyzate substitutes are utilized in its place, the symptoms subside. Early diagnosis, with proper treatment, may prevent permanent cerebral damage.

Mental deficiency may also accompany *glycogenosis* (von Gierke's disease), which is associated with deposition of glycogen in various organs and sometimes involves the brain. Transient hypoglycemia with later retardation has occurred in the children of hypoglycemic mothers.

Gargoylism. Also known as lipochondrodystrophy, or Hurler's disease, this is probably a generalized enzymopathy due to the deposit of a mucopolysaccharide in almost all organs and connective tissue of the body. It is said that the substance deposited in neurones of the brain is a ganglioside.

At birth the infant's head may be enlarged, joint movements are limited, and later the cornea appears clouded. At three months the upper lumbar vertebrae and long bones show deformities by x-ray, and kyphosis is evident. The characteristic features are protrusion of the forehead out of proportion with the stunted body, saddle nose, bushy eyebrows, coarse features, and a deep crease between the thick lips and chin. Abnormal bodies are found in the leukocytes, and there exist both hypermucopolysacchariduria and hyperaminoaciduria. Later in life there develop wedging of the vertebrae, shortened and flexed deformity of the hands, flexion deformities at the hips and knees and enlargement of the liver and spleen. Most children die in their teens.

Hypothyroidism. This condition, either congenital or acquired, may lead to retardation in mental growth. Sometimes recognizable at birth, it usually is not manifest until later months when it may be noticed that the infant is dwarfed, particularly with failure in growth of length. The subcutaneous tissues are thick so that the features are coarse, the skin dry and cold. The child appears dull and puffy. The tongue protrudes and the lips are thick. The forehead may be wrinkled, the hair is thin, and the anterior fontanel is widely open. There is often abdominal distention with associated umbilical hernia, slow pulse, and such neurological signs as ataxia, rigidity, and hyporeflexia. The basal metabolic rate varies from —20 to —50, the protein bound iodine of 4 to 8 micrograms is much below values found in healthy subjects and the uptake of radioactive iodine is reduced. Usually after the age of two the blood cholesterol is elevated, and x-ray studies show recurrent development of ossification centers and epiphyseal union.

In goitrous areas the congenital type may be the consequence of maternal iodine deficiency. The congenital type also includes those cases with absence or hypoplasia of the gland and those with a genetically determined enzyme defect causing inadequate synthesis of thyroxin (biochemical hypothyroidism). In the latter cases, the thyroid appears to be morphologically normal, although a goiter may develop later. However, the degree of mental retardation found in each individual is related as well to the familial occurrence of low, average, or high intelligence and opportunities for education.

Treatment consists in establishing a euthyroid state as early and rapidly as possible without the induction of cardiac decompensation. Dessicated thyroid is as effective as thyroxin and triodothyroxin. Studies have shown that approximately half of those with the most severe types of cretinism commencing before birth and apparent in the first months of life, if treated before the age of six months, attain nearly average intelligence quo-

tients, and less than one-fifth of the group have persisting moderate retardation. Delay in beginning treatment is less disastrous for those with an insidious onset commencing from birth and not clinically recognized until they are over a year of age. It has been suggested that there exists a critical period of brain development in the prenatal or early postnatal life, when irreparable failure may occur as the result of thyroid deficiency.

The neuropathologic findings are reduction in the number of cells in the cortex, failure in myelinization and delays in maturation of fiber tracts and neurons has been reported. The electroencephalogram shows low amplitude and slow alpha rhythm; these are reversible with thyroid medication.

Due to New Growths

TUBEROUS SCLEROSIS. This clinical form of feeble-mindedness, sometimes known as epiloia, is characterized by epilepsy, mental defect, and a butterfly-shaped rash of cutaneous nodules resembling sebaceous adenomas but really consisting of hyperblastic connective and vascular tissue. The disease results from a congenital blastomatous malformation involving the neuro-ectodermal system. The brain shows diffuse disturbances in cyto-architecture and localized neoplastic glial formations.

It is transmitted by a dominant gene with reduced penetrance. Neurofibromatosis, inherited in a similar way, and trigeminal cerebral angiomatosis (Sturge-Weber-Dimitri's disease), which is characterized by the "port-wine stain" or cutaneous angioma of the face, may both be associated with cerebral defect and mental retardation.

Due to Unknown Prenatal Influence

MONGOLISM. This frequent variety of mental deficiency, described by Langdon-Down, was named because the physiognomic features are suggestive of those normally exhibited by the Mongolian race. It is estimated that three to four infants will be mongoloid of each thousand births and that 5 to 10 per cent of all defectives fall into this category.

Clinically the mongoloid is characterized by short stature and a small, round skull, with a flattening both of the occiput and the face. The hair is scanty and coarse. The palpebral fissure is narrow and oblique, with the inner end lower than the outer; a fold of skin continued from the upper eyelid over the inner angle adds to the resemblance to the Asiatic countenance. The tongue is large and fissured, with its papillae hypertrophied, and it is often constantly protruded and withdrawn through the open mouth. The nose is short and broad, with a depressed bridge; the hands are large and stubby, the fifth finger being particularly short and often incurved. The joint ligaments are lax, and the muscles are hypotonic, giving the joints an unusual mobility. The palate is often deformed, the abdomen is large, and the genitalia are underdeveloped. The palm and finger prints are characteristic, as the two main creases across the palm are replaced often by a single crease (simian line). In a tenth of the patients, a congenital heart defect is found. The mongoloid's good disposition and tendency to imitativeness often conceal at first the seriousness of his mental defect. Most mongoloids have an I.Q. between 15 and 40, with an upper limit in the 50's.

Cytogenetic studies by Lejeune in 1959 showed that the somatic cells of patients with mongolism have 47 chromosomes instead of the normal 46, consisting of a trisomy of chromosome 21. It is suggested that during miosis, non-disjunction persists, with the mongolian receiving the undetached segment. The cause of the non-disjunction remains unknown. Statistical studies show clearly that mongolism occurs more frequently in births in older mothers and must reflect abnormal influences acting in utero. By tissue culture growth of leukocytes, and subsequent chromosome counts, it has been possible to establish the diagnosis within a few days of birth.

MISCELLANEOUS CONDITIONS. Other types of mental defect have been identified, as well, to processes of non-disjunction of chromosomes in miosis. *Klinefelter's syndrome*, associated with severe mental defect, which occurs at a frequency of about 1 per cent in institutionalized males, is associated with an abnormal sex chromosomal complement of two X and one Y chromosome. These males are unusually tall and lean and show enlargement of the breasts, with atrophy of the testes and absence of sperm. *Turner's syndrome*, also due to non-disjunction, occurs in females and is associated with the presence of only one X chromosome; it is called the X o variant. Such females lack secondary sex characteristics, and show, in addition to mental defect, other congenital abnormalities, including short stature, "webbed" neck, deafness, and aorta malformation.

Included in other conditions for which no definite etiology has been established are those associated with various cranial and cerebral anomalies. Craniostenosis of various types, hydrocephalus, and hypertelorism fit into the first group. Among the relatively small number of feebleminded persons who exhibit distinctive characteristics of the skull or general bodily conformation, or of brain structure, that entitle them to recognition as clinical varieties are the *microcephalics*. Arbitrarily these defectives, mostly imbeciles or idiots, whose skulls on completion of development do not exceed 17 inches in circumference, are designated as microcephalic. Those of this clinical variety show a peculiarity not only in the size of the head but also in its shape, which is characterized by a receding forehead and a flattening of the occiput. The hair, which is wiry in texture, extends low on the forehead. The scalp is greater in amount than is necessary to cover the cranium, with the result that the excess becomes arranged in corrugations. The chin is usually receding and the stature is short. As might be expected from the limited cranial capacity, the brain of the microcephalic is markedly underdeveloped. Histological defects are the rule, and gross anomalies besides those of size are common.

PSYCHOSES WITH MENTAL DEFICIENCY

It is generally agreed that most of the mental disorders that afflict persons of normal intelligence may also afflict the mentally defective. Sometimes, also, defectives suffer from psychoses of an acute transitory nature, presenting episodes of excitement with depression, paranoid trends, or hallucinatory experiences. The psychoses are often situational in origin.

TREATMENT

Although the limits of development of those aspects of the organism that we call intellectual are for the most part fixed, to a narrow extent intelligence grows by use and atrophies by disuse. It has been found that if identical twins are separated soon after birth and one is provided with educational opportunities definitely superior to the other, he will develop an I.Q. higher than the one placed in a less favorable environment. Even though the intellectual capacity cannot be materially increased, the social capacity can be improved in individuals in whom it is most needed, viz., in the higher-grade defective. It should be remembered that the development of a normal personality requires not only a certain native intellectual endowment but also such emotional essentials as affection, security, social recognition, achievement, and new experiences. So, too, the retarded or defective child should be led to feel that he is loved, approved, and wanted as a member of the family and of groups outside the family. Surrounded with affection, handled with devoted patience, and psychologically stimulated through fondling and play, such a child should acquire the feeling of significance and security essential to the development of a stable personality.

Emotional Problems

The emotional problem created for the parents by the retarded or defective child may be a difficult one, and the manner in which it is met has much influence upon future development. The knowledge that one's child is not developing normally often comes slowly, and the mother may refuse to face the situation and develop a sense of personal shame, failure, and even guilt. Her tearfulness and the father's angered disappointment may leave the child confused, frustrated, and isolated. Again, if he is rejected, emotionally deprived, coerced, and perhaps beaten, the child is restless, insecure, aggressive, and hostile, and perhaps becomes delinquent. Feelings of frustration and futility are more common among parents of the mentally retarded child than among parents of the physically handicapped. The latter can often experience a feeling of compensation in the child's intellectual and emotional growth. Such satisfactions are lacking in the case of the mentally arrested or retarded child, with the result that the underlying problems of the parents are intensified and often expressed in their attitude toward him, with the result that he develops hostility and behavior problems. Many, perhaps most, defective individuals, like normal individuals, have their conflicts regarding their hopes, fears, anxieties, and frustrations. The manner in which these are met by parents and teachers will have much influence on their behavior and social adjustment. Many mentally defective persons are more incapacitated by their emotional difficulties than by their intellectual deficit. As with children of normal intellectual endowment frustrations, humiliations, ridicule, anxieties, emotional deprivations, and insecurities may be expressed in delinquent behavior.

Education and Employment

In the field of education, teachers

should concentrate from the start on those abilities and aptitudes with which the child is most fully endowed. Perhaps nothing is so devastating to the mental health of a defective child as to be offered lessons that are beyond his powers of comprehension.

The social training of retarded children is of immense importance and of far greater significance to them than mere educational attainments. The extent to which they are accepted as agreeable individuals by and in a community is directly proportionate to their social adjustment. This attitude of the community has a direct relation to the mental health of the growing child. If he is accepted, he will feel that he has fulfilled his main ambition of being somebody in the eyes of others. If he is not accepted, he has a feeling of failure and frustration, or grievance and ill will against society, all of which breed discontent and unhappiness, leading to emotional difficulties and maladjustment and perhaps even to delinquency and crime.

Lack of intelligence is not by any means a bar to gainful employment. In many unskilled occupations, what counts in obtaining and retaining a job is not so much skill, literacy, or information as steadiness, reliability, honesty, and the ability to get along well with workmates and the foreman. With happiness will come mental health; and a child who has good mental health, even if he is intellectually defective, is an asset to the community.

It should be considered an obligation of the state to discover, classify, and provide suitable education for all retarded children as early in their careers as possible. In some states an attempt is now made to meet this obligation by requiring an examination of all public school children who are retarded three years or more in their classes and by directing that special classes be provided for such children. Probably with most of these defectives it would be better if they were discovered and assigned to special classes earlier. By assignment to a special class, the child is removed from too difficult a curriculum in which he has no interest, from critical classmates, perhaps from an antagonistic teacher and other humiliating conditions that create feelings of inferiority, destroy a sense of security, and lay the foundations for the easiest method of defense, that of overt, unsocialized behavior and socially maladaptive compensations. Since the child in the special class can compete with his fellows, the undesirable reactions mentioned are not only not stimulated but there is created a feeling of security, self-reliance, satisfaction, and success that has great constructive value in personality formation. Approbation, attention, and praise afford great satisfaction and, within reasonable limits, may produce a desirable, stimulating effect on the individual's effort to fit into a world that is always going to be beyond him. Feeble-minded children should be encouraged to take part with normal children in all those games in which the defective child can compete on equal terms with the normal one.

Institutional Care

In many ways, the first persons who should be selected for admission to the institutions for feeble-minded are children of the moron level for whom special classes are not available or who are deficient in social adaptation. Among the beneficial results of institutional training are an improvement in attitude, stabilization of emotions, and development of habits of industry. It is especially desirable that young, mentally defective children who are beginning to form antisocial habits should be placed in an institutional school before these habits become fixed, particularly if the home environmental influences cannot be modified.

Provision should also be made in the institutional schools for the training of those children of the lowest mental levels. The number of persons who have been trained in the state institutions and placed in the community as useful, often self-supporting, members of society has increased in recent years. It is now estimated that 50 per cent of those admitted to the state schools can be returned to the community socially improved. Such institutions should therefore be looked upon as important parts of the public educational system. There are many who cannot be prepared for living successfully in the community, and yet in the routine, protected life of the institution these individuals become useful citizens.

The problem of treatment of those with moderately severe mental defects is simple and consists largely of physical care and custody. In those with moderate impairment, efforts should be directed at training the child to dress, undress, and bathe himself, to improve his habits of feeding himself, and to curb destructive tendencies, and in teaching him to avoid ordinary dangers, to associate common objects with their names, to pronounce a few easy words, and to express simple wants. At best the object can be merely so to train the child that his care will be less burdensome. Whether this simple training will be undertaken at home or in an institution will depend on many factors, such as the capacity of the mother for training, the size of the family, its economic status, et cetera. In the case of these defective children, the efforts of the mother may usually be more profitably devoted to the rearing of her other children, to the duties of the home, or to such other activities as may contribute to the welfare of her community and the development of her own personality.

With institutional care of the moderately defective child, its family is usually able to make a better economic and social adjustment. From a community point of view, these defective individuals do not constitute an important problem. Their number is small compared to that of individuals with the higher degrees of mental defect, and many die at an early age. They do not constitute a eugenic problem, since the defect is rarely of familial origin, and very few ever procreate.

Some institutionalized defectives are noisy, overactive, aggressive, and destruc-tive. In such cases the phenothiazine derivative often exerts a desirable sedative effect.

Sterilization

Opinions as to the value and wisdom of sterilization of the intellectually defective individuals are not unanimous, but it is no longer regarded as a panacea. Suggested as a means of preventing feeble-mindedness, its eugenic value is much more limited than was at first appreciated. Probably too little is known about the inheritance of mental defect to apply sterilization in any but the lower grades of that condition, in which, in fact, the likelihood of procreation is the least. The legal provision for sterilization applies in most states to those committed to public institutions, but experience shows that a large proportion of high-grade defectives, who of all defectives are most frequently of the familial type, are not committed to institutions. In these, too, the social adjustment is determined fully as much by social and family influence and environment as by the intelligence. Experience has thus far shown that, even when the law provides for their sterilization, only a few of those defectives who are supported by their families are subjected to this operation. Those in the upper levels of the subnormal group are the most highly reproductive.

Contrary to the opinion of many, most high-grade defectives are not prolific, and statistics show that but a very small percentage of male defectives who are committed and subsequently discharged ever marry or have children. Experience indicates that a majority of the detrimental behavior on the part of mental defectives is not their sexual irregularity and reproduction but vagrancy, dependency, and delinquency. Recent studies show that the mortality rate among the feeble-minded is so high that the danger from their unrestrained propagation is thereby reduced much more than has been realized. It is now recognized, too, that society does not need protection from the feeble-minded girl as much as the defective girl needs protection from society.

Many advocates of sterilization forget that it does not increase the patient's sense of social responsibility, that social adjustment is the end sought, and that even if the person is discharged sterilized, but without training in socialized habits, the main object has been lost. Many feeble-minded couples will live a successful, happy life if not burdened with the financial, physiological, and other strains incident to rearing a family, yet many suffer social and economic collapse if obliged to assume these burdens. Much neglect and ill-treatment of children would be forestalled if persons intellectually or emotionally unfit to rear children could be sterilized, but such a measure can scarcely be determined solely on the basis of the I.Q. Its usefulness is more individual than social.

Finally, sterilization as a general policy is a superficial method of approaching the problem of feeble-mindedness, since it ignores the need for special investigation and research as to its cause and prevention.

BIBLIOGRAPHY

Alford, A. F.: Mental health despite mental retardation. Lancet, 1:1233–1235, 1955.

Association for Research in Nervous and Mental Disease. Vol. XXXIX. Mental Retardation. Baltimore, Williams & Wilkins Co., 1962.

Bearn, A. G., and German, J. L. III: Chromosomes and disease. Scientific American, 205:66–76, 1961.

Benda, C. E.: The Child with Mongolism. New York, Grune & Stratton, 1960.

Berry, H. K., Sutherland, B., Guest, G. N., and Warkany, J.: Simple method for detection of phenylketonuria. J.A.M.A., 167:2189–2190, 1958.

Bourne, H.: Protophrenia. Lancet, 2:1156–1163, 1955.

Bradley, C.: Pediatrics, mental retardation and delinquency. J.A.M.A., 157:101–108, 1955.

Dancis, J.: Phenylketonuria and maple sugar disease. Bull. N.Y. Acad. Med., 35:427–432, 1959.

Eustis, R. S.: Specific reading disability. New England J. Med., 237:243–249, 1947.

Gesell, A., and Amatruda, C. S.: Developmental Diagnosis. New York, Paul B. Hoeber, 1949.

Grebler, A. M.: Parental attitudes toward mentally retarded children. Am. J. Ment. Def., 56:475–483, 1952.

Hafemeister, N. R.: Development of a curriculum for the trainable child. Am. J. Ment. Def., 55:495–501, 1951.

Heber, R.: A Manual on Terminology and Classification in Mental Retardation. Monograph Supp. Am. J. Ment. Def., 64:1–111, 1959.

Heller, T.: Über Dementia infantilis. Archiv für Kinderforsch., 37:661–667, 1930.

Holt, L., Jr., and Snyderman, S. E.: Disturbances of amino acid metabolism. Bull. N.Y. Acad. Med., 36:432–450, 1960.

Illingworth, R. S.: Mental retardation in the infant and preschool child. Brit. M. J., 2:1–7, 1955.

Itard, J. M. G.: The Wild Boy of Aveyron. Translated by G. and M. Humphrey, New York, Century Co., 1932.

Kanner, Leo: A Miniature Textbook of Feeblemindedness. New York, Child Care Publications, 1949.

Idem: Emotional interference with intellectual functioning. Am. J. Ment. Def., 56:701–707, 1952.

Kelman, H. R.: The function of a mental clinic for mentally retarded children. Social Casework, 37:237–241, 1956.

Kobayashi, N.: Acid mucopolysaccharide granules in glomerular epithelium in gargoylism. Am. J. Path., 35:591–605, 1959.

Kugel, R. B., and Reque, D.: A comparison of mongoloid children. J.A.M.A., 175:959–961, 1961.

Lee, C. H., Schmid, W., and Smith, P. M.: Definitive diagnoses of mongolism in newborn infants by chromosome studies. J.A.M.A., 178:1030–1032, 1961.

MacGillivray, R. C.: Gargoylism (Hurler's disease). J. Ment. Sc., 98:687–696, 1952.

Masland, R. L.: The prevention of mental retardation. Am. J. Ment. Def., 62:991–1114, 1958.

Menkes, J. H.: Maple syrup disease. Neurology, 9:826–835, 1959.

Milner, K. O.: Delinquent types of mentally defective persons. J. Ment. Sc., 95:989–1112, 1949.

Moncreiff, A., and Wilkenson, R. H.: Further experience in treatment of phenylketonuria. Brit. Med. J., 1:763–767, 1961.

O'Connor, N., and Tizard, J.: The social problem of mental deficiency. London and New York, Pergamon Press, 1956.

Parrotte, I.: Modern trends in education for the educable mentally handicapped. Am. J. Ment. Def., 53:558–561, 1949.

Penrose, L. S.: The Biology of Mental Defect. London, Sidgwick and Jackson, 1950.

Idem: The supposed threat of declining intelligence. Am. J. Ment. Def., 53:114–118, 1948.

Rudy, L. H., et al.: A clinical evaluation of psychopharmacological agents in the management of disturbed mentally defective patients. Am. J. Ment. Def., 62:855–860, 1958.

Sarason, S. B., and Gladwin, T.: Psychological and cultural problems in mental subnormality: a review of research. Am. J. Ment. Def., 62: 1113–1307, 1958.

Stacey, C. L., and DeMartino, M. F., Ed.: Counseling and Psychotherapy with the Mentally Retarded. Glencoe, Illinois, The Free Press, 1957.

Thompson, L. J.: Special disabilities in children with organic brain pathology. North Carolina M. J., 8:224–228, 1947.

Wechsler, D.: The Measurement and Appraisal of Adult Intelligence, 4th Ed., Baltimore, Williams & Wilkins Co., 1958.

Wright, S. W.: Phenylketonuria. J.A.M.A., 165: 2079-2083, 1957.

Chapter Twenty-two

DISORDERS OF PSYCHOGENIC ORIGIN

In the preceding 15 chapters there has been discussion of mental disorders associated with diffuse impairment of cerebral tissue function. It was pointed out that if the brain lesion is reversible, the associated mental reactions are temporary and recoverable, with no residual damage to the personality. On the other hand, if the damage to cerebral tissue is not fully reversible, a variable but permanent impairment of its function, with resulting disturbance of memory, judgment, orientation, comprehension, and affect, will result.

Several of the chapters to follow are devoted to a discussion of disorders that are not associated with any physiological or structural change in the brain so far as is known at the present time. The present belief is that they represent the result of symbolic, emotional, and interpersonal factors acting on the organism. In other words, the group to be discussed includes those in which psychogenic factors are responsible for the malfunctioning of the personality. These psychogenically produced disorders may be divided into four groups:

a. Psychotic disorders;
b. Psychophysiological autonomic and visceral disorders ("psychosomatic" disorders);
c. Psychoneurotic disorders;
d. Personality disorders.

Psychotic Disorders

These disorders are characterized by a varying degree of personality disorganization. To different degrees, too, the patient may break with reality or fail to test and evaluate it correctly. As a result, his capacity for effective work and for adapted relations with other people is temporarily, and in some instances permanently, impaired or destroyed.

Psychophysiological Autonomic and Visceral Disorders

In this group are included disorders in which organ and visceral symptomatology is produced by emotional factors acting through the autonomic nervous system. Such a visceral expression of affect may serve to prevent the individual from becoming conscious of it. Long-continued deranged physiological states of viscera produced in this way by emotional factors may eventually lead to structural changes—to peptic ulcer, for example.

Psychoneurotic Disorders

These disorders represent either a symptomatic expression of "anxiety" or the psychological mechanisms unconsciously and automatically adopted to control it. Material disorganization of the personality does not occur, and there is no gross distortion or falsification of external reality as seen in the psychoses in the form of delusions and hallucinations. General types of psychoneuroses are recognized, the form being determined by the way in which the patient attempts to deal with the threatening danger felt in the conscious area of his personality but arising from the unconscious portion.

Personality Disorders

Disorders in this group are not characterized by mental or emotional symptoms but by developmental defects or pathological trends in the personality. In its classification of psychiatric disorders, the Revised Psychiatric Nomenclature divides personality disorders into three groups:

a. Personality pattern disturbance;
b. Personality trait disturbance;
c. Sociopathic personality disturbance.

In disorders included in this classification, the personality, in its efforts at adjustment to internal and external stresses, utilizes patterns of action or behavior, and not measures or symptoms expressed in the mental, somatic, or emotional spheres.

The first disorders of this psychogenic group to be discussed are those classified by the Revised Psychiatric Nomenclature as psychotic reactions. Such disorders are defined as those in which "the personality in its struggle for adjustment to internal and external stresses utilizes severe affective disturbance, profound autism and withdrawal from reality, and/or formation of delusions or hallucinations."

Chapter Twenty-three

PSYCHOTIC DISORDERS

INVOLUTIONAL PSYCHOTIC REACTIONS

The involutional psychoses tend to fall into two types. One is characterized largely by depression, the other by paranoid ideas. A depression occurring in the involutional period should usually not be included in the involutional psychotic reactions if there is a history of a previous manic–depressive reaction. In spite of the feature of depression common to both manic–depressive and involutional reactions, there are such special physiological and psychological factors in the latter that it is no longer considered to be a modified manic–depressive reaction occurring at a particular physiological epoch.

Involutional Depressive Reaction

The incidence of the depressive type of involutional psychosis is two to three times greater in women than in men. Among first admissions to hospitals for mental diseases it is exceeded in frequency only by schizophrenia, senile dementia, and syndromes associated with cerebral arteriosclerosis.

Age Factors

Although subject to considerable individual variation in the age of incidence, the involutional psychoses occur most frequently in women during the late forties and in men during the late fifties. It will be noted that this is the period when the endocrine and reproductive glands begin to suffer a decrease in functional activity—the age generally known as the involutional period. As the activity of these glands declines, there are extensive changes in the metabolic and vegetative activities of the body. With the cessation of ovarian activity there may be a change in functioning of other parts of the endocrine system, involving an increased irritability of the sympathetic nervous system. Just what part these changes in essential physiological functions play in the genesis of the psychosis is uncertain, but there is much to suggest that they are not so important per se as are their psychological implications. The threat to the personality through the loss of prized biological functions and the imminence of the aging process with all it connotes may be more disturbing to the personality than endocrinological changes. The period is one of psychophysiological stress and one in which increasing threats to an insecure personality are prone to elicit anxiety, depression, and paranoid reactions or both, a period that threatens the security that has been established at a time when the individual can least afford to lose it. It is a period that, in women, has often been anticipated with exaggerated fear.

Prepsychotic Personality

In a significant number of cases of the involutional depressive reaction, there is found a certain general type of personality make-up and of habits of life. Usually the patient was an anxious child with a background of early fundamental insecurity. A review of the patient's previous personality and temperament often shows that she has been a compulsive, inhibited type of individual with a tendency to be quiet, unobtrusive, serious, chronically worrisome, intolerant, reticent, sensitive, scrupulously honest, frugal, and even penurious. Usually, too, she has been of exacting and inflexible standards, lacking in humor, overconscientious, and given to self-punishment. Such persons have been mild, submissive, and sensitive to the moods and feelings of others. They have never been boastful but have depreciated their own worth, which often has actually been high. Not rarely they have been exploited by the selfish. The prepsychotic personality has been marked by a rigidity that represented a neurotic defense, and the patient has been perfectionistic, prudish, and prone to feelings of guilt. The personality has been super-ego dominated. Many involutional patients have been self-effacing and self-sacrificing and have had an exaggerated need for, and dependency upon, the approval of others.

Undoubtedly involutional depression evolves out of a masked neurosis of earlier life. In some instances, hostile and aggressive impulses have been repressed with difficulty. Many psychiatrists consider, in fact, that the prepsychotic personality of the involutional depressive type has been developed as a reaction-formation against aggression. Often the patient's sex life has been suppressed or unsatisfactory. Her interests have been narrow and her habits stereotyped; she has cared little for recreation, has not sought pleasure, and has had but few close friends. Frequently the patient has been a loyal subordinate, meticulous as to detail rather than an aggressive, confident leader. Many have been fidgety, fretful, apprehensive persons. Others have been characterized by caution or indecision.

Predisposing Factors

The age at which the psychosis develops is one when adjustments to new situations and circumstances are no longer easily made. Perhaps life has not brought either the success or satisfaction that hope had cherished. At this period there is a more or less conscious recognition that early dreams and desires cannot now be fulfilled, that the zenith of life has been passed, and that ambition and life's forces are waning. The fact that opportunity no longer exists for repairing old errors or achieving new success creates a sense of frustration and increases the feeling of insecurity. In women, loneliness or fear of a loss of physical attractiveness may be a contributing factor. The high value placed upon youth, beauty, and sex in our culture contributes to the drastic reorientation that must be made. The patient may feel that she is no longer attractive and feminine. At this period of life, some women have a deeply seated resentment, which may be expressed in depression and self-hate.

A rebellion against aging may also tend to promote depression. The transition to another stage of life with its new and difficult problems, both psychological and biological, is not easy. Regrets and a sense of failure contribute to the prevailing mood. Perhaps friends are beginning to die, or children to whom the patient has devoted her life are leaving home and becoming preoccupied with their own lives and families. The patient may feel that she is no longer needed. In some cases, aged parents who formerly represented security but are now dependent on the patient constitute a problem.

An ebbing potency in the male and

the realization of the woman that her most highly prized biological possession, that of childbearing, perhaps long frustrated, is now a lost capacity, is for the patient more than the loss of one of the most fundamental of functions—it is a symbol that both the sources and ends of energy have failed. Sometimes sexual desires, which have previously been suppressed, are perturbingly aroused. Previous reaction-formations prove inadequate, and acquired compensations and other protective mechanisms begin to fail.

As the flush of maturity fades, thoughts of death are suggested and contribute to the anxiety so common in the disorder. With the decrease of physical strength, unconscious forces and old conflicts become relatively stronger and return to threaten and torment. This threat to the ego is ceaseless, and since the source of the danger is hidden and within, any escape from it is impossible. As a result, the apprehension, tension, and unrest of anxiety are intensified. In a certain number of cases, retirement from business means the renunciation of long-cherished interests and a withdrawal of psychic energy. Sometimes a real economic stress or the possibility of becoming dependent upon someone is added to other problems. It is not surprising, therefore, that in the event of some disturbing experience, such as the breaking-up of the home or other threatening change in the life situation, the loss of position, or the death of one upon whom dependence was felt, the psychosis, with its pathological depression, apprehension, ideas of death, and nihilistic and hypochondriacal delusions, is precipitated.

Symptoms

The manifest symptoms of the psychosis are often preceded by a period of several weeks or a few months during which the patient exhibits hypochondriacal trends, becomes irritable, peevish, pessimistic, suffers from insomnia, is perhaps suspicious, shows a disinclination for effort, and may be given to spells of weeping. She is unable to concentrate and shows doubt and indecision. Frequently there is a narrowing of interests and a shrinking from the environment. The patient complains of distressing sensations in the head, eats poorly, loses weight, worries about health or finance, and becomes apprehensive and restless. In a more or less typical case, the most conspicuous symptoms are profound depression, anxiety, agitation, hypochondriasis, and delusions of sin, unworthiness, disease, and impending death.

The patient's appearance becomes one of extreme emotional pain and misery. The fear, apprehension, and agitation increase; the patient wrings her hands, paces back and forth, weeps, may beat her head against the wall, picks at her face, bites her nails, and tears at her handkerchief or clothing. She moans, and in a whining voice constantly repeats, "Why did I do it?" "Oh, God, what will become of me?" or some other stereotyped expression indicating hopelessness and affective distress. The patient may constantly besiege doctors and nurses with inquiries, complaints, or requests for reassurance.

Some patients present a morose depression or a depressive hostility. Misinterpretations and delusions are almost constantly present. Feelings of guilt explain in part both the great emotional depression and many of the delusions. Trifling indiscretions of youth or unformulated sins become the "unpardonable sin." The patient holds herself responsible for the fate of others. She has infected, disgraced, or harmed her family. She is about to be horribly butchered, a fate that she says she deserves, but awaits with intense fear and with pleas for mercy—indicating her ambivalent desire both for death and for life.

The delusion that she is about to be destroyed may be the patient's rationalization of her sense that life forces are declining. Inner distresses and dissatisfactions are rationalized as physical disease and thus produce the hypochondriasis so frequently observed. In this way the patient comes to believe that her intestines are obstructed, that she has no stomach, or that her brain is "dried up." Hallucinations, although less frequent than illusions, may occur. She hears preparations for her torture. Consciousness remains clear, and the patient is oriented, although in some cases the subjective absorption of attention is so great that she may appear to be confused and not thoroughly in touch with her environment.

Some patients are perplexed and bewildered. Depersonalization with feelings of unreality may exist. Food is often refused, sometimes because of a desire for death; at other times this occurs when, because of self-accusatory ideas, the patient believes she does not deserve food; again, refusal may be caused by a belief that the food is poisoned, or by nihilistic ideas that she has no stomach or no intestines. There is no other mental disorder in which suicidal attempts are so common. There is great danger that previous unsuccessful suicidal attempts will be repeated.

Although the patient never has a discriminating insight, she nevertheless usually realizes that matters are not as usual with her mentally. Early in the disorder the poorly understood sense of apprehension and the affective distress are so great, and are recognized as constituting such a contrast to her previous feeling-state, that the patient often expresses the fear she is going to lose her mind. She remains, nevertheless, thoroughly convinced as to the correctness of the idea she expresses. Most patients lose weight and in severe cases become seriously dehydrated. The hands are usually cold and cyanotic. The pulse is rapid and the respirations are shallow. The bowels are constipated and the urine scanty.

The following summary illustrates many of the common features of involutional melancholia.

E. M., a single woman of the early fifties, was admitted to a hospital following a suicidal attempt. She was described as having been a shy, sensitive, and affectionate child. Although in early life she attended dances, she was never known to have had any male friends. She always said she wished to "live alone and not be bothered by a man's company." After coming to America from Ireland at age 23, she secured employment as a domestic. She apparently was well regarded by her employers, to whom she became quite attached and with whom she usually remained for many years of continuous service. She was described as always using all her spare time in "doing little things about the house, darning stockings, cleaning something, and doing ironing." She was conscientious, likable, ambitious, and affectionate, but stubborn and difficult to convince. She was carefully observant of what she considered to be her religious duties and attended church regularly.

On arrival at the hospital, her facies denoted fear and apprehension. Although agitated, she supplied the usual admission data, and when asked if she was married, she at first replied in the affirmative, but a moment later stated that she was not married. Shortly afterward, when seen in the ward, she repeatedly inquired if the place was a jail. Upon being asked the reason for such a question, she replied, "Because jail is the safest place. I hope I don't be killed." She became increasingly anxious, agitated, and apprehensive, and on the day following her admission, she attempted to thrust her head through a closed window. Whenever a physician entered the ward, she approached him and with but little variation constantly repeated: "I am afraid, Doctor. Oh, my God! I am afraid of those men upstairs!" (There were no men in that section of the building.) "Look at those big snakes! Look at those big dogs!"

The patient had always lived frugally and had methodically deposited her savings in a bank, where she had accumulated several thousand dollars. She maintained, however, that her money was all lost and that she was destitute. Several days after her admission the patient was brought before the staff for diagnosis. At that time she showed the same anxious depression and agitation that had characterized her entire hospital residence. Soon after entering the staff room, she asked if the door leading to an anteroom where patients of both sexes were waiting was locked. When asked the occasion for the question, she replied, "I am afraid of the men."

Many of the factors that resulted in this woman's psychosis are comparatively simple and evident. The rigid environment in which she had been reared discouraged a normal interest in those of the opposite sex. That she had repressed any instinctive interest in men was betrayed by her statement that she did not want to be "bothered by a man's company." She became a faithful, conscientious servant, scrupulous as to detail but with an increasing limitation of external interests. Matters continued in this simple but hardly satisfying manner until physical capacity began to decline. The fact that life had not brought all that was desired became more or less vaguely realized; she was also aware that strength was waning and that whatever life had not already brought could never be attained. As physical energy declined with the involutional changes, the repression of material that had formerly been maintained, although with difficulty, began to fail. With their repression weakened, instinctive tendencies that had always been scrupulously denied any conscious recognition, began to threaten from within.

With no escape possible, anxiety, depression, fear and apprehension followed. This fear was projected as one of men, since it was the patient's repressed interest in them which she feared. This sense of danger was rationalized as one of threat to life, while affective and subjective material came to possess the vividness the patient had always associated with sensory experiences, with the result that she heard voices saying she was to be killed. Doubtless the patient's anxiety and depression represented much more than a weakening in the repression of instinctive tendencies of a psychosexual nature; the approach of an age when physical vigor and means of livelihood were declining, a sense of isolation, vague feelings of disappointment and failure and perhaps of guilt, all contributed to a sense of insecurity that added to the affective tension and apprehension.

It will thus be seen that we must not think of the involutional depressive reaction as a circumscribed disease entity resulting from clearly defined bodily changes, but rather, that an individual is being dealt with who usually has long attempted by neurotic defenses to cope with perturbing problems, gnawing conflicts, and resulting threats to security.

Prognosis

Before the introduction of electric shock treatment, about 40 per cent of the patients with involutional melancholia recovered. Convalescence, however, was slow, and those who recovered were frequently ill for two or three years. With the use of electric shock, more than 50 per cent of the involutional melancholia patients show prompt recovery. The more nearly the general manifestations of the reaction approach those usually seen in the depressive phase of manic–depressive psychosis, the better the prognosis. The greater the deterioration of personal habits, the more grotesque the delusions or the hypochondriacal ideas, the greater the occurrence of hallucinations, the more marked the poverty of thought and the tendency to aversion, depersonalization, or rut-formation with its meager affect reaction, the worse is the prognosis. Whining, surliness, and seclusiveness are not favorable symptoms. The more narrow and rigid the prepsychotic personality, the poorer the prognosis.

Diagnosis

Psychiatric disorders that may present features requiring a consideration of differential diagnosis from involutional melancholia are manic–depressive psychosis, cerebral arteriosclerosis, and anxiety states occurring in the psychoneuroses. In *manic–depressive psychosis*, the question of involutional melancholia need not be considered unless the age of the patient is compatible with the latter diagnosis. In that case, there is usually a history of previous attacks either of excitement or of depression. Frequently the manic–depressive has been of a cyclothymic temperament, whereas the involutional depressive has not rarely been of a compulsive type of personality. In the depression of a purely affective psychosis, there is typically a retardation in the flow of thought and in activity. The presence of anxiety, agitation, hypochondriacal and nihilistic ideas, peevishness, and hallucinations points toward an involutional depressive reaction. In this, fear, apprehension, and ideas of impending destruction are more marked. Stereotypes of behavior or speech and admixtures of other schizophrenic symptoms are more consistent with involutional melancholia.

Occasionally the *arteriosclerotic* patient is apprehensive and agitated, but he lacks profound and sustained fear. If the involvement is principally in the smaller vessels, the headaches and unpleasant cephalic sensations may suggest the hypochondriacal ideas of involutional melancholia, but the easy mental fatigability, occurrence of confused periods, slight delay in comprehension, a lessening of initiative rather than a preoccupation, and a slight memory loss should indicate the organic source of the mental disorder.

Although there is often a sustained anxiety of a mild type in *anxiety neurosis*, there is little or no fear except during acute paroxysms. Even then there is no genuine affective depression, and during the interparoxysmal period, affective lability is well retained. In the psychoneuroses, there are no hallucinations or true delusions, and interest in the outer world is comparatively well maintained. In the anxiety of the psychoneuroses, the essential mechanism is a displacement of anxiety from its connection with some emotional dissatisfaction, or from some wish that is not admitted to awareness because of its threat to conscious ideals, to an indifferent idea or situation. In involutional depression, the patient's sense of security is threatened, fear is more intense, and the continued striving in the face of frustration and prospective danger is greater; it is accompanied by pathological depression, and relations with reality may be disturbed. It is quite possible that the foundation of this, as in other depressive reactions, is to be found in a turning inward against the self of aggressive tendencies that can find no other outlet.

Treatment

The patient suffering from an involutional depressive reaction, should usually be cared for in a hospital, particularly since there is no other type of mental disorder in which so large a percentage of patients attempt suicide. The general lines of treatment are the same as those employed in the depressive phase of manic–depressive psychosis, but with particular stress on improving the physical state of the patient, which frequently becomes weakened and impaired. On arrival at the hospital, many patients are badly dehydrated and nearly always undernourished. There must be assurance, therefore, that the patient receives an abundance of liquid and food. If the patient is undernourished, it is often helpful to give her 20 units of insulin 30 minutes before meals. Because of their fear and apprehension, the purpose of any procedure or change from routine should be carefully explained to these patients.

Electroshock therapy is the most effective measure in the treatment of involutional depression. The technique of its application is discussed in Chapter 34. Although there are usually few contraindications to its use, the patient should first receive a careful physical examination. It should not be employed in case of cardiac decompensation. Except for recent fractures, bone disease is not a frequent contraindication. The patient should usually receive from 12 to 20 treatments. Most physicians find it desirable to "soften" the seizure by means of succinylcholine dichloride (Anectine). If the patient is greatly agitated, chlorpromazine may be used for its tranquilizing effect. The antidepressive agents also are now used, perhaps most effectively as maintenance medication after electroshock therapy. Lobotomy is performed today only rarely for this condition.

While estrogenic hormones help to relieve menopausal symptoms such as hot flashes, sweats, tensions, uneasiness and headaches, they are of little or no value in true involutional melancholia. The convalescent patient will frequently be deeply grateful for reassurance and support.

Involutional Paranoid Reaction

A certain number of persons develop a paranoid psychosis during the involutional period. Although never previously psychotic, nearly all such patients are found to have been persons whose prepsychotic personality was characterized by defensive patterns. As in the person who develops melancholia at the involutional period, the life pattern of the one who develops an involutional paranoid reaction has long betrayed an underlying sense of insecurity that she has striven to meet through certain personality traits. Usually it will be found that she has been critical and inclined to blame others for her failures and has seen slights where none were intended. By her associates she was probably regarded as obstinate in opinion, jealous, unforgiving, secretive, unhappy, dissatisfied, given to nursing of grievances, resentful, and suspicious. These defensive character traits prove sufficient support for the personality until the involutional period when, with the added physiological and psychological burdens previously mentioned, they are no longer adequate, and resort is made to the more extreme defensive and compensatory measures provided by the paranoid psychosis with its delusions and misinterpretations. The psychosis seems to merge out of the personality. The delusions usually revolve around ideas of persecution and are well organized, but they lack the fantastic content observed in schizophrenia. Many patients show much bitterness and hostility. The prognosis is less favorable than in melancholia. Electroshock treatment is of limited benefit. The aggressive and disturbed patient may be helped by chlorpromazine.

The following case illustrates many of the features often seen in paranoid involutional psychosis.

A. S. was admitted to the hospital in September, 1946, at the age of 59. The patient was born in Latvia. Little is known concerning her childhood experiences and the emotional climate of the home. She came to the United States in 1906 at the age of 19 to marry a man who had preceded her to this country. She and her husband returned to Latvia in 1913 to visit his parents but because of World War I could not return to America as planned. During that war they were driven into Russia, where they endured intense hardship. Finally they returned to Latvia, where the husband took over his father's farm and attained considerable success and status. At this point the farm buildings were destroyed by fire, and the patient was so seriously burned that she required hospital care for three months. In 1924 they returned to the United States and the husband established an upholstering business in which the patient assisted until the financial depression of the early '30's. The husband then began to drink, and in 1934 he committed suicide by hanging, a casualty discovered by the patient.

About 1940, at approximately 54 years of age, the patient began to complain that people were talking about her, that her son-in-law was maritally unfaithful, that nearly all persons, especially the clergy of a different religious faith, were sexually immoral. She expressed a fear that she would be "signed away for experimental purposes." She stated that a physician who had treated her at the menopause had given her cancer. Finally, after having complained to the police on several occasions that her food was being drugged and that a "society of science" was plotting against her, she was committed.

Following the patient's admission to the hospital, her daughter, in describing her mother's personality pattern, reported that she had always been a meticulous, hard-working person who was critical, suspicious, stubborn, uncompromising and domineering. The daughter described her mother as an immaculate housekeeper who also did "beautiful sewing."

On arrival at the hospital, her sensorium was clear, and she was fully oriented. She was suspicious, and when her abdominal reflexes were tested, she asked if the physician was going to operate on her. At times she became quite agitated and hostile and insisted that she be permitted to leave. Someone, she said, was trying to secure possession of her home and to kill her; she must therefore appeal to the police to help her. She complained that the nurses were trying to compel her to perform unpleasant tasks because they were members of a religious organization that was persecuting her.

Because of an electrocardiogram suggestive of coronary involvement and myocardial damage, it was decided not to give the patient electroshock treatment. After seven months of hospital residence, the patient became much less tense, was pleasant and cooperative, and was regarded as one of the most faithful and capable workers in the hospital cafeteria. Within a year after her admission, she was given freedom of the hospital grounds and was to spend week-ends with friends. Unless questioned, she expressed no delusional ideas. Upon inquiry, however, it was found that there had been no fundamental change in her paranoid ideation. Fifteen months after her admission the patient was permitted to leave the hospital. A year later her employer wrote: "Mrs. S. is cheerful and pleasant and I am very satisfied with her work."

So little is known about this woman's emotional relations with parents and siblings during childhood and any early traumatizing experiences that it is not easy to construct a desirably complete genetic-dynamic formulation of her psychotic personality disturbance. Her daughter's report that the patient was a meticulous, critical, suspicious, stubborn, dominating, and uncompromising person suggests that, because of a basic feeling of insecurity, she had developed these personality characteristics to serve as defenses. In spite of a long series of threats, these defenses proved adequate for many years. Among these stresses and threats were the drowning of a sibling during the patient's childhood (we do not know what feelings this death may have aroused in the patient), an almost fatal burn with its permanent scarring of the body, the enforced expulsion to Russia with the accompanying exposure to hardship and near-starvation, the destruction of the re-established home in Latvia, the return to the United States with the poverty that accompanied the financial depression, the unknown fate of relatives in World War II, the suicide of her husband with its probable but unknown psychological reverberations, the elopement of her daughter, and the development of mild diabetes. The rigid personality traits proved to be adequate defenses until the involutional period, with its various accompanying psychological factors, became so menacing that life-long traits were no longer able to control anxiety-producing threats. As a further defense, therefore, the patient resorted to projection to a reality-sacrificing, or psychotic, degree.

Although the problems that the patient had found too difficult to meet must remain a matter of speculation, one suspects, in view of the nature of her personality traits and the character of her delusions, that a deeply seated hostility, the fear of economic insecurity, and a weakening in the repression of instinctive sex drives may have been important ones.

BIBLIOGRAPHY

Davidoff, Eugene: The Involutional Psychoses. Chap. VIII in Kaplan, O. J., (Ed.): Mental Disorders in Later Life. Palo Alto, California, Stanford University Press, 1944.

Freeman, Walter, and Watts, J. W.: Psychosurgery, 2nd ed. Springfield, Illinois, Charles C Thomas, 1951.

Kalinowsky, L. B., and Hoch, P. H.: Shock Treatments, Psychosurgery and Other Somatic Treatments in Psychiatry, 2nd revised and enlarged ed. New York, Grune & Stratton, 1952.

Malzberg, Benjamin: A statistical study of first admissions with involutional psychoses to hospitals for mental diseases in New York. Psychiatric Quart., 22: Part 1, 141–155, 1948.

Palmer, H. D., and Sherman, S. H.: The involutional melancholia process. Arch. Neurol. & Psychiat., 40:762–768, 1938.

Rogers, Joseph: The menopause. New England J. Med., 254:697–703, 1956.

Tait, C. D., and Burns, G. C.: Involutional illnesses. Am. J. Psychiat., 108:27, 1951.

Titley, W. B.: Prepsychotic personality of patients with involutional melancholia. Arch. Neurol. & Psychiat., 36:19–33, 1936.

Chapter Twenty-four

PSYCHOTIC DISORDERS

AFFECTIVE REACTIONS

The group of affective psychoses constitute those behavior disturbances characterized principally by increased or decreased activity and thought expressive of a predominating mood of depression or elation. Although at the ranges of disturbance the behavioral change is conspicuous, it is seldom bizarre. The abnormalities of activity, affect, and thought seem often to the casual observer to have a plausible relationship to the immediate social environment.

Although the contrasting affective states, depression and elation, had been recognized for many years to occur in the same patient, it was not until 1896 that Emil Kraepelin designated the condition as manic–depressive insanity. He observed the periodicity and favorable outcome of the seemingly opposite stages of disordered affect and concluded they were variations of a single morbid process based upon physiological determinants.

Today, it is known that many patients may have only recurrent depressive reactions without elation; few present the alternation between the two affects. For these reasons, these conditions are subclassified in the nomenclature of the American Psychiatric Association as manic–depressive reaction, "manic type," or "depressive type." There is also designated a separate category of psychotic depressive reaction.

Causes

The not uncommon occurrence of manic–depressive psychoses in the same family suggests that a biogenetic factor may be at least a contributory cause, but this can scarcely be proved or denied. Rüdin has stated that the incidence of manic–depressive psychosis is 25 times as high among the siblings of manic–depressive patients as in the average population. If it occurs in monozygotic twins, both of them will be affected in more than half of the cases. In a German psychiatric clinic to which patients are admitted irrespective of social position, Luxemberger found manic–depressive psychoses to be nearly three times as frequent in the highest social class and four times as frequent in the professional classes as in the general population. This distribution of incidence seems to be similar to that observed by American psychiatrists. In World War II, manic–depressive psychoses were three times as frequent among officers of the American army as among enlisted men. They occur about twice as frequently in women as in men, and the average age of onset in women is younger. The aggressive woman with masculine strivings seems to be especially predisposed. Although these reactions are most frequently recognized during early maturity, more recent clinical observations have shown initial periods of morbid depression with crying commencing in early childhood. The nuclear facets of the personality characteristics defined in the adult patients are then already evident.

Even if constitutional factors exist, mentally dynamic ones are never absent. It is estimated that definite, disturbing life situations exist in about four-fifths of the attacks. In many instances, for example, particularly among persons of middle life or later, one finds that difficulties in adjusting to changes in environment or threats to social, economic, or physical security may serve as precipitating factors in a depressive attack. Some psychiatrists suggest that the disease is caused by disturbances in the chemical, vegetative, or regulatory processes of the body; others believe that these derangements so often seen in this disorder are but part of the total psychobiological reaction of the organism. No histological, biochemical, or biophysical correlates have ever been demonstrated in the brain. The electroencephalogram does not change as the patient shifts from one affective phase to the other.

Frequency

Statistics as to the frequency of manic–depressive psychoses show wide variations. Some institutions for mental disorders report that nearly 15 per cent of the patients admitted are suffering from this form of psychosis; others report 5 per cent only. The smaller figure is probably more nearly correct if those cases are excluded, even though episodic, that are characterized by a disturbance in the integration of thought, feeling, and behavior and by falsification of perception and of reality in response to internal needs, and should, therefore, be regarded as schizophrenic in nature. The experience of psychiatrists in private practice seems to show that many cases are not recognized if they are of mild form or of brief duration. This is particularly true if they assume the form of a period of fatigue or of brief periods of depression lasting perhaps from a few hours to a few days. In such cases the attention of both physician and patient may become focused on alleged or attendant somatic disorders.

Psychopathology

There are two well-defined types or phases of the manic–depressive psychoses: a manic or hyperactive phase, and a depressive phase.

Although the disorder typically assumes the form of psychotic episodes separated by intervals of mental health, a person may never suffer from more than one episode, or again, the disorder may become continuous. These episodes may be in the nature of a manic or of a depressive reaction, but there is no constant sequence or alternation of these reactions. The swings from one phase to another seems to prove the homogeneity of the manic–depressive psychoses.

MANIC PHASE. In his personality make-up the patient whose episodes are of a manic type has usually been a self-satisfied, confident, aggressive, effervescing extrovert, at ease with other people. He has been inclined to scatter his energy over a wide field of interests. His affective attitude has been one of emotional expression and responsiveness. The manic phase or reaction is usually preceded by a simple depression. This depression is of brief duration and mild in degree, often lasting for only a few days and either not noted by the patient's family or not considered significant. This brief period is followed by exhilaration or mild excitement.

Sometimes the attack remains in this attenuated form known as *hypomania*. In this hypomanic state there is an emotionally unstable, increased assertiveness, an air of self-assurance, careless gaiety, breezy affability, self-satisfaction, buoyant self-confidence, and boundless energy. No matter how inhibited the patient may normally have been, he is now irrepressible, demanding, uninhibited, effusive, and often astonishingly unconventional in speech and manner. He is narcissistic, childishly proud, and quite intolerant of criticism. Glib of tongue and genial of hand, the patient is socially aggressive, witty, boastful, flippant, argumentative, spends his money extravagantly, pawns his belongings, is full of ambitious schemes, and starts enterprises that soon fail or that he soon abandons.

Often striking is the frequency of use of direct and indirect quotations, particularized references, and adverbs of degree ("absolutely," "much," "never"). His conversation is directed principally to a recital of events, circumstances, and meetings with others, but it seldom contains statements as to their inner affective meaning to him or as to his personal evaluation of the interactions between himself and others. Thus there is little evidence of introspection but more that of comparing, weighing, and evaluating the performances of others and himself. From this trend, coupled with the many indications of denial and overcompensatory self references, there emerges a self-image toward which the patient appears to be striving.

His excuses and arguments contain a superficial but specious plausibility. His disregard for the truth may carry great conviction to those not previously acquainted with him. The patient is bored with routine, lacks a sustained interest in any activity, and is too busy to submit his impressions to critical examination. Attention is often easily distracted, thought processes are accelerated, and the stream of thought is prone to wander. His manner of speaking has an undertone of emphasis and exaggeration.

Many hypomanic patients are mischievous, boisterous, and full of pranks, indulge in risqué remarks and coarse and unseemly jokes, and make facetious comments about some object, or especially some person, in the environment. They are superficial in their relationships with other persons and insensitive to the latters' needs and feelings. Some hypomanic individuals delight in joking efforts to tease the physician. Unbridled criticism and bluntness of speech, even to the point of impudence, are common.

Without constraint, the manic patient blurts out what he has doubtless long wished to say but has previously been afraid to express. The usual good humor, which is often infectious in nature, frequently continues as long as every whim of the patient is gratified, but it tends to be replaced with anger, caustic speech, and verbal abuse if anyone questions his opinion or thwarts his wishes. In place of this good humor, one occasionally meets with a sustained anger, argumentativeness, irritability, haughtiness, arrogance, sarcasm, and querulousness. Open hostility to members of the family is common. After her recovery, one woman whose hypomanic attacks were characterized by a great outburst of hostility described her psychotic episodes as seeming "like a prolonged spell of anger." In her normal periods, she was a friendly person, anxious to help others, and took great pride in her love for them. (One suspects that this desirable personality characteristic was a reaction formation that served as a defense against a deep-seated hostility.)

Sudden oscillations of emotion are common. In the midst of an exuberance of manner and spirits, the patient may suddenly burst into tears and give expression to some depressive idea, but after a moment be as cheerful as ever. He may likewise change rapidly from irritability to affability. The hypomanic patient may work with great, but capricious, enthusiasm and energy, but his stimulation and expansiveness impair his judgment. He is often so officious and meddlesome that he becomes an annoyance to those about him. He declares that he needs no rest. Although under a constant pressure of activity, he feels no sense of fatigue. He writes numerous letters in which he underscores many words and passages and introduces various parenthetical remarks. The style of composition may be flowery and witty and the script large, flowing, and perhaps graceful. No sooner, perhaps, has he posted a letter than he decides that the mail is too slow for his urgent business so he dispatches a telegram to his correspondent. He discusses with strangers and without reserve matters of an intimate, private nature. The hypomanic is often erotic and, if a man, may indulge in sexual excesses, while a previously chaste and modest young woman may become sexually promiscuous or marry a man far below her social level. Although from custom and convenience the symptoms just described are designated as hypomanic, any attempt to divide the imperceptible gradations of hyperactivity occurring in manic–depressive psychosis into clinical groups is entirely arbitrary.

In a well-developed picture of mania the *affective tonality* is one of eagerness, exaltation, and joyous excitement. The tempo of the whole personality is quickened. The patient's patterns of thinking and behavior reflect his mood. He sings, dances about, whistles, and may be exhilarated to the point of noisy hilarity. He shows an unrestrained playfulness and mischievousness. His elation stimulates ideas of grandeur and perhaps fleeting delusions of wealth and power. The exhilaration may be punctuated with anger, irritability, and even with combativeness if the patient is denied some request or privilege, a granting of which his disturbed state forbids. Again, a well-developed paranoid trend may exist, and the patient may be verbally abusive to the person toward whom, for the moment, he may feel most resentful. Patients with this impure affect are often haughty, demanding, revengeful, sarcastic, and arrogant. They may seem to delight in an unbounded expression of aggressiveness and hostility.

The *stream of thought* is characterized by loquaciousness and rapid association of ideas. Frequently the patient speaks with a crispness and vigor of articulation, with emphatic accents and frequent changes of pitch. His style of phrasing may be pompous, and his speech may assume the character of theatrical declamation. As the hypomanic state passes into acute mania, the pressure of speech develops into a flight of ideas with rhyming, play upon words, and "clang" associations of words having similar sounds but no relation in meaning. Superficially the therapist receives the impression of a great variety of ideas, but if he carefully observes the manic patient's associational products, he discovers that their range is really limited. As a matter of fact, the manic individual evades thinking and is occupied with phonetics rather than meaning. Associations that remind the patient of some overvalued idea or egocentric interest are particularly apt to divert the stream of thought. Although the patient's racing flow of ideas appears illogical and directed by such stimuli as similarity of sound and environmental objects and events, beneath these superficial associations may often be discovered an underlying but limited range of topics toward which associations tend to flow. Without realizing their significance, the patient often makes remarks that afford a hint as to the unconscious motivation of his ideas, since, although apparently devoid of motivation, they are not so in fact. In both sequence and significance, they approach the character of free associations and therefore, like them, are prompted by unconscious and instinctive agencies.

The third of the mental fields in which it has been customary to describe disturbances as taking place is that of *psychomotor activity*. There is an overactivity, ranging from the pressure of occupation described in hypomania to the violent motor excitement of acute mania. In the hospital the patient meddles with ward activities and with other patients; he has numerous suggestions as to how the institution should be conducted. He decorates himself with trinkets and improvised badges and medals. In more excited states, he tears his clothing into ribbons with which he decorates himself in a grotesque manner. He sings, shouts, and assumes dramatic attitudes. He may destroy bed and personal clothing, an activity usually not prompted by malice but by an urge to be busy. A woman ordinarily refined and modest may disregard all former sense of propriety, make indecent sexual proposals, and be obscene in speech. The overactive manic sleeps little and yet does not appear fatigued. He sustains cuts and abrasions to which he pays no attention and for which he will permit no treatment. Infections may occur and complicate the clinical picture. Rarely the patient shows such a pressure of activity that he does not eat and requires tube feeding, although in the usual degree of excitement the patient may bolt large quantities of food with complete disregard of manners.

The attention of the manic is usually much disturbed, the disorder being caused not by any defect in vigility but by lack of tenacity, as a result of which attention is easily distracted. Environmental noises and activities constantly divert his attention. Not rarely he misidentifies persons, being particularly prone to identify a stranger as a former acquaintance because of the fact that he discovers some slight point of similarity but fails to scrutinize the points of dissimilarity. The patient usually remains well oriented, but at times his grasp of his environment may be faulty because of an absence of sustained and discriminating attention.

Hallucinations may occur in manic excitement but are not common and are usually more in the nature of illusions.

Although delusions are not conspicuous symptoms, they often occur, are usually expansive or wish-fulfilling in nature, are fleeting, and not systematized. Ideas of persecution are not rare.

Physically the patients classed as milder cases appear in excellent health. The eyes are bright, the face flushed, the head erect, the step quick, and weight may be gained. In extreme excitement the patient may lose weight because of great expenditure of energy. In greatly overactive states, the patient is usually dehydrated. Pneumonia, acute nephritis, and other infections may be unrecognized because of the difficulty in making a physical examination of a patient so extremely excited. In such cases, the real nature of a superimposed delirioid state may escape recognition. Any real clouding of consciousness in a patient who has been greatly excited should suggest the possibility of a complicating infection.

The following taken from the records of a man who first entered a public institution for mental diseases when 54 years of age illustrates many of the typical behavior reactions of manic excitement:

At ages 35, 41, and 47, the patient suffered from depressed episodes, each attack being from four to six months in duration. In January he became restless and talkative. Early in February he began to send checks to friends, sometimes even to strangers who, he said, might be in need. Ten days later he was sent home from the office where he was employed with the explanation that he was becoming overwrought. A few days after his suspension from work he was admitted to a private institution for mental disorders where he pretended to commit suicide by mercury poisoning. He then drew a skull and cross bones on the wall of his room. After three weeks he was taken home, but a few days later he was committed to a public institution where he bustled about the ward, giving the impression that he had important business to which he must attend.

Occasionally he was seen lying on a bench, pretending to sleep, but in a few minutes he resumed his usual activity. He talked quickly, loudly, and nearly constantly. He was interested in everything and everyone around him. He talked familiarly to patients, attendants, nurses, and physicians. He took a fancy to the woman physician on duty in the admission building, calling her by her first name and annoying her with letters and with his familiar, ill-mannered, and obtrusive attentions. On his arrival he gave five dollars to one patient and one dollar to another. He made many comments and asked many questions about other patients and promised that he would secure their discharge. He interfered with their affairs and soon received a blow on the jaw from one patient and a black eye from another. He wrote letters demanding his release, also letters to friends describing in a circumstantial, inaccurate, and facetious way conditions in the hospital. His letters were interlarded with trite Latin phrases. He drew caricatures of the physicians and the nurses and wrote music on toilet paper. He drew pictures on his arms; on one occasion he secured a bottle of mercurochrome and painted the face of another manic patient. When permitted to play the ward piano, he played piece after piece without stopping, improvising a great deal. A doctor rarely passed through the ward without being called by the patient, who would slap the physician on the back or shake hands effusively and talk until the door closed. At times during an interview his voice became tremulous, tears came to his eyes, and he sobbed audibly with his face buried in his arms. A moment later, however, he was laughing—a manifestation of the bipolarity of emotion so markedly illustrated in this disease.

DEPRESSIVE PHASE. Although a larger percentage of the episodic depressions of this disorder occur in persons who have also a history of manic episodes, in not a few manic–depressives the psychotic episodes are confined to those of a depressive type. In such cases one often finds a rather characteristic type of prepsychotic personality. Many of these individuals whose psychotic episodes are limited to depressive reactions have always been friendly, unobtrusive, timid persons with an underlying sense of insecurity and overdependency. Not a few have manifested sensitive and appreciative emotional responses. Many have been scrupulous persons of rigid ethical and moral standards, meticulous, self-demanding, perfectionistic, self-depreciatory, prudish, given to self-reproach, and sensitive to criticism. Their obsessive-compulsive tendencies have doubtless been defensive mechanisms for handling hostility, which characteristically they cannot express externally. Frequently they have had fixed opinions and set ways of doing things and are habitually apprehensive and fearful. Many have been hesitant and without courage, yet have sought and achieved worthwhile accomplishments. Frequently their greatest emotional need seems to have been that of being loved, accepted, and belonging.

Just as in the manic type of manic–depressive psychosis all degrees of over-activity are found, so in the depressive type one meets with varying degrees of depression. If arbitrarily we describe three degrees of manic activity—hypomania, acute mania, and delirious mania—in the excited phase, so mild depression, acute depression, and stupor may be said to represent the different degrees of depression. One should remember, however, that these arbitrary divisions merge imperceptibly one into the other.

Because of the absence of striking disturbances, the real nature of *mild depression* is frequently not recognized. In fact, it should be borne in mind that various moods that are called normal pass imperceptibly into the different forms of manic–depressive psychosis. Mild depressive phases tend, roughly speaking, to assume one of two general forms: either a period of fatigue, staleness, and inertia, or one during which the patient has physical complaints for which no organic basis can be discovered. Affective depression exists in both forms but does not constitute the chief complaint and consists in a mild downheartedness. Occasionally the onset is characterized by obsessive features. If the depression stands a bit to the fore, the patient's friends may speak of his episodes as "blue spells." The patient lacks confidence in himself, loses his zest for living, feels inadequate and tired, shows a growing aversion to activity, likes to be left alone, and finds it difficult to perform his ordinary duties. Color and joy are gone out of life. Every task seems a burden, and in many cases the patient gives up any attempt to continue his employment. He has doubts and fears, is frequently over-anxious about his family, states he has not provided amply for their future welfare, and has mild ideas of unworthiness. Thinking may be difficult, ideational content becomes confined to a few topics, spontaneous speech is limited, replies to questions are delayed and condensed as much as possible, and the patient is disinclined to reveal his private thoughts. Social contacts are not sought, and the patient may even show an obstinate unwillingness to meet people. Many show a marked indecisiveness, probably indicative of their apprehension of further failure, rejection, and retaliation. Those with an "impure" depression tend to be gloomily irritable, sensitive, and morose rather than sad. They are often stubborn, peevish, and inconsiderate of others and are inclined to project in the form of dissatisfaction and fault-finding.

In the second group of mild depressions, physical complaints are among the most conspicuous symptoms and may mask the depression. There is not merely the loss of weight, coated tongue, disturbed and unrefreshing sleep, and poor appetite observed in depressive states, but the patient has various hypochondriacal ideas. He feels weak and fatigued, worries over trifles, suffers from insomnia, headache, and debility and perhaps from precordial or epigastric distress. Any bodily sensations that may arise on a physical, tension, or anxiety basis become the principal object of the patient's attention. He therefore believes, as often do his friends, that the real disorder is physical and that his downheartedness is the natural result of ill health, whereas the physical complaints are really but the rationalization of a primary affective distress. To the inexperienced practitioner, these depressive episodes may appear to be neurasthenic. Occasionally there is a history of laparotomy or pelvic surgery without a discoverable pathologic condition having been revealed.

The onset of a *severe depression* may resemble the mild depressive states just described, but the initial downheartedness soon passes into a profound affective distress. Posture, muscle tensions, and various physical signs and symptoms present a composite picture indicating depression. The body is stooped, the head flexed, the facies immobile, the forehead furrowed, and the patient looks fixedly downward. Deep vertical wrinkles appear between the eyebrows, the nasolabial folds are marked, and the down-turned angles of the mouth constitute a picture of dejection. The face may have a troubled, perplexed expression. The patient loses weight and appears ill. Perspiration and other secretions are decreased. Muscle tone is decreased, the bowels are constipated, sexual desire is decreased, and the male patient is usually impotent. The sleeping pattern is disturbed in a characteristic way. Although there is usually little delay in falling asleep, the patient awakens much earlier than when he is well. The diurnal severity of his depressive affect also varies

in a customary way in that it is usually most severe in the morning and relents as the day wears on. The depression becomes more profound, and everything is interpreted in terms of hopelessness and despondency.

Occasionally a patient says he has no feeling. Others complain that things seem strange and unnatural—feelings of unreality. They usually recognize that the change, caused by the influence of depressed feeling-tone on perceptions, by the loss of interest in external phenomena, and by the altered affective relationship to them, is in themselves and not in the fundamental nature of environmental objects. Many patients have an indefinite dread or a sense of impending disaster, frequently accompanied by an attitude of submission to their fate. Efforts at reassurance make no impression, and the patient shows no response to appreciative and sympathetic counsel. Some patients manifest a hostile bitterness. A sense of fear is not uncommon and, if intense, consciousness may be clouded and the patient be confused.

The purest type of depression is a *retarded depression*. In this there is an inhibition of the stream of thought and of psychomotor activity. The retarded patient speaks slowly and seems at a loss for words. His replies are brief, frequently monosyllabic, and expressed in a low tone. Not rarely he begins, but never completes, the reply to some inquiry, or else he finishes it only as the examiner moves away. Perhaps he may merely move his lips but fail to utter any intelligible response. Efforts to make decisions result in vacillation or perplexity.

In the psychomotor field, externally directed behavior becomes progressively retarded and inhibited. There is slowness both in initiation and in execution. The patient complains of an inability to carry out suggested activities, and every attempt requires great exertion. Retardation may be so pronounced as to amount to stupor.

In depressive states the patient's ideas tend to represent a projected expression of his inner feelings and a rationalization of his affects. The delusions of both manic and depressive patients seem to be more the reflections of their mood than true delusional experiences, as in schizophrenia. The delusional content of the depressive patient is therefore characterized by self-depreciation, ideas of guilt, remorse, self-accusation, and hypochondriasis. Not infrequently there is a suspicious, paranoid, complaining, and persecutory trend to the patient's ideas. This is particularly the case when the patient's prepsychotic personality was characterized by sensitiveness and feelings of inferiority. Some depressive patients are sullen and morose. Hate is not an uncommon, although at times concealed, constituent of depression. Sometimes the patient may present a hostile, punitive attitude. Resentment and aversion to treatment may be associated. Aversion reactions should not be confused with negativism.

Hallucinations are not conspicuous symptoms in the depression of manic–depressive psychosis, and although they may occur, a persistent falsification of reality in this way should raise the question of a more malignant psychosis, particularly if the hallucinations do not clearly represent the projection of affective distress. Illusionary misinterpretations are frequent—a pounding in the basement is that of workmen constructing the patient's coffin.

The patient usually remains well oriented unless from his affective distress he becomes so preoccupied that attention is impaired. As already indicated, he may be confused if his fear is intense. Depressed patients usually have little or no appetite, and some would starve if not encouraged or forced to eat. Spoon or tube feeding is often necessary. This failure to eat may result from the profound psychomotor inhibition, or from the patient's belief that he is unworthy to receive the food, or from a desire to die. This feeling of unworthiness and the desire for self-punishment often lead to suicidal attempts and occasionally to mutilation of self.

The most intense form of the de-pressive phase is depressive *stupor*. It was probably this type of stupor to which Esquirol gave the name "acute dementia." In this profoundly inhibited state, there is practically no spontaneous motor activity. There is a complete, or almost complete, immobility, with a minimal response to external stimuli. The patient is mute, his sensorium is clouded, and he is intensely preoccupied, often with ideas of death and with dream-like hallucinations. The face is either mask-like or rigidly anxious. Many have to be tube-fed; some soil and wet themselves.

Elderly depressed patients may manifest organic mental symptoms such as confusion, disorientation, and memory defects, which are alleviated or may even disappear with recovery from depression. Not rarely, a depression terminates with a brief hypomanic reaction.

The possibility that crimes of violence may occur with the manic–depressive psychoses is usually considered. Such crimes are not unknown, however, and are more frequent in depressed than in manic states, probably because of the fact that depression may be a result of a weakening in the repression of hate and aggressive strivings. It is reported that of 90 patients confined to the Broadmoor, England, Criminal Lunatic Asylum because of murder committed during affective phychoses, 62 were suffering from depression and 28 from mania at the time the homicides took place. More homicides are committed by depressed women than by depressed men. Usually the victim is not only a member of the patient's family but the one who has apparently been the most loved. It has been suggested that the homicide may be regarded as an extension of the suicidal impulse. If suicide is considered as an act of aggression against self, then the homicide (in depressive patients) might be considered as an extension of aggression to include not only the self but those things that are nearest the self, the victim being almost a part of the self. Perhaps this is the psychopathology manifested when a depressed mother kills both herself and her child.

The following case represents a fairly typical picture of the depressive phase.

E. D., aged 60, was admitted to the hospital because he was depressed, ate insufficiently, and believed that his stomach was "rotting away." The patient was described as a friendly, sociable individual, not quarrelsome, jealous, or critical, and with a sense of humor. He was considered even-tempered, slow to anger, tenderhearted, and emotional.

At 51 the patient suffered from a depression and was obliged to resign his position. This depression continued for about nine months, after which he apparently fully recovered. He resumed his work but after two years suffered from a second depression. Again he recovered after several months and returned to a similar position and held it until two months before his admission. At this time he began to worry lest he was not doing his work well, talked much of his lack of fitness for his duties, and finally resigned. He spent Thanksgiving Day at his son's in a neighboring city, but while there he was sure that the water pipes in his own house would freeze during his absence and that he and his family would be "turned out into the street." A few days later he was found standing by a pond, evidently contemplating suicide. He soon began to remain in bed and sometimes wrapped his head in the bed clothing to shut out the external world. He declared that he was "rotting away inside" and that if he ate, the food would kill him. He urged the family not to touch the glasses or towels he used lest they become contaminated.

On arrival at the hospital, he appeared older than his years. He was pale, poorly nourished, dehydrated, with his lips dry, cracked, and covered with sordes. His facial expression and general bearing suggested a feeling of utter hopelessness. He was self-absorbed and manifested no interest in his environment. When urged to answer questions, there was a long delay before he attempted to reply, but he finally spoke briefly, hesitatingly, and in a low tone. He occasionally became agitated and repeatedly said, "Oh, doctor, why did I ever get into anything like this? Doctor, I am all filled up! I can't get anything through me—what am I going to do? Oh, dear! Oh, dear!" In explaining his presence in the hospital, he said he realized he had been sent by his family because they believed he would be benefited by the treatment, but added, "I don't know how they sent me here when they had not the means. My wife cannot pay for me, and by this time she must have been put out of the house."

After several months the patient began to improve, although hypochondriacal ideas persisted for a considerable period. Finally, when the matter of freedom of the hospital grounds was considered, he seemed in a normal mood and indicated that he was beginning to think somewhat differently concerning his gastrointestinal

tract. At that time he commented, "There's a good deal of life in the old horse yet." A month later he passed into a mildly hypomanic state. He became alert, animated, talkative, exuberant in spirits, and confident in manner. This mildly excited state continued for about two months, when he settled down into what seemed to be his normal mood and state of activity. After a few weeks he was discharged, but several months later he again showed signs of depression and hanged himself before arrangements for readmission had been made.

CYCLIC TYPE. Although the episodes suffered by some patients are always manic or always depressive, those of others may be of irregular sequence in respect to the mood disturbance. Again the episodes of still other patients may be characterized by an alternation of manic and depressive reactions. In some patients there may be no appreciable interval of normality between the alternations; in other cases there may be variable periods free from symptoms.

The following case illustrates the tendency to cycles and how the frequency of recurring mood swings may prevent successful adjustment during a large part of the patient's adult life.

M. M. was first admitted to a state hospital at the age of 38, although since childhood she had been characterized by swings of mood, some of which had been so extreme that they had been psychotic in degree. At 17 she suffered from a depression that rendered her unable to work for several months, although she was not hospitalized. At 33, shortly before the birth of her first child, the patient was greatly depressed. For a period of four days she was in a coma. About a month after the birth of the baby she "became excited" and was entered as a patient in an institution for neurotic and mildly psychotic patients. As she began to improve, she was sent to a shore hotel for a brief vacation. The patient remained at the hotel for one night and on the following day signed a year's lease on an apartment, bought furniture, and became heavily involved in debt. Shortly thereafter Mrs. M. became depressed and returned to the hospital in which she had previously been a patient. After several months she recovered and, except for relatively mild fluctuations of mood, remained well for approximately two years.

She then became overactive and exuberant in spirits and visited her friends to whom she outlined her plans for re-establishing different forms of lucrative business. She purchased many clothes, bought furniture, pawned her rings, and wrote checks without funds. She was then entered in a public mental hospital. Gradually her manic symptoms subsided, and after four months she was discharged. For a period thereafter she was mildly depressed. In a little less than a year Mrs. M. again became overactive, played her radio until late in the night, smoked excessively, took out insurance on a car that she had not yet bought. Contrary to her usual habits, she swore frequently and loudly, created a disturbance in a club to which she did not belong, and instituted divorce proceedings. On the day prior to her second admission to the hospital, she purchased 57 hats.

During the past 18 years this patient has been admitted and dismissed from the hospital on many occasions. At times, with the onset of a depressed period, she has returned to the hospital seeking admission. At such times she complained that her "brain just won't work." She would say, "I have no energy, am unable to do my housework; I have let my family down; I am living from day to day. There is no one to blame but myself." During one of her manic periods, she sent the following telegram to a physician with whom she had become much enamored: "To: You; Street and No.: Everywhere; Place: the remains at peace! We did our best, but God's will be done! I am so very sorry for all of us. To brave it through thus far. Yes, Darling— from Hello Handsome. Handsome is as Handsome does, thinks, lives and breathes. It takes clear air, Brother of Mine, in a girl's hour of need. All my love to the Best Inspiration one ever had."

For the past year Mrs. M., now 59, has been making an excellent home and community adjustment. Her husband has had several cerebrovascular accidents and has required considerable nursing and assistance. She has efficiently met the various responsibilities and family emergencies that have befallen her and has supplemented her husband's pension by baby-sitting. It is altogether probable, however, that she will experience returns either of excitement or of depression.

MIXED TYPES. Psychomotor activity, flow of thought, and affectivity were formerly thought of as independent and more or less separable functions of the mind, which in their positive or negative variations could be combined in various ways as may the letters of the alphabet. Basing his ideas on this conception of a co-existence of manic and depressive elements, Kraepelin described special clinical forms. These he designated as the "mixed" types of manic–depressive psychosis. He conceived of these positive or negative unitary faculties as being capable of arrangement and rearrangement in various combinations. It should be remembered, however, that behavior is a unitary, purposive process, and that it is not the result of a haphazard union of component elements. Kraepelin described such "mixed" forms as agitated depression, manic stupor, unproductive mania, depressive mania, depression with flight, and inhibited mania. The present tendency is to discontinue such artificial classifications.

Of these groups, *agitated depression* most nearly deserves a special recognition, yet this group is really a depressive reaction in which the agitation is simply an expression of anxiety—a persistent expression of the apprehension, tension, and feeling of prospective harm arising from threatening factors deep in the mental life. The great internal uneasiness produces a psychomotor agitation.

Psychotic Depressive Reaction

Not all psychotic depressive reactions should be included among those of a manic–depressive type. In the latter type of depressions, there is usually the history either of previous, perhaps repeated, depressions or of cyclothymic mood swings in which periods of elation as well as of depression may have been of psychotic degree. The depressions of a manic– depressive nature, too, usually develop without obvious cause and in the absence of any experience such as might seem logically provocative of depression. Occasionally one meets with depressions which lack these distinctive features of a manic–depressive reaction. Such depressions arise when the patient has been confronted with a personal situation of great stress. Environmental factors and personal experiences have been cruelly frustrating, have aroused intense feelings of guilt or remorse, or have painfully wounded pride. In these disorders, the reaction to the current situation is a definitely pathological depression, at times associated with gross misinterpretation of reality in the form of delusions, frequently, but not always, somatic, suicidal ruminations or attempts, intense feelings of guilt, and retardation of thought and of psychomotor activity.

Pathophysiology

In recent years, certain physiological functions have been found to be disordered in a high proportion of patients examined during the psychotic phases. Strongin and Hinsie's finding that the rate of salivary secretion is lowered in depression has been confirmed repeatedly. This diminution of salivary secretion has not been correlated with the clinical degree of depression and may persist after improvement. Salivary secretion is easily measured by the methods described by Busfield.

The "sedation threshold," defined by Shagass as the amount of amobarbital sodium in milligrams per kilogram of body weight required to produce a specific inflection in the amplitude of frontal lobe electroencephalographic activity during intravenous injection, is lowered in those with psychotic depressive reactions, again in contrast with other types of psychosis. The threshold for each individual is reproducible over time, and it is not modified greatly by moderate doses of phenothiazines. The techniques of measurement and scales are given in the papers by Shagass and Nymgaard.

Psychodynamics

Various theories have been offered to explain the psychological dynamics of the two contrasting affective reactions of depression and mania. From a theoretical standpoint, it is considered that the capacity for warm social relations existing in the future manic–depressive stem from a satisfying early infantile contact with the mother. Yet it is thought that at that stage of development during which the child commences to evolve the early nucleus of personal identity, the relationship is such that he fails to lay down the basis for resolving the conflicting feelings of tenderness and rage towards a single person. In those with cyclic manic–depressive reactions, it has been suggested that they have failed to construct a unitary identity and shift from partial identifications made with both parents or others who are highly divergent in their personal characteristics and defenses. Thus one of the parents may be submissive and overconscientious, the other outwardly aggressive and dynamic.

At the present time, there seems to be much to suggest that depression should be regarded as a result of anxiety in a person who experienced severe loss, real or fantasied, at an early stage of development. The loss is perceived as rejection, which precipitates anger. Since the feeling of anger cannot be tolerated, it is repressed and turned inward on the self. Although these feelings of anger and hostility are repressed, they cause the individual to feel guilty, unworthy, and depressed.

It well may be that the shift from depression to elation takes place in association with vacillating processes of identification with parental figures. During depression the patient identifies with the maternal figure in a submissive role. At the initiation of the period of elation, he denies the submissive, maternal identification and acts out an intense, acquisitive, sadistic drive with fantasies of strength in which he becomes emancipated, elated, and overaggressive, in imitation of the paternal figure, with whom he is now identified. With the failure of his aggressiveness to accomplish the fantasied aim of revenge, the patient again has to renounce the paternal identification, to deny his aggressiveness, and so he becomes depressed and helpless. These aggressive and assured personality characteristics of the manic are not necessarily related to the parental sex, as in some instances the mother is identified as the striving person who provided for the child the ideal of strength in times of family stress. As one woman manic patient expressed it, "When our family and its fortune was falling apart during the depression, my mother laughed and made light of it—my father withdrew. I have always admired her and sought to be like her when things were bad."

The manic's behavior is essentially a defense of massive denial against the underlying depression. Although he may appear confident and occupy the role of a leader, the manic is basically overdependent. Although he appears out-going and friendly, he is self-centered, actively controlling, and manipulating. These attitudes are based on an emotional need for dependency relationship. When his demands are frustrated, hostility is generated, which must be repressed so that it does not further imperil the dependency relationship. The imperfectly repressed hostility may, in turn, produce depression.

Sometimes an important source of conflict for the manic–depressive patient seems to be that of strong hostility connected with envy, which is repressed and avoided. He is often the best endowed member of the family and has been expected to provide the prestige for the group. This position places great responsibility on him, yet exposes him to the envy of his siblings, or even to envious competition with his parents. The future manic–depressive has grown sensitive to envy and competition, and to counteract the potentiality of suffering the hostility of envy due to his own abilities, he has unconsciously developed the pattern of disparaging himself in order to conceal his full capacity.

Feelings of guilt and reflected depression springing from them arise in various ways. Some repressed wish, for example, is occasionally granted by accident, such as by the death of a parent whose continued existence had prevented the fulfillment of a greatly desired wish. In such a case, a depression may sometimes result because of the feeling of guilt that follows the gratification of the consciously repudiated desire. In general, as already indicated, feelings of guilt giving rise to depression arise not so much from what one has done as from what one has unconsciously wished to do. Depression represents a penance for repressed hatred, aggressiveness, and other repudiated tendencies and impulses that have given rise to feelings of guilt. Guilt, too, may be expressed in terms of self-punishment. There is much to suggest that hostility is the denominator common to both manic and depressive phases. Because of his rigid super-ego, the depressed patient does not permit himself to live out his hostile, aggressive tendencies against others but re-directs them against himself or expresses them in projected form. The influence of pathological feelings of guilt and of hostile impulses turned against the self may therefore find expression in suicide. The fact that feelings of guilt and self-accusation may be assuaged by attaching to others the motives that created them contributes to the paranoid features that may accompany depression. If the release of repressed impulses is particularly threatening, the depression may be accompanied by manifest expressions of anxiety.

The easiest and most natural way by which an ill-defined sense of guilt or of remorse may be rationalized and thereby find the required sense of reality in the consciousness of the patient is by linking it up with some trifling indiscretion of earlier life. This indiscretion is usually found to have been really trivial, although it never enjoyed full approval of the individual's socially determined conscience. All the energy of the affect, tied up with the repudiated wishes and material that have been repressed, usually with difficulty and for a long period, is displaced to this lapse and its ideational representation. This idea receives the displaced affect that both rationalizes and renders concrete the vague feeling of guilt arising from disowned strivings and desires.

Differential Diagnosis

The most difficult problem in the differential diagnosis of manic–depressive psychosis is its distinction from *schizophrenia*. In the typical case, this presents no difficulty, but in many cases there is doubt as to how symptoms should be interpreted. In general the disturbance in personality in manic–depressive psychoses seems to be a quantitative one, a matter of "too much" or "too little," rather than a lack of organization of personality, as in schizophrenia. There is not, moreover, complete agreement among psychiatrists as to how much temporary disorganization of the personality may be considered consistent with the diagnosis of manic–depressive psychosis, or as to how much diagnostic weight should be assigned different symptoms. Behavior may be equally disturbed in the manic excitement of an affective psychosis and in the catatonic excitement of schizophrenia.

In approaching the problem of differentiation, it is necessary first to secure as full a knowledge as possible as to the prepsychotic personality of the patient, to determine whether cyclothymic or schizoid characteristics have predominated, and whether psychobiological energy trends have been directed into extroverted channels and marked by objectivity and realism, or whether they have been of an introverted nature and characterized by subjectivity. In general, this interpersonal contact with the manic or depressive is more conventional and initially is perceived as a close one by the psychiatrist. With the schizophrenic, the interview is felt to be an uneasy one of distance, unfamiliarity, and suspicion. The presence of flight of ideas and of psychomotor activity in the early phases of a mental disorder may not constitute unequivocal diagnostic criteria, since both may exist in reactions that eventuate as schizophrenia. In schizophrenia, there tends to be more incoherence and greater poverty of ideas. The excitement of the schizophrenic lacks the depth of emotional expression that is usually observed in the excitement of the manic–depressive, is less influenced by the reality of the environment, is more episodic and impulsive, tends to be undirected, stereotyped, confined to a limited space, and determined more by hallucinations, delusions, and autistic processes. The more grotesque, and therefore the more primitive or highly symbolized, the ideas, the

more are they to be looked upon as schizophrenic.

The mood of the schizophrenic lacks both an infectious element and that component causing one to feel himself empathically into the position of the patient, who, in general, is less accessible than the manic depressive. The greater the harmony between mood, ideational content, and behavior, the more is a manic–depressive psychosis suggested, while the less the mental processes remain integrated, the more is schizophrenia denoted. Even though it may at first be temporary, the greater the disorganization of the personality, as shown by absence or inappropriateness of affect, by hallucinations, soiling, and apparent noninterpretability of behavior, the more does one expect an ultimate, and for the most part permanent, schizophrenic disorganization. The clinical picture of some young patients initially considered to be suffering from a manic phase of a manic–depressive psychosis changes to one that is clearly schizophrenic in nature. Finally, just as personalities are not cast in standardized molds, so we find there are all sorts of gradations between those reactions that we call schizophrenic and those that we call manic–depressive.

In the depressive phase, there occurs the customary disturbance of the sleep pattern, with early morning awakening and the morning aggravation of depressive affect, anorexia, weight loss, amenorrhea, and impotence. The physiological diminution of the rate of salivation and the low sedation threshold may be used as differential points.

Many hypomanics in whom the emotional exaltation is replaced by anger, resentment, irritability, irascibility, litigious tendencies, and perhaps paranoid delusions were formerly diagnosed as cases of acute *paranoia*. Such hypomanics lack the solitary and asocial tendency usually exhibited by the true paranoid, who presents a more sustained, brooding, sensitive, suspicious reaction pattern. Persons in whom these impure affects replace an exaltation are ones who, prior to their psychosis, were characterized by a tendency to defensive projections. Emotional difficulties may be a negligible factor in the development of an organic condition but a major one in recovery.

In early *syphilitic meningo-encephalitis,* the presenting symptoms may reflect previous personality trends and therefore suggest a manic–depressive psychosis. Neurological signs and serological tests will at once make a diagnosis possible.

The sense of inadequacy, abnormal fatigability, depressive ideas, and apprehension that may accompany mild forms of the depressive or mixed types, particularly in the early stages, are often misinterpreted as symptoms of *neurasthenia,* of a *compulsion neurosis,* or of an *anxiety state.* The more important points of differentiation between the manic–depressive psychosis and the psychoneuroses are enumerated in Chapter 23. In addition to what is there mentioned, it may be remarked that in manic–depressive psychosis, sluggishness of thought and action is more common, the patient is more reticent as to his feelings, and he does not show the eagerness to interview the physician usually seen in the psychoneuroses. Psychogenic causes and processes are usually more easily ascertained in psychoneuroses. Mild but often unrecognized forms of the depressive type are of frequent occurrence, with the result that the number of manic–depressives in extra-institutional life probably exceeds those under treatment in hospitals for mental disorders.

Prognosis and Course

It has already been indicated that the prognosis for a single affective episode is usually to be regarded as good but that recurrences are not uncommon. Perhaps there has been too great a tendency to stress the frequency of recurrence. Of manic–depressive admissions to state hospitals 55 per cent are first attacks, about 25 per cent second attacks, 9 per cent third, and 5 per cent have had more than three admissions.

Another important feature of manic–depressive psychosis is the fact that even repeated episodes usually leave the mind unchanged in its intellectual, affective, and conative aspects, and that a disorganization of the personality does not follow. Not a little of Ruskin's best work was done during his hypomanic states. Occasionally, after a series of attacks, the patient shows impairment of initiative and of judgment and becomes less able to deal with everyday affairs of life.

The most frequent age for the first manic episode is between 20 and 25 years. The average age of onset for first depressive attacks is about 10 years later. The earlier the onset of either type, the worse the prognosis for the occurrence of further episodes. If the first attack be manic in type, it almost certainly will not be the only one; if it be of a depressed type, it may not be followed by a recurrence. Some recent studies give indication that the prognosis is worse when the precipitation of illness is related directly to an actual loss (exogenous cause) than when it is due to covert experiences or factors (endogenous). This information is contrary to previous viewpoints and differs from data on the outcome of schizophrenic psychoses.

The patient's prepsychotic personality traits influence the prognosis as to both duration and outcome. If he has shown himself to be flexible, tolerant, conciliatory, without defensive, compensatory, or other signs of a deep sense of insecurity, and has had varied and wholesome interests, the prognosis is more favorable than if his personality patterns have been of the opposite type. As age increases, there is some tendency for attacks to be depressive rather than manic, perhaps because of the changing outlook on life. (See discussion of etiological factors in Chapter 23 entitled Involutional Psychotic Reactions.)

The duration of manic–depressive episodes is extremely variable. The average duration of untreated manic attacks may be estimated at six months and of depressive episodes at nine months. There is a tendency for depressions to increase in length with advancing age. Many depressions terminate with a brief hypomanic elation. The duration in individual cases may be either much shorter or much longer. One is never safe in predicting the probable duration of a given episode. Some patients may never have more than a single episode; in others a large part of the time may be occupied with recurring psychotic periods. The more frequent the attacks, the poorer the prognosis. The more chronic the illness, the less severe the symptoms. Depression is much more likely to become chronic than is mania. Chronic mania is uncommon before the age of 40. The prognosis is considered less favorable in depressions manifesting a nihilistic hypochondriasis, particularly if accompanied by anxiety.

Treatment

Depending upon the severity of the depressive or manic reaction and its influence upon the patient's capacity to function in his accustomed vocational and social life, initial therapeutic judgments must be made as to the wisdom of urging continuation of work or advising withdrawal, and whether to provide treatment at home or in a hospital environment.

The treatment of mild depressions may, in certain respects, constitute a greater problem than does the treatment of the deep depressions. The friends of the patient suffering from a mild episode of a manic–depressive nature often refuse to believe that he is suffering from a major mental disorder or that he may have suicidal tendencies.

Today, the mildly depressed may be initially treated with an antidepressant pharmaceutical. Of those available, imipramine (Tofranil) has proved to have the widest and most effective application. Given orally in divided doses of 75 to 300 mg. daily and supplemented with appropriate sedation for insomnia, it produces an effective response usually from 3 to 14 days after its initial administration. In other instances, one of the monamine oxidase inhibitors may be tried. The use of these agents and the complications attending their administration are described more fully in Chapter 33. With office or outpatient treatment, the patient should be seen on a schedule of fixed appointments at frequent intervals. A favorable response presents itself usually in a lessening of self-deprecatory and accusatory statements and hypochondriacal complaints, improvement in the sleeping pattern, increased activity, and interest in socialization. Many patients with mild depression may continue at work with treatment by the antidepressant pharmaceuticals.

If a significant change is not evident within two weeks of institution of pharmacologic therapy, consideration should be given to initiating electroshock without further delay.

In more severe cases, in which psychomotor retardation is of such a degree as to impair or make impossible the patient's usual vocational activities, the issue of hospitalization becomes immediately primary. Many families may be unwilling to accept the physician's opinion and advice; this should usually include a recommendation for the use of electroshock therapy. Although most physicians prefer that the patient be hospitalized during this form of therapy, some give treatments either at the patient's home or in the physician's office in the case of mild depressions. If there is little danger of suicide and the family is co-operative, treatment may be attempted at home. However, with the more severely ill, treatment at home is inadvisable unless skilled nursing services are available. An attempt on the part of the relatives to care for the patient is generally unwise, if for no other reason than that they usually either argue with him concerning his fears, constantly attempt to distract him, or urge the patient to rouse himself. With such patients, an organized program that fills the patient's day is desirable. This should be of a type which will not require spontaneity, close concentration, or strenuous activity. The program may include handicraft, walks, reading, games, social and recreational activities, and the encouragement of special aptitudes and interests. Although the patient should not be idle lest he become unduly pre-occupied with his problems and with self-examination, it should be borne in mind that a depressed patient, prompted by his life-long rigid requirements of self, may undertake too much and become more depressed when he finds he falls short of expected accomplishment. Many depressed patients complain of fatigue, but since this type of fatigue is really an expression of mood, it is not relieved by rest. One should remember that the depressed patient's tendency to hypochondriasis has at times led to unnecessary surgical operations. Unless carefully supervised, the depressed patient may not receive sufficient food.

In case of severe depression, treatment in a hospital is certainly wise. In nearly all cases, the use of electroshock therapy is accompanied by a gratifying improvement. Treatments are usually given three times a week. With many patients, 10 or 12 treatments are effective; others require twenty. Approximately 90 per cent of the depressed patients recover with this form of treatment.

If the patient is greatly agitated, chlorpromazine may be employed, either alone or in conjunction with other antidepressants or electroshock therapy, for its tranquilizing effect. He should not receive reserpine, since this drug frequently aggravates depressions.

It is highly important that the depressed patient receive a diet of high-caloric content. Usually it is desirable that he receive milk or additional food between meals. Refusal of food should not be permitted for more than 24 hours before resorting to lavage (tube-feeding). Sometimes after one feeding by this method the patient will, with a little assistance, eat voluntarily. It would doubtless be better if patients who must be tube-fed were to receive nourishment three times in 24 hours instead of twice, as is the practice in many hospitals.

The tube through which the food is introduced may be passed either through the nose or through the mouth. Usually the co-operation of the patient is not sufficient to make the latter route practicable, and so the feeding is most frequently made through the nose, a nasal tube being employed. Feeding in this manner is not devoid of danger. Occasionally death from pneumonia or from gangrene of the lung occurs; this may result from a particle of food having passed into the bronchi during tube-feeding. During the feeding, the patient may lie on a bed in the supine position, or he may sit upright in a chair. Usually the former position is better. In either case, care should be taken to see that the neck is not extended, as the tube is liable to enter the larynx when the neck is in that position. If the patient is resistive, two nurses should assist, each holding a forearm to prevent his seizing the tube. The head may be held by folding a towel about it and grasping it on either side. The tube is lubricated, introduced into the nares, and passed directly backward, not upward. It will often be found that, because of a deviated septum, one side of the nose offers an easier passage than the other.

Sometimes, as the tube passes the pharynx, it is forced forward and becomes doubled up in the mouth. In such a case, it must be nearly withdrawn and again passed. If the tube enters the larynx, choking and coughing are, of course, produced, and air is expelled from the tube. After the tube has been introduced to a distance of about 18 inches, it is well to let the patient rest a moment and to note if he is breathing freely and normally. A little water is then poured into the funnel. If this flows without obstruction and without disturbing the patient's respirations, the food to be given is slowly poured into the funnel and allowed to pass to the stomach by gravity. After all the food has been given, it is well to withdraw the tube an inch or two and pour a little water into the funnel to remove any bits of food remaining near the end of the tube. The tube is then pinched to prevent dripping of any food as the end passes over the larynx; at the same time, it is withdrawn by a quick movement.

A feeding may consist of 24 ounces of

milk or of malted milk, ½ ounce of butter, ½ ounce of cod liver oil, 1 ounce of orange juice, 2 eggs, and 1½ ounces of sugar. Fruit juices, apple sauce, thin cereals, mashed potatoes, and thin vegetable soups may be added to the feeding. Sometimes patients attempt to regurgitate the food given. Such patients should be made to lie quietly on their backs for a period after they have been fed.

Occasionally the hospital physician finds that for a considerable period before admission a patient has not been receiving sufficient food or water. His tongue is dry and leathery, his breath is foul, he appears dehydrated and has a slight tendency to acidosis. In these patients, special effort must be made to have them receive an abundance of fluid. In depressive stupors, attention should be paid to the condition of the bladder and the bowels.

The danger of suicide must be constantly borne in mind, a fact that should be impressed upon both nurse and family. Suicide is more frequent in patients who have shown tension and anxiety. The history of a suicide in the family increases the possibility that the depressed patient may end his life. It is not unusual for a patient to repeat a previous unsuccessful suicidal attempt.

Among the early signs of recovery is a return of self-confidence and initiative. As convalescence proceeds, there should be a gradually increasing participation in occupational and recreational activities. The patient should be relieved of the necessity for making decisions until he is well on the road to recovery. An early resumption of usual duties and responsibilities is to be discouraged. The question as to when the convalescing depressed patient may be dismissed from the hospital is not always easy. The usual opinion is that he should remain in an institution with its simple routine until convalescence is well established. It must be remembered, too, that, because of the increased danger of suicide during convalescence, the patient may require closer supervision during that period than is possible at home. On the other hand, a return home before the depression is entirely cured may sometimes hasten the patient's recovery. He should not resume full duties for several weeks.

MANIA. The question whether the mild forms of excitement or hypomania should be treated in a hospital is not always easy. In the case of the hypomanic, it is often evident to the psychiatrist that prudence requires more control of the patient's activities than is possible in the home. Since, however, there is nothing "unpsychological" in his behavior, the patient's relatives frequently fail either to accept the statement that his exuberance of spirits, pressure of activity, and volubility are evidence of mental disorder, or to appreciate the embarrassment to themselves and the aggravation of the psychosis that may result from the absence of restraining measures. For these reasons, they are frequently averse to the patient's admission to a mental hospital. They often believe that the only requirement for treatment is a change of scenery or an urging of the patient to rouse himself.

The apparently exhaustless energy of the hypomanic may suggest that an outlet for it should be provided. The physician should remember, however, that fatigue produces not tranquility but excitement. The usual desire for almost constant activity must therefore be curbed, although with the production of as little irritation as possible. The hypomanic patient must be protected from his tendency to enter into unwise business or financial schemes. Careful supervision of the patient who is not hospitalized may be necessary lest an increase in sex drive lead to regrettable indulgences. Frequently the prepsychotic personality of the manic has been characterized by a sensitive pride. The physician will therefore carefully guard against the contradictions and arguments that the hypomanic's irritability, unrestrained speech, activity, and resentment at interference with his wishes are prone to provoke.

Generally speaking, chlorpromazine is the therapeutic measure of choice for the treatment of the overactive manic patient; shock therapy, for the treatment of the depressed patient. If the manic patient is so overactive and dehydrated that quick results are desired, chlorpromazine may be administered intramuscularly, but a change to oral administration is soon made. (See Chapter 33.)

Many physicians prefer electroshock therapy to chlorpromazine in the treatment of the overactive manic patient. Sometimes, if the manic patient shows extreme psychomotor activity, he may be given electroshock treatments twice a day for three or four days. This results in considerable confusion, and the frequency of treatments should soon be reduced to three per week. Episodic recurrences of the manic–depressive psychoses are not prevented by electroshock therapy, and the duration of symptom-free intervals is not made shorter by reason of its use.

Highly effective control of chronic and recurrent mania has been reported by the oral administration of 300 mg. capsules of lithium carbonate given four to seven times weekly. The serum lithium concentration must be maintained below levels of 2 mEq per liter, which may be measured with the use of a flame photometer. Lithium therapy is reported to be effective in patients not responding to the phenothiazines and electroshock but without value in the treatment of the depressive phase of the cyclic reaction. However, it may be continued during the depressive phase. Due to its high toxicity for kidney function, it is contraindicated when the function of this organ is impaired, or in heart disease, epilepsy, and the elderly. The most common minor toxic symptom is a fine tremor of the hands. The drug should be withdrawn if diarrhea or vomiting ensue or if tremulousness is very severe and associated with drowsiness, ataxia, or dizziness. Other symptoms of intoxication are thirst and a large output of urine indicating the presence of diabetes.

PSYCHOTHERAPY. This form of treatment has been employed successfully in the treatment of the mild depressive and hypomanic states; some physicians are attempting to examine its usefulness as a preventive for recurrent or cyclic attacks.

Psychiatrists vary greatly in the extent to which they employ psychoanalytical principles in their therapy. Those who use them to only a slight extent may, through a biographical review and by asking the patient to talk freely about significant life events and his reactions to them, analyze the patient's emotional development during infancy, childhood, and adult life. In this way, dynamic factors may be discovered and discussed and an evaluation may be made of the various factors and situations that may have contributed to the specific organization of the patient's personality. Largely by questions that promote their consideration, the patient is encouraged to examine critically definite situations and reactions and their underlying factors. The psychiatrist so guides the therapeutic interviews that the patient discovers and recognizes for himself the factors and situations that have contributed to the disturbance of his personality and behavior. He then synthesizes, or builds up into a logical formulation and relationship, the elements and influences that have been operative in producing these disturbances. It is the hope of the therapist that, through this formulation and a proper evaluation of these different factors, the patient may acquire such a constructive understanding of himself, his assets, shortcomings, and handicaps that a greater inner harmony and a less disturbing environmental adjustment may follow.

Efforts have been made to treat the manic–depressive patient by classical psychoanalytical techniques. It has usually been found that neither the retarded nor the hyperactive patient lends himself to the rigid routine of the customary psychoanalytical process. New efforts have made it evident, however, that modified analytically-oriented psychotherapy is possible for some patients and seems to be beneficial.

Experience indicates that it is not advisable for the psychotherapeutic interviews with the depressed patient to be held four or five times a week, as is frequently to be recommended in the case of the schizophrenic or often with the neurotic. Interviews, with their implied insistence that the patient be productive, held more frequently than once or twice a week seem to cause him to exaggerate his shame and guilt. Because of the high personal standards that the depressive requires of himself, and because of his feelings of impotence and incapacity, therapy may be very difficult if the psychiatrist urges productiveness. Because of his feelings of guilt and shame, the patient is unable to express his underlying sadness and rage. Since he is unable to meet the demands that he feels the therapist expects, pressure by the latter arouses additional feelings of hatred and shame. The therapist does not, however, adopt the passive role usually followed in a more classical form of psychoanalysis.

Other features of this modified analysis are a constant reassurance of the patient that he will recover and a certain directness and openness in dealing with his problems. It will be remembered that in his depression the patient is overreacting emotionally to an actual or fantasied loss of a love object. He is therefore seeking another, or substitute, love object. The process of calm reassurance fits this need symbolically. The patient has also a need to escape from the feelings of guilt caused by his repressed rage in his depression. If, therefore, he reports events that seem to be conducive to the production of rage and anger within himself but has not expressed their emotional connotation, the therapist may verbalize such feelings and state their relationship to other persons involved in the patient's situation. In this way the patient is relieved of the burden of stating his rage or anger and is not exposed to subsequent feelings of guilt for expressing the forbidden emotions. With this elastic, nondemanding, and at the same time, active, interpretive approach, it is at times possible to abort depressions. Some therapists suggest it is better initially to have the depressed patient focus on an experience of recent loss rather than to encourage him to recall the earlier events and interpersonal experiences in his life that determined or reinforced his depressive symptomatology. Dream productions in the depressed patient are often helpful in breaking through to deep-seated associations that give a clearer understanding of his basic longings and conflicts.

Psychotherapy with the hypomanic or manic is difficult. Since such a patient usually identifies with a covertly aggressive, sadistic, and successful member of the family, the therapist must constantly guard against the provocation of rejecting a patient whose behavior seems designed for such a purpose, i.e., of embarrassing significant object relations. It is generally agreed that the conversion of manic or hypomanic symptoms to depressive ones is desirable. Sometimes this is effected by the therapist's simply indicating his doubts as to the soundness of the patient's presumption that he has reason to behave as if he were successful or in control of the situation.

Psychotherapeutically the aim of treatment of patients with the manic–depressive syndrome is to bring them to the point where they can consciously face periodic loneliness and separation without resorting either to submissive depression or revengeful overactivity.

BIBLIOGRAPHY

Bellak, L.: Manic–Depressive Psychosis. New York, Grune & Stratton, 1951.

Busfield, B. L., Jr., and Wechsler, H.: Studies of salivation in depression. Arch Gen. Psych., 4:10–15, 1961.

Campbell, J. D.: Manic–depressive disease in children. J.A.M.A., 158:154–157, 1955.

Freyhan, F. A.: The modern treatment of depressive disorders. Am. J. Psychiat., 116:1057–1064, 1960.

Gibson, R. W., Cohen, M. B., and Cohen, R. A.: On the dynamics of the manic–depressive personality. Am. J. Psychiat., 115:1101–1107, 1959.

Gottlieb, G., and Paulson, G. S.: Salivation in depressed patients. Arch. Gen. Psychiat., 5:468–477, 1961.

Havens, L. L.: Losses and depressions. The relationship of precipitating events to outcome. J. Nerv. & Ment. Dis., 125:627–636, 1957.

Hendin, H.: Suicide. Psychiatric Quart., 30:267–282, 1956.

Kallmann, F. J.: Genetic principles in manic–depressive psychosis. In Hoch, P. H., and Zubin, J. (Eds.) Depression. Proc. 42nd Annual Meet. Am. Psychopath. Asso. New York, Grune & Stratton, 1954, pp. 1–24.

Kolb, L. C.: Psychotherapeutic evolution and its implications. Psychiatric Quart., 30:579–597, 1956.

Kraepelin, E.: Manic–Depressive Insanity and Paranoia. Translated by Barclay, E. Edinburgh, E. and S. Livingstone, 1921.

Landolt, A. B.: Follow-up studies on circular manic–depressive reactions occurring in the young. Bull. N. Y. Acad. Med., 2nd ser., 33: 65–73, 1957.

Lewin, B. D.: The Psychoanalyses of Elation. New York, W. W. Norton & Co., Inc., 1950.

Lorenz, M.: Language behavior in manic patients. Arch. Neurol. & Psychiat., 69:14–26, 1953.

McHarg, J. F.: Mania in childhood. Arch. Neurol. & Psychiat., 72:531–539, 1954.

Norris, A. A., and Clancy, J.: Hospitalized depressions: drugs or electrotherapy? Arch. Gen. Psych., 5:276–270, 1961.

Nymgaard, K.: Studies on the sedation threshold. A.M.A. Arch. Gen. Psychiat., 1:530–536, 1959.

Parnell, R. W., and Skottowe, I.: Towards preventing suicide. Lancet, 1:206–208, 1957.

Rennie, T. A. C.: Prognosis in manic–depressive psychoses. Am. J. Psychiat., 98:801, 1942.

Schou, M.: Lithium in psychiatric therapy. Psychopharmacologia, 1:65–78, 1959.

Shagass, C., et al.: An objective test which differentiates between neurotic and psychotic depression. A.M.A. Arch. Neur. Psych., 75: 461–471, 1956.

Zetzel, E., Nacht, S., and Recamier, D. C.: Symposium on depressive illness. Int. J. Psychoanal., 41:476–496, 1960.

Chapter Twenty-five

PSYCHOTIC DISORDERS

SCHIZOPHRENIC REACTIONS

Although it is relatively easy to describe some of the more striking psychopathology of the schizophrenic reactions, no definition of this mental illness has yet received universal assent. It is one of the commonest of the serious mental disorders, but its essential nature is probably the least understood. Because of the heterogeneity of the manifestations, it may be more accurate to speak of the group of schizophrenias rather than to think of each group of disordered reaction as a single disease entity. There is, therefore, an increasing inclination to think of schizophrenia as a term for a number of somewhat similar patterns of reactions to life situations that the individual has found too difficult to meet.

Symptomatically, the schizophrenic reactions are recognizable through odd and bizarre behavior apparent in aloofness, suspiciousness, or periods of impulsive destructiveness and immature and exaggerated emotionality, often ambivalently directed and considered inappropriate by the observer. The interpersonal perceptions are distorted in the more serious states by delusional and hallucinatory material. In the most disorganized forms of schizophrenic living, withdrawal into a fantasy life takes place and is associated with profound habit deteriorations

in which the usual social customs and personal care are disregarded.

It is generally considered that the schizophrenic personality is incapable of effectively harmonizing his drives and inhibitions through mature adaptations and defenses. He has failed to develop a satisfying concept of his body and a clear or stable self-concept and is deficient in his capacity to assess clearly the realities of the world. Interactions with others are characterized by immature processes of communication and adaptation.

In psychoanalytic terms, the schizophrenics represent those who have failed, due to either somatic or psychogenic forces, to evolve the ego integrative processes or strengths necessary to resolve flexibly conflicts between their (id) drives and over-demanding superego attitudes and aspirations. They are thus defective in the capacity to adapt to the social demands confronting them and to their own drives and they thereby lack a harmonious self-concept and ego ideal with clear goals and motivations. Much of their adaptation is made, instead, through partially satisfying regressive or fixated infantile behavior.

History of Schizophrenia

Although not so called, the clinical picture we now know as schizophrenia has long been recognized. In 1849 John

Conolly (1794–1866) of Hanwell Asylum in England, the champion of "no restraint," stated in his Croonian Lectures: "Young persons not infrequently fall into a state somewhat resembling melancholia, without any discoverable cause of sorrow, and certainly without any specific grief; they become indolent or pursue their usual occupations or recreations mechanically and without interest; the intellect, the affections, the passions, all seem inactive or deadened and the patients become utterly apathetic."

The term dementia praecox (démence précoce) was first used by the Belgian psychiatrist Morel in 1860 in the case of a boy of 14 who previously had always been "first in his examinations, and that without effort and almost without study. . . . Unconsciously he lost his cheerfulness and became sober, taciturn, and showed a tendency to solitude." The boy showed a "state of melancholy depression and a hatred of his father even with the idea of killing him. . . . The young invalid progressively forgot all that he had learned, and his brilliant intellectual faculties entered into a very disturbing period of arrest. A kind of inactivity bordering on stupidity replaced his former activity and when I saw him again it looked as if a transition into an irrecoverable state of dementia praecox was taking place."

Morel interpreted this disorganization of personality as an arrest of development, to be included with mental deficiency as a "variety of intellectual, physical and moral degeneracy" resulting from heredity.

The next step in the history of dementia praecox was Hecker's description in 1871 of *hebephrenia*, although the term had previously been used by Kahlbaum. "The characteristic features of hebephrenia," wrote Hecker, "above all are: its appearance in connection with puberty, the succession or changing appearance of various forms (melancholia, mania and confusion), the very quick termination in a psychic enfeeblement and a characteristic form of final deterioration the evidences of which can be seen in the first stages of the disease." He considered hebephrenia to be a progressive disease of puberty and adolescence.

Another step in the development of the dementia praecox concept was the description of *catatonia*, or "*tension insanity*," by Kahlbaum in 1874. He described catatonia as "that condition in which the patient sits quietly or completely mute and motionless, immovable, with a staring countenance, the eyes fixed on a distant point and apparently completely without volition, without any reaction to sensory impressions, sometimes with a full fledged cerea flexibilitas as in catalepsy." Kahlbaum assumed that catatonia was the symptom of a structural brain disease.

In 1896 Kraepelin offered the proposition that a common denominator exists among such apparently unrelated syndromes as the hebephrenia of Hecker, the catatonia of Kahlbaum, and many paranoid psychoses. By defining dementia praecox as a distinct syndrome, he introduced order into what had been a clinical chaos so far as observation and classification had been concerned.

In 1906 Adolf Meyer began to develop the thesis that dementia praecox is not a disease entity but rather a type of reaction developing in certain personalities as a result of progressive difficulty in adaptation and that the accumulation of faulty habits of reaction lead to a "habit deterioration."

Another landmark in the history of dementia praecox was the introduction by Eugen Bleuler (1857–1939) in 1911 of the term "*schizophrenia*." Following Bleuler's suggestion, there has been an increasing tendency to supplant the designation *dementia praecox* by the name *schizophrenia* (splitting of the mind), since the disharmony or "split" of the psychobiological expression of the organism that we call mind, and the breaking up of a former normal synthesis of thought, feeling, and activity, are now considered more characteristic and distinctive of the reaction than are symptom-complex and outcome as stressed by Kraepelin.

Conceptions of Schizophrenia

Since present conceptions of schizophrenia are largely based upon the formulations of Kraepelin, Bleuler, Meyer, and Freud, a brief presentation of their respective formulations is added.

Kraepelin was not interested in the psychological meaning of the symptoms of dementia praecox, but through his keen observations he gave an excellent clinical description of the disorder and classified it into types (simple, hebephrenic, catatonic, and paranoid). Bleuler and Meyer, on the other hand, greatly advanced the psychiatric understanding of schizophrenia by their interpretation in dynamic terms of the symptomatic manifestations observed.

KRAEPELIN'S FORMULATIONS. As previously indicated, Kraepelin brought together varied mental syndromes that he concluded were manifestations of a single disease entity. To these he gave the name *dementia praecox*, a term previously having a more limited application. He thought these clinical syndromes arose from the same disease process, since they had in common the following features: a beginning in adolescence or early adulthood; a progression toward a similar state of "dementia." Similar morbid processes were, Kraepelin assumed, the causes of the various clinical features. These causes, he believed, might be either a degenerative disease of the brain or metabolic disturbances that produced autointoxication. He believed, too, that injury to the germ plasm might be of significance in its development. Kraepelin was of the opinion that the clinical results of these processes consisted of a weakening of emotional and volitional reactions and a loss of harmonious connections among emotional, volitional, and intellectual reactions. He gave an extremely comprehensive and lucid description of the clinical features of dementia praecox but was critical of any attempt to explain the behavior of the patient on a psychological basis.

BLEULER'S FORMULATIONS. From 1885 to 1897, Bleuler spent many hours each day at the mental hospital in Rheinau, Switzerland, studying individual patients in an effort to understand what, through their symptoms, they were saying or doing. He came to the conclusion that it was misleading to compare even the extreme deterioration of what Kraepelin called dementia praecox with the state of mind of the mentally defective or with that of organic deterioration caused by severe brain atrophy. Therefore the label "dementia praecox" could no longer be considered satisfactory. He pointed out, too, that the patient's psychological reactions to his environment are very complicated and differentiated, quite different in kind from the elementary, simple reactions of feeble-minded persons and those with organic brain disease. Bleuler believed, therefore, that the disease was not one of *de*-mentia, a state of diminished mind, but a disharmonious state of mind in which most contradictory tendencies, thoughts, and potentialities existed together, so that the harmony of the personality was split. According to this conception, the outcome of the disease was not necessarily one of deterioration, as Kraepelin had maintained, and the diagnosis had nothing to do with the course of the disease. Bleuler was the first to point out that it was not only interesting but extremely important to consider seriously and from a scientific point of view the content of the patient's thoughts, of his trends, of his instincts, and of everything that he did. He noticed that if the patient's hallucinations and delusions were thoroughly studied, they could be brought in connection with his life history, with his early hopes and fears, and with his early relationships with parents and siblings.

Prior to Bleuler's time, it was believed that every mental symptom was caused by an underlying physical disorder. Psychological symptoms, such as delusions, hallucinations, mannerisms, and catatonic musculature signs had been looked at in the same way as aphasia, apraxia, or reflex disturbances. Influenced by the firm and prevailing belief that all psychoses, and even neuroses, were of somatic origin, Bleuler hesitated to conclude that all the morbid manifestations in schizophrenia, or that schizophrenia itself, was of a functional nature and could be understood psychologically. He therefore distinguished between primary and secondary symptoms. He designated as primary signs those that he considered were the direct manifestations of a hypothetical somatic morbid process. As primary signs he included a peculiar loosening of the associational links in thinking, a morbid ambitendence and ambivalence that dominated the affective life of the patient, and a tendency to replace reality by fantasy, a quality that was responsible for the various manifestations of autism. Among the secondary symptoms, or those that he believed were of psychic origin, were delusions explainable by the patient's frustrations and hopes, a part of the hallucinations, the mannerisms, the catatonic muscular symptoms, and a large part of the complicated attitudes that others had called deterioration or dementia. He believed that the secondary symptoms were attempts at adaptation to the primary disturbance.

After Bleuler had become convinced of the importance of psychological influences in the morbid picture of schizophrenia, it became clear to him that the disorder should be treated by psychotherapy. He stressed that a sound, strong, and personal relationship between nurse and patient and between physician and patient would exercise a beneficial therapeutic influence on the latter.

In 1897 Bleuler left Rheinau and became professor of psychiatry in Zurich and director of the Burghöltzli Clinic. Here Bleuler and his first assistant, Carl Jung, became acquainted with Freud, who spent a period at Zurich. As a result, Bleuler developed a great interest in psychoanalysis at a time when few psychiatrists had accepted Freud's teachings. He concluded that, to a large extent, schizophrenic symptoms could be understood by the same symbolization that Freud had discovered in dreams and in neurotic developments. Bleuler's conceptions of schizophrenia and the descriptions of his observations were published in 1912. An English translation, *Dementia Praecox or the Group of Schizophrenias*, was published in 1950. Although Meyer, probably justifiably, criticized Bleuler's conception of schizophrenia as assuming an unwarranted dualism of mind and body, this monograph is nevertheless one of the classics of psychiatry.

MEYER'S FORMULATION. Meyer's more dynamic conception of schizophrenia and his naturalistic behavioral approach in its formulation appeared earlier than Bleuler's work. His views were first presented in a symposium on dementia praecox at a meeting of the British Medical Association at Toronto in 1906. He emphasized the clinical picture of schizophrenia, not as an autonomous disease entity, but as a maladaptation logically understandable in terms of the patient's experiences and life history. He emphasized the concepts of habit deterioration and of reaction types. The schizophrenic reaction, he believed, can best be understood as a habit disorganization resulting from a progressive maladaptation, in which there takes place "a substitution of inefficient and faulty attempts to avoid difficulties rather than to meet them by decisive action." The result is disorganization of the personality and final withdrawal from reality. Many of the clinical symptoms represent abortive and "twisted" attempts at balance and reconstruction. He expressed the opinion that the failure to find any structural or physiological changes in neurons excludes an organic etiology, although he believed that an inferior constitution as well as a great variety of pathologic conditions of a physical nature may add to the individual's load of handicaps.

Meyer was one of the first to emphasize that the interest should be not so much in a classificatory diagnosis as in the facts and factors at work in the individual patient and in his assets. Although admiring Kraepelin's description of the reaction, Meyer did not subscribe to his invariably unfavorable prognosis of a progressive intellectual deterioration. As schizophrenic reactions, Meyer would include "disturbances developing in particular constitutional types and expressed in vague, autistic fancy, projections, passivity, paranoid systemization, formal disorders of language and behavior, incongruity of affect and motivity disturbances." He further described schizophrenic reactions as "twists and fundamental or fancy-born incongruities more or less foreign to average, mature, waking life." Because of the close identification of the term schizophrenia with dementia praecox, Meyer preferred the term "parergasia," meaning thereby distorted or "twisted" behavior, performance, or psychobiologically integrated behavior. While etymologically descriptive, this designation has not been generally adopted. His formulation of schizophrenia has contributed greatly to a dispelling of the artificial dichotomy of mind and body and to the establishment of the proposition that mental disorder is a function of biological behavior.

At the present time, the concepts of Kraepelin, Meyer, Bleuler, and Freud are all considered inadequate. There exists a number of new working hypotheses, which will be discussed under the section on etiology.

Epidemiology

The schizophrenic psychoses are recognized in all cultures in which mental disorders have been subjected to thorough study. Cultural forces appear only to modify the clinical phenomenology of these reactions in terms of the content of delusional and hallucinatory material. Thus in Western society, religious and sexual delusions were more common a century ago than in the present. These psychoses occur in all socio-economic strata, although several epidemiological studies have suggested a correlation between higher prevalence of illness and lower socio-economic status.

At this time the schizophrenics are the most prevalent of the major psychoses and constitute now approximately 25 per cent of the first admissions to public mental hospitals in the United States. Due to the chronicity of these reactions, some 60 per cent of the population of state hospitals is made up of patients

with this syndrome. Calculations made from various epidemiological surveys give the morbid risk for the syndrome as 1 per cent. Morbid risk is defined as the total risk of becoming manifestly ill for all persons surviving the age period of 15 to 45 years, when the disease is customarily recognized.

Etiology

In the light of current knowledge, there is reason to believe that the schizophrenic reaction represents a syndrome dependent upon the complex interplay of various biological and social forces. For the individual patient, at best one may identify from the life history one or several forces as most significant for schizophrenic maldevelopment of personality. Among the major influences considered to determine the occurrence of schizophrenia are genetic forces, qualitative deficiencies in the mother–infant relationship, the nature of the later family transactions and psychodynamics, and the social opportunities and stresses outside the family in successive periods of development.

Genetic studies have shown with consistency that if one member of a family is schizophrenic, the risk for siblings and children approximates the range of 7 to 16 per cent, and for parents, 5 to 10 per cent. In families with two affected parents, the risk is calculated at 40 per cent for their children. The most impressive evidence for the influence of a genetic factor is the statistical data of Kallmann obtained from his extensive studies of twins. Kallmann found that if the disorder exists in one of monozygotic twins, it occurs also in the other twin in 85.8 per cent of the cases. However, the expectancy for a dizygotic twin partner is 14 per cent, equivalent to that of siblings. Kallmann interprets his findings to indicate there exists a genetic predisposition to schizophrenia. Among geneticists there is no unanimity of opinion as to the exact mode of inheritance.

Kallmann is of the opinion that the development of schizophrenia takes place only in a predisposed individual as the result of a complex interplay of later constitutional and environmental factors. Various criticisms have been given to studies of twins. It has been pointed out that such studies lack information on the early family experiences of the twins and have not weighed the psychodynamic forces in twin development that are believed to tend towards mutual identification between twins rather than for the growth of separate identities. Until the present there has not been available a sufficient number of instances of well-studied schizophrenics in a monozygotic twin pair separated at birth and reared in different families to distinguish between the relative importance of the genetic factor and that of the family in the evolution of psychosocial maturation. Nor has sufficient emphasis been placed upon studies of those factors that protect one of a monozygotic twin pair from schizophrenia in at least 15 per cent of the cases. It may be expected that important insights would come from examination of the supportive environmental factors useful in reducing the risk of the reaction in the spared twin.

That genetic or constitutional weaknesses exist is suggested as well by data indicating that schizophrenic mothers have a higher incidence of deviant fetal growth in terms of perinatal mortality and malformations in the newborn than mothers from the population at large. Also, careful physical and psychological investigations of groups of children considered to have childhood schizophrenia have shown that a majority present in their motor, postural, sensoriperceptual and conceptual performances indications of delayed or uneven functioning. These impairments are described in greater detail later in this chapter in relation to childhood schizophrenia. Whether these impairments are due to delays in maturation as a consequence of a defect in genetic endowment or to unrecognized brain damage in early life has not been ascertained. Some would exclude from the schizophrenic reactions all children showing such defects.

The range of such impairments in the conditions designated as childhood schizophrenia is wide; a considerable number shows very little evidence of early retardation in development of sensorimotor, perceptual, and conceptual deficit. However, in cases in which studies have been made of the family unit and its functioning, it appears that gross personality disturbances in parents are more likely to be associated with minimal impairment of physiologic growth of the child, and minimal pathology in the parents is found to be associated with maximal physiological retardation in the schizophrenic child. The family transactions induced by the interplay between the child's capacities determined by his physiological equipment and the expectations of the parents then appear to play an important role in the achievement of a healthy unfolding of personality and in the arrest or inadequate development of ego attitudes and functions. Thus a child who, as the result of delayed maturation of motor development, fails to acquire skill in language, walking, and other coordinated movements may set up anxieties in certain parents with high expectancies and investment in his future that are reflected in the parental relationship, the parents pushing the child beyond his capacities while, at the same time, overprotecting him. In other children, without evidence of physiologic deficit, it has been postulated that the parental investment in the child is disturbed from the beginning, as the child represents an expected source for emotional satisfaction, or the living out of gratifications not obtained in life by one or other of the parents. From the studies of childhood schizophrenics, a wide spectrum of disturbed family interactions has been postulated.

Psychoanalytic theory has held that the earliest periods of mother–infant relationship must be deficient, since the adult pathology of the schizophrenic suggests a regressive withdrawal to infantile emotional behavior in the omnipotent behavior, infantile rage reaction, and inability to perceive reality. In partial support of this hypothesis, there exists now only one limited naturalistic study of the mothering process in schizophrenics. Sobel found that the mothering process was impaired in a few schizophrenic women by their affective depression. Such women did not play with and fondle their infants as do other mothers, although they did carry out well the usual procedures for nurturence and bodily cleanliness of the child. Their infants, in turn, appeared irritable and depressed. If such observations are corroborated, it is probable that the restriction of affective and playful stimulation of the infant impedes the development of those early sensations that establish the body percept and the beginnings of ego attitudes of security, trust, and aggressiveness, upon which must unfold the capacities for self-control and later autonomous independence.

It is unlikely that disturbances in the early mothering process alone are capable of explaining the full range of schizophrenic psychopathology, such as the impaired sense of identity often associated with a confused sexual role, the lack of ability to discriminate fantasy from reality, and the defective interpersonal communication processes. These failures of development are more likely to rest on later deficiencies or distortions in the process of personality development.

From the various studies of family dynamics of the past decade, it has been found with significant frequency that schizophrenic patients have spent their childhood in seriously disturbed family groups in which both parents gave evidence of personality disturbance. In the Lidz studies, two-thirds of the families contained one parent who was found to be schizophrenic. Such family groups are unintegrated and relate through conflict in which the parents oppose each other by derogating and defying the wishes of the spouse and by efforts to win the children to their side to obtain from them the emotional support not found in the spouse. In other families, the parental relationship is disordered in that one parent has a serious personality deficit, shown in domineering, brutal,

aggressive, or alcoholic behavior, while the other passively accepts his behavior or is absent when the child is exposed to an unwholesome environment. Such parents often are doubtful of their own sexual roles, some have been homosexual, and others were in conflict over control of incestuous desires.

Caught in such family groups, the children are unable to find those conflict-free periods of personal interactions and play that establish a sense of personal security, ability to share, and to repress effectively hostile, aggressive, and sexual drives. Nor do they find the sources of sound personal or sexual identification. But most important for the understanding of the schizophrenic reaction are the series of events that impair the evolution of mature communication and thought.

Bateson put forward the hypothesis that the origins of the schizophrenic defects in communication rests upon a "double bind" transaction between two persons. Thus the schizophrenic may be seen as fixed in an intense emotional relationship with a parent who, by the contradictions between her verbal remarks and behavior, makes it impossible for the former to discriminate properly or to respond for clarification, as his questioning is treated as a threat to the needed relationship by the parent. A concrete example is a schizophrenic adolescent who, tied to his mother verbally, is encouraged to use initiative in his school work, yet when he attempts to leave the home to visit the library, he is told he must not do so as the parent needs him and will become ill in his absence. Such a "double bind" restricts and confuses the development of clear communication, since the parent's position is inconsistent and also limits the son's helpful socialization with others, from which he might learn progressive social discriminations and develop the potentiality for evolving other healthy relations. Whether the "double bind" is characteristic of schizophrenic families alone or has special features for such families is not known.

Others have also been struck by the

family milieu as the source of the irrationality of thought of the schizophrenic.
Johnson describes the process as taking
place dynamically in that the growing
child repeatedly has been the recipient
of intrafamilial hostility and at the same
time has identified with parents who
themselves excessively use projection,
denial, or conscious lying in their relations within the family. Upon this background there are often found discrete
assaults upon the child, aggressive or
sexual acts, that the child must deny and
repress in order to preserve his dependent
relationship with the parent. Later the
parent reinforces the child's fear and
guilt by utilizing subsequent incidents to
establish the child's responsibility for the
earlier trauma and to escape from his own
culpability. Thus the mounting denial
and repression of his own internalized
rage leads eventually to breakdown, with
psychotic withdrawal or impulsive sexual
and murderous aggressive acts.

The origins of the shyness, limited
sociability, and shut-in life of the preschizophrenic seem to rest in their own
feelings of insecurity as well as in the
needed dependent position they hold in
the life of one or both parents. Failure
to acquire social skills early narrows the
probability of acquisition of emotional
relations with extrafamily members in
adolescence and adulthood; this again
limits the probability of enhancing the
personal skills and perceptual discriminations and sense of personal autonomy
demanded for an effective social and
heterosexual adaptation in adult life.

Although many hypotheses have been
put forward relative to constitutional, metabolic, endocrine, and neurophysiological
factors that might influence or determine
the etiology of schizophrenia, modern
methods of investigation have yet to provide any significant data that have received corroboration, aside from those
genetic studies mentioned previously.

Onset

The age of onset is from late childhood
to late middle age, although the most
frequent age is adolescence and early

adult life. Although uncommon, it is not
so rare in children (3 to 13 years) as
was formerly believed. The more fully
the previous history is taken, the more
frequently there will be found a previous
manifestation not merely of schizoid
traits, but even of phenomena that were
nearly or quite psychotic in nature. The
high incidence during adolescence is not
unnatural.

There is probably, however, no specific
relationship between schizophrenia and
puberty, which is normally a period of
turbulence, of emotional cross-currents
and of struggle to adapt emergent, maturing urges to the demands of a restraining world. At that time, the individual is
precipitated into a critical emotional
period without preparation or understanding. He is perplexed by new problems, particularly those pertaining to
sex, religion, vocation, and social relations. He may be plagued by a desire for
independence or crippled by a too prolonged dependence. Self-consciousness,
sensitiveness, moodiness, vague yearnings,
sudden outbursts, defensive attitudes, the
tendency to indulge in strange fancies, to
project inadequacies, and to be irritable
are traits often particularly marked in
adolescence, and frequently, especially in
its early course, similar characteristics are
met with in schizophrenia.

Psychopathology

Although there is a striking contrast
between a normal, well-integrated individual and the person reacting with a
malignant form of schizophrenic psychosis, there is frequently no abrupt transition from the schizoid type of personality
to the manifest psychosis. Certain dishar-
monies of thought, of habits, and of interests may have long existed. In adolescence there may have been a tendency
to loneliness and perhaps to slight depressions. Colorfulness of personality may
seem to have been lost. There may have
been a vagueness of thinking, a blandness
of affect, a tendency to projection of
topics touching a special personal sensitivity and perhaps a tendency to be jealous of those more happily adjusted. Even

the person in the so-called "early" stage of schizophrenia has frequently been mentally sick for a considerable period before reaching the mental hospital, although the patient's family has not usually appreciated the nature of significance of any personality change. The *mode of onset*, except in the catatonic type, is often a gradual evolutionary process, and there may be a transitional "preschizophrenic" phase of a year or two. At this early stage there may be no single feature that is pathognomonic of the disease. In some instances, the early symptoms are more suggestive of a psychoneurosis than of a psychosis. A common early symptom is an aloofness, a withdrawal behind barriers to an area in which, if access to it could be gained, would be found loneliness, hopelessness, hatred, and fear. Frequently the patient seems preoccupied and dreamy; his friends may speak of him as appearing "far away." He does not empathize with the feelings of others and manifests little concern about the realities of his life situation. His plans for his future are often vague and unrealistic.

The schizophrenic suffers from a feeling of rejection and from an intolerable lack of self-respect. The characteristic way from which he protects himself against insult is by withdrawal from emotional involvements with other people. The resultant isolation is a protection against painful human relationships, but the loneliness contributes further to his feelings of rejection and hence to further withdrawal. The patient no longer trusts or confides in anyone. Instead of mingling with others, he remains at home, where he may sulk in his room and show an increasing indifference to members of his family, to accustomed interests, and to the demands and opportunities of his environment. It seems as if a fear of interpersonal contact had driven the patient into a state of regression and withdrawal. There may be a seemingly unexplainable deterioration in work. There are shallowness of affect, a paucity of emotional responsiveness, and an impairment in richness and variety of emotional expression.

A loss of appreciation of conventional values is noted. An insidious change in mood and outlook takes place.

Acquaintances may attribute to laziness the patient's listlessness and loss of spontaneity, of ambition, of interest in competition with his group, and of sustained effort in pursuit of former goals. An irritable discontent is common. The patient easily feels slighted and may begin to believe that others are talking about him. He may become ill at ease, restless, taciturn, and unapproachable, and wonder what interpretation others are putting on his behavior. A superficial attitude of superiority is not uncommon. Less heed is paid to social amenities and social requirements, while former loyalties and affections become blunted. The patient becomes disregardful of, and even resistant to, conventionality. Frequently he becomes neglectful of personal care and cleanliness. Ruminations on sexual topics are usual. The patient may feel that something wrong or unusual is going on in his environment. Mysterious meanings are discovered until finally misinterpretations and suspicions may cause him to move from place to place. For a few weeks or months the new environment may be free from any suggestion of hostility, then the patient begins to feel that people are watching him or conspiring against him. Odd mannerisms or ways of acting may appear, but they cause the patient no concern.

Some patients express undue worry over their physical condition. This is especially suggestive of an approaching schizophrenia, when the complaints are unusual or unlikely. The patient may add that he feels he should build himself up by means of dieting and exercise. The early schizophrenic is often preoccupied with abstract speculations or with metaphysical ponderings on such subjects as creation and causality, or with religious doubts, mysticism, and meaningless problems. A young truck driver who had but a seventh grade education wrote an essay entitled, "The Imperative Mind." In the very early stages, a few patients recognize that their ideas of reference and other abnormal mental experiences are un-natural; they may wish to know the mean-ing of their experiences and to understand their problems. Occasionally they may have some appreciation of the causes that have led to their illness. At this time they may be willing to discuss their problems. Later this desire is lost, and the patient becomes inaccessible, while in many the desire never existed. During these early stages, before the construction of an elaborate symbolic system that becomes accepted as reality, the conflicts are much less disguised, and it may often be possi-ble to discover the problems that the patient is living out in the drama of his psychotic behavior. Occasionally the pa-tient may show some sensorial confusion during the first few days of an acute episode.

In that group of schizophrenics now designated as "ambulatory," these indi-cations of social withdrawal are less evi-dent. Their dubious relationship to life is expressed in doubts as to their aims, difficulties in making decisions as to their future, the means to get on or to find a central interest. Although at times they may appear to be driving and busy, their actions are performed to prove them-selves. The adolescent may date to "prove" that he can gain the attention of others as his peers do. Marriage be-comes a means of "proving" that one is a man or woman or that one can "love." The relationship with children is a means of establishing the fact that one can be a mother. All activity is representative of an autistic dramatization without full affective contact with the realities of life, as though there is a continuous screen between the inner person and those with whom he relates. The existence has an "as if" quality; it is split from reality.

Sometimes the onset is sudden and precipitate. During adolescence, the loss of an only friend precedes the gross indi-cations of schizophrenia. Such a friend may have been the only outlet from a turbulent home life. The loss of the friend forces the future patient again to seek satisfaction in the family. This arouses increasing anxiety, and eventually

panic ensues when the adolescent consid-ers, or is unable to control, his hostility, sexuality, or his deepening despair be-cause of being forced backwards into an isolated, lonely, unhappy life of day-dreaming, hating, and fearing.

DISTURBANCES OF AFFECT. As we pass from this initial, and what might be called premonitory stage, or stage of in-cubation, to the manifest psychosis, an apparent *poverty and a disharmony of feeling tone* appear. The dulling of finer feelings and an insidious narrowing of in-terests noted in the incipient stages be-come progressive. The patient is unable to feel and regulate emotions properly. There is a withdrawal of feeling or affect from external realities back into the self. As the disease progresses and the emo-tional impoverishment increases, the pa-tient becomes indifferent, not merely to those sentiments and subjective values that make life worth living for the person in mental health, but, apparently existing at a vegetative level, he may be uncon-cerned as to fundamental comforts and needs. A few patients show, not a burned-out affectivity, but a definite, prevailing one, such as euphoria or depression. These feelings, however, usually lack depth or focus. The persistent mood, or emotional rigidity, has no relation to ex-ternal circumstances or experiences.

Another disturbance of affect is one in which emotional expression is unre-lated to reality. This is manifested by an emotional disharmony, often first exhib-ited by inappropriate smiling or laughing and silly giggling. Frequently the dishar-mony is between mood and conscious idea; there may, for example, be but little subjective feeling of depression even when ideas of despondency are expressed. At times experiences and ideas that should evoke a certain emotional response will produce its opposite—an emotional disconnection or dissociation. The pa-tient, for example, may with a silly laugh speak of the death of his beloved mother. Whenever there is a display of affect by the schizophrenic, it seems unnatural and stilted, lacking in any infectious quality and often it arouses feelings of uneasiness or estrangement in the observer. At times one notes capricious, fitful, apparently causeless changes in affect and mood. This inferior affective capacity, the deterioration and impoverishment of emotional expression, and the inappropriate emotional responses to situations constitute one of the important ways in in which the personality is disorganized or split, and attest the aptness of Bleuler's designation of schizophrenia.

One of the most generally accepted hypotheses advanced as an explanation of this serious disturbance in the affective life of the patient is that the affect, contrary to first impression, is not lost or destroyed but is withdrawn from the conscious, perceptive aspects of the patient's life, from matters of objective reality, and is attached to complexes and other material in the unconscious. The affect is hidden, because it is fixed to highly personalized subjective constellations of ideas. According to this theory, the disorganization of affect appears all the greater because it is associated with, and determined, not by one constellation of unconscious ideas, but by many complexes, among which there may be active conflict and discord. Since the affect is attached to and determined by material that is inaccessible, the emotions appear out of harmony with the contents and expressions of consciousness, although they are really in harmony with the psychic material to which the affect is attached and by which they are governed. The emotional disturbance in schizophrenia is more a displacement than a deterioration.

The emotional apathy of the schizophrenic individual may perhaps be theoretically explained in a somewhat different manner. One way by which the normal person may deal with difficult and threatening situations is by minimizing or ignoring them. It is conceivable, therefore, that the patient defends himself by building a wall of indifference around himself. Although this blunting of feeling may have arisen as a mechanism of defense against a troublesome situation in the inner world of the patient, it irradiates and becomes a general behavior pattern of the personality.

When interest and affect are withdrawn from the conscious, familiar material with which they were formerly connected and are attached to the content of the unconscious, a state known as *depersonalization* may exist. The patient has feelings of vagueness, of unreality, of detachment, or of being a spectator of life instead of taking part in it. He feels himself changed throughout in comparison with his former state. As a result, he no longer acknowledges himself as a personality. His actions seem mechanical and automatic. The patient does not believe he is another personality (transformation of personality) but has rather a sense of loss of the limits of his own personality with its directive ego. The identification of one's own personality may become indistinct or confused. It seems to the patient that he no longer has any internal self to which he can refer forces and influences. In his attempt to rationalize this sense, the patient may come to feel that parts of his body or his mind seem strange and as though they do not belong to him. He may develop more nihilistic ideas and believe that he no longer has a body, that there is no world, or that he is dead. In addition to this change of self, the environment may seem unnatural and appear to have lost its character of reality. States of unreality are probably closely related to thought block, feelings of stupidity, fugues, dream states, and other involuntary withdrawals.

From what has been said, it will be seen that there is rarely a dominant affect in schizophrenia as is the case in manic–depressive psychoses. On the contrary, there are numerous inharmonious affects arising from conflicting desires and complexes, or the affect may be fixed to or absorbed by fantasies, by elaborate symbolic systems, and other products of the unconscious. The result is an inconsistency of affect that contributes to the peculiar disorganization of personality that characterizes the schizophrenic patient.

Among the disturbances of affect in

schizophrenia, hypochondria is occasionally met with. This preoccupation with the body and various subjective feelings provide a meaningful purpose as the schizophrenic loses contact with others in his social environment. The patient may then express toward his own body the same attitudes he has held towards others and use the same ego defenses. These feelings of guilt, due to hostile sexual drives, can be centered on his genitals and lead to preoccupations with defects in genital functioning. He may express these preoccupations in such bizarre terms as "electric currents" in the genitals or as a sense of shrinking of the body. Modification of the body concept is common in the schizophrenic reaction in the early stages. In some instances, other body parts come to represent the genital areas through the process of displacement. Later, in some instances the patient's guilty anxiety becomes so great that he is lead to carry out mutilative actions against his own body in those occasional fantastic acts of personal dismemberment.

ATTENTION AND IDEA ASSOCIATION. One result of the schizophrenic's loss of capacity for attachment of energy and interest to external objects and reality and of his autistic preoccupations is a *narrowing of attention*. Interest, and therefore attention, is centered on subjective creations, on matters within and not without the patient. This lack of attention and of concentration gives rise to the misleading impression that the patient is intellectually impaired, whereas he is intellectually inert. The replies of the schizophrenic individual are often trivial and uninformative because interests and energy are directed toward material not accessible to ordinary questioning. *Paralogia*, a condition in which the patient's reply shows that the question has been understood, but in which the answer is erroneous, is caused by the dereistic thinking to which the schizophrenic patient is particularly given.

Although active attention (concentration), as just indicated, is often disturbed, yet passive attention is much less affected,

with the result that, even if the patient is living in a world of fantasy, he is still able to maintain a contact with reality sufficient for certain practical needs, yet often too inadequate for a socialized adjustment. Schizophrenics may be perplexed but rarely suffer from disturbances of the sensorium and therefore from confusion in the correct sense of the term.

Normally, *associations of ideas* follow one another with a definite logical connection, progressing to an ultimate completeness of thought, but in schizophrenia they may be shortened, fragmented, and otherwise so disturbed as to lack logical relationship. Although the disturbances of associations in schizophrenia do not become particularly marked until serious disorganization of the personality has taken place, frequently one finds that long before any manifest psychosis developed the patient showed a loosening of the associational links in thinking. Later the patient may speak in generalities and abstractions that are difficult to grasp—a dereistic type of verbigeration rather than communicative talk. The use of eccentric, metaphorical expressions is not uncommon. Doubtless the communications of the schizophrenic patient are nearly always self-meaningful, although often their significance is not grasped by others.

One of the earliest symptoms observed by the psychiatrist may be a certain inconsequence of ideas and a thought sequence that is erratic. There is a slight irrelevancy as if the patient has missed the point. In the more disorganized schizophrenic reactions, there is a tendency for associative connections to become more involved, incongruous, and at times so broken or incomplete that the patient's utterances become fragmentary, disconnected, illogical, or even unintelligible. The train of thought may not be pursued to its logical goal, with the result that thinking becomes diffuse and disorganized. Cause and effect may be interchanged. If aware of his disordered thinking, the patient may say that his thoughts are suddenly taken out of his head. Irrelevance in replies to questions, a feature that, when consciousness is clear, is particularly suggestive of schizophrenia, may be quite striking. Probably, however, irrelevance is not irrelevant to the patient and would be relevant to the listener if the latter had clues to the semantic significance of the patient's autistic productions. Set phrases may come to be used repeatedly as stereotypes. The thought productions of the schizophrenic person often become characterized by vague and unusual symbolism. It is believed that the disordered thought productions tend to express, by condensation, the various problems that concern the patient. Speech may show a curiously distorted use of language varying from a stilted and formal phraseology without apparent substance to a "word salad" of nouns and verbs having practically no articulated structure or even without apparently meaningful connection. Doubtless there was earlier a significance that became lost. Affectations in manner of speech are often observed. The patient may show a "flight into intellectualism." The following is taken from a schizophrenic production entitled "Equalitized Metabolic Demention Metabolism."

"Improper wave length—wave length changes, later visible death. That is a moving trollysis similar to circulation of life action. Born high focussating action may die through wave length charge and still live until visible death takes place.

"Education comes from radiation of action. Anyone can study all science in a compositive way. It takes a compositive mind to be able to understand. Can tell compositive minds by stromonized conception. The mind at birth takes on a birthification, becomes environmental by the radiation to it. Metabolism to dimension differ in every person is of actions of metabolism and dimension balancing. . . ."

How the thinking of a formerly well-trained mind may become disorganized in schizophrenia is illustrated in the following intellectualized rumination taken from a letter written by a man who had had a scholastically brilliant college career and after graduation had spent two years at Oxford as a Rhodes scholar.

"I'm too utterly weary from battling with my financial–religious and general–religious problems to be able to survive any shock of learning that unhintably hard-won progress supposed to have been earned in the fraternal-religious problem is illusory. For that would wreck me—in my critically exhausted condition—with horror lest humanity—contrarily from being faith-imbued joy-multipliers of Revelations All Embracing God or Unfathomably Progressive Universe—are duped victims of God's opposite faith deluding us—with illusions of immortality, a Heavenly Father and of progress—into accommodation as evil-absorbers of His unconvertible and endless agonies and struggle."

The explanation for the disorders in the thinking of the schizophrenic is found in the great extent to which associations are directed by internal perceptions and association unrelated to occurrences in the immediate environment—that is, reality. Because of their origin in the unconscious, associations are broken, are led into bypaths, are fragmented, incongruous, do not progress, or are joined through common affects rather than through conscious, logical connection, with the result that various forms of incoherence follow. When the connections appear particularly loose, we speak of the schizophrenic's thought as being "scattered." This means that the unconscious connection of ideas is unusually marked.

Many schizophrenics appear to show a poverty of associations and of ideas, presumably because of preoccupation with material having its source largely in the unconscious and also because of the accompanying narrowing of attention. To be ascribed to these two conditions, as well, are the casual and trivial remarks and replies of the schizophrenic so peculiar to the disorder as to have important diagnostic significance.

Elements in repressed constellations of ideas may produce various ellipses, short-circuitings of ideas, and even neologisms. These words of his own making are condensations and symbolizations of complexes with affect. Within their concealed meaning are compressed the condensations of words that refer to persons or things intimately related to the individual's particular conflict or psychic experience. The use of neologisms by the mental patient always suggests a schizophrenic psychosis.

In connection with disturbances of associations, mention should be made of the fact that in early schizophrenia a fairly typical flight of ideas may occur, which later tends to develop into inconherence.

Blocking may occur as associations approach painful conflict material. It results, perhaps, from a threat that repressed material is approaching awareness. It tends to arise largely in connection with special topics, whereas neutral topics may be handled as usual.

The thinking of the schizophrenic seems directed from the unconscious, and associations and symbols are molded and directed by affective constellations and instinctive undercurrents. They then rise into consciousness where as dereistic thinking they constitute a type of thought much like that of dreams in which one finds active the processes of symbolism, displacement, and condensation. Dereistic thinking is of the pleasurable "primary process" type of early life that tends to falsify reality, to disregard realistic, logical, and scientific thought. It is not corrected by the logic of experiences or by the demands of the external world. Vigotsky, a Russian psychologist, believed that an impairment in the function and formation of concepts is the most important deterioration of thought occurring in schizophrenia. Frequently there is an impairment of abstract thinking as demonstrated by the patient's interpretation of proverbs.

DELUSIONS. The dominant *ideational content* of the schizophrenic is often delusional in nature. Because the satisfactions sought by his beliefs are so highly disguised by their symbolism and because the needs in response to which the *delusions* have been created are often not apparent, the delusions of the schizophrenic often appear grotesque and meaningless. His delusions are never meaningless, however, but are specific and adapted to his peculiar psychological needs and situation and are in keeping with his particular life experiences, although they are conspicuously disregardful of reality. Although it is often difficult to ascertain, there is always a relevance in the schizophrenic's ideas and symbols to the problems and purposes of his personality. In referring to symbols, attention may be called to the fact that if he has artistic ability, he may show symbolic condensations in his drawings or paintings.

The tendency of the schizophrenic's delusions to be grotesque, to be loosely organized, to center around themes of persecution, of grandiosity and of sex, to arise from autistic sources and yet to be expressed in a relatively clear setting is shown in the following letter addressed by a patient to one of the male physicians connected with the hospital in which she was under treatment:

"Dear Dr.———

"My Plan," or as mother used to call you, "The Little Plant," or else one little Plant for I was the other Plant, called "Tant." Will you please see that I am taken out of this hospital and returned to the equity court so I can prove to the court who I am and thereby help establish my identity to the world. Possibly you do not remember or care to remember that you married me May 21, 1882, while you were in England and that I made you by that marriage the Prince of Wales, as I was born Albert Edward, Prince of Wales, I am feminine absolutely, not a double person or a hermaphrodite, so please know I am England's feminine king—the king who is a king.

Your first duty is to me, and if you do not intend to do the right thing, helping me to get out of here, stop the thefts of clothing, money, jewelry, papers, letters, etc., etc.; you will please let me know so I can make some absolute change and further demand of the nations my release.

1874 Building was to have been a palace for my mother, father, myself and you, that is, if you are the one I married—so why not get busy and furnish it up as such when I go abroad. Make my trips (our trips?) short and return to America on important matters and have the right place to hold court. You and Dr. Black can take me to the equity court where I prove up my individuality and this must be done.

> Sincerely,
> "Tant"

Queen of Scotland, Empress of the World, Empress of China, Empress of Russia, Queen of Denmark, Empress of India, Maharajahess of Durban, "Papal authority" as a Protestant.

In the early stages of schizophrenia, the delusions may not be fixed, and the patient may at times be in doubt as to his ideas of reference or as to the hostility of his environment; later he becomes convinced that his delusions are real facts. At the onset of his psychosis, the schizophrenic may have obsessive ideas that prove to be the early stages of a process that later becomes frankly one of externalization and projection.

Delusions in the schizophrenic often serve rather effectually in subjectively reorganizing his life situations and in dealing with such problems as thwarted trends and drives, frustrated hopes, biological inadequacies, feelings of insecurity, disowned qualities, gnawing feelings of guilt, and the affective constellations and other contents of the unconscious. In no other type of mental disorder are the patient's problems, wishes, and conflicts so thoroughly dramatized and symbolized in fantastic form. This fact and the schizophrenic's impairment of his ability to appreciate and test the reality of his fantasies tend to the creation of extravagant and bizarre delusions. The role of fantasy was well expressed by Macfie Campbell: "Fantasy is called on to supply what real life has denied, but the fantasies are not woven into a structure which is compatible with a normal social adaptation." There is a tendency to a reversion to belief in magical cause and effect. Some patients in their schizoid withdrawal show no evidence of delusional ideation.

HALLUCINATIONS. In no other form of mental disorder do *hallucinations,* or the projection of impulses and inner experiences into the external world in terms of perceptual images, occur in the presence of clear consciousness so frequently as in schizophrenia. Their mechanism is not unlike that of hallucinations in other abnormal states, but they tend to be more highly disguised in nature and to constitute a primitive form of adjustment and therefore are of much more serious significance than is their presence in delirium or in dissociative states. It is not difficult to conceive of highly significant material in the schizophrenic's inner life as assuming hallucinatory vividness. It is but a step from the figurative "voice of conscience" to its audible perception. Unconscious material and unadjusted tendencies break through and create sense perceptions, perhaps highly symbolized, in response to psychological needs and problems. Disowned desires and feelings of guilt are projected as auditory hallucinations that, as the voice of conscience, accuse and criticize. The patient, incapable, because of his disorganized ego, of recognizing the origin or significance of his hallucinations, believes in the reality of these projected images, accepts them at face value, and reacts in accordance with what he has accepted as reality. He can no longer distinguish between subjective and objective experiences, with the result that he tends to alter reality with hallucinations and delusions. But not all the hallucinated material of the schizophrenic is accusatory. Oftentimes, as recent studies have found, the auditory perceptions are comforting, provide companionship, **advice,** judgments, and even sexual gratification. These hallucinated perceptions may be identified frequently by patients as representing the voices of significant persons in their lives (parents, lovers, friends) and appear to serve as a substitute for those persons. The accusatory and affectional components thus appear to represent both the actual and the desired elements in the lost personal relationship. Frequently the onset of hallucinatory experience takes place when the individual actually has lost a significant relationship or, through the isolation or the illness or hospital, is deprived of that relationship.

The schizophrenic may find his hallucinations so serviceable that he is unwilling to relinquish them, with the result that they come to constitute one of his cherished means of adjustment, and he becomes occupied, not with a real, but with a hallucinatory world, protected from the disturbances of reality. His hallucinations may be said to collaborate with delusions in the development of the same theme, the one by means of image symbols, the other by ideas.

But little need be said in the way of description of hallucinations in schizophrenia. They are more frequently auditory than of any other sense. Visual hallucinations are not particularly frequent and tend to be limited to acute phases of the psychosis. During their early occurrence, hallucinations are often accompanied by considerable emotional tension and may have a disturbing and disquieting influence on the patient. As time passes, they may cause but little concern and exert less influence upon behavior.

IMPULSE AND CONATION. Among important symptoms of schizophrenia are the *disturbances of impulse and conation,* of action-tendencies or the striving aspects of the personality. Many of these odd, unexplained, and sudden activities grow out of a lack of harmonious association and integration of strivings, affects, and wishes—the existence of incompatible and frequently, also, of changing objectives.

The capricious, impulsive behavior of the schizophrenic is to be looked upon as a result of an ambivalence of impulse, a contradiction of conative tendencies. The concept of ambivalence, or contradictory manifestations of impulse, of idea, or of affect, was greatly stressed by Bleuler, and considered by him to be a fundamental symptom of schizophrenia. It rests upon the principle that the true meaning of an idea, impulse, or affect is to be found in the exact opposite of that manifestly expressed. Many psychiatrists believe that the conscious rejection and denial of expression of a desire, notwithstanding its indirect and unrecognized expression through projection in the form of hallucination or delusion, is a manifestation of the principle of ambivalence. At any rate, we find in schizophrenia a peculiar association of contradictions in mental or personality expressions. Ordinarily our behavior represents a compromise, a working harmony among diverse desires, a resultant of the contrast-

ing considerations, forces, and motives prompting us. In schizophrenia, on the contrary, the two conflicting impulses, one, many believe, of conscious origin, the other of unconscious origin, control behavior in erratic sequence, or even struggle simultaneously to direct it. There is a failure of integration of motive forces. Ambivalence may be manifested by an unstable blending of love and hate, with sudden unaccountable shifts in affection and hostility, leading sometimes to impulsive episodes. Occasionally unpredictable suicidal impulses result in the unexpected death of a patient. Impulsive self-mutilation is not rare, especially in case of an adolescent masturbatory struggle.

At times a schizophrenic may consciously resist a certain impulse, but he may nevertheless carry it through into action. Unconscious and dissociated tendencies acting in this way give the patient a feeling of being forced or controlled. This feeling of being forced permits the entertainment of thoughts or the indulgence in behavior that the socially determined standards of the individual would not permit but for which, with his feelings of being forced, the patient no longer recognizes any responsibility.

ANERGIA. A common disturbance of activity in the schizophrenic is an avoidance of concrete or spontaneous activity, a loss of initiative and purpose, and the development of a state of inaction sometimes designated as anergia. Energy is withdrawn from externality. This deterioration in habits of activity may perhaps best be considered as a loss of interest in, and a retreat from, the world of reality, one of the means adopted by the schizophrenic in renouncing the world with which he cannot cope. Instead of being realistic, his behavior tends to become autistic and regressive. Although the normal person secures his satisfaction by expending his energy in relation to the world of reality, such a way gives no satisfaction to the schizophrenic, whose interest and strivings are progressively withdrawn from the outer world.

The ego weakens and the patient secures his satisfactions through flight into unreality and fantasy and by means of a symbolic gratification of insistent strivings and primitive impulsions. Sexuality may be chaotically organized and may manifest an admixture of various tendencies.

NEGATIVISM AND SUGGESTIBILITY. Another disturbance is negativism, which may manifest itself in a perversity of behavior in the form of antagonism to the environment, in opposition to the wishes of those about him, and, in more marked cases, in mutism, rejection of food, refusal to swallow, or even to void urine. Presumably the patient may feel that negativism is a "safe" way of expressing hostility.

Although it is quite the opposite of negativism in certain of its objective manifestations, one occasionally meets with a *pathological suggestibility* that seems to have for its object the same purpose that negativism may have—a lessening of disturbing contacts with reality. It is less disturbing for the reality-evading patient blindly and passively to accept and follow whatever the environment suggests than it is actively either to oppose or to initiate contacts with reality. He may, therefore, show an automatic obedience to verbal directions without reference to their appropriateness or significance. Instead of answering a question, he may repeat it in a parrot-like manner—echolalia. Again, he may at once imitate the movement of a person in his immediate environment — echopraxia. Obediently to follow the suggestion of the environment involves neither initiative nor responsible contact with others and often seems to express a mocking hostility toward them. The waxy flexibility of the catatonic represents this passive acquiescence to suggestions to a degree that may lead the patient to ignore physical discomfort or pain, accompanied usually by a marked disregard of his environment.

Among the disturbances of activity, mannerisms and stereotypies occupy a large place in the clinical picture. Schizophrenia mannerisms are of a wide variety. They may consist of affectations of manner, speech, gait, et cetera. Others consist of grimaces, sniffing, blowing out the cheeks, wrinkling of the forehead, tic-like movements, or elaborate methods of performing certain activities and constituting a sort of ritual. Some patients assume certain postures for years. Sometimes the lips are puckered and held protruded in what is known as "snout cramp." In general, the schizophrenic's attitudes, gestures, and actions, like many of his verbal communications, appear unintelligible. The bizarre behavior of the schizophrenic has, however, a meaning for him, although its purpose and value are often obscure to others because of condensation and symbolization.

CONSCIOUSNESS AND INTEGRATION. In schizophrenia there is relatively little impairment of consciousness, orientation, or memory, although, because of lack of interest, it is sometimes difficult to test these functions. The time sense of schizophrenics appears impaired. Many are unable to estimate units of time with accuracy, and others state their age as that when their illness or hospitalization first occurred. One often secures incorrect replies in answer to questions as to orientation but these are because of negativism, the habit of giving casual replies in order to avoid troublesome reality, or occasionally they are due to a lack of attention associated with a certain falsification by hallucinations and delusions. Forgetting, inattention, distraction, and imaginative thoughts are used by normal persons as expedients to overcome a disappointment; these are used by the schizophrenic patient, not as substitutive reactions, but as if he were in a rut of least resistance.

Because of the disturbance in the integrative functions of the personality, leading, as it were, to a disturbance in fusion of cognitive, affective, and conative mental elements, the schizophrenic is often described as demented. This, however, is not correct, as there is no irreparable impairment of cognitive and intellectual functions. This does not mean that judgment, the capacity for making conceptual inferences, is not impaired. Rather there has occurred a disorganization of personality or a failure of even development of the ego functions of personality. The patient not only has no appreciation of the disorganization that his personality has suffered, but his concepts as to personal welfare and social relationships and purpose are rendered faulty and unreliable by his introverted tendencies and his distortion both of physical and social reality through delusions and hallucinations.

RESPONSE TO PSYCHOLOGICAL TESTS. The performance of Stanford-Binet and similar intelligence tests by disorganized schizophrenics differs both qualitatively and quantitatively from that of subnormal persons of the same mental age level. In normal persons and in the mentally deficient, the age levels at which failures and successes are intermixed are grouped fairly closely around the determined mental age level, but in disorganized schizophrenics, as in persons suffering from many other psychoses which have led to deterioration, there is usually a spread of failures and successes at a number of age levels above and below the determined one. This phenomenon is known as "scatter."

Because of its value as a means of revealing basic personality traits and structure, the Rorschach test is often employed as an aid in the study of known or suspected schizophrenic behavior. The detection of distinctive schizophrenic features in a Rorschach performance is a complex procedure because of the many variations in the schizophrenic syndrome itself. There is no set or definite pattern, and a diagnosis of schizophrenic characteristics is largely made from inference. Variation in form of responses, contamination of ideas, bizarreness, withdrawal, environmental rejection, and poor affective control are a few of the indicators of the Rorschach test suggesting possible schizophrenic disorders. Each case is an individual problem in itself. The information derived from the Rorschach test is only as reliable as the examiner who administers the technique; in skilled hands,

it is of value in detecting a preschizophrenic process.

PHYSICAL CHANGES. The more disorganized and disturbed schizophrenics sometimes show certain *physical concomitants*. One of the most frequent of these is general disequilibrium of the autonomic nervous system. This is shown by cold, bluish hands and feet, blotchy skin, and widely dilated pupils, which, when tested by a strong light, may contract momentarily but quickly dilate again. Sometimes patients in a catatonic stupor who persist in standing about in an immobile manner develop a striking edema of the lower extremities. Attacks of vertigo and of hysteriform and epileptiform seizures may occur, more frequently in the early stages. Many patients lose weight during the acute phases of the disease. Those who enjoy a favorable outcome of a schizophrenic episode often show a marked increase in weight during convalescence; however, an increase in weight without a coincident mental improvement usually denotes an unfavorable prognosis.

Malnutrition and tuberculosis have been accompaniments of chronically hospitalized schizophrenics. With improved hospital management, active screening and segregation of the tubercular, and the use of appropriate chemotherapy, these complications may be prevented.

Types of Schizophrenia

In formulating his concept of dementia praecox, Kraepelin classified his cases into different varieties, depending on the predominant symptomatology. Although classification according to reaction type continues to be made, it must be recognized that numerous patients show the psychopathology considered characteristic of the individual groups. More is to be gained by studying each patient, evaluating his central pathology, the deficits in his life experience, and the dynamic forces inducing his particular psychopathology, and by erecting a pertinent and individualized therapy than by attempting to categorize his illness in a vague classificatory division. Since these types or divisions are widely used, they are delineated in this section.

SIMPLE TYPE. In this type the most marked disturbances are of emotion, interest, and activity. If hallucinations occur, they are rare and fleeting, and delusions never play an important role. The disorder is usually gradual in its onset and assumes the form of an insidious change and impoverishment of personality, the significance of which is not understood by the patient's friends. In adolescence a youth who has perhaps shown much promise begins to lose interest in school or occupation, becomes moody, irritable, and indolent. His goals are no longer realistic. Shallowness of emotions, indifference or callousness, absence of will or drive, and a progressive meagerness of inner resources betray the withering of personality that constitutes the most prominent feature of this type. Neither criticism by others nor chagrin of parents appears to cause concern. Appreciation of esthetic and moral values is lost. The required period of training or apprenticeship in preparation for a profession or a skilled occupation is not completed. Many become irresponsible idlers, vagrants, tramps, prostitutes, or delinquents. In the milder cases, the social maladaptation is less serious, but the patients are considered to be neighborhood eccentrics and, although intellectually unimpaired, are capable of performing only some simple routine task under supervision. The patient remains uninterested in his environment and unimpressed by responsibilities.

A. R. was committed to the hospital when 21 years of age following his arrest for window-peeping. In describing his childhood characteristics, the patient's family stated that he "was always a little hard to understand," but was a quiet boy who never entered into rough games. His school record was excellent and he always stood high in his class. At age 17, when in the fourth year of high school, he was obliged, because of a long illness of his father, to leave school and secure gainful employment. He secured work with a large manufacturing company where he soon came to be considered the second best operative on a certain type of machine. For two years he worked steadily, seemed ambitious, and appeared to have a normal and wholesome, but not marked, interest in girls. At age 19 he gave up his position,

showed no interest in securing another, and when asked if he worked replied, "What do I want to work for? I have a father and sister working and they are enough." He appeared quite self-satisfied and felt that he should have a position of importance.

At about this time he was first arrested for peeping into women's bedrooms. Through the influence of his father, the charge was dropped. He became careless of his personal appearance and remained unoccupied except for occasional periods, when he set up pins in a bowling alley. A year later he was again arrested but again was released on the intercession of his father. He came to say little unless addressed and grew antagonistic toward his father and sister. He would remain out until midnight and then come home, eat a large meal, read until 2 a.m., and sleep until noon. Finally, after his third arrest for peeping, he was committed to a hospital for mental disorders.

On arrival at the institution, the patient was found to be of asthenic physique and slightly effeminate in appearance. His emotional responses were shallow and inadequate. He showed no concern over his situation, laughed about it in a silly manner, and referred to his offense as "just a foolish idea." His hospital residence was characterized by apathy, preoccupation, and inactivity. During the summer he would at times take part in the patients' baseball games, but in winter he refused ground privileges. He never expressed any delusions and denied hallucinations. At times he would be seen, apparently much preoccupied, walking alone about the hospital reservation, laughing to himself.

Such a case illustrates how an individual is unable to complete the transition from adolescence to maturity with its adult heterosexual and social adjustments. There seemed to be a certain innate limitation to the personality. Interest became largely withdrawn from the actual world, energy was absorbed by the subjective life, and there was a diminished response to social demands. This does not mean that life situations and events or psychological reactions to mental events were not dynamic factors in the patient's personality disorganization, but it shows that, as often happens in the schizophrenic, it is difficult, even by attempts at mental exploration, to discover and evaluate these elements.

HEBEPHRENIC TYPE. The onset of this type is insidious and usually begins in early adolescence. Occasionally the onset is subacute and is characterized by a depression that suggests an affective reaction. Usually, however, affective reactions are shallow and inappropriate. Silliness, giggling, and incongruous or inappropriate smiling and laughter are usual. Hallucinations, which are frequent, often represent the projection of repressed instinctive urges. The ideational content tends to take the form of fantasy or of fragmentary bizarre delusions rather than of elaborate or systematized beliefs. Associative processes are loose, speech is incoherent, neologisms are common, and posturing and mannerisms are frequent. Regressive features are prominent, wetting and soiling are common, and the patient eats in a ravenous, unmannerly fashion. The patient comes to lead a highly autistic life; he becomes bafflingly inaccessible and greatly introverted and withdrawn. The final disintegration of personality and habits is perhaps the greatest of any of the types of schizophrenia.

One of five children, Theresa was her mother's favorite. Greatly petted and babied by her mother, she always remained dependent upon her. She was described as having been a pretty child with a rosy complexion. She early became aware of this fact and enjoyed dressing up and strutting about to display her good looks. In spite of these signs of vanity, she was timid and shy and would blush in a self-conscious way when she realized that people were noticing her. In childhood she did not play freely with other children; "she thought herself above other children," and is described by her sisters as having in later years "a rather good opinion of herself and her abilities," and by her neighbors as "high hat."

Soon after leaving school at age 16, she began to work in a bleachery, where she remained until shortly before her commitment. She never had any girl chums and did not participate in the activities of other girls at her place of employment. Her attitude was one of "proud distance." While she was still in school, there were several boys who were quite friendly toward her, but her sister said she could not remember any instance when the patient had any male callers or associates after she grew up, although she gave much attention to her clothes and personal appearance, obviously in the sister's opinion, in an effort to attract the attention of young men. Her family described her as devoid of humor, sensitive, jealous, stubborn, willful, and easily angered. She became more seclusive, had "melancholy spells," became preoccupied, and paid less attention to her environment, and when addressed she would ask in an indifferent way, "What did you say?" She also became irritable and critical, particularly of the wife of her brother, with whose family she lived.

About six months before commitment to the hospital at age 32 she "began to grow thin and nervous" and became careless about her work, which deteriorated in quality and quantity. She believed that other girls at her place of employment were circulating slanderous stories concerning her. She complained so indignantly that X., an attractive young man employed in the same industrial plant had put his arm around her and insulted her that her family demanded that the charge be investigated. This showed not only that the charge was without foundation but that the young man in question had not spoken to her for months. The family, however, had not suspected mental disease until six days before her commitment, when she returned from her work. As she entered the house that evening, she laughed loudly, watched her sister-in-law suspiciously, refused to answer questions, and at sight of her brother began to cry. She refused to go to the bathroom, saying that X. was looking in the windows at her. She ate no food and the next day declared that her sisters were "bad women," that everyone was talking about her, and that X. had been having sexual relations with her, that although she could not see him he was "always around." In her hallucinatory experiences she heard X. say, "Aren't you going to fire her? I've had her. She don't know it." The patient became resistive, was afraid of being killed, and at times said, "I'm dead." She stated that she was being poisoned, saw her dead mother, and heard her speak.

As the patient became noisy, did not sleep, and ate but little and only then when spoon-fed, she was committed to a private institution. Here she was unco-operative, silly, grimaced, and whiningly repeated, "Oh, mama! mama! I want to see my father before I die." She heard voices outside her window and at night would come to the door of her room several times saying, "What is it all about? Oh, mama!" Her associations became loose; she took no interest in the care of her person or in other patients but would stand for hours with her back against the wall, her head thrust forward, fingering her hair, and unobservant of her environment.

After a residence of four months in the private institution, the patient was transferred to a public hospital. As she entered the admitting office, she laughed loudly and repeatedly screamed in a loud tone, "She cannot stay here; she's got to go home!" She grimaced and performed various stereotyped movements of her hands. When seen on the ward an hour later, she paid no attention to questions, although she talked to herself in a childish tone. She moved about constantly, walking on her toes in a dancing manner, pointed aimlessly about, and put out her tongue and sucked her lips in the manner of an infant. At times she moaned and cried like a child but shed no tears. As the months passed, she remained silly, childish, preoccupied, inaccessible, grimacing, gesturing, pointing at objects in a stereotyped way, usually chattering to herself in a peculiar high-pitched voice, little of what she said being understood. At an interview 18 months after her hospitalization, she presented an unkempt appearance, was without shoes, sat stooped far over, smiled in a silly manner, and presented a picture of extreme introversion and regression. During the attempted interview, she rarely spoke, although she occasionally replied, "I don't know" in an entirely indifferent manner and apparently with no heed to the question. The nurse reported the patient as seclusive, resistive, idle, and with no interest either in the activities of the institution or in her relatives who visited her.

CATATONIC TYPE. The catatonic type is characterized by phases of stupor or of excitement, in both of which negativism and automatism are prominent features. There may be alternation between little or no movement on the one hand to an explosive overactivity on the other. Frequently, however, a given catatonic episode may present but one phase, either stupor or disorganized overactivity, throughout its course. Again, there may be an admixture of symptoms usually thought of as belonging characteristically to one or the other phase. The most frequent age of appearance is between 15 and 25. Of the various types of schizophrenia, catatonia most frequently has a somewhat acute onset and is most frequently precipitated or preceded by an emotionally disturbing experience. The prognosis for a recovery with reintegration of personality after a catatonic episode is more favorable than in other types of schizophrenia, although after a period, perhaps after several episodes, there is a tendency for the catatonic type to pass over into states approaching the hebephrenic or paranoid, with permanent disorganization of the personality.

Catatonic stupor. Catatonic stupor, or the stupor phase, is often preceded by depression, discontent, or emotional fermentation. The patient is inclined to be uncommunicative, and his reactions become increasingly characterized by failing interest, inattention, preoccupation, emotional poverty, and dreaminess. Mute, stuporous, and with mask-like facies, the catatonic may occasionally keep his eyes closed but more frequently he stares fixedly and blankly downward.

He may stand almost immobile, seldom shifting his position during the whole day. The skin of his feet may become turgid and engorged, with swelling of unsupported parts. Another catatonic may spend the day sitting on the edge of a chair or crouching on the floor. With his implicit loss of reality sense, he denies the world and actively resists the environment. He opposes any effort to move him from attitudes and positions, often constrained and peculiar, that he has assumed and may maintain for months. The patient refuses to dress or to eat, although occasionally, if he thinks he is unobserved, he will eat greedily. Saliva, urine, and bowel contents are often retained. He may not only soil clothing but even exhibit an apparent purposefulness in his annoying disregard of all cleanliness in his habits of excretion.

Gestures, grimacing, and grinning are common. The hands may be held tightly clenched and other muscle tensions may be maintained. Occasionally the physical manifestations of catatonia show some points of similarity to parkinsonian akinesia and rigidity. Catalepsy, either flexible or rigid, may be present. In this state, the patient initiates no spontaneous movements but maintains the postures into which he is passively impressed. Through automatic obedience, the patient may carry out any verbal instructions, regardless of their absurd or even dangerous nature. He shows no avoiding reaction to feinting motions before the eyes, to pinpricks, or to other painful stimuli. Although giving no indication whatsoever that he is at all aware of what is going on about him, the patient really registers the events of his environment, and when he begins to speak again, he may give a surprisingly full account of incidents occurring in his stupor.

In spite of the apparent ideational poverty, there seems to be every reason to believe that ideas and representations are by no means absent, but rather are centered about a dominant ideo-affective constellation. Perhaps an analogue to catatonic stupor may exist in the unapprehending, impassive response with which profound, overwhelming bereavement or catastrophe may at times be met. Both this reaction and the catatonic stupor of the schizophrenic may serve as methods of meeting situations too difficult to be met by active, resolute measures. The stupor may be thought of as a protective withdrawal from contact with surroundings that seem threatening. Again, the stupor may be compared to a retreat into an intense, trance-like preoccupation or reverie.

After a period of extremely variable duration, the patient may slowly, or at times suddenly, emerge from this profound generalized inhibition. Occasionally catatonic rigidity and negativism may terminate in response to affective stimuli. The opposite occurrence, the sudden sinking into a stuporous akinesia following an apparently trivial physical or mental event, is more frequent. Interest, affect, and behavior may return more or less closely to normal, or the patient may pass into a state of catatonic excitement.

CATATONIC EXCITEMENT. Catatonic excitement is characterized by an unorganized and aggressive motor activity. It is not accompanied with emotional expression and is not influenced by external stimuli; it is apparently purposeless and stereotyped and is usually confined to a limited space. Of all schizophrenics, the excited catatonic most frequently shows impulsive and unpredictable behavior. Without warning or apparent cause, he may suddenly attack an inoffensive bystander or break a window. He destroys his clothing, remains nude, and disregards all excretory cleanliness. Negativism is usually marked. The flow of speech may vary from mutism to a pressure suggesting a flight of ideas. Attitudinizing, mannerisms, stereotypies, and grimaces are frequent. The patient may react to terrifying or ecstatic hallucinations of sight or hearing. Mystical experiences are not uncommon. Hostility and feelings of resentment are common. The patient may be sleepless, appear delirioid, refuse food, and become dehydrated and exhausted. There is often a rapid loss of weight. On rare occasions the acutely and extremely excited catatonic may collapse and die. Usually no pathologic condition sufficient to explain the cause of death is found at necropsy. In such cases, therefore, the death is ordinarily said to be a result of "exhaustion syndrome."

Probably acute catatonic excitement is often the same as the reaction that Kempf termed *acute homosexual panic*. The great activity is often accompanied by fearfulness and auditory hallucinations that accuse the patient of homosexual practices or inclinations. As previously noted, he is often assaultive.

Meyer considered that catatonia is a psychobiological reaction. Hohman, his former assistant, quotes him as describing it as "closely related to what is seen in hypnotic states and in mystical fancies, and like stages in religious symbolism and feelings of submission to influence by mystic power." When the problems of life are too great, we naturally seek death, but we are deterred from suicide by the instinct of self-preservation. Many psychiatrists, therefore, look upon catatonic stupor as a profound regression, a dramatization of death. Attention is called to the similarity between catatonia and the instinctive immobility reaction exhibited by certain animals when confronted with a life-threatening situation.

The case of A. C., aged 32, will illustrate many of the features observed both in the excited and the stuporous phases of catatonia.

The patient's father was stubborn and self-willed, his mother was excitable and temperamental. At seven years of age he went to live with his grandparents. The grandfather, whose "word was law," suffered from epileptic seizures and subsequently died in a hospital for mental diseases; he had no understanding of the child's point of view. His seizures greatly frightened the boy. The patient was a seclusive, day-dreaming, timid, shy, and sensitive, but stubborn and self-willed, child. He still remembers with resentment how his father whipped him before another boy whom he would not thank for an apple. He was uninterested in the play life of other children and spent his time either in the town library or in his own room, where he made various toys that he guarded jealously from other children, allowing only his sister, his sole confidante, to share them. At age 17 he was graduated from high school, where he had learned easily but had taken no part in extracurricular activities.

His occupational history was without significance except that his early promise of success as a draftsman and designer of airplanes and motors had not been sustained and that for eight years prior to his commitment he had earned practically nothing. At age 20 he married.

Two months before commitment the patient began to talk about how he had failed, had "spoiled" his whole life, that it was now "too late." He spoke of hearing someone say, "You must submit." One night his wife was awakened by his talking. He told her of having several visions but refused to describe them. He stated that someone was after him and trying to blame him for the death of a certain man. He had been poisoned, he said. Whenever he saw a truck or a fire engine, the patient stated that someone in it was looking for him in order to claim his assistance to help save the world. He had periods of laughing and shouting and became so noisy and unmanageable that it was necessary to commit him.

On arrival at the hospital, the patient was noted to be an asthenic, poorly nourished man with dilated pupils, hyperactive tendon reflexes, and a pulse rate of 120 per minute. In the admission office he showed many mannerisms, lay down on the floor, pulled at his foot, made undirected, violent striking movements, again struck attendants, grimaced, assumed rigid, attitudinized postures, refused to speak, and appeared to be having auditory hallucinations. He was at once placed in a continuous bath where, when seen later in the day, he was found to be in a stuporous state. His face was without expression, he was mute and rigid, and paid no attention to those about him or to their questions. His eyes were closed and the lids could be separated only with effort. There was no response to pinpricks or other painful stimuli.

On the following morning an attempt was made to bring him before the medical staff for the routine admission interview. As he was brought into the room supported by two attendants, he struggled, grimaced, shouted incoherently, and was resistive. For five days he remained mute, negativistic, and inaccessible, at times staring vacantly into space, at times with his eyes tightly closed. He ate poorly and gave no response to questions but once was heard to mutter to himself in a greatly preoccupied manner, "I'm going to die—I know it—you know it." On the evening of the sixth day he looked about, apparently astonished to find himself in the bath, and asked where he was and how he came there. When asked to tell of his life, he related many known events and how he had once worked in an airplane factory, but added that he had invented an appliance pertaining to airplanes, that this had been stolen and patented through fraud and that as a result he had lost his position. He ate ravenously, then fell asleep, and on awaking was in a catatonic stupor, remaining in this state for several days. He gradually became accessible, and when

asked concerning himself, he replied that he had had a "nervous breakdown following the physical breakdown." He referred to his stuporous period as sleep and maintained that he had no recollection of any events occurring during it. He said, "When I was in the tub I didn't know anything. Everything seemed to be dark as far as my mind is concerned. Then I began to see a little light, like the shape of a star. Then my head got through the star gradually. I saw more and more light until I saw everything in a perfect form a few days ago." Two days later he admitted that he could remember having seen the examiner while in the bath. He rationalized his former mutism by a statement that he had been afraid he would "say the wrong thing," also that he "didn't know exactly what to talk about." From his obviously inadequate emotional response and his statement that he was "a scientist and an inventor of the most extraordinary genius of the twentieth century," it was plain that he was still far from well.

PARANOID TYPES. The features that tend to be most evident in this type or phase are delusions, which are often numerous, illogical, and disregardful of reality, hallucinations, and the usual schizophrenic disturbance of associations and of affect, together with negativism.

Frequently the prepsychotic personality of the paranoid schizophrenic is characterized by poor interpersonal rapport. Often he is cold, withdrawn, distrustful, and resentful of other persons. Many are truculent, have a chip-on-the-shoulder attitude, and are argumentative, scornful, sarcastic, defiant, resentful of suggestions or of authority, and given to caustic remarks. Sometimes flippant, facetious responses are covering an underlying hostility.

The paranoid type tends to have its frank appearance at a somewhat later age than the other forms. It is not common until after adolescence and occurs most frequently after 30 years of age. The patient's previous negative attitudes become more marked, and misinterpretations are common. Ideas of reference are often among the first symptoms. Disorders of association appear. Many patients show an unpleasant emotional aggressiveness. Through displacement, the patient may begin to act out his hostile impulses. His grip on reality begins to loosen. At first his delusions are limited, but later they become numerous and changeable. In the early stages, too, their character usually indicates more clearly the particular psychological needs or experiences that they are created to meet. Occasional remarks may supply fragmentary disclosures of the patient's preoccupations. Rejected tendencies are ideationally projected instead of undergoing repression. Delusions of persecution are the most prominent occurrences in paranoid schizophrenia, but expansive and obviously wish-fulfilling ideas and hypochondriacal and depressive delusions are not uncommon. With increasing personality disorganization, delusional beliefs become less logical. Verbal expressions may be inappropriate and neologistic. The patient is subjected to vague magical forces, and his explanations become extremely vague and irrational. Imaginative fantasy may become extreme but take on the value of reality. Repressed aggressive tendencies may be released in a major outburst; some inarticulate paranoids may manifest an unpredictable assaultiveness. Many paranoid schizophrenics are irritable, discontented, resentful, and angrily suspicious and show a surly aversion to being interviewed. Some manifest an unapproachable, aggressively hostile attitude and may live in a bitter aloofness. Auditory hallucinations usually occur, and the voices are most frequently threatening or accusatory in nature. The patient may show varying degrees of tension and may be subject to upsurges of rage that he seems unable to control. As personality disorganization proceeds, affective responses become increasingly flattened. Mannerisms, apathy, and incoherence are common. In general, paranoid schizophrenia may be regarded as a projective, regressive, defensive type of reaction.

The following is in many respects a rather typical case of paranoid schizophrenia.

A. B., a physician, 38 years of age, was admitted in 1937 to a public hospital for mental disease following his arrest for disturbing the peace. Specifically, he had frightened his neighbors by hurling objects at imaginary people who, he said, were tormenting him, by beating the air with ropes, and by breaking glass in the apartment that he and his wife occupied.

The patient was born in the Ukraine. Little is known of parental characteristics. His mother is described as being "sweet and good-natured as long as things went her way, but she would have violent outbursts of temper, during which she would throw dishes and break glasses when aroused." The patient, the youngest son, is said to have been "the favorite of the whole family. He was spoiled, given his own way, and invariably the other children would be whipped for the misdemeanors of which he was guilty."

When 16 years of age, the patient came to the United States, where he continued his studies. After graduation from college, he entered medical school. His medical course continued satisfactorily until the third year, when he failed to pass a pathology course, which until that time had been one of his best subjects. For some reason, not stated in his history, he was dismissed from the first medical school he entered, but later was admitted to a second one, where he repeated the third year and was graduated.

Upon his commitment to the hospital, his wife described his personality traits as follows: "He has always been a deep thinker. Lately, however, he cannot concentrate. He is rather aggressive and is the type who insists upon imposing his own ideas on everyone else. He thinks that people have to agree with him. He is stubborn and argumentative. This trait was even referred to in his college yearbook. He is an independent thinker and is very bright. He had big plans for the future. He was formerly quite extrovertive until the last few years, when he refused to go out and mingle with people."

Soon after beginning his internship, trouble developed between the young physician and the chief resident. The former was compelled to resign but secured appointment in another hospital and completed an internship. Following this, he went to Vienna to pursue graduate work in ophthalmology, otolaryngology, and bronchoscopy. After his return to the United States, he entered private practice and was apparently successful for the first four years, although, because of various difficulties, he changed locations on several occasions. For some reason not stated in the history, but presumably because of beginning mental disease, the patient gave up his practice and became a medical officer in a Civilian Conservation Camp. He soon began to complain that the commanding officer was "against" him. He made frequent applications of cocaine to his nasal mucous membrane, not, he said, because he was a cocaine addict but in order to neutralize the effects of chloral hydrate, which was being sprayed upon him. After a few months he was released from his Camp appointment. He then began practice in another city, but as he believed that the spraying of chloral hydrate continued there, he remained but two months and then returned to his original place of practice. He met with but little success, as the same ideas of persecution persisted. According to his history, too, "He became forgetful and neglected his cases. He had lapses of memory and seemed to be preoccupied with his own thoughts."

The patient's wife described him as having usually preferred the company of men, "but he has quite a history as far as the opposite sex is concerned." While studying in Vienna, he became involved with a widow and married her. Two weeks after their marriage he discovered, he alleged, that his wife was unfaithful to him and was "a member of a gang of dope peddlers who tried to involve young medical students in their racket." He then returned to the United States. The following year he married again, but the couple lived together for only three months. Three years later the date was set for his third wedding, but he did not appear at a party scheduled to precede the wedding. A quarrel with the expectant bride followed, but finally the wedding took place. Soon he began to object to his wife's talking with other men and accused her of infidelity. On two occasions when she had not even been absent from home, he insisted he had seen her on the street with other men.

Four months before his commitment the patient awoke his wife and told her she must leave the house permanently the following day. He insisted that she was not his wife any longer and the next day asked if she had made her plans to leave. In view of the failure of three marriages, his accusations of infidelity in at least two of them, and his preference for the company of men, the probability at once suggests itself that at least some of the patient's personality difficulties arose from unrecognized homosexual tendencies. Further support to this assumption is added by the fact that, during the psychiatric examination after his hospital admission, he remarked that certain physical complaints from which he was suffering suggested sexual perversion. Doubtless, too, the fact that for several years he had consumed a half pint or more of alcohol daily may be of corroborative significance.

As the patient's mental disorder progressed, he developed a great wealth of delusions. He stated that he was "the link between the living and the dead," that he was a "universal medium," that a certain physician called on him by mental telepathy for added strength and skill in surgical operations. He believed that someone was hiding in a trunk in his house and so he fired several bullets into the trunk. He accused his brother of spraying him with chloral hydrate from the third floor of his house. He therefore sat behind a closed door waiting for his brother, and upon hearing a noise, shot through the door. He grew a beard because his face, he said, was being changed in subtle ways by outside influences, adding that if he wore a beard, his true identity would be known. Following his admission to the hospital, he often spent long hours in his room where he could be heard pacing the floor, moaning, or making a noise

like a dog, striking his head with his fist, or pounding the wall. When asked the reason for his behavior, he explained that he was suffering tortures because people abused their powers of mental telepathy and were directing those powers toward him. He spent nearly all the day in his room where, during the fourth and fifth years of his hospital residence, he would frequently be heard shouting, screaming, and uttering noises that the attendants described as resembling the howling of a wolf. In explanation of these noises, the patient stated that there was a woman spiritualist who, in some way through persons in the hospital, was exerting a peculiar spell on him, and that by making these noises, he could drive the spirits away. His thought processes became progressively disorganized.

Thirteen years after his admission to the hospital, he wrote his ward physician a 10-page letter which he concluded as follows: "In view of the facts and their significance, and in view of the connection of tendencies and the contingent and pertinent effects, and in view of my physical condition brought about by the connected and sustained tendencies and actuating reasons behind them, I shall not consider it a mere negligence, or merely a form of criminal negligence, or merely an ethical vice, but I shall consider your interference with the anatomical and physiological requirements of my health as an outright, deliberate, well-accounted for and reasoned out criminal and dastardly endeavor at homicide."

As the years passed, he was rarely to be seen on his ward but remained in his room, where most of his days were spent in writing and reading. When approached, he was hostile and resentful in attitude. He was, however, less aggressive and less abusive in speech. As frequently happens in the paranoid schizophrenic, his prolonged institutional residence had produced a lessening of tension but little or no modification of thought content.

SCHIZO-AFFECTIVE TYPE. Less frequently seen are cases of mental disorder characterized by recurring episodes that continue to show admixtures of schizophrenic and affective symptoms. The mental content, for example, may be so reality-disregarding that it seems schizophrenic, whereas the mood is one of pronounced elation or depression. Again, the affective features may stand to the fore, but the patient's behavior may be so bizarre that it must be regarded as schizophrenic. In some instances, the prepsychotic personality may have been strongly schizoid or, on the other hand, outgoing and well-socialized, yet the clinical features of the psychosis may be quite at variance or inconsistent with the early personality pattern. It is not uncommon to see depressions in schizoid individuals who, in addition to the depression, show a great deal of anxiety and many neurotic patterns. Such patients are usually refractory to treatment.

Stanley Cobb suggests that schizoid and affective psychoses are variants of one general disease. He offers the opinion that, although in typical cases these two types of psychoses are quite different and easily separated as to classification, they are the extremes of a continuous series of variables. If cases with purely manic–depressive symptoms are put at one end of the series and those with purely schizophrenic symptoms at the other, the space between can be filled in with a long series of cases that are mixtures. Near one end will be examples of depression or mania with "schizophrenic coloring"; near the other, schizophrenia with depressive elements or cyclic mood changes. Cases in which the symptoms are entirely schizophrenic but run in cycles are well known. In the mid-zone of this series are those cases that can scarcely be diagnosed as either schizophrenic or cyclothymic and so are called schizo-affective. Perhaps, as has already been suggested, instead of being variables in a "disease," the variations in clinical symptoms represent admixtures of affective and schizoid components in the basic personality structure.

PSEUDONEUROTIC TYPE. Hoch and Polatin have described what they term *"pseudoneurotic schizophrenia,"* a condition frequently seen in private practice and only occasionally in the public mental hospital. As the name implies, the dynamics are psychotic in character, although the symptom picture, at least in the early stages, is neurotic. The pseudoneurotic schizophrenic usually shows a mixture of anxiety and of phobic, obsessive, depressive, and hypochondriacal symptoms. The underlying schizophrenic disorder is hidden by a façade of neurotic manifestations. Hoch and Polatin speak of the symptomatology as a pan-neurosis. A diffuse anxiety does not leave any life-approach of the patient free from tension. Practically everything he experiences influences this anxiety, and although he tries to force pleasurable experiences, he does not derive pleasure from anything. The neurotic manifestations constantly shift but are never completely absent. The true neurotic is usually anxious to describe his symptoms in minute detail and presses his physician with his explanations. The pseudoneurotic schizophrenic's explanations are vague, indistinct, and often contradictory, and are repeated in a stereotyped manner without details. The organization of the patient's sexuality is often chaotic. Some of these patients have brief psychotic episodes. About one-third of the patients with this misleading neurotic overlay gradually go on to a frank psychosis, although with less regression than that observed in the usual schizophrenic. Many of these patients have previously received unsuccessful psychotherapy.

Schizophrenia in Childhood

There has been much controversy as to whether childhood schizophrenia is the same as adult schizophrenia or whether it is a reactive pattern, reactive in particular to a cold emotional climate in the home during the first two years of life.

ETIOLOGY. It must be said that the causes are obscure. Theories of etiology range all the way from a psychogenic cause based on early disturbance in the mother–child relationship to a deterministic concept rooted in genetics. Bender, who has had an unusually wide experience with childhood schizophrenia, is impressed with the importance of constitutional or, at least, biological factors. She believes that it results from "a developmental lag of the biological processes from which subsequent behavior evolves by maturation at an embryological level, leading to anxiety and secondarily to neurotic defense mechanisms." In her opinion, the fundamental pathological process is a diffuse encephalopathy for which no confirming anatomical evidence is described. Although the etiology is still debatable, there is an increasing belief that schizophrenia is the result of an interaction of constitutional and psychological factors. Perhaps childhood schizophrenia is not a separate and distinct clinical entity but rather a group of related and overlapping clinical syndromes.

Thus W. Goldfarb and others have found that the range of children diagnosed as schizophrenic includes several general clusters. On the one hand, there are those with predominant evidence of neurological or neurophysiologic disturbance who were brought up in families found by psychosocial studies to provide adequate sources for identifications and skill in communications and social awareness. On the other hand, there is a cluster of such children who show little evidence of neurological defect who were reared in disturbed families that provided inadequate roots for the growth of personal identification, communication, and perceptual and conceptual clarity.

Diagnostically these children show impairment in ego functioning. The development of a clear body image, sexual identity, and ability to conceive clearly time and space is impaired. They tend to use preferably the sensory information available from the contact receptors—touch, taste, smell—rather than the distance receptors—sight and vision; thus they limit their capacities for anticipation and generalization and their ability to find a personal identity. It is probable, then, that a goodly proportion of the small children classified as schizophrenic might more properly be considered to be suffering from the personality disorders associated with organic brain damage. Some so classified undoubtedly fall into the group of mental deficiencies.

DIAGNOSIS. The diagnostic criteria specific for childhood schizophrenia are not definitely established. There is undoubtedly a wide variety of clinical pictures. Bender points out that some schizophrenic children are regressive, retarded, blocked, inhibited, mute, autistic, withdrawn, physically asthenic, unsocial, and unable to relate. Others develop overfast, have an exaggerated intellectual brilliance, and are overactive, precocious in language development, and excessively abstract in their thinking. In her experience, any severe psychoneurotic disorder in a child before puberty, whether it is obsessive–compulsive, so-called hysterical, or severe anxiety, is a reactive response to a deep, inherent, threatening disorder, most often schizophrenic in nature.

The older the child, the more does the clinical picture resemble that seen in adults. In such a child, therefore, we may see not only withdrawal and loss of contact and affect, but also hallucinations and delusions. The last two symptoms do not occur below 8 years of age. In the older patient, the onset may be insidious or acute, the insidious type being more frequent. It may be difficult to date the beginning, although retrospectively it is often remembered that peculiarities may have been noted. It is characterized by a general reduction of interests in play and other activities. There is a gradual loss of affective contact with people, accompanied by regressive phenomena. Some patients show a tendency to brooding or to obsessive rumination on some topic ordinarily not of interest to a child. Some patients become aggressive and destructive. Many appear to be feeble-minded and are committed to an institution for mental deficiency. Any great improvement is unusual. Children having an acute onset have usually not been previously regarded as abnormal. Shortly before the appearance of acute features, there may have been an impairment of ability to concentrate, with an accompanying drop in quality of school work. The child may then begin to mumble to himself, sleep poorly, maintain odd postures, show diminished or rigid affect, become inaccessible and extremely restless, and perhaps scream and kick. Usually improvement takes place after several weeks but with a reduction of emotional and ideational expression. Subsequent acute episodes are usual, each one followed by increased personality disorganization.

The psychological problems that the child is attempting to meet with his schizophrenic reaction are those naturally accompanying, or appropriate to, childhood and are therefore different from those of adolescence or adulthood. They are also appropriate to the particular developmental period within childhood at which the onset of the disorder occurs. The symptom formation will therefore be related to the problem that has created the anxiety. In other words, much of the symptom formation is determined by the way in which the child deals with his anxiety. Bender is of the opinion that the principal problems, particularly in the small child, are those of self-identity and therefore of relating to the rest of the world and to body function and of relating to objects, for example, to play material, food, or clothes. In somewhat older children, there may be the problem of relationship to a parent, particularly the mother or siblings, or early childhood sex problems. Mental mechanisms that are normal for early childhood become points of fixation, become exaggerated by repetition, become mingled with other mechanisms, and are carried into later periods of personality development, where they constitute the psychotic symptoms of the schizophrenic child.

EARLY INFANTILE AUTISM. In 1943 Kanner described a syndrome beginning as early as ages 2 or 3 years and characterized by an extreme withdrawal and obsessiveness. To this syndrome he gave the name "early infantile autism." Because of its similarities to, and its differences from, childhood schizophrenia, its categorical place presents a challenging problem. The striking disability in interpersonal relations and the severe obsessive–compulsive mechanisms are the pathognomonic features of autism, but the peculiarities of language and thought, although somewhat different, share the general features of schizophrenia. This early autism occurs more frequently in boys than in girls. The psychotic nature of the illness becomes apparent before the end of the first, and certainly not later than during the second, year of life.

Affective contacts with mother and other persons and the ability of the child to relate himself in the ordinary way to people and situations should normally be well established by 2 or 3 years of age. In early autism there seems to be an inability to form affective ties, with a resulting lack of responsiveness. Almost invariably it is found that the parents of these children are intelligent and successful, often professional persons in good economic circumstances, but obsessively preoccupied with abstractions of a scientific, literary, or artistic nature. The family life is of a cold, formal type, and the child has received extremely little fondling, cuddling, or warm, genuine parental affection. The behavior of the mother toward the child is mechanical and does not convey love.

When a child with early autism is brought to a psychiatrist, his parents have usually assumed that he is severely feebleminded. The autistic child 3 or 4 years of age usually does not talk, does not respond to people, and often has temper tantrums if interfered with. He has little ability to empathize with the feelings of others. His autistic and impenetrable aloneness shuts out anything that comes to the child from outside. If he attempts to form sentences, they are usually for a long time mostly parrot-like repetitions of word combinations that he has overheard, often long previously. He frequently refers to himself as "you" and to the person spoken to as "I." Although the child has no interest in people, he has a good relation to objects and may play happily with them for hours. He has an obsessive urge for a maintenance of sameness. Furniture must continue to be arranged in the same manner and the routine of life must be unchanged.

Although the extreme withdrawal and limited responsiveness of the autistic child suggest that he is feeble-minded, it will usually be found that he has average or even superior intellectual potentiality. The facial expression is often serious and perhaps tense but is usually strikingly intelligent. Frequently those who speak have an extensive vocabulary and a surprising rote memory.

Many of these children continue to function in an emotional vacuum and, for all practical purposes, remain feeble-minded all their lives. Some of them, through permissiveness and emotional stimulation, attain a normal intelligence quotient, become able to pay attention to persons, and to accept and return affection. They may even participate in environmental activities, although they often remain "peculiar."

Perhaps the primary psychopathological mechanism in infantile autism may be described as a disturbance in social perception, analogous to, but more complex than, perceptual difficulties at the sensory–motor level. The question has been raised if there may not be, parallel to intellectual inadequacy, a syndrome of affective inadequacy.

Follow-up studies of autistic children show that by 15 years of age one-third have achieved a moderate social adjustment. About half of those who possess a meaningful language by the age of 5 show further improvement, whereas only rarely does the child without ability to communicate verbally by that age show significant subsequent improvement.

DIFFERENTIAL DIAGNOSIS. Childhood schizophrenia must be differentiated from mental deficiency, organic brain disease, familial dysautonomia, severe neurotic disorders (especially anxiety and obsessive-compulsive states), and behavior disorders based on disturbance in interpersonal relationships.

Course and Prognosis of Schizophrenia

Although the onset of gross schizophrenic disorganization often occurs suddenly, careful examination of the patient's developmental history shows that there have been many indications of personality disturbances in earlier years. More often the diagnosis is made at the time family members no longer are capable of adapting to the progressive disturbance in behavior that which has proceeded insidiously over a number of years. Earlier, the indicators of childhood schizophrenia have been described. In the O'Neal and Robins follow-up of children seen in one clinic, those who became schizophrenic had more infectious diseases during the first two years of life, more hearing problems, difficulties in locomotion, and physical disfigurements than normal children have. The boys were often spoken of as having a feminine appearance. Also, the presence of antisocial behavior antedated the schizophrenic reaction in half of those who were later so diagnosed. They were physically aggressive, incorrigible, and given to vandalism and pathological lying; they also had more phobias, feelings of depression, unhappiness, and paranoid trends than other children.

Granted that schizophrenia can perhaps best be regarded as a special type of maladjustment that usually shows a tendency to be progressive and is therefore to be looked upon with apprehension, a permanent disorganization of the personality does not invariably follow. Indeed, it is now the opinion of many of the closest students of schizophrenia that acute, rather clearly psychogenic schizophrenia may at times disappear, without leaving any injury to the personality. Formerly its incurable nature and progressive course were implied in the definition of the disease, and a favorable outcome was considered presumptive evidence of an error in diagnosis. Of course, the occurrence of an obviously schizophrenic reaction should make the physician exceedingly careful in predicting that a permanently inferior type of adjustment will not be sustained. In recent years, too, there has been an increasing recognition that the episodic nature of a psychosis and the occurrence of symptom-free intermissions may not exclude its schizophrenic nature.

Occasionally one observes a schizophrenic episode of a mild, fleeting nature, with no subsequent recurrence. In many instances, however, the favorable outcome should be characterized as "social recovery" rather than as "cured," or as full recovery. By this it is meant that the patient is able to return to his previous social environment and to previous or equivalent occupation, but with minor symptoms and signs, such as irritability, shyness, or shallowness of affective responses.

From what has been said, it is evident

that in any given case the effect upon the personality and future adjustment of the appearance of a schizophrenic reaction may be quite uncertain. In some cases the course is continuously progressive; in others it is intermittent. More frequently it is a question of remissions and relapses in which, although from the first interests and habits tend to be undermined insidiously, there occur periods of adjustment at a lower level for a considerable period of time. It is estimated that 40 per cent of the schizophrenic patients who enter public mental hospitals or clinics recover or improve; the other 60 per cent fail to improve or ultimately suffer that permanent, malignant disorganization of personality somewhat inaccurately designated as deterioration. Of committed patients who improve sufficiently to be released, about 80 per cent leave the mental hospital within the first year of residence. The expectancy of recovery falls with each year of continued illness. Roughly, about one-third of those patients who are hospitalized during the first year of their illness make a fairly ·complete recovery; one-third get a bit better and become able to return to outside life but remain damaged personalities and may have to return to the hospital from time to time. The remaining third will require indefinite hospital care.

This differentiation of the schizophrenias by course of illness has lead to a tendency to separate schizophrenia into "process" and "reactive groups." In the former are those usually who pursue a persistently chronic and disorganized course and seldom, if ever, make a social adjustment outside hospitals. Langfeldt separates the two groups under the designations of schizophrenia and schizophreniform psychoses. From his studies, he considers that those showing at the beginning emotional blunting, with lack of initiative and peculiar behavior, as well as those paranoid persons with depersonalization and derealization experienced as an influence from outside the self will fall almost invariably into the group of patients with poor prognosis.

The age of onset is not of prognostic significance except that relatively late age offers a less favorable prognosis. Sex has no prognostic significance. Since onset in adolescence sometimes has seemed to occur after loss of a friendship, a study done to examine such relations suggests that one indicator of prognosis for the adolescent schizophrenic is the range and quality of his friendships. It has been found that those who pursue a course of chronic deterioration and hospitalizations have either none or very few adolescent friends. Such friendships are seldom lengthy and, if severed, are infrequently replaced. Usually the friend is either much older or younger, and the interaction between the patient and the friend is infrequent and is limited to a single form of activity. A lack of participation in group activities also expresses the same deficit in establishing interpersonal contacts beyond the family.

As highly desirable and important as it is, it is not yet possible, with our limited knowledge concerning the factors and processes involved, for the psychiatrist, when confronted with acute schizophrenia, definitely to predict what the future course of the particular psychosis will be. In making a prognosis the physician will consider, among other factors, the patient's past record of ability to derive satisfaction from occupation, wholesome group and social activities, and his record of constructive interpersonal relationships. There are certain facts, however, that may serve as general guides in suggesting an opinion.

It will usually be found true that, if the psychosis represents an insidious development and unfolding of a previous schizoid personality, the prognosis is unfavorable. Many such psychoses represent the culmination of a long period of unsatisfactory adaptation. The better adjusted the patient's prepsychotic personality, the more directly and confidently the patient has been accustomed to meet the problems and difficulties of life, the richer his interests, the more definite an external precipitating situation, and the more rapid the onset, the better the prognosis. The existence of anxiety and of an easily ascertained emotional problem makes the prognosis more favorable. With the presence of features such as those just mentioned, "spontaneous" recoveries, i.e., without therapeutic efforts by a physician, are not uncommon. A slow, insidious withdrawal is apt to lead to an irreversible disorganization of the personality. If the ego was not strong enough to withstand routine difficulties, the prognosis is not good. If it broke only after overwhelming stress, the prognosis is better.

The prognosis is not influenced by the intelligence or previous education of the patient. Those with high personal aspirations for success often do poorly. An apparently "mild" case need not be an early one or of favorable prognosis. The presence of a well-marked affective element is of hopeful significance, although hypochondriasis is not desirable, particularly if these are predominantly self-accusatory. Self-condemnatory hallucinations have a more favorable connotation and seem related to the patient's willingness to accept some responsibility for his behavior. The presence of cyclothymic factors in the personality background renders the prognosis more favorable. The persistence of hallucinations after an initial emotional tension has subsided is not a favorable indication. If the psychosis has existed for a year without clear-cut signs of improvement, a favorable outcome is scarcely to be expected, although it is by no means unknown.

Previous remissions should lead one to expect that a given episode will be followed by improvement. The longer the interval between attacks, the better the prognosis. In many cases of schizophrenia, regression is an important mechanism, so attempts are often made to base a prognosis on the depth of regression manifested by the patient. Infantile posture and behavior, although often of unfavorable significance, should not outweigh other considerations in forming an opinion as to prognosis. It may be parenthetically commented that the physician whose psychiatric experience has been confined to institutions tends to develop an unwarrantably pessimistic attitude in prognosis. Until recently, the mortality rate among institutionalized schizophrenic patients was estimated to be twice as high as in the normal, community population.

A word should be said as to the prognosis in the different types. In catatonia, the prognosis is relatively good if the onset has been stormy and the episode is still acute. Many of these patients are restored to their prepsychotic level of adjustment for varying periods, at times for several years. The prognosis in the simple form, with its insidious marasmus of the personality developing in the absence of unusual environmental and experiential stresses, is poor. A certain number, sheltered by some normal member of the family, maintain a colorless, uneventful existence, while others become paupers, hoboes, or petty criminals. The course of the hebephrenic form tends to be one of dereistic regression and of progressive disorganization, although occasionally remissions occur before the final disorganization of personality.

The question as to whether the paranoid type of schizophrenia ever recovers is sometimes raised. The reply to this depends somewhat on a definition of terms. Undoubtedly remissions occur, and these may be looked upon as social recoveries, but they are rarely to be judged as psychological recoveries, even though the patient's adjustment during the interval is well socialized and there are no distortions of reality in response to subjective needs. In general, surly and bitter attitudes indicate the presence of a malignant process.

Finally, both for the sake of stating the opinion of one of the greatest students of schizophrenia as to the prognosis and for emphasizing the responsibility of the physician who undertakes the care of the early case of schizophrenia, the conclusion of Bleuler must be quoted: "Although a certain number of patients become deteriorated with every treatment, and others improve even in apparently severe cases, the treatment will decide in more than one third of schizophrenic cases whether they can become social men again or not." The more individualized and personalized the care and treatment, the greater the recovery rate.

Diagnosis

At times perplexing similarities are observed between schizophrenia and the psychoneuroses, between schizophrenia and other biogenetic major psychoses, particularly the manic–depressive ones, but rarely between schizophrenia and organic mental disorders. It is doubtful, too, if there is any definite demarcation between psychoneurotic and schizophrenic reactions. Again, the distinction between schizophrenic disturbances of the personality and those of the psychopath or character neurotic may be very difficult. Extreme caution should be exercised in declaring that an isolated symptom is conclusive evidence of schizophrenia, and in evaluating a symptom, the clinical setting in which it occurs should be carefully examined. Neither should the eventual outcome be the most important determinant in diagnosis.

Many of the differential points among schizophrenic patients, hysteria, and dissociative reactions are discussed in Chapter 28. In addition to what is mentioned there, attention should be called to the fact that the onset in hysteria is usually more sudden and that a psychological motive is more apparent. In schizophrenic stupor, one does not discover the expression of an emotional state. In dissociative stupor, on the other hand, one may note an expression of perplexity, fear, elation, or some other affective state. The history of an insidious change in interests points toward schizophrenia. Not only are the symptoms of hysteria and of dissociation more sudden in onset, but they are more paroxysmal. The symptoms of hysteria are influenced more obviously by certain persons in the environment. Whereas the hysteric desires attention, the schizophrenic is more apt to have periods when he is preoccupied, detached, and apathetic. The hysteric uses conventional, intelligible symbols,

while the schizophrenic uses individual or archaic ones. One can feel himself into the psychic life of the hysteric and of some dissociative states, but with difficulty, if at all, into that of the schizophrenic.

In the early stage of schizophrenia, the differentiation from obsessive neurosis may be difficult. Sometimes schizophrenic reactions result from the release of primitive impulses that had previously been kept under control by the aid of obsessional symptoms. In schizophrenia there is usually more rumination and less tension than in the obsessive neurosis, as the patient who suffers from the latter has a strong conscious resistance to his obsessions and compulsions, a resistance that is lacking in the schizophrenic, who is not particularly disturbed by them. Often the schizophrenic, in the early phases of the disorder, expresses hypochondriacal complaints. His hypochondria lacks, however, the dramatization seen in the psychoneuroses.

Frequently one of the most difficult differentiations in mental disorders is between schizophrenia and manic–depressive psychosis. Doubtless this is a result, in part at least, of the fact that many people are not pure schizoid or pure syntonic types but rather are personality alloys and are characterized by admixtures in their personality. In addition to what is said in Chapter 23 on affective reactions, attention may be called to the fact that the onset of schizophrenia tends to be more insidious and the excitement in schizophrenia is more frequently paroxysmal, while that of the manic is more sustained; the mood of the schizophrenic rarely possesses the infectious quality seen in the manic–depressive. The delusions of the depressed schizophrenic are more grotesque than those of the depressed manic, and he is less distressed by them. Illogical remarks and incongruous statements suggest schizophrenia.

The difficulty in differentiating between these two disorders arises largely in the earlier stages of schizophrenia. With recurring episodes, the schizophrenic nature of symptoms previously doubtful becomes more apparent, with the result that confusion with manic–depressive symptomatology no longer exists. It rarely happens that a psychosis that is apparently schizophrenic in its early phases proves subsequently to be of a manic–depressive reaction type. The reverse, however, is common. There are, nevertheless, many cases of mental disorder, the recurring episodes of which continue to show a mixture of schizophrenic symptoms and of affective ones, especially depression and anxiety.

There is usually no difficulty in distinguishing schizophrenia from epilepsy. Occasionally, nevertheless, the schizophrenic suffers from epileptiform or syncopal attacks that to the inexperienced observer strongly suggest the seizures of epilepsy. In that case, careful inquiry should be made as to whether the seizures or the mental symptoms appeared first, and the nature of the seizure should be observed; in schizophrenia it lacks the definiteness in type and the genuine disturbance of consciousness occurring in epilepsy.

In discussing the diagnosis of schizophrenia, mention should be made of what is often spoken of as chronic alcoholic hallucinosis. The permanent persistence in the chronic alcoholic of auditory hallucinations in a setting of clear consciousness, frequently with systematized delusions, was formerly considered as a symptom of an alcoholic psychosis. Many psychiatrists now believe that such cases are really schizophrenic reactions.

Adolescent psychoses do not belong in any special classification of their own, yet their capacity for variation in duration, intensity, and form frequently cause them to present difficulties in diagnosis. At that period one may alternatively see phases of anxiety, behavior disorder, affective disturbance, or schizophrenia. In retrospect, truancy and other forms of delinquent behavior have preceded the onset of a disorder that is subsequently diagnosed as schizophrenia. The adolescent schizophrenic frequently shows a more lively emotional response than is usual in the adult and also less incongruity of affect.

The symptomatic emphasis in adolescent schizophrenia is usually on social withdrawal, on disorders of activity, interest, and speech, and on peculiarities of manner. It must be acknowledged, however, that it is not always easy to differentiate the emotional disorders of adolescence from incipient schizophrenia. That period is normally one of emotional turmoil and instability. Much that would be regarded as pathological in later life may then be but a temporary exaggeration of normal tendencies. The adolescent, with his self-questioning and perturbing heart-searching, may verbalize his disruption of emotion and impulse without being schizophrenic. Adolescent maladjustments among shy, withdrawn personalities with feelings of inadequacy or inferiority, with evident internal conflict and family tensions, particularly with one or other parent, are not uncommon. Poor socialization, lack of motivation, and a brooding sense of inferiority may be merely a retarded ability to integrate the new emotional drives and experiences of adolescence. Such symptoms may, however, be those of an incipient schizophrenia.

Treatment

The treatment of schizophrenia, particularly in its early stages, is undertaken with far less pessimism than formerly. Its success depends to no small degree upon the therapeutic initiative, energy, and effort of the physician, although the results will be small if the psychotic methods of thinking and feeling have become habits and established forms of adjustment. In early cases, the remission rate after treatment is about twice as high as is that of remissions occurring spontaneously.

MENTAL HYGIENE. Since it has been said that schizophrenia becomes manifest for the most part only after a prolonged period of incubation, the question naturally arises as to whether a disease so disorganizing to the personality can be prevented. The goal of the modern mental hygiene movement, with its child-guidance clinics and its school and college psychiatrists, is not merely to prevent or correct faulty attitudes and the less malignant maladjustments of childhood or adolescence, but to promote healthful patterns of feeling and thinking and to prevent the establishment of subterfuges and substitutions that result in imbalances of personality and may finally culminate in the major psychoses, of which schizophrenia is the most important. How far the rapidly-growing preventive psychiatric movement will be able to modify the various factors that lead to a schizophrenic adaptation is as yet entirely unknown. In the light of the knowledge now available, however, the body of principles included in the term mental hygiene seems to constitute the most rational means of preventing the malfunctioning of the personality known as schizophrenia, and the shy, retiring, seclusive, unsociable child and those exhibiting antisocial activities should receive careful guidance designed to promote socialization and a wholesome adaptation between the growing personality and its environment.

EARLY STAGES. Ideally, treatment of the schizophrenic should have begun before obvious symptoms of a mental disorder are manifest. Unfortunately, this rarely occurs. The patient only occasionally seeks treatment himself, and his family, unable or unwilling to recognize that he is mentally ill, does not refer him to a psychiatrist.

Following the initial examination, decision usually must be made as to whether the patient should be treated in an out-patient department or office or admitted to a hospital. If behavior has been disturbed and promises to threaten later social acceptance, prompt admission for hospital treatment is indicated. Again, some form of hospital care is advisable when the patient is living in a home in which the family attitude is argumentative, critical, domineering, or rejecting. Social isolation at home or in a lodging and lack of vocational and social skills may suggest the advisability of day or night hospital care.

PHARMACOLOGICAL THERAPY. Whether the decision is to commence treatment on an out-patient or a hospital basis, the first therapeutic move is to provide relief of anxiety and its attendant reflections in the psychotic symptom-complex.

Phenothiazines. Administration of one of the phenothiazine derivatives is today the immediate method of choice. *Chlorpromazine,* the first of these agents to be introduced, probably is the preferred drug for the majority of patients. There are no standard rules for the administration of chlorpromazine or its analogues. For the mildly disturbed schizophrenic, initial oral dosages of 25 to 50 mg. three to four times daily may be tried for several days to ascertain the patient's tolerance and idiosyncratic responses. The drug may then be administered in doses of 100 or 200 mg. three or four times daily if the patient's condition seems to indicate this amount. Many patients may be maintained on a dosage of 400 mg. daily for indefinite periods. Some have received total daily doses of 1000 mg. or more without ill effect. If the patient is acutely disturbed when first seen, a 50 mg. dose of chlorpromazine may be tried by intramuscular injection; the drug is again given at this level, or in 100 mg. doses, every three or four hours.

Chlorpromazine is indicated for all types of schizophrenia. It is of particular value in the treatment of those patients who show tension, psychomotor overactivity, agitation, impulsiveness, aggressive outbursts, destructiveness, and antagonistic, paranoid reactions. Administration of chlorpromazine to the acutely ill schizophrenic patient frequently results in the disappearance of hallucinations and delusional ideas within the first two weeks of treatment.

The longer the schizophrenic has been ill, the less chance there is that the use of chlorpromazine will be followed by recovery. The best results are secured with patients who have not been ill for more than two years. Among these, the results will depend largely on the clinical manifestations, the degree of improvement being much greater in the over-active, disturbed patient, who improves to a degree that he becomes amenable to occupational and other activity therapies and, hopefully, to some degree of psychotherapy. Although most over-active schizophrenics who have been hospitalized for long periods of time show some improvement, not more than 5 to 10 per cent of those who have been hospitalized for more than five continuous years become well enough to leave the hospital, and an appreciable number of these will have to return at a later time. The problem of the care of the chronically ill, over-active patient who does not improve sufficiently to leave the hospital will be greatly eased by chlorpromazine, however. Delusions and hallucinations may persist, but usually they are no longer disturbing to the patient. The sullen, sarcastic, and antagonistic patient is less irritable and frequently becomes quiet, co-operative, and accessible.

Of the various types of schizophrenia, the acute paranoid forms appear to respond most favorably, followed by the acute catatonic. The behavior of the chronic catatonic patients and the hebephrenic is less modifiable, although lessening of aggressive and impulsive actions usually follows the use of this drug.

Certain other phenothiazines are reported to be more effective in modifying some forms of disturbed behavior than chlorpromazine. Thus trifluoperazine (Stelazine) is said to be particularly beneficial for the withdrawn, apathetic, and depressed schizophrenic. It is administered by giving initially oral doses of 5 mg. three or four times daily; this dosage may be increased to total daily levels of 60 to 80 mg. Thioridazin (Mellaril) serves as effectively as the other phenothiazines but is less likely to produce the general run of toxic side effects. Perphenazine (Trilafon) is indicated for those patients likely to be exposed to the sun, since its usage has not been associated with the skin photosensitivity noted with chlorpromazine and other derivatives. More complete descriptions are given of the pharmacological actions, dosage ranges, and side and toxic effects of these agents in Chapter 33, Pharmacological Therapy.

Reserpine. Tranquilizing effects similar to those produced by the use of chlorpromazine may be obtained by the administration of reserpine. Its greatest usefulness in schizophrenia is, therefore, in the case of the tense, overactive, combative, hostile, and threatening patient. Its effects, however, are less prompt than those secured by chlorpromazine. Like the latter drug, reserpine may be given intramuscularly or by mouth. The dosage should be individually adjusted. The initial dose may be 1 mg. given intramuscularly twice a day. After three days, the intramuscular dose may be increased to 2 mg. At that time the patient may also receive 1 mg. twice a day by mouth. After one week, intramuscular administration may be stopped and the oral dose increased to 4 mg. twice a day. Usually this dosage is not increased, although some physicians increase it to 4 mg. or 5 mg. twice a day if side effects do not appear.

In spite of its greater toxicity, chlorpromazine is more widely used than reserpine. Many psychiatrists are of the opinion that chlorpromazine is more effective than reserpine in the treatment of schizo-affective and paranoid schizophrenias.

Combination therapy. Combined reserpine–chlorpromazine therapy may be beneficial in chronic deteriorated schizophrenic or in chronic schizophrenic patients in whom apathy and withdrawal are prominent. Their combined use is often advisable in patients who have failed to respond to chlorpromazine alone or in schizophrenic patients in whom long-term maintenance therapy is anticipated.

PSYCHOTHERAPY. In addition to the relief of anxiety and its attendant symptoms, the psychiatric therapist will be concerned with the establishment of a treatment regimen that provides over time opportunity for development of a more stable and adaptive personality. He will be particularly mindful of those weaknesses of ego identity and function that characterize the schizophrenic and will attempt to ascertain in his growing knowledge of the patient's development whether these defects are due to lack or deprivation of socializing experiences or the consequence of isolation and withdrawal as the result of psychological conflict and associated emotional turmoil.

It is necessary, then, to consider, in the long term planning for treatment for the schizophrenic, the day-to-day social milieu in which he lives as well as his needs for specialized psychotherapy. Measures must be taken to strengthen his ego through restructuring the environment so that he comes in contact with other healthy persons whose interpersonal contact provides a ground in which he may develop trust, assurance, and, hopefully, some personal autonomy. The possible identifications with others than family members will clarify his confusion about his own social and sexual identity. The therapeutic milieu must be stimulating physically so as to provide an increasing awareness and perception of his own body and its functions, upon which may be established a satisfying and realistic concept of his body and its actions. Furthermore, this environment must provide a structured and stimulating social world so that there may be ingrained the sense of time and satisfactions in completeness of action and so that he may avoid the inevitable consequences of isolation. It must be emphasized that isolation leads to reduced awareness of perceptual stimulation from within and without and results in reexperiencing and becoming preoccupied with thought processes divorced from ego control, followed by regressive infantile thinking processes and hallucinatory satisfactions.

Therefore, if the patient is to be treated as an out-patient, arrangements should be made for the psychiatrist to see him on a regular schedule of appointments, with a clearly understood recognition that improvement with insight will not be quickly gained. The frequency of appointments for treatment designed to modify and improve ego function should not be less than twice weekly and often must be more. The psychiatrist should aid his patient to decide if he is to continue to work or attend school, or to limit his strivings in other directions. The patient should be cautioned as to the toxic side effects of the pharmaceuticals prescribed.

Many psychotherapists believe that the primary problem of the schizophrenic is not his anxiety about others and a consequent narcissistic withdrawal, often dating back to childhood, but fear of his own hostile, destructive tendencies. Although preoccupied, suspicious, and anxiety-ridden because of the negative impulses he feels in himself, the schizophrenic can often, at least in the early stages of his illness, be helped to relate himself to people. Frieda Fromm-Reichmann stressed that, although the schizophrenic longs for interpersonal contact, he equally fears such a closeness. Thus in office psychotherapy, careful consideration must be given to the extent and readiness of each patient to engage in social relations with others. In many instances, aid must be provided to the withdrawn patient through planning with social service agencies and workers.

For the more seriously disturbed, hospital care is advisable. The good hospital not only protects the patient from a threatening family, social, or vocational environment but provides healthy substitutes for erecting new identifications and sources for resolving conflicts as well as learning social skills previously weak or defective.

Thus, the hospital psychiatrist and many other special therapists and patients of both sexes offer opportunities to the patient for testing and establishing less anxiety-ridden relations with others. In turn, these opportunities allow the potentiality for reducing the confusion of personal and sexual identity so characteristic of these patients. The well-regulated and structured activity of a therapeutic institution provides arrangements for the reestablishment of the patient's ego, allowing him to make clear-cut discriminations between himself and the environment and to refix his concepts of time and space. The use of recreational aids and physiotherapies is dynamically important in stimulating bodily activity that under-lies the development of sound and satis-fying body ego.

One attempts to stimulate the patient's interests and redirect them to things out-side himself, detach his emotions from sub-jective material, inculcate healthful, so-cialized habits, and abstract him from his spiritual isolation. Among important aids to these ends and to the gaining of satisfaction from adaptive behavior are forms of occupational therapy chosen to meet his emotional needs. Recreation, games, music, and congenial companion-ships all have a common objective of promoting interpersonal relationships. Occupational therapy not only helps to re-establish contacts with reality, but through personal contact with the ther-apist frequently brings a therapeutic emo-tional relationship. Probably, in fact, the most important tool that the occupa-tional or other auxiliary therapist brings to the treatment situation is a genuine warmth, understanding, flexibility, and objectivity.

Although not a few patients become permanently isolated in their own autistic lives in spite of every effort at treatment, the degree of improvement is, broadly speaking, directly proportional to the at-tention and treatment that they receive. There is usually a tendency to a progres-sive introversion and habit-deterioration. A constant effort should therefore be made to keep alive or re-establish an affective contact with reality and prevent the patient from drifting into a state of inactivity and indifference. He should be encouraged to participate in congenial ac-tivity, and his environment should pro-vide as many as possible of those things of life that interest and satisfy the person in mental health. Treatment in institu-tions should undoubtedly be socialized to a greater extent than is now the case. In no instance should the patient be lost in the obscurity of chronically ill persons in a ward. It has been said that the pic-ture seen in chronic and hopeless insti-tutional cases is one-third a result of dis-ease, while two-thirds is a reaction to an unfavorable and unsuitable environment.

The ideal hospital would provide what the home cannot, in addition to the ad-vantages that the patient would have re-ceived had he remained in the home.

In 1939 Myerson described what he termed the "total push" method for the treatment of the institutionalized chroni-cally ill schizophrenic. The patient is ap-proached with stimulating and activating procedures from as many sides as possible. Measures that tend to arouse the patient from his automatized isolation are vigor-ously employed day by day. An attempt is made not to emphasize the separation created by the patient's illness, but to create as nearly as possible an atmosphere like that of the general community. Daily, weather permitting, the patient is taken for walks. Sustained, active efforts are made to overcome the inertia of the pa-tient and his resistance to participation in games and exercise. Classes in bowling are organized, and a game room is pro-vided.

As patients improve, they participate in dancing, music, craftsmanship, and gen-eral occupational therapy. Physiothera-peutic measures, such as showers, douches, and massages, are utilized daily. Diet is liberal, and small doses of insulin are often employed. Stress is placed on keeping the patient properly dressed in attractive clothing; the male patient is shaved regularly, and fingernails and hair receive careful attention. Praise in the presence of the group and reward under the same circumstances are liberally uti-lized as motives. The relationships de-veloped between patient and the worker are of therapeutic value. Also, an effort is made to provide the patient with op-portunity for experiencing a sense of be-longing. A constructive release of hostility is encouraged, a sense of personal worth is fostered, and opportunity for social interaction is facilitated. The participa-tion of the nurse and aide in these highly-organized activities improves their morale and promotes a greater interest in the welfare of the patient.

Myerson's "total push" therapy was directed to the chronic "deteriorated" schizophrenic. This "deterioration" is largely the result of rejection by others, of the patient's belief that the world is basically hostile, and the great failure of his environment to meet his emotional needs. All too often his hospital life is spent in idleness or futile routine. His surroundings are drab, his communications are not understood, and he feels isolated from those assigned to care for him. He feels chronically frustrated in his search for a way of relating comfortably to the hospital environment and as a result becomes more deeply withdrawn.

Stanton and Schwartz have made interesting contributions to the conception of schizophrenic deterioration as a psychosocial adaptive pattern. They found it was possible to discern meaningful patterns in the occurrences in a mental hospital. They studied, for example, the symptoms of soiling and wetting, so common in chronic deteriorated schizophrenics. They pointed out that the term "incontinence" is a misnomer if by that term is meant loss of sphincter control. The so-called incontinent schizophrenic patient, Stanton and Schwartz discovered, discharges his excreta in a highly controlled manner. There are some situations in which wetting and soiling rarely, if ever, occur. On the other hand, they may take place in a specific constellation of circumstances under the pressure of an emotional need. One patient, for example, who was extremely fearful of human contact found that people left her alone when she had soiled. Another patient who craved the attentions of a mother figure soiled herself to compel attentions from a nurse.

Special Forms of Treatment

INTENSIVE PSYCHOTHERAPY. In recent years there has been an increasing use of psychotherapy, either as a supplementary or as an exclusive measure, in the treatment of schizophrenia. Although psychoanalytical techniques such as are usually employed in the neuroses have never been satisfactorily successful in the treatment of schizophrenia, yet modifications have now been evolved that may successfully maintain many patients at a functioning level of social adjustment.

The establishment of a working relationship with the patient is essential to successful therapy in the schizophrenic. The relationship of the patient to the therapist is of a different quality from that seen in neuroses. It is exceedingly fragile and is subject to withdrawal on the basis of any suspicion or indication that there is a limitation of interest on the part of the physician. Breaking through to obtain the trust of the suspicious, withdrawn, highly sensitive, and perhaps disturbed patient requires infinite patience and tolerance. Rarely can the physician confine his contacts with the patient to set office hours. He must be available whenever periods of great anxiety occur. In the early stages of treatment, the patient's verbal communications may be incomprehensible to the physician, and some form of communication between the two must be established. At this stage, the therapist does not attempt to have the patient, as would be done with the neurotic, form an association with the verbalizations he is producing. Rather does the therapist listen and try to relate the patient's verbalizations to the feeling-tone of the particular interpersonal events that are reported to have preceded the distorted communications or are observed to occur in close temporal relationship. Then, when particular communications are heard, the therapist may interpret the patient's feeling directly and make it possible for him to appreciate that he is understood and will not be hurt. The patient must find in the therapist a sustaining source of security on the emergence of anxiety and hostility.

The therapist must be constantly alert to his own behavior and of its possible meanings to the patient. For this reason, the therapy is conducted with the patient facing the therapist. The patient has a continuing need to check his reaction through visualizing the gestures and moves of the therapist. The latter must see himself as an active participant with his patient and must be free to disclose his own feelings and the meanings of his actions in order to clarify the patient's frequent distortions of the situation.

Contrary to the usual custom in the analytical therapy of the neuroses, the analysis of dreams is not advised. Preoccupation with dream analysis perpetuates the schizophrenic's propensity for withdrawal into fantasy living. What he needs is to face continually the emotionally toned events of everyday living and to learn socially adaptive methods of accepting them. Usually, too, the primitive impulses of the schizophrenic are so evident in their overt pathology that dream analysis will provide but little additional information. In contrast with earlier attempts to resolve delusional and hallucinatory experiences through analysis of their content, this is now recognized as unsatisfactory procedure in the therapeutic process. Rather, efforts are made to derive an understanding of the interpersonal situations that precipitate the patient's expressions of delusional and hallucinatory material and the significance of the psychopathology in terms of the affect produced in such situations. Frieda Fromm-Reichmann described this technique in some detail.

It should be remembered that there are limitations in the psychotherapy of the schizophrenic patient. Complete resolution of the schizophrenic process, fixed through indelible deprivations or traumata of early life, is rarely obtained, even by therapists of the greatest experience and patience. If, in an effort to reach the ideal, the enthusiastic psychiatrist presses his patient beyond his capacity, he may do him incalculable harm. The therapist must, of course, continue indefinitely a supportive, though distant, therapeutic relationship when the patient indicates the need.

In not a few schizophrenics, a "spontaneous" remission or recovery occurs. In such cases, the therapeutic agent usually remains unknown. In many instances it would appear that improvement followed because, for some years, the patient was able to make contact with some individual—perhaps a nurse, aide, or even some other patient—in his environment, and that through this interpersonal relationship the individual became a bridge toward reality.

Group psychotherapy. Group psychotherapy has proved useful for many schizophrenic patients. It has been administered in conjunction with individual therapy or as the sole psychotherapeutic measure. It is most likely to have value for the schizophrenic with major deficit in group living and for those inhibited in individual psychotherapy.

INSULIN COMA THERAPY. The history of the therapy of schizophrenia has been characterized by the use of various methods that temporarily had enthusiastic proponents but failed to stand the test of time. Insulin shock therapy has been largely superceded by the effectiveness of the phenothiazine drugs in recent years. The details of its application are discussed in Chapter 34.

The percentage of remissions following insulin therapy depends largely on the previous duration of the psychosis. The recovery rate is by far the greatest in patients who have not been ill for more than six months and are thus those most likely to improve without the aid of specific therapies. Patients who have been sick less than one year will, under insulin treatment, do twice as well as those who have been sick more than one year. Full remission in patients who have been ill for more than two years is rare. Combined insulin and electroconvulsive therapy may succeed in cases in which the two treatments given separately have failed. Insulin therapy in paranoid forms produces better results than in hebephrenic or simple types. Treatment is not followed by any change in the prepsychotic personality.

ELECTRIC CONVULSIVE THERAPY. Because of the simplicity of its application, its fewer hazards, and the need for a smaller group of specially-trained personnel, there has been a tendency to substitute electric convulsive treatment for insulin therapy if some form of shock therapy is desired. There continues to be some controversy as to the relative results secured in schizophrenia by insulin and shock therapy. It would seem probable that a slightly larger number of full remissions is secured by insulin therapy, yet many psychiatrists believe that if electric shock treatment is prolonged and intensive, with at least 20 treatments, it is as effective as insulin. Of the subtypes of schizophrenia, catatonic excitement and acute paranoid forms respond best to electroshock treatment. The results are naturally best when affective features are present and the assets of the prepsychotic personality are good. Patients who relapse after each of two successive courses of treatment have been kept on a maintenance treatment regimen of one or two treatments a week. The use of electroshock as a maintenance treatment has been largely discontinued since the introduction of tranquilizing drugs.

Manfred Bleuler, who, like his distinguished father, Eugen Bleuler, has been a devoted student of schizophrenia, is doubtful if permanence of improvement after either electroshock or insulin coma is greater than after schizophrenic remissions without them. He adds: "Cures effected by shock treatments will be achieved preferably in the case of schizophrenics who would be expected to improve without them on the basis of a wavelike-acute course, administered in the light of personal history prior to illness and of family relationships. In fact, shock therapies seldom produce lasting cures in schizophrenics whose personal psychodynamics, chronic course and family constellations would necessitate from the very beginning an unfavorable prognosis. . . . Shock (electric and insulin) are probably not causal treatments. They subdue and improve the patient and accelerate his cure. They facilitate human contact and, thereby, psychotherapeutic accessibility."

PREFRONTAL LOBOTOMY. This form of treatment will not be employed unless all others have failed. If it is to be employed, it should be used before emotional deterioration is advanced. If, after two or three years of active treatment that has included psychotherapy, tranquilizing drugs, and coma therapies, the patient has shown no improvement, frontal lobotomy is usually to be recommended. Best results are secured if the patient's original personality was relatively well organized. Patients who show persistent tension, excessive motor activity, resistiveness, destructiveness, or combativeness are the most suitable subjects for this treatment. In such cases, one may at least reasonably expect that improvement will be obtained in adaptive behavior in simple situations as well as in social and ward behavior and in work activity. Mood level will be more desirable, and aggressive tendencies will be reduced. However, if the schizophrenic process has progressed to a chronic and general personality disorganization, marked by persisting emotional dulling, loss of contact with people, widespread delusions, and emotional disintegration, the results of the operation are disappointing. In fact, very few patients are helped if the disease has existed for 10 years or more. Hebephrenics rarely respond favorably. Catatonic excitement usually responds well to lobotomy, as do paranoid schizophrenic states.

BIBLIOGRAPHY

Arieti, S.: Interpretation of Schizophrenia. New York, Robert Brunner, 1955.

Bateson, G., Jackson, D. D., Haley, J., and Weakland, J.: Toward a theory of schizophrenia. Behavioral Science, 1:251–264, 1956.

Beck, S. J.: The Six Schizophrenias. Research Monographs, No. 6, New York, American Orthopsychiatric Association, 1954.

Bender, L.: Childhood schizophrenia. Psychiat. Quart., 27:663–681, 1953.

Idem, and Helme, W. H.: A quantitative test of theory and diagnostic indicators of childhood schizophrenia. Arch. Neurol. & Psychiat., 70: 413–427, 1953.

Idem, and Freedman, A. M.: A study of the first three years in the maturation of schizophrenic children. Quart. J. Child Behavior, 4:245–272, 1952.

Bleuler, E.: Dementia Praecox or the Group of Schizophrenias. Translated by Zinkin, J. New York, International Universities Press, Inc., 1950.

Idem: Textbook of Psychiatry. Translated by Brill, A. A. New York, Dover Publications, 1951.

Brody, E. B., and Redlich, F. C.: Psychotherapy with Schizophrenics. New York, International Universities Press, Inc., 1951.

Conolly, J.: The Treatment of the Insane Without Mechanical Restraints. London, Smith, Elder & Co., 65, Cornhill, 1856.

Ehrentheil, O. F., and Jenney, P. B.: Does time stand still for some psychotics? Arch. Gen. Psych., 3:1–3, 1960.

Eisenberg, L.: The autistic child in adolescence. Am. J. Psychiat., 112:607–612, 1956.

Idem: The course of childhood schizophrenia. Arch. Neurol. & Psychiat., 78:69–83, 1957.

Idem, and Kanner, L.: Early infantile autism. Am. J. Orthopsychiat., 26:556–566, 1956.

Fish, B.: The detection of schizophrenia in infancy. J. Nerv. & Ment. Dis., 125:1–24, 1957.

Fisher, S.: Some observations suggested by the Rorschach test concerning the "ambulatory schizophrenic." Psychiat. Quart. Supplement, 29:81–89, 1955.

Freeman, T., Cameron, J. L., and McGhee, A.: Chronic Schizophrenia. New York, International Universities Press, Inc., 1958.

Freyhan, F. A., and Bleuler, E.: Concept of the group of schizophrenias at mid-century. Am. J. Psychiat., 114:769–779, 1958.

Fromm-Reichmann, F.: Principles of Intensive Psychotherapy. Chicago, The University of Chicago Press, 1950.

Idem: Notes on the development of treatment of schizophrenics by psychoanalytic psychotherapy. Psychiatry, 11:263–273, 1948.

Idem: Psychotherapy of schizophrenia. Am. J. Psychiat., 111:410–419, 1954.

Goldfarb, W.: Childhood Schizophrenia. Cambridge, Massachusetts, Harvard University Press, 1961.

Gregory, I.: Genetic factors in schizophrenia. Am. J. Psychiat., 116:961–972, 1960.

Hanfmann, E., and Kasanin, J.: Conceptual Thinking in Schizophrenia. New York, Nervous and Mental Disease Monographs, 1943.

Hecker, E.: Die Hebephrenie. Virchow's Archiv f. pathol. Anat., Physiol., und klin. Medizin, 52:394–431, 1871.

Hoch, P. H., and Polatin, P.: Pseudoneurotic forms of schizophrenia. Psychiatric Quart., 23: 248–276, 1949.

Horwitt, M. K.: Fact and artifact in the biology of schizophrenia. Science, 124:429–430, 1956.

Jackson, D. D. (Ed.): Etiology of Schizophrenia. New York, Basic Books, Inc., 1960.

Johnson, A. M., Giffin, M. E., Watson, E. J., and Beckett, P. G. S.: Observations on ego functions in schizophrenia. Psychiatry, 19:143–148, 1956.

Kahlbaum, K.: Die Katatonie oder das Spannungsirresein. Berlin, August Hirschwald, 1874.

Kalinowsky, L., and Hoch, P. H.: Somatic Treatments in Psychiatry. New York, Grune & Stratton, 1961.

Kallmann, F. J.: Heredity in Health and Mental Disorder. New York, W. W. Norton & Co., Inc., 1953.

Kanner, L.: Early infantile autism. J. Pediat., 25:211–217, 1944.

Idem: Problems of nosology and psychodynamics of early infantile autism. Am. J. Orthopsychiat., 19:416–426, 1949.

Kasanin, J.: Language and Thought in Schizophrenia. Berkeley, University of California Press, 1944.

Kety, S. S.: Biochemical theories of schizophrenia. Science, 129:1528–1532, 1959.

Knight, R. P.: Borderline states. Bull. Menninger Clin., 17:1–12, 1953.

Kolb, L. C.: Psychotherapeutic evolution and its implications. Psychiatric Quart., 30:579–597, 1956.

Kraepelin, E.: Dementia Praecox. Translated by Barclay, R. M. Edinburgh, E. & S. Livingstone, 1919.

Langfeldt, G.: Diagnosis and prognosis of schizophrenia. Proc. Royal Soc. Med., 53:1047–1052, 1960.

Lidz, T., Cornelison, A., Parker, B., Fleck, S. and Terry, D.: The intra-familial environment of schizophrenic patients: II, Marital schism and marital skew. Am. J. Psychiat., 114:241–248, 1957.

Lidz, T., Cornelison, A., Terry, D., and Fleck, S.: Intra-familial environment of the schizophrenic patient: VI, The transmission of irrationality. Arch. Neur. & Psych., 79:305–316, 1958.

Lidz, R. W., and Lidz, T.: The family environment of schizophrenic patients. Am. J. Psychiat., 106:332–345, 1949.

Lidz, T., Parker, B., and Cornelison, A.: The role of the father in the family environment of the schizophrenic patient. Am. J. Psychiat., 113: 126–132, 1956.

Meyer, A.: Fundamental conceptions of dementia praecox. Brit. M. J., 2:757–759, 1906; J. Nerv. & Ment. Dis., 34:331–336, 1907.

Idem: Dynamic interpretation of dementia praecox. Am. J. Psychol., 21:385–403, 1910.

Idem: The nature and conception of dementia praecox. J. Abnormal Psychol., 5:274–285, 1910.

Idem: Constructive formulation of schizophrenia. Am. J. Psychiat., 78:355–364, 1922. (The preceding articles will also be found in: Winters, E., Ed.: The Collected Papers of Adolf Meyer, Vol. II. Baltimore, Johns Hopkins Press, 1951.)

Modell, A. H.: An approach to the nature of auditory hallucinations in schizophrenia. Arch. Gen. Psych., 3:259–266, 1960.

Morel, B. A.: Traité des Maladies Mentales. Paris, Victor Masson, 1860.

Myerson, A.: Theory and principles of the "total push" method in the treatment of chronic schizophrenia. Am. J. Psychiat., 95:1197–1204, 1939.

O'Neal, P., and Robins, L. N.: Childhood patterns predictive of adult schizophrenia: a 30-year follow-up study. Am. J. Psychiat., 115:385–391, 1958.

Proceedings of Association for Research in Nervous and Mental Disease: Vol. XXXIV, Neurology and Psychiatry in Children, Part VI: Symposium of juvenile schizophrenia. Baltimore, Williams & Wilkins Co., 1954.

Rosenthal, D.: Confusion of identity and the frequency of schizophrenia in twins. Arch. Gen. Psych., 3:297–304, 1960.

Sands, D. E.: The psychoses of adolescence. J. Ment. Sc., 102:308–318, 1956.

Sobel, D. E.: Children of schizophrenic patients: preliminary observations on early development. Am. J. Psychiat., 118:512–517, 1961.

Idem: Infant mortality and malformations in children of schizophrenic women. Psychiat. Quart., 35:60–65, 1961.

Stanton, A. H., and Schwartz, M. S.: The Mental Hospital. A Study of Institutional Participation in Psychiatric Illness and Treatment. New York, Basic Books, Inc., 1954.

Wahl, C. W.: Some antecedent factors in the family histories of 568 male schizophrenics of the United States Navy. Am. J. Psychiat., 113: 201–210, 1956.

Whitehorn, J. C., and Betz, B. J.: A study of psychotherapeutic relationships between physicians and schizophrenic patients. Am. J. Psychiat., 111:321–331, 1954.

Zilboorg, G.: Further observations on ambulatory schizophrenias. Am. J. Orthopsychiat., 27:677–682, 1957.

Zubin, J., et al.: A Biometric Approach to Prognosis in Schizophrenia. In Hoch, P. H., and Zubin, J. (Ed.): Comparative Epidemiology of the Mental Disorders. New York, Grune & Stratton, 1961, pp. 143–203.

Chapter Twenty-six

PSYCHOTIC DISORDERS

PARANOID REACTIONS (PARANOIA AND PARANOID CONDITIONS)

Paranoia is a chronic mental disorder of insidious development and is characterized by persistent, unalterable, systematized, logically reasoned delusions. General demeanor, talk, and emotional and behavior reactions remain unaltered except as they are influenced by delusioned beliefs, which become the uppermost and guiding theme of the patient's life and may therefore seriously impair discretion and judgment. The term was first used in 1863 by Kahlbaum to designate various persecutory and grandiose states. That the most conspicuous symptom is in the field of thought is indicated by the etymology of the name applied to mental disorders of this type ($\pi\alpha\rho\grave{\alpha}$, beside, in the sense of altered or changed, and $\nu o\hat{v}s$, intellect or reason).

Etiology

There seems to be convincing evidence that the causes of paranoia and paranoid conditions are psychological. Among these psychological causes may be ambitious but frustrated strivings; a need for defense of the personality against undesirable tendencies and repudiated impulses; feelings of insecurity, guilt, or other anxiety-producing factors; a continued failure to achieve overvalued goals; or a need for enhancing prestige or self-esteem. Specific traumatic life experiences may serve as contributory factors. In a significant number of cases it will be found that the paranoiac comes from a family that has been severely authoritarian, harsh, and cruel. Frequently a parent, usually of the same sex, has been a hostile, controlling person who rejects the child and, through accusations, produces fear, anxiety, feelings of inadequacy, and a self-image of the "bad" child, which, however, he does not accept. In many, perhaps in most, cases there has been an early overidentification with the parent of the opposite sex. As a result of his emotional experiences and frustrations, patterns of hatred and aggression are frequently established; these, however, the child must endeavor to repress because of fear of his parent. As is frequently observed, parents whose personalities were warped through unwholesome attitudes and relationships with their parents may affectively distort those of their own children. Early affective frustrations may lead the child to a withdrawal from social contacts and to a resulting feeling of rejection. This may stimulate resentment and contribute a paranoid element to the developing personality that may finally culminate in the paranoid psychosis. Sometimes self-pity or sibling rivalry seems to facilitate the establishment of paranoid tendencies.

Even as a child, the future paranoid individual usually shows troublesome trends that make it difficult for him to participate in congenial play with other children for more than brief periods. He is often a lonely, unhappy, brooding, insecure child, lacking friends with whom he can share confidences and exchange perspectives. It will frequently be found that he is suspicious, stubborn, secretive, obstinate, and resentful of discipline. When crossed, he is apt to be sullen, morose, peevish, and irritable. As adult life is approached, the early personality characteristics become accentuated. The future patient becomes increasingly sensitive about the attitude and behavior of others, "builds mountains out of molehills," and may believe that others wish to do him injury. He is lacking in a sense of humor, is egotistic, self-confident, self-assertive, sarcastic, derogatory, querulous, embittered, and resentful. Usually the paranoid person has always been critical, demanding, inflexible, biased, mistrustful, impatient and often defiant of conventions. Characteristically he has been argumentative, uncompromising, and aggressive. Interpersonal relationships are difficult. He approaches others with a "chip-on-the-shoulder" attitude. The drive for achievement may be intense and may impel him to seek goals that are beyond his capacity. Intolerant of criticism and unable to accept suggestions, he readily criticises and belittles others. Meticulous and precise, he is in some respects highly efficient but is jealous and unadaptable. He needs to demonstrate his superiority. If in a position of authority, he may be a petty tyrant.

At times one meets persons handicapped by such *paranoid personality* characteristics that, however, never develop further. In others these characteristics become gradually and insidiously intensified until the patient is clearly psychotic. In the same problems and factors are to be found the sources both of the paranoid personality and the paranoid psychosis.

The latter represents a progressive, developing continuance of the former. In some instances, as in other paranoid reactions, repressed homosexual impulses seem to be the source of the psychopathology.

The mental mechanisms and reactions observed in paranoia are but exaggerations of ones noted constantly among persons who are not thought of as psychotic. In everyday life, fear and insecurity are expressed in such disguises as pettiness, oversensitiveness, irascibility, never-ending bickering, overcompensation, seclusiveness, selfishness, or cynicism. Even caution may develop into suspiciousness. Many people are at times inclined to feel slighted, to think that their merits are unrecognized, to blame their environment for what are really dissatisfactions with self, or perhaps in part to fulfill their wishes in fantasy. Daily we meet those who are unable to recognize and admit their faults and defects. Real or imagined injuries to pride tend to result in feelings of resentment and bitterness of variable duration. The well-defined paranoid personality often seems to display a remarkable genius for detecting in the ordinary run-of-life situations just those tiny slights, inadvertencies, or trifling disparagements that others overlook but that he builds up into crucial issues, not altogether imaginary but vastly overemphasized.

The paranoid personality may be overaggressive and see an aggressor in everyone around him. This makes him feel that his war against the world is waged in self-defense. A rebellious, superior attitude may serve to bolster self-esteem and prevent a realistic but intolerable self-evaluation. Not rarely the paranoid individual treats others as projections of certain of his own unconscious trends. As a result, his statements, manner, and behavior alienate friends and create enemies. The fact that he thereby incurs the hostility of others and is therefore often rejected and isolated adds more fuel to the psychopathogenic fire. Affective states may for a time give rise to false references to one's self and lead to rationalization and to the suspension of reflective logic, although the ideas thus affectively determined do not continue to multiply and spread as in paranoia. One must agree with the English psychiatrist, Crichton-Miller: "For every fully developed case of paranoia in our mental hospitals there must be hundreds, if not thousands, who suffer from minor degrees of suspicion and mistrust; whose lives are blighted by this barrier to human harmony; and who poison the springs of social life for the community."

In the paranoid personality, we meet with an exaggeration of the common tendency to ascribe responsibility to others, to repudiate aspects of the personality that do not measure up to the standards the individual has set for himself, to obtain satisfaction through compensatory strivings, to maintain self-esteem by constructing emotionally satisfying but irrational explanations for his own failures, and to attribute hostile or aggressive motives to others. Disappointments, humiliation, or injuries sustained may accentuate a paranoid tendency and even appear to precipitate a paranoid psychosis. The causes of paranoia are, then, to be sought in the need for protecting particularly vulnerable aspects of the personality, in the craving for a recognition greater than attainment can command, in the particular mental conflicts of the individual, and in frustrations and vague fears, and in a need for relieving one's own anxiety over guilt by blaming someone else.

Many cases of paranoid psychoses seem to derive from the mechanism whereby guilt-inspiring impulses are repudiated by projection to a persecutor. As we study the behavior of individuals and the methods by which they meet conflicts within and blows from without, we often find it difficult to say when the expressions of a paranoid personality become the symptoms of a paranoid psychosis. Anomalies of character become continuous with the psychosis, both, to a large degree, going back to the needs and problems of the personality and to the habitual techniques or patterns that the individual has adopted in attempting to meet such irregularities.

Formerly there was a tendency to subdivide the permanent paranoid reactions into definite disease entities. Kraepelin looked upon paranoia as a fixed type of disease resulting exclusively from internal causes and characterized by persistent, systematized delusions, the preservation of clear and orderly thinking and acting, and the absence of hallucinations. Intermediate between paranoia and paranoid schizophrenia he recognized an entity he called paraphrenia, differing principally from paranoia by the fact that the delusions lack the logical systematization of the latter disorder. The delusions are more apt to be extravagant and, in addition, hallucinations are present at times. Not for many years, if at all, is there any deterioration of general interest or of personality. Kraepelin's paraphrenia corresponds rather closely to the psychoses included in the present official classification under the title, "Paranoid State." It would appear, however, that there is no sharp line of distinction between "Paranoia" and "Paranoid State." Rather do the paranoid-reaction psychoses constitute a continuous transition with imperceptible gradations in respect to the following: the extent to which affect is adequately and appropriately responsive to individual experience and environment; the extent to which delusions are systematically organized; the correctness of evaluation of reality; the extent to which subjective mental material is symbolized and projected in terms of such sensory experiences as hallucinations; and finally, the extent to which psychobiological integration is disturbed and personality disorganized. In all these respects, the distintegrative processes become greatest as the schizophrenic pole of the paranoid series is approached.

True Kraepelinian paranoia is much less frequent than are paranoid reactions having a wide variation of schizophrenic features associated with them. The difference in final outcome of the psychoses in the inclusive paranoid-reaction group is one of degree of preservation of personality. Except for the fact that paranoid reactions accompanied by such markedly schizoid features as to place them among the schizophrenias will not be included in this discussion, there will be no attempt to draw lines of distinction between so-called "true" paranoia and the other paranoid reactions that through a long course of evolution have come to represent a permanent type of life adjustment. Practically, whether one considers those paranoid reactions that are comparatively free from schizophrenic features as cases of paranoia or of paranoid state is a matter of opinion and not important. The fact that the paranoid reactions, represented at one extreme by paranoia and at the other by paranoid schizophrenia, seem to form a continuum and to merge imperceptibly one into the other is what may be expected; since types of personalities do not fall into sharply defined categories, neither are there fixed and exclusive mental methods by which individuals meet their emotional conflicts, their limitations, and the experiences of life.

Psychopathology

As previously noted, there is no clearly defined point at which the personality marked by the characteristics previously described should be called psychotic. Perhaps the criterion should be the degree to which reality is distorted and adjustment disturbed. The paranoid tendencies rarely become so extreme as to justify a diagnosis of paranoia before the age of 30. The disorder is more common in men. As already indicated, the presenting symptom of paranoia and of paranoid states is a rigid, persistent system of delusions. At times the patient's delusions may take their origin in some actual fact. On cross section, his behavior and thought content may be deceptive, and a severe disorder be camouflaged by a seemingly normal surface. On longitudinal section, however, the paranoid theme is discovered. The content of paranoid ideas varies widely and is determined primarily by the particular psychological needs they are created to fulfill, and secondarily by the type of rationalization that will appeal to the ideas and beliefs current in the patient's environment.

The patient's own inclinations are mirrored in the particular motives and intentions attributed to others. His rationalizations are vigorously defended, and he exhibits a convincing earnestness in his efforts to win others to his delusional beliefs. The patient may rationalize so plausibly that his friends accept his allegation that specific individuals, rather than himself, are responsible for his difficulties. His superior intellectual endowment may remain unimpaired. Some paranoiacs become aware that the credibility of their delusions is questioned and therefore attempt to hide them. The patient's judgment may be defective only in relation to his delusional system, which often develops slowly and ultimately becomes intricate and complex. The dominating ideas tend to be those of persecution, of expansive grandiosity, or of those containing both themes.

As *persecutory* trends develop, the patient attributes hostile or aggressive motives to others, nurses his grievances, and becomes increasingly secretive. In the earlier period of his psychosis, he may be hypochondriacal and uneasy. He may become depressed, gloomy, spiteful, vindictive, and given to morose rumination. Frequently he manifests a self-righteous resentment against others. Misunderstandings and misinterpretations develop into delusions of persecution.

The tendency of the paranoiac to seek for ulterior motives on the part of others or to misinterpret events is illustrated by the case of a woman who, soon after graduation from a law school, the faculty of which had awarded her the annual prize for the greatest improvement in scholastic work during her professional course, sued the school for damages, alleging that the awarding of such a prize was for the purpose of representing her as having been more poorly fitted than her associates for the study of law. (Doubtless the same sense of insecurity that led to her psychosis determined also her choice of law as a profession.)

In his effort to control his hostile impulses in which the genesis of his paranoid reaction is often to be found, the patient projects them and experiences them as being directed against himself. Filled with hate, he feels and believes that he is the victim of persecutors, who, in fact, are but the objects upon whom he has projected his own hate. The mood of many paranoiacs is one of sustained sullenness. Ideas of reference appear: there is a hidden meaning in what is taking place in his environment; cryptic significances are read into casual remarks and events; slights and indignities are imagined; far-reaching significance is attached to trivial details in the behavior of others. Vague feelings of fear tend to increase suspicion and the patient's malevolent trend of thought. Although in the case of the "normal" person incredulity, indignation, and anger often help to prevent the individual from becoming aware of qualities, strivings, and tendencies that offend self-esteem, these defensive reactions are used much more by the paranoid patient. Delusional ideas extend: the patient believes that people spread lies about him; persons tamper with his mail, accusing remarks are overheard; hostility and jealousy are observed on every hand; business plans are thwarted; he is the victim of a conspiracy, and the agents of malevolent social organizations pursue him, persecutors seek to conceal their identity by various disguises. He may become depressed and even suicidal because he feels overwhelmed by an environment with which he cannot cope.

In the persecutory as well as in other forms of paranoia, there is a central delusional theme that pervades the whole life of the patient, who is quite incapable of criticizing the pseudologic he employs in supporting this dominant idea. His premises are not scrutinized, and present events, regardless of their relevancy to the prevailing idea, are interpreted wholly with reference to it. Affect determines the patient's logic. Incidents of the past receive a new interpretation and are fitted into the framework of present persecution—a process known as retrospective falsification. As a result, the delusional system constantly extends, and the most commonplace incidents, because of their affective interpretation with reference to the prevailing idea, become events of the greatest importance. In all paranoid reactions, the patient, always confident that he is right, clings obstinately to his opinions, since his inner sense of insecurity cannot permit him to feel otherwise. He maintains his delusional misinterpretations, too, by continually overemphasizing the inferred or implied meaning and by discarding the obvious and real content of a statement or action.

A not uncommon form of paranoia is the *litigious* type. Although it will usually be found that this type of paranoiac individual was always stubborn, insistent upon his "rights," and with many defensive mechanisms, the litigious activities frequently do not appear until after some legal experience that eventuated less satisfactorily than the patient desired. Because of his dissatisfaction, the patient initiates further but ill-advised legal action. He always fails to see that he has not proved his case. Every new litigation brings further controversies and new grievances for which the patient feels prompted to seek redress. His attempts to secure it, however, result in fresh feelings of injustice. Fundamentally, it is often not a question of law and justice, as the patient insists, but of attempts to put others in the wrong, to show that he was right, that he is superior, in order that thereby his sensitive insecurity may be strengthened and the weak points of his personality may be protected.

In the *exalted* type of paranoia, the ideas of grandeur may appear after a long preceding stage of persecution, or at times the grandiosity may be present practically from the beginning of the psychosis. Ideas of invention constitute a frequent form of grandiosity. Patients with such beliefs usually neglect their usual method of livelihood and devote their time to the drawing of plans and the construction of models. At times the patient claims that models are completed but that enemies prevent him from securing a patent; again, he is on the point of perfecting the machine. In either case, the patient frequently claims to utilize some force or to attain some objective contrary to the accepted laws of science. In this type of disorder, the patient may have a sense of mission and pursue his impracticable goal with more zeal than discretion. Others have expansive ideas of noble birth. Frequently the grandiose patient attempts to play the role that his ideas have assigned him. If, for example, he believes he is a religious leader, he may wear long hair and a beard and affect an air of humility—an air that often disguises but poorly a repressed hatred.

The exalted beliefs in some paranoid states are of a religious nature. The patient is the chosen one of God, is Christ, prophesied the war, has supernatural powers. Some establish new religious sects and secure adherents; others proclaim themselves leaders of a new order but are so bizarre in belief and behavior that they fail to secure followers.

Occasionally paranoia assumes an *erotic* form. The patient believes that some woman of title or wealth whom he may have casually seen or met is in love with him. He writes her affectionate letters and perhaps poems. Her failure to reply to them is intended solely to test his love. Items in the newspapers, the flight of the birds, and various events are disguised recognitions of her present and acknowledgments of her love. Such patients may become annoyingly persistent in their attentions and threatening in their manner.

Among common causes for the commitment of paranoid patients are homicidal or suicidal attempts, the writing of anonymous letters to persons in authority, litigation, or persistent statements that they are the victims of a conspiracy.

Psychodynamics

Although disparity between achievement and ambition, early experience heavily loaded with affect, vague or subconscious feelings of dissatisfaction or irritation with self, injuries to self-evaluation, as well as various other needs for defense may act as dynamic agents and lead or contribute to a fixed paranoid reaction type, there is much to suggest that in some, but by no means all, cases repressed homosexual impulses may be a genetic factor. An increasing number of psychiatrists, have come to believe that unadjusted psychosexual tendencies in many instances bear a relation to paranoia. The persistence of homosexual impulses, unrecognized consciously, may doubtless be caused by more than one factor, but, characterized as the homosexual is with his infantile survivals and mother imprint, there seems good reason to believe that if, at puberty, an inhibitive maternal overpossessiveness impedes the maturation of the psychosexual aspects of her son's personality, these may remain fixated and never attain a mature heterosexual development.

Assuming that there is a relation between this fixation, or incomplete evolution of the personality, and homosexuality, how does the latter lead to paranoia? According to Freud, it is through the mechanism of projection by which the original but repressed and therefore consciously rejected affect is reversed and transferred to the homosexual object. Because it is consciously inadmissible, the patient's "I love him" is changed to "I do not love him; I hate him," which, to be acceptable, requires projection as "He hates me" and is elaborated into "I am persecuted by him."

An abnormally high percentage of paranoids do not marry. This is not only because of a basic homosexual orientation but also because of the fact that their chronic hostility and anger make them undesirable as partners. If the paranoiac does marry, the marital life is so full of discord that it frequently ends in divorce.

The "true" paranoiac is often a person of superior intellectual endowment, but his energy is so largely expended in repudiating desires that do not wish to be recognized as such, in compensatory efforts whereby self-esteem may be enhanced, and in striving for satisfactions that life has not supplied, that social relations become disturbed and constructive achievements are nil. The fact that life has failed to bring the success and satisfactions to which the native intelligence of the patient would ordinarily have entitled him undoubtedly tends to aggravate his defensive reactions. As already indicated, a large percentage of cases of paranoia occur among people of superior intelligence. This is perhaps because the person of superior intellectual endowment finds rationalization and projection to be readily available and satisfactory mechanisms of defense. The more promptly and passively the individual gives up the struggle for self-esteem and for recognition, the more nearly will the reaction approach the schizophrenic, regardless of the native intelligence, while the more active and sustained the struggle, the more likely is the result to approach paranoia.

The following case presents, in some respects, many of the characteristic features of paranoia:

P. G. was committed to a hospital for mental diseases because of his peculiar religious ideas and rites, one of them being the practice of going about nude. The patient's parents were strict in their moral principles and rigid in discipline. All the paternal siblings were teachers except the patient's father, who was a farmer and who was always dissatisfied with his lot, often expressing the wish that he could "get away where he could read and study and reform the world." The patient had one sister, also a brother who was older and stronger and who used to "lord it over" the patient. His association with his sister was close, and shortly before leaving home as a young man he suggested to her that if she would not get married, he would not do so either, and they would live together.

As a child he was described as sensitive and fearing criticism. "Because he was not strong, he was somewhat of a sissy," the sister stated. At school he was a ready scholar and completed the equivalent of two years of high school work. If he received less than 90 in his grades, he felt disgraced. Prior to his marriage at age 26 he had paid little attention to persons of the opposite sex. At that age he married his landlady, a woman of 66, "as a humane act"; this was his characterization of the match when he entered the hospital. When questioned concerning his sex life, he stated that men had aroused him sexually more than women, for whom he had no sexual desire. He took part in homosexual practices on only a few occasions. When asked if he thought his religion had helped him in repressing his homosexual tendencies, he replied, "I do not think so, I know

it." He acknowledged that he derived pleasure from exposing himself to other men, although he claimed that his practice of going about nude was a health measure permitted by his religion and not for the purpose of satisfying exhibitionistic impulses—doubtless a rationalization of socially prohibited inclinations. When questioned concerning his social life, he had, he said, "a distinct aversion to secret organizations"—perhaps an unconscious defense against his homosexual tendencies, since such organizations, made up as they usually are of individuals of one sex, serve to provide a sublimated and socialized outlet for homosexual trends, although the psychological basis of these bodies is also one of narcissism and compensation.

During his early adult life, the patient became interested in various unusual religious cults (probably an effort to obtain a feeling of security), although this striving did not result in such a serious disturbance in thought and behavior as to lead to his being considered psychotic until after he was 40 years of age. He described himself as suffering at about that period from "lack of initiative, inability to concentrate, general weakness, anxiety about the future, irritability, and hypopotency of the heart." Doubtless this represented a stage of subjective analysis often occurring in the disease. He addressed a prayer to the "Diety" asking for aid and threatening to commit suicide if it were not forthcoming. Almost immediately it was "revealed" to him, not through a voice or visible signs but "simply through thought process," that he was to establish a new religion to take the place of Christianity, one that would be more comforting and satisfactory. He called his new religion "Omnivitism" and spent day after day writing "a set of mottoes instead of commandments, a set of actions and ideals, prayers, verse, comment on principles, affirmations and denials, suggestions regarding services, and miscellaneous dissertations." When questioned as to the specific teachings of his religion, little but vague generalities was to be secured. "It teaches," he said "that all forms and phases of existence are essential factors of one all-sufficient existence that is called 'Omniad.'" He had tracts printed and distributed them widely, setting forth "the rule of Omnivitism, which is to teach according to his needs."

About this time he began to go to isolated spots and to walk about nude, explaining that he was taking "sun baths." Gradually he made few attempts to retire from sight when taking his "sun baths," particularly after one occasion when he derived considerable enjoyment from the fact that he was seen by the occupants of two automobiles that passed while he was unclothed. Finally, after having been warned on repeated occasions by the local constable that he must not continue his exhibitionistic practices, the patient was committed to a hospital for mental disorders.

On arrival at the hospital, the patient was pleasant and smiling but obviously exalted, with an air of self-satisfaction and superiority. He was a small man of rather effeminate physique, his hair reached nearly to his shoulders, and his beard was long, his appearance strongly resembling the traditional picture of Christ. He accepted his detention philosophically, expressing the opinion that it was what one in his position must expect— a sort of martyrdom in a worthy cause. He had, he said, founded a religion "more up to date" than that of Christianity and one that would supplant the latter and dominate the world; it had been revealed to him that by 1940 it would have been substantially established. Further, in 1948, the patient was to have been President of the United States. This, he added, was in accordance with the prophecy of Sir William Hope made on the day of Washington's birth. On that day he foretold that a new nation would arise in America and the part that would be played by Washington, and that finally there would come a ruler whom he characterized as "six plus added six—great, good and wise," at the same time referring to "a star that on his way shall shine." This prophecy, the patient said, referred to him, since there were six letters in each of his names, while his sister was the star, since it was she who had invited him to come to their old home. In an old novel, too, the patient claimed he had found the following: "There will come in the western continent a greater man than this world has seen since this civilization began. It will not be through the ignorance of the people that this man will be carried into the White House. In some respects this man will be the intellectual and philosophical leader. He will be to the world what Mohammed was to Arabia, Columbus to the New World, Moses to the Jews, Plato to the Greeks, etcetera— yet he will be greater than all and more powerful for good." This. the patient said, referred to him.

On psychometric examination by the Stanford-Binet scale, the patient was found to have an intelligence quotient of 115. It is interesting to note that in ability to see logical relationships, language ability, and constructive visual imagery he attained an 18-year level, but on practical judgment in social situations he graded at a 9-year-and-1-month level. In describing his attitude toward the examination, the psychologist recorded that he seemed to enjoy the opportunity of demonstrating his intellectual endowment, that he frequently laughed in a superior and condescending manner, that he exhibited great precision of speech, and delighted in showing off his large and unusual vocabulary. On several occasions, in a tolerant and somewhat condescending manner, he criticized the examiner for her use of words.

The patient's paranoid system was associated with too great disorganization of personality and disturbance of reality evaluation to permit the diagnosis of paranoia, but may properly, we believe, be regarded as a paranoid state rather than paranoid schizophrenia. The patient

was unable to secure a satisfying adjustment to a sense of biological and social inadequacy, to a fundamental homosexuality, and doubtless to other conflicts. However, instead of investing the external world with his own unrecognized but repudiated trends and feelings, he organized his emotional constellations into ideational systems that afforded a satisfying but unsocialized adjustment. The compensatory feelings of superiority developed to meet the subconscious feelings of inferiority and doubtless of guilt (arising from an imperfectly repressed homosexuality) were rationalized into grandiose delusions.

Other factors, too, presumably contributed to the life pattern of the patient's personality and his desire for high personal value. It may well have been that the dissatisfactions with self and the vaguely defined strivings owed their origin in part to absorption from the early family life, since we learned that his father was dissatisfied with his lot and wished to "study and reform the world." The fact that he was "lorded over" by a stronger brother presumably led to feelings of inadequacy and contributed to the psychological need for the artificially-obtained feeling of security and self-esteem. To have been taught that school grades below an unreasonably high standard constituted a disgrace tended to lead the boy to form ambitions that, with his limitations of personality and opportunities for training, inevitably resulted in wounds to pride and vanity.

Among the traits of childhood were sensitiveness and fear of criticism. His slightness of physique called for compensation, and a certain degree of biological deviation and the failure to emancipate himself emotionally from his older sister, who perhaps served as a mother surrogate, served to fix the development of his personality at a homosexual level. His exhibitionistic practices are doubtless also to be explained on the basis of arrest in psychosexual evolution. His egotistic wishes prejudiced his judgment and led it to disregard the usual criteria of reality, thereby both preventing a correct perspective and destroying the capacity for self-criticism.

Folie à Deux

Inasmuch as the clinical features are nearly always paranoid in nature, mention may be made at this point of an induced or communicated form of psychosis described by Lasègue and Falret in 1877 to which they · gave the name *"folie à deux."* Identification is usually an important mechanism in its production. This is a mental disorder in which mental symptoms, particularly paranoid delusions, from which one of two persons intimately associated with each other, usually for years, is suffering are communicated to and accepted by the other. Most frequently such a dual psychosis involves mother and daughter, two sisters, or husband and wife. The person suffering from the primary psychosis is usually the dominant individual, while the one who develops the secondary or induced psychosis is of a submissive and suggestible type, dependent upon and having a close emotional attachment to the infector. As misinterpretations, illusions, and ideas of persecution increasingly disturb the infector, he persuasively relates his convictions and psychotic experiences to the weaker person or infectee, who comes to accept and react to the systematized delusional ideas of the first. It will often be found that both persons have been poorly adjusted individuals having a narrow range of interests, of the same general background and environment, and facing perhaps the same situation. The induced ideas must be acceptable and usually offer some satisfaction to the person infected. In nearly every instance the delusional ideas are dropped by the recipient if he is removed from association with the dominant person. The usual setting of the disorder is one in which the two persons concerned live in comparative seclusion. It is more frequently found . among women. This is probably because they tend to be more isolated within the domestic circle. They are, on the whole, more passive, submissive, and suggestible,

and their outside interests and ambitions are more likely to be restricted or frustrated.

Diagnosis

At times psychiatric literature contains references to "acute paranoia." Although descriptively this is a good term, it is somewhat misleading, since it will be found that the episodes thus classified are fundamentally affective in nature, being hypomanic attacks of manic–depressive psychosis in which the usual emotional exaltation is replaced by irritability and anger. The patient is aggressive, haughty, hostile, and complaining. In paranoia there is a greater tendency to project and to rationalize one's affective state than in the usual manic episode. The true paranoiac is more restrained both in behavior and in speech, and his ideational content is characterized by a more sustained and dominant idea than is the more excited manic with his fleeting charges. As the affect subsides, the delusional ideas of the acute paranoid episode are dropped, but they are not corrected, and the patient remains without insight as to the beliefs he formerly expressed with great conviction and feeling.

There is often discussion as to whether a given paranoic syndrome should be classified as one of paranoia, paranoid state, or paranoid schizophrenia. The general factors that determine the place of a paranoid reaction in this imperceptibly graded series of paranoid psychoses have already been indicated. In addition to what has already been said concerning the mechanisms and symptoms to be observed in making a diagnosis in this paranoid group, it may be helpful to bear in mind that the greater the logical systematization of delusions and the less the patient's relations with reality are disturbed, the more nearly does the psychosis approach traditional paranoia. The greater the extent to which repressed material comes through to consciousness in the form of hallucinations, the more bizarre the delusional system, and the more regressive and disorganized the form of adjustment, the more nearly does it approach paranoid schizophrenia. Although anger and hatred are common in all the paranoic disorders, yet as time progresses there is an increasing tendency for the schizophrenic patient's affect to "burn out." The paranoid schizophrenic patient lacks the intensive drive for achievement usually seen in paranoia.

Often there is difficulty in deciding whether a person whose behavior is governed by, and indicates a thorough contact with, reality, who has suffered no dilapidation of affect or of personality, and who is not hallucinated, but who constantly employs projection and other defensive measures should be considered as suffering from paranoia or as a paranoid, but not psychotic, personality. Here, too, an imperceptibly graded series is dealt with, ranging from a mild and perhaps justifiable sense of injury and a belief that merits are not recognized, at one pole, to the exaggerated delusions of persecution or of grandeur of true paranoia at the other. At one extreme is a reaction that would not, except to the psychopathologist, be regarded as abnormal. When this reaction becomes so intensified as to warrant a diagnosis of paranoia may also be a matter of opinion, since paranoia is essentially an exaggeration of mechanisms observed daily. In general, if the exaggerated reaction is continuous, if the beliefs through which it manifests itself cannot be corrected, if they disclose an inadequacy of logic, and particularly if they tend to spread and to reveal that the affective and conative forces are sustained and have great energy, then the reaction must be looked upon as psychotic. The psychiatrist will not forget that paranoid tendencies may be channeled and expressed in many eccentricities and fanatical ways.

Prognosis

It is doubtful if a case of traditional paranoia ever recovers. In those cases in the paranoid series that most nearly approach paranoid schizophrenia, a remission may rarely occur, but in these, also, the ultimate prognosis is poor. In true paranoia there is little or no general per-

sonality disorganization, and the patient's conduct usually remains within the bounds that society will tolerate. For this reason, a large proportion of such cases do not enter a hospital for mental disorders. In the community the individuals are often looked upon as "cranks," but as they usually do not act without reflection, show a certain amount of self-control, and limit themselves to legal means of redress, they avoid commitment much more frequently than do those with paranoid conditions that approach the schizophrenic pole of the series. The latter are less sociable, less industrious, and less restrained by social custom and law.

An analysis of the causes of death in the psychoses shows that a larger percentage of paranoid patients than of any other group of biogenetic psychoses die of degenerative circulatory disease.

Treatment

As already indicated, the more nearly the paranoid psychosis approaches "true paranoia," the less frequently is hospitalization required. Unless his behavior is too disturbing socially, it is well for the patient with this disease to remain in the community, since interference and restraint embitter him and lead to an extension of his delusional system and to a stimulation of his hatred. If the paranoiac is considered dangerous, commitment, of course, becomes imperative.

To determine when he has become dangerous is not always easy. A careful evaluation of the patient's history will usually indicate the extent to which delusions may be expected to control behavior. If delusions have exerted an important influence on behavior and if they are directed toward particular individuals, this estimate should be made. The willingness and the degree of objectivity with which the patient will discuss his delusions are important. The character and intensity of his emotional reaction will greatly aid in deciding the questions as to the hazard entailed in the patient's liberty; the greater the overt hostility, the more imperative is his removal from society. Many times the patient will discuss the extent to which he believes he is justified in protecting himself or his interests or in securing redress. An indication can thus be obtained as to the probability of acts of violence.

Whether the patient is to be treated as an in-patient or out-patient, the therapist must keep clearly in mind certain expectations relative to the transference. The paranoid is generally suspicious and distrustful, considers himself unloved and incapable of giving affection, and has usually come to believe through long experience that what is conveyed by the spoken word does not reflect the actual intent of those with whom he has been closely related. He has a need to see himself as a center of interest and activity as a means to sustain a façade of importance that protects him from suffering hurt by his deep sense of personal inadequacy, shame, or humiliation.

Treatment, then, should initially be as permissive as possible. The physician should maintain an open, courteous, considerate attitude, coupled with scrupulous truthfulness and good faith. Recalling the essential pathology, attention should be paid to the patient's delusions, but no attempt should be made to criticize or convince the patient that he is in error as to his conclusions. Such efforts only produce a further lowering of self-esteem and arouse greater compensatory deficiencies or outright acts of destructive hatefulness. Nor should any efforts be made to convince him that he is among friends who are kindly disposed to him, or that he has a warm and attractive personality himself. All forms of ingratiation should be avoided, as they will be interpreted as evidence that the patient is again related to persons similar to those whom he believes have betrayed him in the past. The physician's attitude to the delusions will not imply agreement, however. It will imply rather, "I can understand how you feel, but it does not seem so to me." The physician will make his role and his position clear and hold them firmly.

The patient's anxiety and tension should be relieved by the administration of a phenothiazine as described in the previous chapter. With these measures, it is surprising that many paranoid patients will, if allowed the opportunity, commence exploration of their problems in psychotherapy. Such a patient should be allowed to follow his own leads, and when occasions arise, the physician may offer tentative and alternative hypotheses as to the determining factors that the patient provides to explain his delusional interpretations of his relations to others, his failures and successes. By such means, creation of doubt may be created in the patient's concept of his relations with others. Later, more direct confrontations may be used, and realistic appraisal of his interpretations may be provided.

As for the homosexual trends, oftentimes these are regressive fantasies due to fear of rejection or lack of success in relating to women. Sometimes they are representative of impotency, which is the outcome of the deep lack of security of the patient. Sexual fears will be dealt with, then, in terms of the patient's anxieties in relation to those of the opposite sex rather than by humiliating remarks or interpretations concerning homosexuality. The patient should be advised that from time to time he is likely to become suspicious or distrustful of the psychotherapist and also advised he should speak of it when he has this experience so that the underlying reasons may be clarified.

This therapeutic approach, which consistently allows a deeper examination of reality without exposing the patient to shame and enlightment and, at the same time, strengthens the patient's satisfaction in achievements within the limits of his capacities, has been of aid in bringing about satisfactory social adaptation.

BIBLIOGRAPHY

Bleuler, E.: Affectivity, suggestibility, paranoia. Translated by C. S. Ricksher. Utica, State Hospitals Press, 1912.

Bonner, H.: The problem of diagnosis in paranoic disorders. Am. J. Psychiat., 107:677–683, 1951.

Cameron, N.: The development of paranoiac thinking. Psychol. Rev., 50:219–233, 1943.

Dewhurst, K., and Todd, J.: The psychosis of association—folie à deux. J. Nerv. and Ment. Dis., *124:*451–459, 1957.

Freud, S.: Certain neurotic mechanisms in jealousy, paranoia and homosexuality. Internat. J. Psycho-Analysis, *4:*1–10, 1923.

Idem: Psychoanalytic Notes upon an Autobiographical Account of a Case of Paranoia. In Collected Papers, Vol. 3, London, Hogarth, 1925.

Greenberg, H. P.: Crime and folie à deux: review and case history. J. Ment. Sc., *102:*772–779, 1956.

Kahn, E., and Richter, H. G.: Sensitivity. Am. J. Psychiat., *96:*609–622, 1939.

Kretschmer, E.: Der sensitive Beziehungswahn. Berlin, Julius Springer, 1927.

Lasègue, C., and Falret, J.: La folie à deux ou folie communiquée. Ann. méd. psychol., *18:*321–355, 1877.

Novey, S.: The outpatient treatment of borderline paranoid states. Psychiatry, *23:*357–364, 1960.

Rosen, H., and Kiene, H. E.: Paranoia and paranoiac reaction types. Dis. Nerv. System, *7:*330–337, 1946.

Idem: The paranoiac officer and the officer paranee. Am. J. Psychiat., *103:*614–621, 1947.

Salzman, L.: Paranoid state—theory and therapy. A.M.A. Arch. Gen. Psychiat., *2:*679–693, 1960.

Waelder, R.: The structure of paranoid ideas: a critical survey of various theories. Internat. J. Psycho-Analysis, *32:*167–177, 1951.

Wolff, S.: Folie à trois: a clinical study. J. Ment. Sc., *103:*355–363, 1957.

Chapter Twenty-seven

PSYCHOPHYSIOLOGICAL AUTONOMIC AND VISCERAL DISORDERS

"The sorrow which has no vent in tears may make other organs weep."

Henry Maudsley

The reactions included under the caption of psychophysiological autonomic and visceral disorders comprise those that are more frequently referred to as "psychosomatic disorders." Anxiety leads to disturbances that are predominantly physiological rather than symbolic. The expression of affect being through viscera, its feeling or subjective part is repressed and therefore largely prevented from becoming conscious. Neither is its expression under full voluntary control or perception. The long-continued and exaggerated physiological expression of anxiety may eventually lead to structural change in the organ or viscus through which it is expressed. The physiological and the organic are secondary to vascular disturbance, smooth muscle dysfunction, and hypersecretion or hyposecretion of glands, innervated largely by the sympathetic and parasympathetic divisions of the autonomic nervous system.

The tendency, however, to delineate only such psychosomatic disturbances as those that are expressed through the path-ological mediation of the autonomic nervous system is not in keeping with the structural or functional organization of the organism. Furthermore, it tends to provide a too narrow interpretation of psychosomatic interrelations and their disturbances. The broader concept used here is to classify as psychosomatic all those disturbances involving the organs of internal economy, of instinctual function, and of the body image as a whole. Thus are excluded the involvement of organs subserving the human relationship to the external world. It is evident that the internal organ systems located within the body cavities are largely controlled through the connections of the central nervous system and various metabolic and hormonal feed-backs. The organ systems that have direct contact with the external environment are used for the intake and elimination of needed bodily substances and for procreative activity (respiratory, gastrointestinal and genital apparatus) and are controlled in part at their orifices by the voluntary nervous system and also by the autonomic through the integrative activity of the central nervous pathways. Here is seen initiation of the functions by utilization of the voluntary nervous system followed by increasing degrees of automatization through the sympathetic and parasympathetic innervations.

In the instances of the body image disturbances, the total organism is involved and not a single organ or series of organs. Excluded, then, from the area of the psychosomatic disorders are dysfunctions of the central nervous system subserving the external relations of the individual, his perceptual and conative activities, communicative systems, orientations in space and time, and his capacity to organize and integrate the information provided him from the outside world. It is clear that the borderline between the disorders subsumed under the body image and those of the integrative functions of the nervous system in contact with the external world may not be sharply delimited and subtly merge with personality growth.

The concept of psychosomatic medicine, criticized by many, has provided one of the great contributions of psychiatry to medicine during the past quarter of a century in its re-emphasis of the human factor in illness and in the wider appreciation of the personality–illness relationship and of the influence of psychological factors in the genesis of somatic symptoms, and even of somatic disease. Prior to this re-emphasis, there had been an unfortunately increasing tendency for medicine to look upon the patient as "the uninteresting vehicle of a fascinating disease process." Influenced by psychiatry, medical science has in recent years increasingly adopted a more comprehensive point of view and has to a greater extent come to realize that the pathology of disease is that of the living, integrated human organism and not merely of cells and tissue. It is now recognized that many factors cannot be studied by the usual methods of medicine or described in terms of physiology. These factors, nevertheless, may disturb the functioning

of the organism as greatly as those agencies that are revealed by the microscope or the test tube. Such factors can be ascertained only through "an intimate understanding of the patient as a whole man or woman with a home and anxieties and economic problems and a past and a future and a job to be held or lost."

It has become clear, too, that mechanisms invoked by the human personality to deal with problems of adjustment to its environment may either underlie or modify many disease processes. The physician should therefore focus his attention on the patient himself, including his emotional life—not merely on his physical complaints. He should remember that physiological processes and the psychodynamics of emotions are intimately bound up, the one affecting the other. He must aim to discover and understand the interrelation and interaction of psychological and organic factors in the development and course of illness. The physician's concern, then, should not be limited to infections and physico-chemical deviations determined in the laboratory. As an editorial writer in The Lancet* has pointed out, there is danger that the student's perspective may be distorted in the ward atmosphere of intensive, largely mechanical, investigation in which the minutiae and the rarities of disease receive so much attention and its human significance so little. He adds that by the time the student enters private practice, his mind is often cast in the mold his teachers have given it and that as a result a cardiac murmur may always seem to him more important than an overpossessive mother who may so warp her child's personality development that his mental health and social adjustment are permanently impaired.

Because chronic emotional states frequently associated with physiological malfunctions are often closely related to the everyday problems of living, the physician or psychiatrist makes a careful and extended look into the whole development and experience of the patient. Home life and its jealousies and frustrations, work-

* The Lancet, *152*:413, 1947.

ing conditions frequently involving the boredom of constant repetition or a perpetual striving for security or achievement, with the attendant drives for prestige or comradeship in relation to those in authority or to other persons, are common problems, yet ones that may lead to a variety of symptoms that have no organic basis. Cumulative problems of interpersonal relationships produce a large share of the tensions and anxieties that beset the human being and upset his physiology. Lack of emotional satisfaction in one's life may act likewise. Anxiety reactions to situational difficulties and crises seem particularly prone to be expressed in psychosomatic symptoms. The psychiatrist inquires, therefore, for personal situations that may give rise to anxiety, hostility, aggression, guilt, bottled-up resentment, smoldering discontent, and other disturbing emotions and unwholesome attitudes that may act as the cause or as an aggravating factor in the production of much ill health manifested at the somatic level. All too often it will be found that the sickness has developed in an effort to find a solution for the difficulties that occur in human relationships. Frequently the nature of a body disorder can be appreciated only when psychological happenings, as well as physical disturbances, are investigated. The patient's feelings, his personal relationships, his life situation, and his reactions to his environment should be subject to the same painstaking scrutiny as his physical body and its symptoms. If a good life history is taken, much time and expense can often be saved in diagnostic studies. Sometimes a temporal relationship can be established between the onset of the apparently physical symptom and some emotionally disturbing event. Again, it may be possible to identify experiences of early life that seem highly relevant to adult attitudes and diseases. Ruesch makes the observation that the psychosomatic disorders as organ reflections of psychological tension are most common in the middle class, with its greater burden of self-required striving, conforming, and repressing. There seems, also, to be a greater tendency for emotionally introverted persons to show somatic complaints than for those who are extroverted.

Physical symptoms are the presenting ones and so dominate the clinical picture that their mental source is not superficially recognizable. The neurotic patient rarely complains of his anxiety, depression, resentment, or sexual tension, but rather of his disorder of bodily functions, such as anorexia, vomiting, backache, headache or palpitation.

Psychosomatic medicine does not, strictly speaking, include psychological reactions that the physically-ill patient may develop in response to his illness, but these may, in themselves, be of great significance to him and constitute an important disabling factor in his illness.

Psychosomatic medicine deals with several groups of patients: (1) In the first group, are those who suffer from various physical symptoms but who do not have a bodily disease that may serve as a cause for the symptoms. As the result of the failure to recognize that such illnesses are of emotional origin, they have often been called "functional." (2) In another group of psychosomatic disorders, a physical disease exists, but the original, causative factors were of an emotional nature. The pathological condition resulting from the action of the emotional causes reaches a point where it is no longer reversible. (3) In a third group of psychosomatic disorders, the patient does have actual organic disease, but certain of his symptoms do not arise from this disease but from mental factors, perhaps from anxiety arising from some situation in relation to other persons. In disorders of this type, the disability is often out of proportion to the physical disease. The physician must look further than the organic pathologic condition for an explanation of all the symptoms and the total disability. Since the same symptom may be a result of structural pathology, of personal pathology ("functional"), or of a fusion of both, the physician must make a thorough investigation of both physical condition and personality. Unless he does so, he may overlook any psychosomatic components in organic disease and will make a diagnosis of "functional" by a process of exclusion only. If, moreover, the physician makes a diagnosis by exclusion only, he is in no way prepared to prescribe rational and adequate treatment. This can be outlined only if he has a knowledge of the psychological stresses and situations to which the patient's physical symptoms represent a reaction. Most patients with psychosomatic reactions do not have such frank symptoms of the psychoneurosis as compulsions, phobias, and anxiety states.

Types of Reaction to Psychological Stresses

In previous chapters, we have observed that life experiences, especially those involving meaningful, anxiety-producing human relationships, may be productive of such emotions as fear, rage, resentment, guilt, grief, sadness, and loneliness, and that as a consequence a psychosis with its disorganization of personality or its disturbance of reality evaluation may follow. Chapter 28 shows that in some instances such experiences, with their resulting psychopathology, lead to anxiety states and to various defensive and substitutive reactions known as psychoneuroses. In this chapter, we shall attempt to show how in other persons life experiences, with their resulting anxieties, hostilities, insecurities, fears, and emotional tensions and attitudes, are expressed not in neurotic symptoms but in physical symptoms and organ-dysfunctions—in other words, how physical symptoms may develop in reaction to psychological stress. Physiological changes are set up by autonomic nerve impulses generated as a result of emotional conflict or tension.

In previous chapters, we have seen how emotional forces may affect perception, thinking, feeling, and behavior. In this chapter, emphasis will be placed on the influence of emotions on physiology. A simple and familiar illustration of the fact that emotions may influence physiological processes is the flow of tears associated with the emotion of grief; another is the quickened heart action associated with anger. Cannon and others showed that various physiological changes, such as those of secretion, muscle tension, and circulation, which are under the control of the vegetative nervous system, may be produced by emotions. The chronic emotional state stimulates a response of the vegetative nervous system with resulting physiological malfunctions that, if persistent, tend eventually to produce pathological changes. Such an influence of emotional factors on physiological functions was well demonstrated by Wolf and Wolff in their patient with a gastrostomy with herniated gastric mucosa. It was found that pleasurable emotions of appetite led to some increase in secretion and vascularity of the mucosa, with increased motility of the stomach wall. Sadness, discouragement, and self-reproach led to prolonged pallor of the mucosa and hyposecretion. Anxiety produced hyperemia, hypersecretion, and hypermotility. Aggressive feelings, including resentment and hostility, led to a great increase in secretion and vascularity and to some increase in motility.

The same investigators showed also, in the case of portions of exposed colons in fistulous patients, that situations productive of conflict, resentment and hostility were associated with hypermotility and hypersecretion of the enzyme lysozyme and of mucus. In some patients, with sustained hyperfunction during anger and resentment the appearance of petechial hemorrhages was noted. Dejection and fear were associated with hypofunction of most of the large intestine. The fact that emotions may influence physiological functions and dysfunctions is now well established by both clinical and experimental observation. That a patient suffering from physical disorder, especially if it is of a serious and progressive nature, is very prone to develop some psychological response to it is equally well known.

Processes of Origin and Symptom

The psychophysiological responses may be interpreted as the inappropriate perpetuations of organ reactions adaptive to, or protective against, some stress in human life experience. As has been shown in previous chapters such reactions include not only those caused by assault by other organisms and physical agents, but also those consequent to man's capacity to interpret symbols as indicative of danger derived from his past experiences, including the threats resulting from necessary conformity to family and cultural mores, that in themselves lead to deprivation of certain innately desired satisfactions. In response to the stress imposed by various threats and conflicts, organ reactions, in conjunction with various feelings and attitudes, occur to assist in adaptation or to prepare for emergencies to protect the individual. The perpetuation of the organ reactions beyond the period of stress leads to sustained responses that are inappropriate and may end in tissue damage.

The psychosomatic symptom represents the physiological concomitant of an emotional state. In the acute emotional state of rage, for example, it is a normal vegetative process for the blood pressure to be raised. This rise in blood pressure will subside if the angry man releases his emotional tension by physical or verbal attack on the object of his anger. If, however, a persistent, inhibited aggression (chronic rage) continues, the patient's emotional tension does not subside, his blood pressure does not become less, and he suffers from "essential" hypertension. In other words, a chronic emotional tension has activated bodily changes resulting in vascular hypertension. The physical symptoms of some cases of hypertension are therefore of psychosomatic origin. If a chronic emotional tension acting through the vegetative nervous system stimulates muscular or secretory activity of the gastrointestinal tract, then the psychosomatic symptom will be referable to that system. The physiological expressions of anxiety may then be interpreted by the patient as "stomach trouble." Through introspection, these self-diagnosed conditions may be exaggerated.

There is a difference of opinion among psychiatrists as to whether there is a correlation between type of personality and type and locus of psychosomatic disease, or a correlation between certain emotional constellations and the vegetative innervations and responses. Most psychiatrists now agree that the conception of Dunbar of a personality constellation specific to each psychosomatic disorder has no sound foundation. Alexander and others stress rather the specific nature of the conflict situation. Other psychiatrists are of the opinion that the organ system affected by the emotionally acting influences is determined not by psychological factors, but by an inherited tendency to respond somatically to stress and conflict in a fashion consistent for himself. This view, presented by Wolff, differs from the earlier ideas of inherited or acquired systemic or organic weaknesses.

In Chapter 28, reference will frequently be made to the assumed fact that many mental symptoms, such as phobia, compulsions, and various others, represent defenses at the psychological level against repudiated impulses, hostilities, and other psychopathogenetic material. It is, perhaps, a pertinent analogy to think of the "functional," psychosomatic symptom as also a defense, expressed not at the psychological level, but at the physiological level through the mediation of the vegetative nervous system. The psychosomatic symptom alone, however, does not fully account for the patient's distress. More influential is the underlying anxiety that gave rise to the symptom and threatens to break through failing defenses. In a way, therefore, the psychosomatic, "functional" symptom may be considered as an emergency measure to prevent the patient from being overwhelmed by anxiety. He may consciously want relief from his neurotic, defensive symptom. The psychosomatic patient, like the neurotic, has likewise an unconscious resistance to the relinquishing of measures that are largely or in part defensive. In his endeavor to stress a purely somatic origin of his symptoms and to deny even the possibility of psychological causes, the patient may seem to protest too much. His conscious negation of such an origin amounts to an unconscious acknowledgment. One objective in therapy is to help the patient to understand the relation of his symptoms to the particular personality difficulties and maladjustments that are a source of anxiety.

If the physician fails or refuses to recognize the importance of emotional factors in illness, or by a useless repetition of previously negative examinations he continues to search for an organic pathological condition, the patient becomes even more convinced that his trouble is organic. The doctor's attitudes may, too, be important factors in perpetuating or provoking illness. By his tone of voice, gestures, et cetera, his own anxiety may readily be transferred to the patient. If some incidental pathological condition is found, the patient's anxiety becomes fixed on the system in which the pathologic condition, often unimportant, is found. In emotional disorders misidentified and mistreated as organic diseases, the patient's troublesome symptoms, instead of improving, tend to become chronic.

TYPES OF PSYCHOPHYSIO-LOGICAL REACTIONS

It has been pointed out that emotional conflicts produce anxiety that through prolonged action on the vegetative nervous system may seriously disrupt the autonomic regulation of the body, with resulting manifestations of symptoms referable to various visceral vegetative organs. These symptoms tend to be manifested in disturbances of certain systems, particularly the cardiovascular system, the gastrointestinal tract, the endocrine system, the respiratory tract, the skin, and the genitourinary system.

Because the resulting symptomatology is so definitely referred to viscera, many of these disorders were known as "organ neuroses." If the emotionally generated autonomic impulse produced physiological disturbance of heart action, the disorder was known as a "cardiac neurosis." If the disturbance was of the stomach, it was known as "gastric neurosis." Clinical experience shows that at times an individual may successively or simultaneously have disorders affecting several organ systems. For the purposes of classification, the dysfunctions are separated into those of various systems.

Cardiovascular System

For various reasons, perhaps largely because it is generally regarded as the most important bodily organ and because the idea of sudden death is often associated with it, anxiety, under conditions creating prolonged tension, may readily become attached to the heart. It has been demonstrated that stress invoking anxiety tends to increase the heart rate, cardiac output, and blood pressure, as well as cause changes in the rhythm and the electrocardiogram. Dejection and despair are associated with diminution in the cardiac rate and output and lowering of the blood pressure. With anxiety and resentment, exercise tolerance is impaired. Such functional derangements may become the neurotic focus, particularly if associated with injudicious comment or procedure by the examining physician, or if some suggestive but not significant symptom adds contributive influence. The majority of persons who have symptoms referred to the heart region do not have organic heart disease.

Symptoms

Common psychosomatic symptoms associated with cardiac neurosis are pain in the heart region, palpitation, arrhythmia, shortness of breath, fatigue, faintness, and insomnia. For the most part, these symptoms are somatic manifestations of anxiety. The clinical picture known as *neurocirculatory asthenia*, or effort syndrome, and characterized by breathlessness, easy fatigability, palpitation or heart consciousness, trembling, fainting, giddiness, headache, and fear of effort, is not of organic but of psychosomatic origin. The term "effort syndrome" is a misnomer, since the symptoms of the syndrome are not confined to effort. The term "effort intolerance" has been suggested as more appropriate. To a varying degree, the symptoms of anxiety co-exist and assume the form of bad dreams, apprehensiveness, sweating, depression, trembling, and a tense restlessness. The disorder was first described by Da Costa during the War Between the States. During World War I it constituted a major problem among English soldiers since, because of its supposedly organic nature, it called for discharge from military service. As a result, it became widely induced by suggestion. It is most frequently seen in persons who remain dependent and immature emotionally. Weiss, probably with much justification, emphasizes that there is no constitutional or physiological deficit in the cardiovascular system. The symptoms described in many instances represent the physiological expression of the hyperventilation syndrome that is precipitated by situations that arouse acute anxiety or fear in the individual. This condition, although not always the physiological source of the "effort syndrome," is readily recognizable and is described later in this chapter under the heading of Respiratory System.

Anxiety is the most frequent pathological mental symptom in cardiac patients. Sometimes excessive dependency needs or needs to control the environment may prolong an invalidism for secondary gain. As in the case of other disabling illnesses, the patient may use his invalidism to escape from some emotionally troublesome situation and may be reluctant to relinquish this defense as he improves physically. Again, the threat of his illness may be so intolerable to the patient as to lead to an irrational and rebellious denial of its existence.

Emotional decompensation may occur after surgical procedures, such as mitral commissurotomy, with sudden increase in physical capacity associated with expectations of increased activity. Those patients who have become dependent through long invalidism or have utilized the illness to avoid anxiety-provoking situations are most prone to respond to the surgical procedure in this manner.

Treatment

The treatment of mental disorders associated with disturbances of the circulation will be directed largely to the cause of the disturbance. In those associated with heart disease, this will, of course, include rest and proper cardiac stimulation, particularly with digitalis preparations. Sedatives may be necessary, but hypnotics should be avoided lest a drug delirium develop.

As may be inferred from what has already been said, the internist has been prone, in heart disease as in many other organic diseases, to forget the importance of associated emotional factors. With cardiac function already greatly disturbed by a serious somatic lesion, a load of anxiety added from the psychic side may be sufficient to throw the balance in the direction of decompensation. If a patient is found to have frequent breaks in compensation when there is but relatively slight damage of heart muscle, a search should be made for complicating psychic factors the elimination of which may determine the course of the illness. From the standpoint of the psychiatrist, the most important problem is the handling of the patient's anxiety. Frequently he is deeply threatened by his symptoms and by the implications, often irrational, conveyed by the diagnosis. The physician should utilize his knowledge of psychopathology in dealing with the lowering of personality defenses that may occur in the face of fear of possible impending death. A strong, dependable, and constructive doctor-patient relationship should help the patient in handling both intrinsic and extrinsic tensions and the emotionally disturbing life situations that frequently exist.

In heart disease, particularly in coronary thrombosis, the physician should seek to dissipate the patient's fear of the disorder as an incapacitating or fatal ailment. Unwarranted fear is too often fostered by the gloomy predictions of the physician.

Hypertension

Vascular hypertension is not, of course, a specific disease but rather a systemic reaction that may be induced by a variety of causes. The cases of primary interest to the psychiatrist are those in which a major factor is emotional tension operating through the vegetative nervous system to cause vasoconstriction. Some psychiatrists are of the opinion that the unrealized inner tension that often accompanies hypertension is to be attributed to the mobilization of excessive rage in the face of a threat to the dependent relationship of the hypertensive patient. This emotion is seen as partly repressed and suppressed and inadequately discharged through verbal or motor activities. The personality of many hypertensive patients is one of outward serenity and affability, but it covers conflicting attitudes of readiness for aggressive hostility with needs to conform in order to maintain often strong dependent attachments. However, hostility is not peculiar to hypertension. Many hypertensives are neurotic, with strong perfectionistic and compulsive tendencies. It must not, of course, be assumed that psychodynamic factors are the only ones that contribute to essential hypertension.

Some patients with early hypertension suffer also from gastrointestinal symptoms, head discomforts, and fatigue. Such symptoms cannot usually be accounted for on the basis of the hypertension itself but are presumably a result of the same emotional factors that contributed to, but did not cause, the hypertension. With the patient's discovery of the hypertension, the "blood pressure phobia" may dominate the clinical picture. No final statement can yet be made concerning the influence of psychological factors in the production of essential hypertension. There is much reason to believe, however, that many of the symptoms attributed to hypertension are of emotional origin. Investigation of the life situation and psychotherapy will often make the patient a more contented and effective person, even though the hypertensive disease itself is not significantly influenced by psychotherapy.

Migraine

Although the conspicuous feature of migraine is the episodic and usually unilateral headache, the syndrome consists of a widespread neurovascular dysfunction and other somatic symptoms accompanied as well by disturbance of mood in individuals of a driving perfectionistic personality.

SYMPTOMS. Before the onset of headache, there exists for some hours or days evidence of mood change, associated with increased variability in the contractile state of the blood vessels, particularly of the head. Irritability or moodiness at this time is often associated with flushing or pallor of the face due to contraction or dilatation of the extracranial blood vessels. Visual phenomena, including scintillating scotomata, unilateral or homonymous hemianopia, occur in about 15 per cent of the patients in the hour or two preceding the headache due to vasoconstriction of the retinal vessels. As these symptoms disappear, the typical throbbing unilateral headache ensues, usually located opposite to the side of the perceived visual disturbance. The headache is due to vasodilatation of the common carotid and external carotid arteries and may be relieved by pressure upon them by the actions of vasoconstricting pharmaceuticals. With the persistence of vasodilatation for several hours, there occurs edema or tenderness in the vessels, which become incompressible and less amenable to the actions of vasoconstricting drugs. Also at this time, redness or tearing of the eye and swelling of the nasal mucosa, and, in some patients, painful contraction of the neck musculature follow. With some patients, nausea, vomiting, fluid retention, and other variant phenomena are associated or may represent minor variants of the migraine attack.

ETIOLOGY. The migraine sufferers tend to come from ambitious, highly-conventional families that attach great significance to attainment and in which children are required to conform to strict behavior patterns that limit the direct expression of aggression by either physical or verbal activity. Failure to conform threatens the family attachment. Thus hostile feelings toward parents or other respected or loved persons are repressed. Consequently, the arousal of rage or hostile wishes leads to conflict and anxiety, and this condition acts as precipitant for the pathophysiologic neurovascular response. Migrainous patients often disclose in psychotherapy hostile fantasies toward siblings and other family members. Frequently they have fantasied smashing the head of the person toward whom they have felt hateful. The arousal of sexual drives, which in turn are rejected by their overly strict superego, may lead again to the secondary emergence of rage and consequent precipitation of headache. The personality of the majority of those with migraine is one expressive of consideration to others, controlled, outwardly calm, and the individual is often thought of as an effective driving and perfectionistic person. Just prior to the migraine attack, some personality traits and moodiness more directly expressive of the concealed rage may become evident. There is frequently a family history of migraine, and women are affected more often than men.

TREATMENT. Treatment for the migrainous attack is directed to symptomatic relief by providing a vasoconstricting agent. The administration by mouth of 1 mg. of ergotamine tartrate and 100 mg. of caffeine sodium benzoate (available in tablet form as Cafergot) repeated at 30-minute intervals up to six doses usually effectively relieves or aborts the headache. If the patient is nauseated or vomiting, a subcutaneous injection of 0.25 or 0.5 mg. of ergotamine tartrate may be given.

When the migrainous episodes are so frequent or so disturbing as to affect the general life adaptation of the sufferer, psychotherapy is indicated. Treatment should be directed to allowing more direct and constructive expression of the rage and aggressive drives and to reducing the exaggerated superego demands.

Tension Headaches

Tension headaches are precipitated in other individuals of essentially the same personality make-up by similar emotional conflicts, or they may complicate the migrainous state. The tension headache typically produces diffuse and sustained aching pain in the forehead, back of the head, shoulders, and neck. It is frequently encountered as the somatic component of a chronic anxiety state or in those whose personality characteristics and development are described in Chapter 28. Hence the pain is due to prolonged and sustained contracture of the cervical musculature.

Symptomatic relief from these headaches may be obtained with the use of drugs relieving anxiety and by muscular relaxants. Meprobamate, 400 mg., may be prescribed with barbiturate medication, such as sodium amytal, repeated at 3-hour intervals. Again, the frequent or prolonged occurrence of such headaches indicates the prescription of dynamic psychotherapy to allow recognition of conflict and modification of the underlying pathological structure of the personality.

Both types of headaches are to be discriminated from those due to other physical illness, as well as those symbolic complaints of head pain or peculiar head sensations seen occasionally in the schizophrenic that represent in some way derogatory inferences to intellectual functioning or doubts as to social or emotional capacities. Patients with such a concept frequently speak of their complaints in vague and bizarre manners, in contrast to the usual stereotyped descriptions of headache provided by those with an organ illness or neurovascular or neuromuscular dysfunction involving the head and neck.

Gastrointestinal System

It is not surprising that the gastrointestinal function provide the most frequent focus of psychosomatic syndromes. In life experience, the first contact of the infant with another person comes in relation to the nursing process. The infant here experiences his first relief from physical discomfort and tension through the intake of milk. The satisfaction of relief from hunger through this experience becomes strongly associated with feelings of well-being in maturity. On the other hand, deprivation of food or its irregular presentation is associated with feelings of tension and rage. Compounded with the somatic disturbance and the attending emotions are the gradually developing perceptual processes in relation to contacts with the mother and mother surrogates.

In addition to the growing awareness of the dependent relationship on the mother with its satisfactions and frustrations coming as they do through feeding, there is also the similar interpersonal conditioning that takes place through the eliminative activities of the lower end of the gastrointestinal tract. Here again the infant is brought to eliminate and retain fecal matter in terms of relating to the mother.

Thus it is seen that the satisfactions gained through the early sucking process are associated with the emotion of being loved and the development of feelings of security and satisfaction. On the other hand, the bowel training process again provides opportunity for the feelings of approval through cleanliness or of stubbornness through retention and constipation. Frustration of the pleasures of feeding mobilizes aggressive activity in the form of biting, taking, greed, and envy. Again the process of eating is surrounded both in the family and in the culture with many opportunities for pleasure and conflict in interpersonal reactions. This is less apparent in respect to eliminative processes, which are usually solitary.

The symptoms of gastrointestinal disturbance through anxiety may extend from anorexia, nausea, "nervous indigestion," vomiting, belching, distress from gas, and epigastric pain to problems of diarrhea and constipation. Many patients complain also of fatigue. Frequently the abdominal pains and discomforts are attributed to "chronic appendicitis," and the patient is subjected to surgery. This is soon followed by a recurrence of symptoms. In other cases the gall bladder is removed. Spastic or mucous colitis with diarrhea and constipation represent another phenomenon of this disturbance of the gastrointestinal tract. In addition, obesity and anorexia nervosa may be considered psychosomatic expressions of this system.

Peptic Ulcer

Not only the clinician but also the lay person is aware that functional gastric symptoms are commonly produced by worry, business reverses, family quarrels, and other emotionally-disturbing experiences. Similarly, it is recognized that psychogenic factors are of importance in the etiology of peptic ulcer. It is still unknown whether the physiological disturbance in secretory and motor functions produced by emotionally-generated autonomic activity results in the formation of ulcers. It is possible that the motor disturbances result in spasm of the pylorus and therefore cause prolonged retention of the acid content of the stomach. Also, the blood supply of the stomach may be affected by the excitation of the autonomic nervous system.

At any rate, the ulcer syndrome is now among the most frequently encountered of psychosomatic conditions. It is of interest that the incidence of peptic ulcer has significantly changed within the past half century in western European societies. At one time it was extremely prevalent in women, but now it occurs chiefly in men. The change in the sex ratio is unexplained. Recent pediatric studies have shown that such ulcers occur as well in children. Peptic ulcer is much more frequently seen in those subject to depressions and alcoholism and is uncommon in the schizophrenic.

Saul has indicated that peptic ulcer may occur under a number of circumstances. It may be seen as an acute transient reaction in the face of unusual stress. Such stresses may be the serious threats of military life, or, on the other hand, internal inhibition may lead to frustration, mounting tension, and consequent psychosomatic expression through the gastrointestinal tract. In addition, there is a group of individuals in whom dependency longings are so exaggerated that they may not be satisfied or are bound to remain ungratified because of the ordinary demands of living. These are individuals with essentially infantile personalities.

Many psychiatrists, including Alexander, consider that the type of conflict situation has a determining significance in regard to the peptic ulcer psychophysiologic reaction. It is asserted that patients with this condition are basically dependent, that the exaggerated aggressive, ambitious, and independent "go-getting" attitudes that are noted superficially are a reaction to the underlying basic dependency needs. On the other hand, this type of conflict is not exclusively associated with the peptic ulcer syndrome. It has been pointed out that the description of the ulcer patient as a self-sufficient, independent, and overly-responsible person is not always appropriate, and many of them are overtly irresponsible, dependent, and inactive. There is some evidence to suggest that the dependency-independency conflict is only one variable in the induction of peptic ulcer. The ulcer patient is usually hypersecretory, as judged from the sustained high levels of serum and urinary pepsinogen. Only in individuals with such evidence of hypersecretion who also present psychodynamic conflict does ulcer develop. Studies of women with peptic ulcer have recently shown that the onset is often related to surgical procedures or other events that have threatened in reality or in fantasy their sexual functioning. Since threat to the sexual functioning may also simultaneously be seen as a threat to the dependency relationship of the patient, the production of ulcer symptoms may well be related to the conflict situation described by Alexander.

From the therapeutic point of view, the psychiatrist may seldom function suc-cessfully as the therapist for these patients. There are on record some excellent therapeutic results from prolonged psychoanalysis, but whether these outcomes exceed the frequency in patient groups treated by medical measures alone has not been demonstrated. It may be recommended that the repressed dependency needs of the patient be gratified directly or indirectly without inducing shame, guilt, or resistance. This can be done by environmental manipulation, including vacation, enlisting the support of key figures in the patient's environment, or by strengthening the patient–physician contact through regularity and frequency of visits. In those individuals with an infantile personality, the facing of the conflict by psychiatric treatment may well lead to serious depression and a more disturbing personality reaction than that accompanying the primary ulcer symptomatology.

Mucous Colitis

In this disease we meet with a group of symptoms into which anxiety-producing problems are not infrequently translated. Among these symptoms are constipation and the discharge of mucus-containing stools. Shreds of membrane are discharged in masses or mixed with soft or liquid fecal matter. The patient complains of indigestion. The appetite is poor and capricious, and the patient resorts to an increasing restriction of diet in an attempt to find one that will not cause discomfort. Distention of the stomach, belching, flatulence, heaviness or pain after eating, nausea, and other gastric symptoms are common. Many patients are asthenic and show diminished output of energy. In many cases this physiological disturbance appears to be in response to anxiety, guilt, sensitivity, overconscientiousness, and resentment. It is common for the symptoms to be attributed to various alleged causes varying from chronic prostatitis to gallbladder disease. All too frequently the patient is advised to have colon irrigations or an operation. It is stated that mucous colitis is responsible for the removal of more undiseased appendices than any other cause.

Ulcerative Colitis

A relationship between periods of emotional stress and the onset or exacerbation of symptoms has been recognized in those with ulcerative colitis. Quite frequently the attacks commence three or four weeks after a sudden, unforeseen threat to the patient's security, commonly in the form of bereavement through death, separation, rejection, disillusionment, loss of a part of one's body, or changes in psychological status, such as graduation, failures at school or at work, and other causes of diminished self-esteem. Although those patients who have been studied psychiatrically often appear to be highly intelligent, their emotional lives suggest impaired capacity for appropriate affective experiences. Yet they seem keenly perceptive and sensitive to the emotional responsivity of others. With ambivalent human contacts, they respond to loss with depression and rage, accompanied by disorganization of bowel function. Many patients whose primary affective need was the protective care of a maternal figure were disturbed through their early conditioning in relationship to dominating, hostile, or rejecting mothers, so that they expected humiliating rejection. Again, in the family setting physical symptoms often had signified preferential care. With emerging hostility or rage toward the wanted person, such patients frequently responded with guilty fear of retaliation. It has been noticed that both men and women with ulcerative colitis, when referred for psychiatric treatment, have shown considerable evidence of disturbance of psychosexual development.

Treatment of the patient with ulcerative colitis must generally be carried out by the physician or internist. The psychiatrist's contribution initially is that of assisting in or advising the establishment of a solid dependency relationship that will again provide the patient with a feeling of mastery over himself and his environment. Dramatic interruption of attacks of colitis have been obtained by some psychiatrists through assuming a simple supportive and protective role for the patient and demanding little. Margolin goes so far as to establish what is termed an anaclitic therapy, in which the patient is regarded as a helpless infant and is encouraged to regressive behavior. Here the therapy is somatically directed. It is generally recognized that intensive psychotherapy or analytic therapy is not possible during the acute phases of the illness. Others have criticized analytic therapy even in later stages of the illness as implying too extensive a commitment of the therapist to the patient's emotional and psychological demands. Some patients are unable to accept extreme solicitude and sympathetic behavior because of their own personality make-up and their expectation of further rejection. On the other hand, the effort of Lindemann to restore the patient's former equilibrium in a dependency relationship through attempting to replace the lost supportive figure may fail if the patient's expectations in such a role are not fulfilled.

There is evidence from carefully controlled follow-up studies by Daniels and his colleagues that those patients who receive intensive dynamic psychotherapy over time more effectively manage their symptoms and present other evidences of improved social, sexual, and emotional functioning compared to patients who receive little psychotherapy. At the same time, such treatment does not modify significantly the lesions in the colon as visualized by the proctoscope. In this series of patients, a high proportion was schizophrenic, and the severity of the illness and ultimate prognosis for those with this personality disorder was much less hopeful than for those with other types of personality organization.

Obesity

Obesity has been understood largely from the standpoint of an increased drive to eat. Both physiological and psychological studies have directed the unraveling of this source of pathological drive. It now appears, from the physiological demonstration of two hypothalamic areas subserving separately the act of feeding and the accomplishment of satiation, that over-eating must be recognized as a much more complex problem than a simple increase in a drive to provide satisfactions of a need. In the laboratory, diminution in the capacity for satiation through specific brain lesions causes hyperphagia without increase in hunger.

As our knowledge of the physiological processes underlying feeding behavior and satiation have enlarged, so also has that pertaining to the parental influences on personality growth that affect the development of eating behavior. For the majority of patients, these latter factors are probably the major determinants in the obese syndrome. Without their recognition and consideration, the treatment of the overweight patient often fails and in some occasions leads to serious disruptions of personality functioning.

What constitutes obesity or overweight is not well defined. As Bruch has made clear, the changes and fluctuations in weight measured over a period of time provide a better index of weight disturbance than the percentage of weight excess computed from the standard height-weight tables. Stability in weight, then, is recognized when the individual maintains a relatively constant poundage without concern over dieting. Some individuals maintain weight curves close to the average but only through a perspective on life that is fixed on maintenance of weight through dieting, a measure that for them is abnormal. The study of the extended temporal weight curve provides important clues for the treatment of the obese person who is seeking help.

With evidence of many fluctuations up and down, with or without medical supervision, inference may be made that additional attempts at weight reduction will be unsuccessful, since the previous failures and successes have not been comprehended in their fullest meaning. Here a study of the weight changes in relation to the total personality functioning, which includes an estimate of the sense of well-being and adequacy of perform-

ance in the individual's spheres of life action, becomes as important as the weight changes. Stability in weight is a reliable guide to estimate whether the obese person is adapting well to his life experiences. This is particularly so during childhood and adolescence. A degree of overweight in these periods, if stable, becomes disturbing only when the growing person is involved in a ceaseless struggle owing to family and cultural pressure, enhanced in Western society in these times by the insistence on slimness as a desirable bodily trait.

In recent years the statistical evidence that overweight contributes significantly to increased death rates resulting from circulatory disturbance has been strongly challenged by new information and analysis. Yet the health emphasis on weight reduction continues. It is accepted in many medical circles that a weight 20 per cent above the standard for a particular age and sex constitutes pathological overweight. The concept, although useful in the clinic in detecting individuals at the extremes of the weight curves and providing clues pertaining to pathological disturbances and their changes, fails to do justification to the genetic and constitutional differences in individuals. It is perhaps wiser to think of a "preferred weight" for the individual as Bruch does.

The development of obesity often occurs in a family setting in which the parents compensate for their own life frustrations and disappointments through their attachment to the child. In most instances the mother is the dominant family member and holds the obese child or children by anxious overprotection, including a pushing of food. The mother frequently has high expectations for achievement for the child, achievement to compensate for the failures of the parents and those of their children. The child is not cared for as an individual with particular problems that require emotional support, and, as the aims of the parents are predominant, the child fails to develop personal independence or self-esteem. Often the mother's attitudes reflect her own early sufferings and hardships coupled with resentments to her family's and her own childhood experiences. Toward herself she appears self-pitying, yet intent on saving her children from similar experiences. In many instances the obese child is not a wanted child. He is often one who has passively accepted the indulged role without rebellion because of his own demanding attitude, which cannot be met outside the home. On the surface, the obese individual, as a child and as an adult, is most frequently seen as submissive and unaggressive. Yet this is not really the case. His demands are met in the family setting by the balance provided through the food expression of love and satisfaction. The overweight adult often is unable either to notice the existence of hunger contractions or to estimate as well as others the amount of his food consumption. Bruch has recently suggested that there occurs through the family feeding processes a distortion of the perception of the growing child's bodily sensations that prevents them from properly identifying and responding to hunger and satiation appropriately. This takes place by the parental figure telling the child how he feels and forcing food as a means of alleviating the parent's anxiety but not in relation to the bodily demands of the child. This perceptive distortion is considered by Bruch as crucial for the understanding of developmental obesity. Also contributing to the condition is the greatly limited physical activity of the obese person.

When exposed to social frustrations with their consequent arousal of hostility, the overweight person seeks his satisfaction in over-eating and by this means symbolically obtains an expression of his aggression, as if the food represents to the patient evidence that he is the best loved. Oftentimes the over-eating is done at night time in association with insomnia and is then accompanied by morning anorexia. There is some indication that the uptake of glucose by the tissues in the obese is accelerated in periods of anxiety. If this is the case, satiation might well not occur physiologically.

In time, the obese body image also comes to have high emotional significance, as it often represents the desire to be strong and powerful and actually, in life, provides satisfactions. The child is conspicuous and may receive attention through this source, even though denied it by other socially more acceptable means. Loss of weight becomes difficult not only because of inability to face the physical discomfort of hunger, but also because of the symbolic loss of love and revenge that eating had provided, and later because of fear of loss of the power symbolically represented by the obese frame.

With the concept of specialness and power that the obese child develops from the maternal association and later attaches to his size, the psychological life becomes filled with grandiose daydreams, particularly in those persons who daily suffer defeat in their major aspirations. These fantasies are usually conscious and not deeply repressed as in many with psychoneuroses. The fantasies differ from those of the psychotic because the obese person has awareness of their unreasonableness. Obesity at a later stage then becomes, in itself, the rationalization for failure. In some, the overweight is used as a means of escaping the anxieties requisite for the pursuit of a creative social existence. The overweight person's attitude toward himself is further complicated by his felt rejection by family and friends because of his obesity, particularly since he has a deep need to be accepted as he is.

Sexual maturation is complicated for both the overweight boy and girl. In many fat men, there is marked lack of interest in women and failure to establish heterosexual relations. Yet homosexuality seems rare. The clear concept of the man as a masculine personality is often lacking. Overweight women are usually outgoing with men and succeed in establishing marriage relationships.

The term "reactive obesity" has been used by Bruch to separate out those problems of overweight that occur suddenly after a psychologically traumatic incident in persons who have not previously been evidently stout. Yet indications from the study of such persons show they have previously reacted to stress with overeating, and the family patterns and personality development are very similar to those with "developmental obesity." Most frequently the incident leading to reactive over-eating has been either the death, or the anxiety associated with the possible loss, of a close and significant person. Among those who may be considered as reactively obese are individuals who have for periods been deprived by starvation. Obesity has been frequently observed in those who have spent long periods in prison camps, deprived of love, happiness, and recognition and have substituted eating for satisfaction.

The satisfactions of over-eating appear protective in some with incipient psychoses. Not infrequently such a person develops a full-blown psychotic state when undertaking to lose weight by dieting. This is particularly so in the schizophrenic, while in the depressive individual we most frequently encounter anorexia with weight loss. A number of patients over-eat and become overweight, sometimes with reversal of depressive mood to manic behavior.

The psychology of the obese person, as discussed, explains the usual failure of medical therapies to effect continuing change in the overweight state. Since simple loss of weight in those with developmental obesity threatens their psychological defenses, symbolized by the satisfactions of eating and the personal concept of strength in size, the failure to obtain gratifications either through fantasy or through becoming slender results in relapse. Before yielding to the wish of the overweight patient or of his parents for treatment, it is necessary to determine whether the desired change is likely to threaten the physical and psychological balance of the individual. The threat to physical health in terms of later cardiovascular disease appears to be overemphasized, and the physician and psychiatrist should take into account possible serious psychological and emotional disturbances that may result from efforts at weight reduction.

Successful treatment of the obese person requires a knowledge of his total personality, also that the goal of treatment be directed beyond the mere reduction of weight. With young people, these aims are not likely to be obtained unless the parent in the parent–child symbiosis that led to the over-eating is also willing to participate in the treatment, even in some instances to the point of undertaking simultaneous psychotherapy. When psychotherapy is utilized, it is unwise to attempt weight reduction initially and then discontinue therapy at the point the patient has attained an ideal weight. The timing of the dieting, in association with psychotherapy, needs careful consideration. The nature of the diet and its palatability are important. There is again a growing appreciation that exercise, coupled with diet, is important in reducing weight and maintaining a slender figure. Since inactivity, like over-eating, is often an essential facet of the personality of many obese individuals, a simple medical authoritarian approach is unlikely to increase the exercise of the sick patient. In individuals in whom eating provides the major satisfaction in life and other gratifications are not available, psychotherapy is often not successful.

Anorexia Nervosa

A somewhat uncommon psychophysiologic gastrointestinal reaction is that known as *anorexia nervosa*. The presenting symptom of this reaction is a persistent lack of appetite, or rather disgust for food, with vomiting if it is forced. The disorder was first described in 1868 by Sir William Gull and given the name anorexia nervosa in 1874. In a classical paper, he called attention to its neurotic peculiarities. The reaction occurs largely in young, single women. Most patients are intellectually superior and in personality characteristics are introverted, stubborn, selfish, perfectionistic, and overly sensitive, and manifest compulsive and self-punitive behavior.

In addition to the loss of appetite, there is an extreme emaciation with a remarkable preservation of bodily vigor that, as Gull pointed out, cannot be reconciled with inanition caused by constitutional disease. Other symptoms are amenorrhea, constipation, low metabolic rate, dehydration, dryness of skin, falling of hair, and restless activity. Roentgenographical gastrointestinal studies are negative, and no evidence of pituitary disease is demonstrable by roentgen ray examination.

There is often a preceding history of obesity and over-eating, with a feeling of shame at being fat. Usually there are unhappy home relations, often taking the form of hostility between mother and daughter. There may also be sibling rivalry and jealousy. In a striking number of cases there is a history of frustration in heterosexual adjustment. In some cases, a pregnancy fantasy seems to have prompted the patient to begin to diet.

Probably, however, the neurosis can have many varied conscious and unconscious psychological roots. Some psychiatrists point out that the patient seems to achieve both primary and secondary neurotic gains through the reaction. They suggest that, through working out her hostilities and by provoking the environment to acts of punishment that alleviate a sense of guilt, a primary or internal gain is obtained. The illness brings, too, a secondary, but unconscious, gain in the form of desired attention, affection, and sympathy from the family. In some instances it seems to lead to a diversion of family notice from a supposedly more popular sibling.

Care must be taken not to confuse anorexia nervosa with Simmonds' disease, which results from insufficiency of the anterior lobe of the pituitary, or Sheehan's acute pituitary neurosis, which occurs secondary to pregnancy and parturition.

Treatment consists of psychotherapy, with an associated effort to improve the total adjustment of the personality. During treatment, reference to the anorexia should usually be avoided. Intimate personal attention at meals, including spoon-feeding, may be effective in getting the patient to eat normally. Small doses of insulin are advisable. Some patients may require tube-feeding. Removal from the family environment may be advisable.

Musculoskeletal System

Rheumatoid Arthritis

Psychiatric interest in rheumatoid arthritis stems from the repeated observation that the onset or exacerbation of the illness has been related to a period of emotional stress. The patient with rheumatoid arthritis has often been described as an individual who is composed emotionally, seldom expresses his feelings overtly, and appears to derive gratification from being of service to others. He is usually active physically and intellectually and is inclined to outdoor and competitive sports. His dependence on others is masked. The majority of such persons were brought up in families in which the mother was the domineering parent, while the father was gentle and compliant. This led to a strong dependency, with fear of the maternal figure and, in girls, a competitive relationship toward the father and brothers. Control of the intense hostility is accomplished through neuromuscular activity, domineering position, ability to control the environment, and overevaluation of physical functions.

The precipitating events leading to the arthritis have ranged from the death of the mother and threat of the father to remarry, separation or rejection from husbands or other important figures, to birth of a child, miscarriage, or disappointments in the personal relations of the patient. It is believed that the common factor in these various events has been an unconscious increase in the feelings of resentment, rebellion, and hostility associated with guilt that had been previously handled through self-sacrificing activity and service to others. In a number of patients exacerbations of rheumatoid arthritis have occurred following the suppression of feelings of grief on the loss of an important family member. Sometimes such exacerbations are seen as anniversary reactions to the loss, associated with feelings of depression.

There is a frequent association of rheumatoid arthritis with duodenal ulcer. Although it has been stated that individuals with psychoses seldom suffer from rheumatoid arthritis, yet in a study of a number of arthritic patients by psychoanalytical technique, covert psychotic defenses were noted, and in the course of treatment several became overtly disturbed.

At the time of onset of rheumatoid arthritis, or during emergencies, the therapy is essentially one of management of acute illness by the internist, with restoration of the patient's sense of security. The psychiatrist's assistance at this time is most effective as a consultant and advisor unless the patient has been in psychiatric treatment previously. Here active support without too rigid control of therapeutic needs is important. Patients with rheumatoid arthritis do poorly in classical psychoanalytical treatment. They respond best to activity on the part of the therapist and for a long time accept activity, rather than words, as security. Psychiatric therapy may be of assistance in those in whom tissue damage is extensive and the extent of disability exceeds the impairment of neuromuscular function. Many patients with this illness deny their need for help, yet with the establishment of a regular regimen of therapeutic interview arranged on the authority of a physician, they often do well over long periods of time on little more than supportive treatment. Only in occasional instances can the patient be freed from his often unrecognized hostile identifications with lost persons.

Respiratory System

Hyperventilation Syndrome

Subjective symptoms resulting from overbreathing are frequently not recognized by either the psychiatrist or the internist. Hyperventilation is the common physiological means by which the subjective disturbance noted in the usual acute anxiety attack takes place. It may be induced by any condition producing fear and not uncommonly occurs in the course of other personality disturbances when anxiety becomes manifest. Its recognition is of importance since in the medical clinic the afflicted patient is often considered to have heart disease, angina pectoris, asthma, or other respiratory disease, or even painful lesions presumed to be a result of spinal cord disease. In the psychiatric clinic, many patients have been exposed to a time-wasting therapy in which efforts were made to interpret the symbolic meaning of the subjective phenomenon produced by overbreathing.

The sufferer usually does not recognize that he is overbreathing. The increase and the depth and rapidity of respiration may be so slight that they go unobserved. It is well known that an irregular respiratory rhythm occurs in anxious individuals and is accompanied by sighing and yawning. Furthermore, these respiratory disturbances, if sufficiently prolonged, lead to reduction in the alveolar air and the carbon dioxide tension of the arterial blood with a fall in the blood bicarbonate. Consequently many physiological systems are altered. The acid-base equilibrium is disturbed, the urine composition and volume are affected, circulatory changes take place, and neuromuscular and electroencephalographic alterations ensue. It is not surprising that subjective disturbances take place.

The initial subjective feelings resulting from overbreathing are light-headedness or giddiness. If overbreathing continues, the individual has the sensation that he is about to faint, he may perspire profusely, and, if walking, his gait may seem unstable. There then follows a sensation of air hunger or shortness of breath and feelings of pressure in the thorax. Some patients speak of palpitation or of pain in the heart; others describe a bandlike feeling about the chest. With mounting anxiety over presumed lack of air, many consciously increase the depth and rate of breathing, thereby exacerbating the initial cause of the subjective symptoms.

The more commonly recognized symptoms of hyperventilation consist of tingling paresthesias in the fingertips, perioral region, or toes, followed by tetanic contractions. If overbreathing persists over a sufficiently prolonged period, disturbance of awareness may result, associated with pallor, vasomotor collapse, rapid, irregular, and weak pulse, and ending, in many instances, in loss of consciousness or in convulsions.

In those instances in which the psychiatrist sees a patient who complains of attacks of breathlessness, palpitation, and dizziness or perspiration, consideration should be given to the symptomatology as representative of episodic attacks of hyperventilation precipitated by acute situational anxiety. Such patients frequently are able to define well the situations in which the attacks occur and provide excellent descriptions of disturbing interpersonal contacts, with arousal of unbearable feelings of hostility, resentment, or sexuality. Not infrequently the attack of hyperventilation takes place as the consequence of a disturbing dream or nightmare. The diagnosis of a hyperventilation syndrome as the source of the symptoms of the individual patient may be easily determined by requesting the patient to overbreathe for a period of two minutes in a sitting position.

In order to carry out this test effectively, it is frequently necessary to provide a brief demonstration of what is required, also strongly to encourage the patient to continue overbreathing, as many will attempt to desist after 30 seconds of hyperventilation. At the end of this test the patient may be asked to describe his subjective symptoms. If he is unable to elaborate them spontaneously, the psychiatrist should inquire as to the presence of giddiness, breathlessness, palpitation, shortness of breath, perspiration, and pins-and-needles sensation. The patient then may be asked if he identifies the subjective sensations of overbreathing as those that he has suffered in the episodic attacks of which he complains. Not infrequently the neurological symptoms that occur in the course of this disturbance are unilateral. In general, the carbon dioxide combining power of the blood and the blood calcium are unchanged. However, in those instances in which chronic hyperventilation exists, venous alkalosis has in some instances been demonstrated. Occasionally with chronic, persistent hyperventilation, a compensatory acidosis, with reduction in blood carbon dioxide, has been reported.

Hyperventilation may result, not only from sudden emotional stress and anxiety but also in the course of febrile illnesses, high altitude anoxemia, high external temperatures over a long prolonged period of time, and occasionally in the course of encephalitis.

In some sufferers, the reduplication of the characteristic symptom complex by means of requested hyperventilation provides immediate and continuing relief of symptoms. On the other hand, in those individuals who have clear-cut evidence of chronic anxiety usually associated with phobic symptoms or with depressive or schizophrenic personality disorders, the demonstration of the physiological source of the symptomatology is effective only in providing an intellectual interpretation of the acutely disturbing symptoms and not in providing them with continuing relief. In these instances, it is recommended that the patient receive psychotherapy. In the course of such treatment, a modification of the personality structure that predisposes to the eruption of anxiety precipitated repetitively in particular situations may be brought about. The following case report provides an example of the need for psychotherapy in patients who present the hyperventilation syndrome.

A 57-year-old-woman who had been under medical care since her menopause at the age of 50 was referred for psychiatric treatment. At the onset of the menopause she had complained of headaches, nausea, tremulousness, and cold sweats. Her blood pressure was usually about 180 systolic, 90 diastolic. She made regular visits to her physician, who treated her with diet and Theominal. The patient did well for a period of 5 years until her treatment by this physician was abruptly terminated by her husband.

The patient was brought for psychiatric treatment 2 years later by her husband, who stated in her presence that he could no longer stand her "huffing and puffing." In the intervening 2 years he had taken her to several other physicians for her increasingly frequent and severe attacks of apparent shortness of breath. The patient described these as occurring only in the morning upon awaking. She would then seem short of breath and soon become dizzy and weak. She next suffered from palpitation, followed by tingling and numbness about the mouth and tips of the extremities. The attacks had increased in frequency to one daily. Each morning they prevented her husband and daughter from going to work and kept her from preparing the breakfast and doing the housework. The patient had been advised to "snap out of it," and had been given sedatives and ammonium chloride without avail.

The only abnormality observed on physical examination was a slight elevation of blood pressure. She was requested to hyperventilate and it was demonstrated to her that her symptoms could be reproduced by this procedure. The patient was considered to have essential hypertension complicated by attacks of hyperventilation resulting from chronic anxiety.

From spontaneous remarks made by the patient at this time, it was learned that during the period of overbreathing she was concerned about dying— not the possibility of her own death, but the death of her husband. She spoke of the recent death of her brother from heart disease and cancer, she went on to state that her children had now grown up and no longer needed her and she commented that the family had threatened to place her in a hospital for mental disorders. Her past history indicated that the patient was a driving, energetic woman who had been completely immersed in her family. It was inferred from her remarks about death that she harbored repressed resentment toward her husband, who showed little sympathy with her during the initial interview. It soon seemed apparent that situations arousing repressed hostility toward her husband and family, feelings that were unacceptable to her as a conscientious person, and threats of separation from her family induced the acute anxiety attacks manifested by overbreathing.

It was learned that the patient had married her husband suddenly after having been jilted. At that time, too, she had given up an excellent job. Her own daughter had been jilted some 6 months prior to the consultation. The patient described her husband as self-centered, buried in his work, disinterested in social life, and disparaging in his attitude toward her church and recreational activities. He was seen and advised to spend more time with his wife.

In four subsequent visits she was encouraged to ventilate her unacceptable feelings concerning her family and husband. She commented on the fact that she wished to resume typing and playing the piano. She was frank in speaking of her anger toward her husband for his years of indifference.

obstinacy, and ridicule, culminating when he forbade her to continue to attend the doctor who had helped her so well throughout the menopause. The patient was encouraged to plan activities outside the home that might help to make her less dependent on the family. The patient responded quickly. Within 6 weeks she was free of overbreathing attacks, did not require medication, and had returned to her house work. She then decided that further treatment was unnecessary, since her immediate symptoms had been relieved.

This case illustrates several important factors in the management of the hyperventilation syndrome. First, the patient was made aware of the physiological mechanism underlying the attacks by having her hyperventilate. This test also made her realize that her symptoms were regarded as significant in themselves. Second, a series of simple psychotherapeutic discussions allowed the patient to express herself freely concerning her emotions and attitude toward her family. This discussion of her feelings, interspersed only with a few directional questions related to possible anger and resentment, relieved her of her symptoms. Third, this patient was an excellent choice for brief psychotherapy as she gave a history of previous satisfactory adjustment at home, at work, and in marriage.

Asthma

That a relationship exists between emotional arousal and the precipitation of an asthmatic attack has been a matter of comment since the time of Hippocrates. Despite the fact that it is generally conceded that the asthma occurs in individuals with a constitutional predisposition, there are now on record many cases in which the attacks were initiated by events other than the presence of a specific antigen. The well-known instance of "rose asthma" is representative of this type of induction, in which the patient regularly had an attack when she was brought into contact with roses but also had asthma when she was shown a papier-mâché rose. Other similar precipitating instances are recorded in which patients have their asthmatic attack at a regular hour each day, when they hear a particular song or type of story, or react on hearing comments about a parent, or visit the parent's grave. The attack has been thought of as symbolic of a conflict, or as a sign but not a symbol of the conflict to which the patient responds as a conditional reflex. In some surveys of allergic patients as many as 75 per cent were found to have an emotional component influencing their attacks.

The asthmatic personality is often one of irritability and quickness to respond, coupled with lack of confidence, submissiveness, and anxiety. It has been noticed that there is an unusually strong maternal dependency that arouses conflict when aggressive or sexual drives threaten that relationship. The exaggerated dependency drive has arisen either through the relationship of the child to a rejecting mother or through too early urging by the parents that the child assume independence, a pseudo-independent façade thus being forced. The attack has been thought to represent symbolically both a protest against separation from the mother and also the wish to re-establish this relationship through crying; thus it is considered equivalent to a repressed cry. Others have stressed the relationship of the asthmatic attack to arousal of repressed conflicts relating to bodily odors, particularly concerned with excretions and secretions and thereby presumably involved in early childhood rearing relative to cleanliness and dirtiness. There is evidence to show that asthmatics show significantly greater blocking of associations on exposure to various odors than do other groups.

In addition to medical care to prevent and also treat the acute seizure, many asthmatics may profit by psychotherapy particularly directed to resolution of the dependency problem, which is often associated with repressed hostility. It has been found that children with asthma frequently respond promptly on separation from their parents. Permanent improvement for such children requires, as well, effective counseling and psychotherapy for the involved parents.

Endocrine System

Diabetes Mellitus

Among the more striking examples of the influence of emotional disturbances on somatic functioning is that observed in certain patients suffering from diabetes mellitus. Personality factors and the consequent emotional responses to the treatment regimen of this condition relate to almost all the issues pertaining to the therapy of diabetes. The psychiatrist may make a major contribution in the treatment and management of those difficult patients with "brittle diabetes." Psychosomatic investigations in recent years have clearly elucidated the disturbances in glucose metabolism and in variations in ketonemia resulting from changes in the emotional state of the individual.

It has been suggested that the onset of diabetes is often related to periods of severe emotional distress after such experiences as disruption of the home, or frustration associated with long periods of grinding work. Although the inquiry into the personality structure of the diabetic has failed to demonstrate a uniform personality picture, many psychiatrists have emphasized the passivity and immaturity with which diabetic patients look for attention and affection. Psychoanalytical studies of a few patients suggest that certain diabetics are frustrated when their demands for love and attention cannot be met. Others have stated that the psychological trauma derives from reactivation of dependency needs by new exposure to rejection and deprivation through the loss of another person.

On the physiological side, it has been shown that urinary and blood glucose levels are elevated following periods of emotional stress and that the glucose tolerance curves may be modified at such times. In general, the glucose tolerance test has been found to indicate a higher degree of diabetes when the individual is feeling more hostile and depressed, and it approaches the healthy curve when the patient feels accepted and cared for. It has been shown that an increase in ketone bodies in the blood stream may occur in similar situations; also, that with increasing diuresis, the diabetic may lose sugar, ketones, and chlorides, with depletion of fixed base and a rapid fall of glycogen in the blood stream. Such physiological changes, associated with the metabolic defect, lead to acidosis and may precipitate coma, particularly when the anxious patient neglects his diabetic regimen, as frequently takes place.

Since the customary regulation of diabetes requires both a control of the diet and the administration of insulin, the management of the disease is often complicated by the fact that the symbolic significance of the feeding process and its relationship to provision of emotional support through love may modify the therapeutic indications. It is particularly true that the giving of food and its deprivation become paramount in those homes where tension exists between parents and a diabetic child. The illness magnifies the difficulty between the child and the parent. Those parents with perfectionistic, aggressive attitudes may bring their children to good control of the diabetes but with the creation of a behavior difficulty. On the other hand, parents who pity themselves or blame the child and reject it may foster poor control of the diabetes.

The need to limit food often becomes a battleground between the child and parents and the child and physician. This is particularly so since the giving of candy or of food is often a token of approval in the family. The child has an excellent weapon that he can use against rigid punitive parents by refusing to eat when he is denied his wishes. Other children, under treatment for diabetes mellitus, finding themselves starved for food or affection, express their hostility through eating as they wish and then lying convincingly. Thus the rigid dietary management insisted upon by the physician and the family often leads to rather serious emotional disturbance in the child, with concomitant change or modification of the glucose metabolism and probable ketosis, or to psychological conflicts that deter the proper acceptance of the therapeutic needs of the illness. In such instances, the psychiatrist is needed as a means of working through the emotional conflict of the child with the parents, in assisting the parents to understand the child's problem and occasionally in providing advice to the internist in regard to the personality reactions of the child and the need to modify the dietary regimen and insulin requirements in conformity with the emotional problem that exists.

Due to the fact that this 16-year-old-lad had been hospitalized nine times in a general hospital for diabetic acidosis or coma during the preceding 6 months, he was referred for psychiatric consultation. There was a history of diabetes commencing 3 years previously, when his mother noticed he had lost weight and suffered abnormal thirst and frequency of urination.

Previous to the onset of the diabetes the boy had been able to engage in all activities with friends of his age. He withdrew from his contacts with other children following the commencement of his treatment due to their teasing of him as "diabetic kid" and "sugar blood kid." His physicians advised him that if he did not care for his diabetes by restriction of diet and proper use of insulin, he might lose a limb or his sight or be subjected to overwhelming infections if he were hurt. His diabetic treatment proceeded well during the first year under the care of a firm, insistent, older physician. However, difficulties arose when this physician retired and the patient transferred to another more permissive doctor. In view of the inability to control him under general medical care and as the result of the psychiatric consultation, it was decided to hospitalize him in a psychiatric nursing unit.

On admission the patient advised that his problem was simple. He stated he was a compulsive eater and that all he had to do was learn how not to eat. When his mother was consulted, she appeared anxious and expressed feelings of depression and hopelessness in regard to the patient. She described her deep feelings of guilt toward him but explained she was unable to cope with his rebelliousness. Her three other children were obedient. She stated that he seemed to awaken at all hours of the night and had taken to stealing food, frequently failed to give himself insulin injections, and strongly resisted the mother's attempts to administer them. He refused absolutely to perform the urinalysis, and he falsified reports to the clinic physician. He told his mother that he would rather have cancer and die than continue with the diabetes. He was openly aggressive toward her, and when angry he threatened to refuse to take insulin the next day. His relationship with his father was similar to that with the mother.

The mother admitted that she constantly argued with the patient to persist with his diet and to take the insulin as prescribed. At the same time, she forbade mention of the diabetes at other periods. The father saw the patient's diabetes as a severe blow, as he had long hoped that the patient would be able to assume the financial support of the family. The father described his discontent in the marriage and accused the mother of forcing him into marriage. The patient was born as an illegitimate child. However, approximately 2 years later, the parents married following the mother's second pregnancy. The father spoke of his resentment toward his very active son because of his noisy play and admitted frequent beatings of the boy.

The developmental history revealed that the patient was a feeding problem from birth onwards. He cried frequently at night and was awake for most of the day. Following an early circumcision, he developed projectile vomiting. Throughout his childhood he was a poor eater and required small feedings eight to ten times daily. His mother held and fed him until he was 3 years of age. With the birth of his sibling, there was evident rivalry and hostility. Since the father worked at night, this boy had slept in the mother's bedroom until the onset of the diabetes.

It was formulated that this young patient had suffered early affective deprivation that established an exaggerated need for a dependent emotional relationship. Also, the early feeding pattern had formed a demanding need for satisfactions that were not being met through the restricted and rigid diabetic dieting. In addition, it was considered that the boy was fearful of expressions of hostility due to the threatening relationship with the father and the threats provided him by the physicians in charge of his case. In reaction to his exaggerated dependency needs, he had developed an air of defiance. It was accordingly arranged that on admission to the hospital he would be allowed a permissive diet, with the privilege of controlling his own utilization of insulin, and that treatment should be conducted by a relatively firm male physician.

The patient was seen twice weekly in psychotherapy over a period of one year. Initially he was grandiose, defiant, and a braggart, both in relation to other patients on the ward and during treatment hours. Much anger was expressed toward his father, and he suffered mood swings. Some 10 weeks after admission, he burst into tears while describing an incident in childhood when his father had locked him in a room. At this point he verbalized the reasons for his hostile feelings towards his mother and simultaneously was defiant toward the nurses on the wards. Many fears were then expressed relative to mutilation and death that were traced to the father's early threats of bodily harm.

Following a home visit, when he had an argument with the father, he developed a stuporous condition simulating a diabetic coma on return to the hospital. This was recognized as a hysterical dissociation; it was treated conservatively and later studied in psychotherapy. In the course of a succeeding therapeutic hour, he acted out his rage toward the father relation to the therapist. When no harm resulted, there were no further recurrences of the dissociated activity, diabetic coma, or acidosis. He was discharged home to his family, continuing on the permissive diet and personal control of insulin.

Control of diabetes with evident improved relationship and understanding between the patient, parents, and sibling were evident in follow-up visits extending 2 years after his discharge from psychiatric hospitalization. The diagnosis was character neurosis with diabetes mellitus, juvenile type.

Adult diabetics who repeatedly go into acidosis are usually individuals who are seriously disturbed. Such individuals either give up all dietary control or cease taking insulin as a means of expressing their depressive and suicidal drives. Although this is the case in the majority of instances, other persons are precipitated into states of acidosis by serious transient emotional disturbances. Sexual difficulties are common in both men and women with diabetes. Diabetic women are concerned over child bearing, while diabetic men are frequently impotent. Childbirth itself may activate regressive cravings for care and affection in diabetics of either sex. The new child may be seen as a rival for the affection of the husband or wife. Thus the dependent cravings of the patient may be magnified, with resulting feelings of anxiety and depression that disturb the metabolic balance or lead to despair and diminished motivation for control of diet. Obese diabetics who are addicted to sweets or to over-eating are likely to over-eat when anxious in spite of threats of physicians concerning their future health if they fail to adhere to the diabetic regimen. Here, again, the need for psychiatric aid becomes important.

Hyperthyroidism

The most important of the endocrine glands as related to psychosomatic medicine is the *thyroid*. Although as early as 1803 reference was made to the occurence of sudden fright preceding hyperthyroidism, yet not until relatively recently has the possibility that emotional troubles may play an important part in the cause and course of the disease received adequate attention in the treatment of thyrotoxic states. This recent knowledge is detailed in Chapter 12 of this book.

Skin

A recognition of the importance of psychological factors in many dermatoses is by no means recent. Sydenham (1624–1689), for example, writing of the "hysteric diseases," described angioneurotic edema affecting one leg. Since the skin is an organ subject to the direct influences of the autonomic nervous system and the indirect effect of endocrine activity, as well as subject on the body surface to compulsive contact or self-inflicted damage representing unconscious conflict, the means of expression of the psychological disturbance vary greatly from one type of lesion to another. In the past few years, with the increasing recognition of psychological factors in the genesis of somatic diseases, the dermatologists have emphasized a high degree of association between various skin diseases, such as pruritus, neurodermatoses, hyperhydrosis, and other reactions, and evidences of difficulties in adjustment of personality to stressful life situations. Some dermatology clinics have reported that psychiatric factors were found to be of significance in over 75 per cent of their patients.

In cases of the dry type of neurodermatitis, it has been considered that excoriation of the skin is more fundamental than the pruritus usually complained of by these patients. The itching often represents a voluptuous or tantalizing sensation. Events that produce the emotions of anger, with depression and feelings of guilt, generally precipitate the exacerbation of the cutaneous eruption. The family constellation is often that of a hostile dependent maternal relationship, in which itching and scratching symbolize anger at the mother figure handled masochistically due to guilt.

In the exudative type of neuroderma-

titis of children (atopic dermatitis), there has been found evidence of maternal rejection. Here the emotional disturbance is thought to be expressed primarily through a psychophysiological mechanism that induces vesiculation. In urticaria the psychodynamic explanation is very similar to that of asthma, with the lesions precipitated by situations that induce resentment and frustration resulting from a threat to an important dependency relationship. With pruritus of the anogenital area, repression of various sexual conflicts has been observed. Dermatitis factitia has been recognized for many years as psychologically determined. Sadomasochistic mechanisms associated with the need to maintain a gratifying passive dependency again underlie the self-infliction of the lesions in many such instances.

Various methods of treatment for the neurodermatoses have been devised. Frequently separation from the significant family members brings about clearing, with recurrence noted on return to the family. The following case report represents a trial with a brief psychotherapeutic method of the type recently described by Seitz.

The patient, a 46-year-old retired policeman, was seen with the chief complaint of a skin rash. The onset of his dermatitis occurred 25 years previously when, shortly after his marriage, he noted the gradual appearance of a diffuse scaling eruption of the scalp. Some time later he developed redness and scaling in the groin, and a more or less generalized eruption, especially around the sides of his neck and in the creases of the knees and elbows. The rash was intensely pruritic, and the patient frequently scratched until he bled. Two years prior to admission, the eruption became generalized. No relief was obtained from steroid therapy and a multitude of other medications. Because of a life-long history of emotional problems, he was referred for psychiatric consultation.

The patient was the second of six children. His father was described as a strict disciplinarian who beat the children regularly with a cat-o'-nine-tails. Until 17 years of age, the patient was not allowed to stay out in the evening without his father's permission, and if he arrived home late he was beaten.

The mother was described as a warm, understanding person who was affectionate with the children but showed little love toward her husband. The patient's older brother was a fireman, who had retired 10 years previously following an acute psychotic episode. The other four siblings appeared to be in good health. The patient explained their good fortune with the statement, "By the time they arrived, my father had mellowed."

The patient's early development was unremarkable and his progress at school was average. He remembered that he was never able to express anger and never disobeyed his father's detailed instructions.

As an adolescent the patient was a shy, sensitive boy who was self-conscious and avoided social relationships with girls. There were exaggerated guilt feelings over masturbation. When confronted with social situations that were threatening, he would turn to drinking. He stated, "I had a terrific inferiority complex and liquor helped me to overcome it."

Since a civil service position offered a secure position and pension, he joined the police force at the suggestion of his father. When 20 years of age, he married in the hope of getting away from home. From the first there was marital difficulty, and he began to drink a quart of liquor daily.

Fourteen years before psychiatric consultation, the patient, during a riot, was struck on the head and sustained a concussion necessitating a brief hospitalization. Following his discharge he became tremulous and complained of extreme nervousness. His alcoholic intake increased in an effort to alleviate the pruritus, his anxiety, and the constant fear that he was about to die. He was discharged from the police force with a pension and the diagnosis of post-traumatic psychoneurosis.

During the subsequent two years he separated from his wife and child, lost contact with his family, and lived with an alcoholic woman who was suffering from cirrhosis. There were several episodes of delirium tremens, and he was hospitalized for alcoholic neuropathy, hepatic cirrhosis, and hematemesis.

Eight years prior to this consultation and following the death of his female companion, he was warned by a physician that if he continued drinking he would probably not survive another year. He discontinued drinking, was reconciled with his wife, and his dermatitis cleared, leaving only a few eczematous patches. He returned to work as a law clerk, attended church regularly and, in his own words, "became a model citizen." He maintained a rigid routine involving difficult hours of work. He dressed meticulously and attempted to do a perfect job at the office.

During the past two years his rash again became generalized and intensely pruritic. His wife informed him that, while asleep, he scratched as if he were intent on killing himself. He was admitted to a hospital in the hope that separation from his family and job would help in the treatment of his skin condition.

When seen in psychiatric consultation, he appeared as a well-groomed, neatly-attired, middle-aged man, alert and accurate, who spoke of his past experiences with obvious embarrassment. His memory was good, and he was well oriented, with an average intelligence and a normal fund of knowledge. He seemed anxious to please the interviewer and stated that he needed psychiatric help. During consultation he scratched freely. He volunteered that scratching usually brought him great relief and, at times, a satisfaction not unlike that of sexual pleasure. When psychotherapy was suggested, he quickly agreed. It was explained that he would be seen once a week for a period of 10 weeks by the psychiatrist in the out-patient department and that immediately preceding the interview he would be seen by the dermatologist for a brief examination.

During the first two interviews, an anamnesis was obtained, with particular emphasis on his current activity. He discussed the present fear of his father and the avoidance of situations that would bring him in contact with him. His wife frequently accused him of being a coward because of this, but he could not admit his fear to her. He described his wife as a stubborn, outspoken woman who was usually the disciplinarian with his 17-year-old boy. When he attempted to punish his son, his wife became outraged and pointed out to him how good it was of both of them to accept him back eight years ago. He nevertheless denied that there was friction in the household and stated that, in many ways, they were an ideal family. His son had recently been arrested on a minor charge, and it was suggested to the patient that perhaps he was failing as a father by not setting limits for the son.

During the third visit it was noted that the scratching had increased, and there was no improvement in the skin condition. He stated early in the interview, "I followed your advice and asserted myself with the boy but was careful not to become angry." His wife had been angry with him, but he pacified her by taking her out for a drive. He admitted that he dare not express anger toward her for fear she would leave him. Scratching was frequent, especially when his fear of expressing anger was discussed. His wife insisted upon knowing what was going on in therapy. He resented this but felt he could not refuse to tell her. He was told that it was not necessary to tell her, and he appeared to have considerable anxiety over this.

At work he was accused by a colleague of being a perfectionist; he admitted being angry at this criticism. When it was suggested that he deal more directly with the problems confronting him at work and at home, he scratched and talked of his extreme loneliness. When the patient attempted to discuss early experiences and relationships, he was referred back to current areas of conflict.

At the fourth interview, his skin condition was much worse, and he was unable to attend work. He had purchased two suits of clothing without consulting his wife, who usually accompanied him. He made some rather feeble attempts to tell his wife that he preferred shopping without her but felt that it was unsuccessful. He turned to the interviewer and asked, "Doc, tell me, what do you do when you become angry?" There was a fantasy of telling off a co-worker, and he remarked that recently he felt resentful and angry, wondering if his increased scratching was related to this.

At the time of the sixth interview, his skin remained unchanged. He expressed his fear of losing control of his anger and appeared more aware of his current problems. He talked of his helplessness and became angry with the interviewer for not being of more help to him.

With the seventh interview, his skin looked considerably better. He had informed his wife that he was the boss around the house and, following a minor altercation with his son, had told him that he was "not yet dry around the ears." He appeared surprised that his wife was "snapping to," and that his son was spending more time around the house.

In the ninth week, his skin improved remarkably. He related an incident with pride in which, when his wife refused to prepare breakfast for him, he had advised her that she had better behave herself, ordered her to the bedroom, and had intercourse with her. That evening he took her to the movies and noted that she was affectionate.

He remarked that during the previous week he had been able to tell his employer that too much of the work fell on him and that this should be changed.

Treatment was terminated after twelve visits. The patient was seen in dermatology clinic two months later. His skin had cleared completely except for a small area of dermatitis behind the knees. He was feeling well, had no difficulty sleeping, required no medication, and was much satisfied with the changes in his relations with his family and employers.

Genitourinary System

As a consequence of the close anatomical relationship of the sexual and excretory organs and the prolonged exposure of the growing child to the conflicting biological drives and the attitudes of his family and society to excretory patterns and sexual behavior, it is no wonder that in no other system, except perhaps the gastrointestinal, are disturbances of function so common. During development, ideas pertaining to urination, defecation, and sexuality become associated with feelings of shame, disgust, guilt, fear, and hatred. On occasion the anatomical–physiological functions of these organs are not properly discriminated and the result is confusion of function and attitude. Although such attitudes are often caused by faulty and deficient education, in many instances they represent a symptomatic expression of a general personality disorder that requires for their solution skilled psychiatric treatment. Even though urologists and gynecologists have become increasingly aware that the majority of such disorders are the consequence of personality maldevelopment and educational defects, far too many men and women continue to be subjected to unnecessary surgical and physical procedures that usually only serve to fix a conviction of physical illness, thus impairing the effective potentiality of the indicated forms of treatment.

In men, the common psychosomatic symptoms are impotence and premature ejaculation. Frigidity, dysmenorrhea, dyspareunia, premenstrual tension, the drive for abortions, and other castrating operations are the common expressions of psychopathology in women.

Impotence and Premature Ejaculation

Various degrees of impotence may be recognized, extending from complete failure to obtain an erection with no interest in coitus, a partial or inadequate erection with limited interest, periodic failure of erection coupled with limited libido, ability to establish erection but lack of sexual gratification with ejaculation in coitus, and premature ejaculation.

For the successful completion of the sexual act, there is needed a certain sexual drive (libido), an attractive partner, a situation that provides freedom from distraction and anxiety, allowing in turn erection, penile insertion, and the muscular activity that provides penile friction and stimulation to mount to eventual ejaculation accompanied by a distinctive pleasure and climactic orgasm.

Impotence, then, may follow when there is either lack of attraction to the partner or when the coital environment is threatening or distracting. Much more commonly, however, are those often unconscious and conflictful loves, due either to persisting infantile attachments to the mother, sister, or some other important succoring woman in early life, or to instances of latent homosexual attachments. Again, anxiety may prevent potency due to underlying hostilities toward women stemming from childhood experiences in which the opposite sex is perceived as critical, punitive, and capable of damaging the male genitals. Guilt, anxiety, or shame may lead to impotency in which the sufferer fears disapproval by parents or society, has unconscious wishes to damage the partner, or considers exposure of his body or his sexual performance as subject to ridicule. Also, fears of contacting venereal disease or of dying sometimes inhibit potent behavior. Impotency is a common accompaniment of the depressive reactions in which it often is obscured by the symptoms of backache, which serves to prevent efforts at coitus.

To establish the diagnosis of psychogenic impotency, a careful history must be taken that will determine the situations in which failure at intercourse has occurred. Particular attention should be paid to the attitude toward the partner, the environment of the coital acts, the frequency of sexual relations, attitudes toward and desires for various forms of precoital stimulation, and a study of the attitude of the partner. Note should be made of any fantasies that take place during intercourse. Some men undertake relations while thinking of another partner or are dissatisfied in the belief that their partner will disallow precoital stimulation of various kinds when they desire it; others find themselves impotent only with certain women. As an example, a man may be unable to have satisfying successful relations with his wife, yet may be potent with prostitutes or in extramarital affairs. Those who use intercourse as a means of defense against unconscious homosexual fears are likely to fail. The attitude of the partner is most significant. If the woman is domineering or competitive with men, her persistent derogation of her husband or lover may not only induce but also perpetuate the impotence.

Impotency due to such illnesses as multiple sclerosis, syphilis, diabetes, or other disorders involving the sacral segments of the spinal cord, the lumbar parasympathetic outflow, or the lumbar sympathetic chain should be excluded by general medical and neurological examination. In psychiatric patients treated with phenothiazines, impotency may be a toxic effect of drug administration.

Aside from those occasional instances in which the symptoms may be rectified by simple advice relative to disturbing situational conditions, such as attempting intercourse in the parental home or bedroom or avoidance of an unwanted partner, the indicated treatment is psychotherapeutic and preferably with psychoanalytic orientation. In most cases of failure of erection, the patient should be advised initially to avoid intercourse and failure as a means of preventing further lowering of self-esteem. Such advice is probably unnecessary and unwise in the instances of premature ejaculation, in which more frequent attempts may reduce the anticipatory tension. When impotency is a symptom of depression, the patient may be advised that the symptoms will disappear with subordinance of the affective disorder, which should, of course, be treated appropriately in its own right. Relief of the symptom is less likely in the elderly or in those cases in which the sexual partner is consistently intimidating or threatening.

Non-Specific Urethritis

This condition, frequent in young men, in some instances probably represents a psychosomatic response to continuing sexual fantasies, perhaps associated with excessive secretion from the urethral glands. It may be complicated by a secondary non-gonococcal infectious process.

Menstrual Disorders

With the regular fluctuation in hormonal control that maintains the menstrual cycle throughout the child-bearing period, there occurs parallel shifting in emotional state. At the onset of the cycle and coincident with the gradually rising production of estrogen, there occurs an active drive to heterosexual contact with the biological aims of copulation. This phase is commonly one of emotional well-being and may be recognized in the behavior, conscious activities, and desires of healthy women. If the drives of the phase remain ungratified, tension with irritability and restlessness betray the frustration. On the other hand, in the inhibited or immature woman the activated heterosexual drive of this period may be defended against by hostility toward men. With ovulation, there occurs readiness for conception, and the behavioral tendencies just commented upon reach their height.

Relief of tension takes place after ovulation, when both estrogen and progesterone are secreted take place simultaneously. At this time according to Benedek's description, there occurs a shift from the heterosexual to a receptive-retentive phase, which, in neurotic young women, may bring out infantile wishes to be cared for as a child. This may be expressed through increasing need for attention or dissatisfactions due to lack of care.

Coincident with the fall in horomonal production in the premenstrual period, there generally follows a depressive mood, with inclination to bodily complaints, preoccupations, and emotional regression with less control. At the onset of menstruation, and associated with the sudden decrease in hormonal production, tension and excitability again decrease. Overdetermined responses to this recurring cycle of psychophysiologic preparation for sexuality and conception constitute the basis for many of the menstrual disorders.

PREMENSTRUAL TENSION. This seems to occur in several forms. In one it is first noticed with menarche and persists throughout the menstrual period; in the second, it commences initially several years after the menarche. In the former, sexuality and menstruation have been presented to the developing girl in a derogatory way by her mother. The feminine role is derogated by her, sexual activity is presented as immoral or disgust-ing, and the menses are spoken of as illness. The menarche is experienced by girls identifying with these mothers as a messy, unwanted event that they complain about as sickness and for which they often demand excessive care. Such young women live in a hostile, dependent relationship with their mother, who herself is living in marital discord. With the delayed form of premenstrual tension, there is more likely to be found guilt over sexual temptations or transgressions in recent life experiences. However, there is a greater initial acceptance and pride in the female experience of menarche.

DYSMENORRHEA. Severe dysmenorrhea and the less well-recognized condition of *pelvic pain*, which may be related to vascular congestion, seem to occur also in women ambivalent to their sexual and feminine role in life due to early anxieties, doubts, or lack of healthy identification and training for feminine sexual, maternal, and home-making roles.

AMENORRHEA. Although amenorrhea may be the consequence of delayed sexual maturation due to hypogonadism, it may also occur as a defense against sexuality. It is seen as well in depressions in women and, similar to the impotence of depressed men, disappears when recovery takes place. Menses cease also with *pseudocyesis* when, influenced by the wish for and fear of pregnancy, certain immature women present themselves for examination with many of the signs of the condition, including distended abdomen, changes in the breast, and increase in weight. The majority of women with pseudocyesis have dependent hysterical personalities who seek to preserve a marriage in which they perceive themselves as unwanted unless they bear children. On some occasions, sexual relations have not occurred.

MENOPAUSE. Menopausal symptoms again represent a complex of physiological and psychological responses to which the mature woman usually adapts more effectively than those who have neurotic or psychotic personalities or in those whose sexual and maternal functions have been frustrated. With the diminution of hormonal secretions, neurovascular control becomes labile, and there result episodic periods of perspiration, flushings, tension, or moodiness. Associated may be increasing anxiety and agitation, with exaggerations of all personality defenses. The prescription of synthetic hormones will alleviate the physiologically determined symptoms but not those aroused as the consequence of growing awareness of fading opportunities to fulfill the primary biological functions of womanhood or those secondary to loss of parental responsibility, where grown children are separated from the home and deprive the mother of satisfaction in their immediate care.

Frigidity, Dyspareunia, and Infertility

In considering the response to sexual intercourse, it must be kept in mind that the climax of coitus in women is not analogous to orgasm in the male. Even the anatomical structure of the feminine genital tract differs from that of the male. Sensory cells similar to those found in the glans penis are confined largely to the clitoris, with some located in the labia minora and lower vaginal muscles. The vagina is homologous with the penile shaft and therefore cannot respond to sexual stimulation in the same way as the phallus. This widely-held notion and the expectation of many women of rapid and climactic orgasm similar to that of men is probably incorrect. For satisfactory sexual relations, women must find themselves with a desirable partner, devoid of anxiety and guilt, and must then be provided with appropriate stimulation in order to achieve a slower but more enduring gratification. Many women believe they are frigid due to misconceptions about feminine arousal.

Frigidity is related to fear of injury in intercourse or of pregnancy and may spring from envy and hostility to men. Unfulfilled expectations of their sexual response arouse in some women feelings of shameful inadequacy or rage at their partner. Less anxious women and those who accept a more giving and passive role are often gratified even without full clitoral stimulation and orgasm. Dyspareunia and vaginismus are the consequence of the same anxieties and fears that impair sexual satisfaction in women. It appears likely that infertility also has its origins in suppression by central mechanisms of ovulation through persisting anxieties and doubts of pregnancy and child-bearing.

In these conditions, analytic psychotherapy is the indicated treatment. It is more likely to prove beneficial in those whose inhibitions are due to unconscious feelings of guilt, disgust, or repressed hostility than in women with a strong maternal fixation and infantile personality make-up.

Reactions to Abortion, Sterilization, and Contraception

Those medical and surgical procedures that prevent or deprive women and men of their reproductive function are bound to produce psychological conflict and emotional disturbance. Since the ideal concept of healthy human growth carries within the attainment of adult status that of sexual maturity, including both the capacity to conceive and bear children, measures that prevent the realization of these aspirations are likely to arouse feelings of sadness, shame, inadequacy, envy, and hostility toward the more fortunate, including those who are seen as responsible for the frustration. Furthermore, anxiety and depression are mobilized, with their attendant defenses. Such emotional responses may be expected and do occur more frequently in those who have not attained the satisfaction of marriage and the bearing and rearing of children. It is not surprising that women are more frequently disturbed than men following surgical operations on the genitalia, since marriage and the maternal function play a significantly greater role in the realization of a satisfying self-concept than the attainment of fatherhood.

The physician and psychiatrist today are even more frequently called upon to make judgments pertaining to therapeutic abortions, sterilization, hysterectomies, and the use of contraceptives. Medical and surgical skills have decreased the frequency of indication for therapeutic abortion for such illnesses as heart disease, tuberculosis, and diabetes. At the same time, the number of abortions performed on the recommendation of psychiatrists has increased rapidly in the past two decades, both abroad and in the United States. Although there is little difference in the recognized indications for therapeutic abortion on the grounds of physical disease, the range of indications on social–psychological grounds varies tremendously from country to country throughout the world. In some states and countries, therapeutic abortion may only be recommended legally when the life of the mother is threatened by the pregnancy coming to term. In other countries, notably the Scandinavian, therapeutic abortion may be recommended for economic, social, and psychological reasons. In these countries, there has been brought to light much information from the careful studies of the emotional responses of women who have been recommended for and denied abortions that they requested. The insistent biological urge to conception shines through clearly. In Ekblad's series, over a third of the women who were not sterilized at the time of abortion became pregnant again. A number do so consciously, and in short periods after the abortion. As high as a fifth of the women allowed therapeutic abortions later expressed regret for accepting the procedure, although in a tenth these personal reproaches were of short duration. Although it seems that these unfavorable psychological sequelae are seldom severe, when one considers the advisability of allowing therapeutic abortions liberally to all women, there remains a substantial group of women who react with severe and continuing psychopathology. Undoubtedly in this group are those with persisting personality disorders that have not been leavened by the satisfactions of conception and motherhood.

Solution of the clinical problem confronting the psychiatrist called upon to determine whether abortion or any sterilizing procedure should be performed demands not only a full knowledge of the life experiences, expectancies, and personality weaknesses of his patient, but also awareness of the legal status of therapeutic abortion and sterilization in his community. From the study of many psychiatrically ill patients, the conclusion is inescapable that those women who do not wish to bring a particular conception to birth seldom make a satisfactory mother for that child. The experienced clinician, however, will not easily accept the initial verbal declaration of patients that they do not want to bear; in some instances these declarations are made to gain or regain love and attention or may be compliant demands made at the request or insistence of a consort who does not wish to bear his responsibility for the child.

Experience does not show that pregnancy and birth of the child influence adversely the course of the schizophrenias, manic–depressive illnesses, or the majority of the psychoneurosis but they may be the precipitating factor for a period of serious ego decompensation. Even women who have a postpartum psychotic reaction often go through later pregnancies without ego disorganization. Suicidal threats are used frequently to force recommendation for abortions. Here again, experience has shown that its execution is uncommon when the mother is allowed to go to term. If suicidal attempts have been made previously when a psychotic disorder is known to exist or when previous postpartum personality disorders have occurred, there exist grounds for psychiatric considerations for therapeutic abortion. The eventual psychiatric recommendation must rest not only upon the personality of the patient and the past sexual and maternal satisfactions, but on her needs for future stability. Allowing the birth of a child, even in the face of a physical illness, is indicated for the future preservation of mental health for certain women. In such instances, however, all arrangements must be made to assume the needed medical and psychiatric care both through term and beyond parturition.

Although the use of contraceptive devices is increasingly accepted, for many, sexual conflicts are complicated by this very fact. In assessing the sexual complaints of individual patients, both the wishes and attitudes of each partner should be explored toward the use of contraceptives. In some instances, the type of contraceptive device may impair sexual gratification, as, for example, in the limitation of frictional stimulation experienced by some men with the use of condoms or in the feeling of disgust or lack of spontaneity induced by the use of a diaphragm in certain women. Again, family or religious training may contradict the use of such devices, and yet fear of pregnancy may induce their trial and so lead to guilty anxiety. No less difficult are those interpersonal conflicts in which the responsibility for the use of the contraceptive is foisted upon an unwilling partner as a means of expressing hostility or neurotic dependent demands and intimidating the partner by denying sexual relations when he or she complains or fails to accept this responsibility.

Both physician and psychiatrist should be fully acquainted with the various types of contraceptive measures that may be prescribed as well as the commonly-accepted views of various religious groups toward their application. With the recent introduction of an effective oral contraceptive (ethynylestradiol 3-methyl ether, and norethynodrel) in tablet form, it is possible to offer a widely acceptable and safe method of preventing conception that should prove highly useful in preventing untimely pregnancy in those with disorders of personality. This preparation (Enovid) is given as a single 5 mg. tablet daily for 20 days, commencing on the fifth day after the beginning of the menstrual period. The tablets are then stopped and menses occur in three or four days. Then the cycle of administration is started again. The less intelligent and those unconsciously desiring pregnancy are less likely to follow the above

instructions. To date, no psychological complications have been reported from the taking of this estrogen preparation.

Nervous System

Disturbances of the Image of the Body

Although our modern conceptions of the body-image derive from the studies of Schilder, the knowledge of phantom phenomena, which demonstrate so strikingly the validity of this concept, extend well back into medical antiquity. They were known to Ambroise Paré and surgeons before his time. They were the subject of study by Weir Mitchell over a century ago. It is now recognized that, with growth, the individual develops a total perception of his own body as well as certain attitudes toward his physical self that many consider the core structure in the development of the ego. The body percept slowly evolves through the multiple sensory experiences of the infant in the discovery of his body parts. The various sensory impressions conveyed by means of kinesthetic, visual, and tactile apparatus to the cortex lead to an expanding and growing perception of body awareness, presumably organized and integrated in the parieto-temporal cortex of the brain.

In addition to this physiological substratum acquired over the years by postural, tactile, and visual percepts, each individual attaches to this appreciation of body surface and its various parts attitudes with emotional overtones that derive from his early experiences in the family and as a result of the parental evaluations of his physique. The attitudes are ingrained through verbal remarks, non-verbal indications, and the expressions of valuation pertaining to desirable physical traits and attainment. The comparison of his own physique with that of his parents and peers and the emphasis on the differences play a large role in the body-image of the growing child. The parents imply that the child's body and its parts are good or bad, pleasing or repulsive, clean or dirty, loved or disliked.

Thus, in some families in which physical strength and physical accomplishment are emphasized, a boy's attitude toward his body is determined to a large extent by the parents' feelings and attitudes toward development of his limbs and muscles. In a similar manner, the parents or the culture may over-emphasize physical beauty or particular physical attributes in girls. The American cultural over-emphases are evident in our advertising and writing.

It may be mentioned that certain families and ethical groups tend to derogate various body parts that have sexual significance. This, in turn, reflects in part on both conscious and unconscious conceptions of body parts in certain individuals. The loss of a hand, for example, may have a very different meaning to a violinist than to a professor of history, and a resulting disturbance or disorganization of the personality be therefore much more apt to result in the former. Lesions in parts of the body that psychologically represent organs of marked value for the personality—such as eyes, breasts, sexual organs—may be highly disturbing, even though the disease, objectively considered, is not serious. Disturbances of the personality rarely follow operations upon the appendix or other organs not invested with deep emotional value. On the contrary, psychiatric complications following operations upon highly valued ones, such as the reproductive organs, are not uncommon.

Disabling physical handicaps, such as crippling, blindness, and deafness, which put the patient at a disadvantage with his fellows, may have profound effect upon emotional health. The sensitive, even paranoid, reactions of the deaf, at times more disturbing to the individual's social adjustment than the deafness itself, are familiar observations. In girls, particularly, a serious physical handicap may produce mental problems that completely overshadow the defect.

Because of the high evaluations placed upon their biological functions and because any conditions that adversely affect these functions may seriously jeopardize their personal, economic, and social security and happiness, women are particularly subject to fears and emotional conflicts when such functions are disturbed. Lack of attractiveness, or physical defects that preclude offers of marriage, an inability to bear children, the loss of physical charm through age or disease, the presence of conditions that make discontinuance of marital relations necessary, or the approach of the involutional period may constitute problems to which emotional adjustment is difficult or impossible within the limits of mental health.

For the clinical psychiatrist, disturbances of the body-image will be observed in association with many of the major psychoneurotic and psychotic disorders. However, there are certain expressions of primary body-image disturbance of particular interest that may be recognized as separate entities. Among these are the various phantom phenomena and the efforts on the part of the individual to adapt to these phenomena, as well as such conditions as neurasthenia and hypochondriasis.

Phantom Phenomena

Phantom phenomena are considered the expression of the enduring concept of the individual's body-image persisting after loss of a body part. It is significant that phantoms have not been noted in those with absence of a limb resulting from a congenital defect or from infantile amputations. The phantom is not explainable, then, on the basis of wish fulfillment or "gestalt" psychology. The observation of a phantom limb after amputation occurs in some 98 per cent of amputees. Such phantoms are initially perceived as consisting of the whole extremity. Usually the distal portion of the phantom, such as the hand or foot, is most conspicuous. As time passes, the phantom appendage tends to shrink and may eventually disappear into the stump. Movements of the amputation stump may induce the impression of movement of the phantom extremity provided kinesthetic sensation remains in the stump.

Three kinds of sensory phenomena may

be noted in the phantom limb. In all patients with a phantom, there occurs a mild tingling, the basic phantom phenomenon, which may be regarded as dependent upon the function of the sensory–motor cerebral cortex. A stronger momentary pins-and-needles sensation may occur in the phantom by touching neuromas in the stump; this sensation is dependent upon functional activity of lower spinal centers. Also included under the second type of sensory phenomena are sensations referred into the phantom in the presence of disease of other organs, such as referred pain of cardiac origin. Referred sensations into the phantom may be elicited by deep pressure on the amputation stump, less often with algesic skin stimulation, and least by tactile stimulation.

The third type of painful sensory disturbance in the phantom is the common cause of the amputee's referral for psychiatric or neurologic consultation. Questioning usually reveals that the patient is concerned about sensations that he describes variously as "twisting," "burning," "pulling," or "itching." In most instances, the symptom is intermittent. It is more often annoying than agonizing. The introspective, observant amputee notes its aggravation by stimulation of the stump, sometimes by micturition in those who have lost a leg, by changes in weather, and in many instances by emotionally disturbing incidents.

Although limb phantoms are common, mammary, penile, rectal, and nasal phantoms are rare. Phantoms of the bladder and rectum have rarely been observed in paraplegic patients, while those of the flaccid penis and erect penis are more frequent. The existence of phantom images of other internal organs is not generally accepted as occurring, although it has been suggested that the occurrence of phantom pain in the abdomen may explain the recurrence of peptic ulcer pain in the patients who initially report the disappearance of such pain after vagotomy.

The admission by an amputee of a limb phantom should be regarded as a healthy psychological response. Subsequent to an amputation, the healthy individual slowly reorganizes his body image by means of the new sensory experiences related to the changed body form. The persistence of a physical defect irritating the afferent nerves from the amputated part will delay this reorganization and may cause pain.

The healthy amputee accepts his defect, resumes his family position, returns to his occupation, and, with an adequate stump, makes use of an appropriate prosthesis. On the other hand, those who complain of persistent or intermittent pain in a phantom incapacitating them for a return to life in society, in whom the painful symptom does not conform to the recognized descriptions of the sensations resulting from irritation of known structures, with referral into recognized areas of nervous distribution, and in whom there is resistance to the acceptance of a prosthesis or poor family, marital, or occupational adaptation, are usually suffering a serious personality disturbance. Such disturbances, though rare, occur as amputation leads to an upsurge of anxiety owing to the distortion of the patient's concept of his body and therefore of himself and his relations with others. This distortion requires readaptation in relation to others and to society. Also, hostile feelings may emerge in the amputee toward those people with whom he identifies, on whom he is dependent, and whose rejection he now apprehends. The painful symptom thus may symbolize the need for, and apprehension relative to, a possible loss of dependency.

Kolb found that in many instances the amputee with the painful phantom has identified in a hostile way with another amputee significantly related to him in his early life. In those amputees with a hysterical personality make-up and identification with another amputee, the fantasy life often discloses superstitious rationalization to explain the existence of the phantom phenomenon. The rationalizations are concerned with the loss and the fantasied disposal of the amputated part. In association with these fantasies, the amputee attempts to master his grief and mourning over the loss of the amputated part. He desires to have the part disposed of tenderly and respectfully as if the whole body were to be buried.

The neurotically over-determined painful symptom has been relieved by a variety of psychiatric therapies, including suggestion, hypnosis, narcotherapy, electroshock, lobotomy, and more recently by the tranquilizing drugs. The therapeutic procedure of choice must be determined on the basis of the over-all personality disturbance observed in the individual patient. The following report illustrates an acute emotional disturbance associated with the phantom phenomenon.

A 14-year-old boy came to clinic complaining of a "knot in his leg." He said he had bumped the lower part of his right leg against a step one month previously.

On examination a hard, fixed, tender mass was noted in the middle third of the injured part of the leg. Roentgenograms showed a primary malignant tumor involving the anterolateral cortex of the right tibia. Three days later, amputation of the right leg was performed through the lower third of the femur. The pathologist reported an osteogenic sarcoma of the tibia. The patient complained of pain in the phantom right leg shortly after recovery from the anesthesia. Within two days after operation, large doses of narcotic agents were being employed in an attempt to relieve him of pain. By the ninth postoperative day, the patient was complaining bitterly of a burning pain, was over-active, thrashed about in bed, and spoke of jumping out of a window. Special nurses were required at this time, and psychiatric consultation was requested. The patient was found to be fearful, disoriented, and confused. Administration of all drugs except morphine was discontinued in order to alleviate the mild toxic delirious state.

The next day the patient was rolling about in his bed, with his eyes closed, apparently oblivious to those about him. He cried out repetitiously, "Help me, help me. Do something for the pain." It was believed that frightening rationalizations as to the origin of the phantom contributed in part to the state of painful panic. The boy was therefore asked if he were aware of the feeling of a phantom limb after operation. Surprisingly, the boy immediately became silent, opened his eyes, and responded affirmatively. Under questioning he stated that a year previously one of his school teachers had casually discussed amputations with his class. The teacher told the class a story of a man who had undergone an amputation, after

which a severe stinging pain developed in his phantom limb. The story went that the limb was disinterred and that ants were discovered burrowing into and stinging the amputated part.

When inquiry was made as to what disposition the boy believed had been made of his own amputated extremity, he stated that he thought it was being burned. He was reassured and informed otherwise. The complaint of pain and his wild overactivity subsided to a large extent immediately after this interview. It was possible to discontinue the use of all morphine within 24 hours and to discharge the patient's special nurse shortly thereafter.

Complete relief of his pain, however, required four additional hours of psychotherapy. It was learned that the boy had been severely upset by his mother's death from cancer of the breast five years previously. The boy never spoke of his mother after her death but was morbidly inquisitive whenever anyone became ill and would inquire of his father if the person were about to die. The mother had undergone amputation of the breast. The latter hours of treatment brought to awareness the boy's repressed hostility toward his mother, with whom he identified as an amputee and his ambivalent feelings toward his father.

When he was dismissed from the clinic 25 days after operation, the boy had no pain, did not require medication, was active on crutches, and was eager to have a prosthesis fitted. A year later his stepmother wrote that he was without pain and was wearing a prosthesis. He had returned to school, was doing well in his studies, and had been elected to a class office.

Neurasthenia

The concept of neurasthenia has undergone many manifestations, and one might say abuses, since the term was first introduced by Beard in 1867 to describe a condition caused, he believed, by an exhaustion of the nerve cells through depletion of their stored nutriment. Probably the term should be dropped altogether and some of the clinical syndromes formerly included under it should be assigned to the anxiety reactions, some to conversion hysteria, and some included under the category of psychophysiological asthenic reactions. The present tendency is to assign to the last group most of the symptom complexes formerly classified as neurasthenia.

General fatigue, with its feeling of overwhelming exhaustion and of diffuse "nervousness," is the predominating complaint in the reaction that should be regarded as a response to emotional conflicts and their attendant anxiety. The causes therefore are psychological. It is no longer believed that "neurasthenia" is caused by a generally impaired or exhausted physical state, as a result of which the nervous system is drained of its energy in the manner of a partially discharged battery of low voltage. Some complaints seem to be disappointment reactions, while others appear to be the expression of sexual dissatisfaction or conflicts. Sometimes repressed hostility or other anxiety-exciting factors produce the reaction. In other instances, the asthenic reaction seems to arise from constant failure, frustration, and disappointment. Boredom, monotony, and absence of goals may serve as contributory causes. It will be found that many patients have had a difficult childhood, with little interest or affection from their parents. The existence of family or social problems should always be considered.

SYMPTOMS. The premorbid personality of the patient with psychophysiological asthenic reaction has usually been characterized by dissatisfaction and by a sense of being thwarted and rejected. The premorbid characteristics often merge so insidiously into the symptoms of the reaction that no definite time of its onset can be stated. As already indicated, the asthenic reaction patient has a long-continued subjective sensation of overwhelming exhaustion. Any exertion, either mental or physical, seems too great. An exaggerated degree of attention is paid to the bodily organs and their functions. The patient may complain of dizziness, of a feeling of pressure on the head, and perhaps of pain at the nape of the neck. There is an intolerance of noise, bright lights, and cold, and complaints about muscae volitantes are common. Associated gastrointestinal discomfort is frequent. Indigestion, constipation, and diarrhea may occur.

Palpitation, extrasystoles, and tachycardia, symptoms of an associated anxiety state, increase the alarm of the patient. Vasomotor instability is frequent so that the skin is at times flushed and again sweating or cold. Patients with this vasomotor instability wrap themselves in mufflers and are in constant fear of catching cold. Complaints of "fallen stomach" or "loose kidney" are common. The sexual functions of the male are disturbed; impaired potency, nocturnal emissions, and failures at intercourse are common. The significance of these symptoms is magnified, and the patient greatly distressed. Women with asthenic reaction often suffer from dysmenorrhea. Paresthesias and hypesthesias are common.

The patient may suffer from broken sleep and disturbing dreams. In the morning he awakes with a feeling of exhaustion. As the day progresses, the patient feels better, and in the evening he may be comparatively free from his sense of exhaustion. He complains of poor memory, but this defect is a result only of preoccupation and lack of concentration. Many patients are shy, awkward, and irritable, lack confidence, and exhibit irresolution, indecision, and irascibility. They are pessimistic and lack initiative and ambition. Asthenic patients are often critical, whining, dissatisfied, envious, and resentful. A tendency to projection is not uncommon. Some patients develop a complaining attitude and may appear to take pleasure in finding fault with and annoying others. Moderate depression is the rule. Varying degrees of anxiety are present.

The neurasthenic is characterically preoccupied with his bodily weakness and a multitude of minor subjective physical perceptions that are overlooked or disregarded by the active and healthy person. He comes to rationalize his failures and dissatisfactions, which are accompanied by underlying emotions of rage, guilt, and anxiety as to these subjective perceptions, and, in turn, they allow much in terms of secondary gain through attention and consideration by others not available through socially-constructive adaptations. The persisting underlying anxieties feed back into the various systems mediating psychophysiologic responses and continually maintain the opportunity for bodily preoccupation, with the psychological defenses of weakness, lack of strength and persistence, and help-lessness. Many patients with predominant neurasthenic defenses have been reared in families in which somatic symptoms or illness were used in a similar manner by parents or siblings. Thus the symptom choice rests often on the process of iden-tification.

DIAGNOSIS. One of the most impor-tant differentiations to be made is to dis-tinguish the asthenic reaction from the depressive form of manic–depressive psy-chosis. Many mild cases of this psychosis do not come to the attention of the psy-chiatrist, and the patients are considered by the general practitioner to be suffering from neurasthenia. Manic–depressive psy-chosis occurs in more definite episodes, with intervals free from symptoms of mental disorder, while the asthenic reac-tion is a more continuous, or at least prolonged, process, and the patient, even when comparatively well, is solicitous as to his health. The chief complaint of the neurasthenic is of weakness and shifting physical ailments, which he is eager to discuss on every occasion, whereas that of the manic–depressive is depression. Al-though the neurasthenic is apparently de-pressed, his emotional manifestations and responses are well marked and even ex-cessive, whereas the depression of the affective psychosis remains unchanged by experience or environment. Sometimes it is difficult to distinguish early schizo-phrenia from the asthenic reaction. The schizophrenic does not usually have so great a variety of physical complaints, which sooner or later become obviously delusional. The neurasthenic lacks the listless apathy and the indifference to external circumstances usually manifested by the schizophrenic. The neurasthenic, unlike the schizophrenic, is not given to day-dreaming.

Neurasthenic-like symptoms first mani-fested at middle age should arouse the suspicion of neurosyphilis. Experience suggests that some cases of chronic bru-cellosis have been diagnosed as neuras-thenia. Thiamine deficiency may produce an asthenic reaction syndrome character-ized by generalized feelings of weakness,

fatigability, poor appetite, poor sleep, various somatic complaints, and subjec-tive difficulties in concentration and memory.

TREATMENT. The treatment of the asthenic reaction is psychotherapeutic. Usually encouraging results are limited to relatively early cases.

Psychophysiological Symptom versus Conversion Hysteria

Since both conversion hysteria and psychophysiological symptoms arise from emotional factors and both produce "functional" physical symptoms, it might be suggested that they are essentially the same psychodynamically and physiologi-cally. This, however, is not at all the case. The psychophysiological symptom is pro-duced by the fact that emotions may in-fluence the autonomic nervous system, with resulting stimulation or inhibition of the function of a visceral organ. It represents the disturbed physiological re-sponse of a vegetative organ to psycho-logical stress and tension acting through the vegetative nervous system. Physio-logical changes are set up in an organ by autonomic nerve impulses generated as a result of emotional conflict or ten-sion. The effects of the emotions are seen especially in secretion, vascularity, and motility of viscera. In some cases, the prolonged disturbance in the function of an organ may lead to structural changes that may threaten life. In con-version *hysteria*, the symptom is not pro-duced through the vegetative nervous system but is the symbolic expression, either through the voluntary neuromus-cular or through the sensory-perceptive systems, of emotionally charged psycho-logical content. The reaction of these last two is not consciously voluntary and does not follow the traditional pattern of physiological responses in the body. Conversion hysteria is quite effective in alleviating anxiety, hence *la belle indif-férence* is often associated with it. The secondary gain obtained by the psycho-somatic patient from his symptom is ei-ther absent or less conspicuous than in the hysteric patient. Hysteria does not produce visceral changes. Basically the only similarity between hysterical symptoms and psychophysiologic symptoms lies in the fact that both are responses to psychological stimuli. Yet both hysteric symptomatology and psychophysiological disturbance may be observed in the same individual, particularly when the conversion response is removed through treatment or is only partially effective in allaying the anxiety consequent on conflict.

Diagnostic Errors

The patient who is reacting with psychophysiologic symptoms thinks that these constitute his illness and does not understand that the essential difficulties are his conflicts and anxieties and his inability to establish order, peace, and security in his personal life. Although the patient can scarcely be expected to recognize that mental or personality disorders may manifest themselves in terms of the soma, yet the physician must not forget that organs may react to anxiety in many ways. Unless he remembers that psychogenic illness may masquerade under the guise of physical symptoms, also that mental illnesses are not ordinarily secondary to physical disease, he will inevitably make many errors in diagnosis and treatment. As Bennett points out: "The sick man's personality must be judged along with the physical and laboratory data." Because much mental illness is either not recognized or is not treated properly, many maladjusted persons go from doctor to doctor and receive treatment that only aggravates their personality problems. If emotional disorders are misidentified or mistreated as organic diseases, the tendency of such disorders will be not toward recovery but toward chronicity. If, too, some incidental organic pathologic condition is found, the patient's anxiety is very apt to become fixed on the system involved. It should be remembered, also, that repeated tests and examinations tend to fix the idea in the patient's mind that he must certainly have a "physical" illness, probably a mysterious one. He will then even more resist the idea that emo-

tions may have had any part in the production or perpetuation of his illness. Bennett found that 150 patients who finally came for psychiatric treatment had been diagnosed and treated for a deplorably large number and variety of organic diseases, most of which did not exist. The histories of these patients as a group revealed 496 medical treatments, 244 surgical procedures, and 71 miscellaneous therapeutic attempts. Most of these patients were suffering from involutional melancholia or psychophysiological ailments. "After proper psychiatric therapy was instituted the percentage of complete and social recoveries was excellent." Except when symptoms are acute, surgery should be avoided in the neurotic person until emotional factors have been investigated.

EMOTIONAL COMPONENTS OF PHYSICAL ILLNESS

The preceding part of this chapter has been devoted to a discussion of psychophysiological illnesses. Such illnesses may present a great variety of physical symptoms and complaints referable to the viscera through the action of emotional tension upon the vegetative nervous system. Broadly speaking, emotions may, in such disorders, be regarded as the cause of physical disturbance or distress. Conversely, in a general way, organic physical illness may be provocative of emotions that may greatly complicate the somatic disability. Mental and emotional factors may pathologically influence component organs of the body; disordered organs may induce mental and emotional factors that disturb the function or adjustment of the organism as a whole. Although not strictly relevant to psychophysiological disorders, the remainder of the chapter will deal with emotional factors and problems incident to physical illness. Their importance in medical practice is so great that an awareness of personality–illness relationship should be constantly in the physician's mind.

A knowledge of the personality and its

development and structure affords a greater awareness of its role in illness. The manifestations of a physical illness are frequently much colored by the patient's personality. Many persons who already have a well-defined disease of chronic nature experience exacerbations or complications of it in relation to severe life stress. The course and outcome of the organic process may be greatly influenced by the mental attitude of the patient. Illness, therefore, of a clearly-established physical nature is often attended by important psychological concomitants that, because of their importance both in prognosis and treatment, should be recognized by the physician. A patient suffering from serious and progressive physical disorder is very prone to develop some psychological response to it. Among such psychological responses may be repression, denial, or perhaps exaggeration of symptoms through a desire for pity and attention. At times the damage suffered by the emotional life and mental health of the patient through somatic illness or disability may be more serious and permanent than are the physical results of the organic lesion. It is therefore not only illness or disability in itself that is of psychiatric importance, but also what a particular ailment means to a particular individual. This matter has been discussed earlier under the body-image.

Many fears and exaggerations of the importance of disease arise from feelings of guilt, particularly from a sense of guilt concerning early sex activities or indiscretions. A slight indisposition may be attributed to a regretted lapse and may be magnified into disabling or fatal illness and regarded as a just desert.

ATTITUDE TOWARD ILLNESS. The attitude that the patient manifests toward his disability should be taken into consideration. The patient must adapt himself not only to his disability, but also to the idea of his disability. Faced with physical disease, the patient may readily accept or even suggest that his disability is of mental origin. He may neglect his symptoms or deceive himself as to their seriousness. On the other hand, the patient whose disability is of psychic origin seeks for a physical basis. Instances in which the patient consciously desires cure from a physical disability but unconsciously wishes that the symptom may continue are not uncommon. The patient sincerely believes that he desires to be cured but unconsciously clings to his disability with a tenacity that may defeat the physician's therapeutic efforts. The motives that delay the recovery may be various—self-punishment, self-importance, revenge, or protest. For various psychological motives, too, certain patients may welcome or request surgical operations. With some patients, surgery may be an attention-gaining device, with others a means of punishing themselves for feelings of guilt or of escaping responsibility or irksome drudgery. If psychic or emotional components accompany definite physical disease, a failure to treat them also will often tend to prolong convalescence or encourage a reaction of chronic invalidism. If the physician concentrates his attention on symptoms without an adequate attempt to ascertain or remove their causes, he may aggravate or permanently fix them.

SOCIAL ENVIRONMENT. Factors arising from the patient's social environment or from interactions between the patient and his social setting may be important in the causation of illness and require consideration in its diagnosis and treatment. It is not always easy to determine if his symptoms are to be attributed entirely to his disease or in part or even largely to his personality disturbance or to his environment. A study of an unselected series of patients who consulted the out-patient clinic of a large general hospital showed that in 65 per cent of these patients there were adverse social conditions related to their illnesses. In 35 per cent of these cases there were emotional reactions that were largely responsible for their illnesses. The physician should remember that in the general hospital, conditions and situations may constantly arise that tend to produce various stresses and tensions and thereby promote unhealthy mental reactions or physical complaints, perhaps with visceral disturbance. Among them may be protracted convalescence, awareness of incurable or crippling disease, fear of death, conflicting medical statements or advice, the misinformation and misguided advice of other patients, and other factors.

PSYCHOLOGICAL NEEDS. Every specialty is accompanied by procedures or situations heavily weighted with elements potentially disturbing to emotional life or personality. In ophthalmology, for example, the bandaging of both eyes during a prolonged convalescence in a darkened room may precipitate a panic reaction of a delirioid nature. In gynecology, there may be problems connected with contraceptive practices, illegitimate pregnancy, or the occurrence of cystoscopy addiction. In urology, psychiatric problems connected with impotence, frigidity, dyspareunia, or premature ejaculations are common. It would be a happy combination if as much effort were expended in the psychological treatment of preoperative fear and apprehension as there is in the search for a drug to alleviate them. In surgical disorders, a fear of mutilation or disfigurement or of loss of vital structure of capacity may threaten the patient's sense of security. Although frequently this results merely in an apprehensive preoccupation, it may lead to anxiety, depression, mild panic states, or exaggerations of previous personality tendencies. In many other medical situations, too, the associated psychiatric problems may be more disturbing than the physical symptoms. It is essential that positive evidences of emotional difficulty be followed up just as faithfully as indications of physical damage.

Convalescence from a serious physical illness often constitutes a psychiatric problem. The patient may be reluctant to give up the luxuries of the sick room and the unconscious secondary gain of illness. He may be resentful as the warmth of feeling and interest previously manifested by his family seem to lessen. More frequently, the family may insist on continuing to be protective and the patient on being babied, with the result that regressive personality characteristics persist. He may even create new symptoms as they are needed. The longer the patient defers his return to his responsibilities, the harder it is to come back, and the more firmly are fixed any unwholesome personality reactions that have been established. His convalescence and rehabilitation may be largely dependent on his adjustment to an existing emotional problem.

PERSONALITY PATTERNS. Frequently the manifestations of the patient's illness are determined more by his personality characteristics than by the nature of the etiological agent producing the disease; he experiences his illness in accordance with his personality make-up and established types of reaction to stress. These patterns are brought particularly into the foreground in the case of chronic disabling illness. Some patients accept their handicap in a spirit of apathy and refuse to make any active effort to overcome their handicap. They may regress to a dependency pattern. In some instances, the reaction may be one of depression and anxiety; again, there may be a greater feeling of optimism and well-being than may rightly be expected. The patient may attempt to maintain a feeling of health by means of psychological mechanism. If the patient feels that there is an implication of inferiority, abnormality, or incurability associated with his disease, he may, through brooding and resentment, develop various compensatory and defensive reactions, perhaps of an aggressive nature.

Among the psychological concomitants of chronic illness, the physician should remember the unwholesome effects that may result from the continued presence in the family of a member suffering from prolonged disability, particularly if the patient reacts to his disease with irritability, aggressiveness, or in some other unpleasant way, or if the responsibility for for his care means the frustration of deeply cherished desires on the part of some other member. At times, too, chronic invalids suffer more from diseased family relationships that have grown out of the disability than from the disease itself.

Whatever the individual's physical disability may be, a certain amount of anxiety is added to the burden imposed by the disease or injury itself. The clinical picture may therefore be directly influenced by this anxiety and the particular reactions of the patient to it.

It is hoped that the discussion presented in this and previous chapters will lead the student to recognize that psychiatry should be integrated with medicine in all its branches and that artificial distinctions between body and mind should be obliterated. Man is a biological organism but one whose life expressions are determined not merely by physical, chemical, physiological, and neurological factors, but by mental, emotional, and social ones. At times one group of factors, again another group, plays the more important role in the etiology, diagnosis, development, and management of sickness. At no time can one group be disregarded; frequently a reciprocal relationship exists.

BIBLIOGRAPHY

Aldrich, C. K.: Psychiatry for the Family Physician. New York, The Blakiston Division, McGraw Hill Book Co., Inc., 1955.

Alexander, F.: Psychosomatic Medicine. New York, W. W. Norton & Co., Inc., 1950.

Association for Research in Nervous and Mental Disease: Life Stress and Bodily Disease. Vol. 29, 1950.

Bartemeier, L. H.: The attitude of the physician. J.A.M.A., 145:1122–1125, 1951.

Benedek, T. F.: Sexual functions in women and their disturbance. In Arieti, S. (Ed.): American Handbook of Psychiatry. Vol. I:727–748. New York, Basic Books, Inc., 1959.

Bennett, A. E.: Faulty management of psychiatric syndromes simulating organic disease. J.A.M.A., 130:1203–1208, 1946.

Berle, B. B., and Javert, C. T.: Stress and habitual abortion. Obst. & Gynec., 3:298–306, 1954.

Bibring, G.: Psychiatry and medical practice in a general hospital. New England J. Med., 254:366–372, 1956.

Brown, E. B., Jr.: Physiological effects of hyperventilation. Physiol. Rev., 33:445–471, 1953.

Bruch, H.: The Importance of Overweight. New York, W. W. Norton & Co., Inc., 1957.

Idem: Conceptual confusion in eating disorders. J. Nerv. & Ment. Dis., 133:46–54, 1961.

Calderone, M. S. (Ed.): Abortion in the United States. New York, Hoeber-Harper, 1958.

Cannon, W. B.: Bodily Changes in Pain, Hunger, Fear and Rage, 2nd ed. New York, D. Appleton Century Co., 1929.

Carryer, H. M.: The role of hyperventilation in functional disorders. Proc. Staff Meetings Mayo Clinic, 21:267–361, 1946.

Cobb, S.: Emotions and Clinical Medicine. New York, W. W. Norton & Co., Inc., 1950.

Cohen, S. I., Silverman, A. J., and Magnusson, F.: New psychophysiological correlates in women with peptic ulcers. Am. J. Psychiat., 112:1025–1026, 1956.

DaCosta, J. M.: On irritable heart: A clinical study of a form of functional cardiac disorder and its consequences. Am. J. Med., 61:17–52, 1871.

Daniels, G., O'Connor, J. F., Karush, A., Moses, L., Flood, C. A., and Lepore, M.: Three decades in the observation and treatment of ulcerative colitis. Psychosom. Med., 24:85–93, 1962.

Dekker, E., and Groen, J.: Reproducible psychogenic attacks of asthma: A laboratory study. J. Psychosom. Res., 1:58–67, 1956.

Ekblad, M.: Induced abortion on psychiatric grounds. A follow-up study of 479 women. Acta. Psychiat. et Neurol. Scandinav. supp., 99:1–238, 1955.

Fortin, J. N., Wittkover, E. D., and Kalz, F.: A psychosomatic approach to the pre-menstrual tension syndrome. Canad. M.A.J., 79:978–981, 1958.

Frazier, S. H., Jr., Faubian, M. H., Giffin, M. E., and Johnson, A. M.: A specific factor in symptom choice. Proc. Staff Meetings Mayo Clinic, 30:227–244, 1955.

Gidro-Frank, L., Gordon, T., and Taylor, H. C., Jr.: Pelvic pain and female identity. Am. J. Obs. and Gyn., 79:1184–1202, 1960.

Gosling, R. H.: Peptic ulcer and mental disorder. II. J. Psychosom. Res., 2:285–301, 1958.

Grinker, R. R., and Robbins, E. P.: Psychosomatic Case Book. New York, The Blakiston Co., Inc., 1954.

Gull, W. W.: Anorexia nervosa. Lancet, 2:171–176, 1868. (The address in medicine delivered before the annual meeting of the British Med. Assn., at Oxford.)

Gutheil, E.: Sexual dysfunctions in men. In Arieti, S. (Ed.): American Handbook of Psychiatry. Vol. I: 708–726. New York, Basic Books, Inc. 1959.

Halliday, J. L.: Psychosocial Medicine. New York, W. W. Norton & Co., Inc., 1948.

Harvey, W. A., and Sherfey, M. J.: Vomiting in Pregnancy. Psychosom. Med., 16:1–9, 1954.

Hinsie, L. E.: The Person in the Body. New York, W. W. Norton & Co., Inc., 1945.

Hollander, M. H.: The Psychology of Medical Practice. Philadelphia, W. B. Saunders Company, 1958.

Kay, D. W. K., and Leigh, D.: The natural history, treatment and prognosis of anorexia nervosa based on a study of 38 patients. J. Ment. Sc., 100:411–431, 1954.

Kolb, L. C.: Disturbances of the Body-Image. In Arieti, S. (Ed.): American Handbook of Psychiatry. Vol. I:749–769. New York, Basic Books, Inc., 1959.

Kroger, W. S., and Freed, S. C.: Psychosomatic Gynecology. Philadelphia, W. B. Saunders Company, 1951.

Kubie, L. S.: The central representation of the symbolic process in psychosomatic disorders. Psychosom. Med., 15:1–7, 1953.

MacLean, P. D.: Psychosomatic disease and the "visceral brain." Psychosom. Med., 11:338–353, 1949.

Miles, H. H. W., and Cobb, S.: Neurocirculatory asthenia, anxiety and neurosis. New England J. Med., 245:711–719, 1951.

Panel Discussion: Problems of Hypertension. J. Am. Psychoanalytic Assn., 1:562–574, 1953.

Reiser, M. F., and Bakst, H.: Psychology of cardiovascular disorders. In Arieti, S. (Ed.): American Handbook of Psychiatry. Vol. I: 659–677. New York, Basic Books, Inc., 1959.

Rosen, H. (Ed.): Therapeutic Abortion. New York, The Julian Press, Inc., 1954.

Ruesch, J. et al.: Chronic Disease and Psychological Invalidism. Berkeley and Los Angeles, Univ. of California Press, 1951.

Saul, L. J.: Psychosomatic aspects of peptic ulcer. Samiksa, 7:225–235, 1953.

Schonfeld, W. A.: Gynecomastia in adolescence. Personality effects. A.M.A. Arch. Gen. Psychiat., 5:46–54, 1961.

Seitz, P. F.: Dynamically oriented brief psychotherapy: Psychocutaneous excoriation syndrome. Psychosom. Med., 15:200–242, 1953.

Stein, M., and Ottenberg, P.: Role of odors in asthma. Psychosom. Med., 20:60–65, 1958.

Stearns, S.: Some emotional aspects of the treatment of diabetes mellitus and the role of the physician. New England J. Med., 249:471–476, 1953.

Stunkard, A. J., and Wolff, H. G.: Pathogenesis in human obesity. Psychosom. Med., 20:17–29, 1958.

Sullivan, A. J., and McKell, T. E.: Personality in Peptic Ulcer. Springfield, Illinois, Charles C Thomas, 1950.

Tuft, H. S.: The development and management of intractable asthma of childhood. A.M.A. J. Dis. of Children, 93:251–254, 1957.

Wall, J. H.: Anorexia nervosa. Bull. New York Acad. Med., 32:116–126, 1956.

Weiner, H., Thaler, M., Reiser, M. F., and Mirsky, I. A.: Etiology of duodenal ulcer. I. Relation of specific psychological characteristics to rate of gastric secretion (serum pepsinogen). Psychosom. Med., 19:1–10, 1957.

Weiss, E.: Emotional Factors in Cardiovascular Disease. Springfield, Illinois, Charles C Thomas, 1951.

Idem, and English, O. S.: Psychosomatic Medicine, 3rd ed. Philadelphia, W. B. Saunders Company, 1957.

Wheeler, E. O., White, P. D., Reed, E. W., and Cohen, M. E.: Neurocirculatory asthenia. J.A.M.A., 142:878–889, 1950.

Wittkower, E., and Cleghorn, R. A. (eds.): Recent Developments in Psychosomatic Medicine. Philadelphia, J. B. Lippincott Co., 1954.

Ziskind, E.: Psychophysiologic Medicine. Philadelphia, Lea & Febiger, 1954.

Chapter Twenty-eight

PSYCHONEUROTIC DISORDERS

The psychoneuroses comprise a relatively benign group of personality disturbances that are often described as being intermediate, or as forming a connecting link, between the various adaptive devices unconsciously utilized by the average mind on the one hand and the extreme, often disorganizing, methods observed in the psychotic on the other. Hysteria, for example, is often but an exaggeration or caricature of comparable protective mechanisms observed in everyday life.

Psychoneurotic personality disorders arise from an effort to deal with specific, private, internal psychological problems and stressful situations that the patient is unable to master without tension or disturbing psychological devices caused by the anxiety aroused. Many psychiatrists, therefore, regard anxiety as the common dynamic source of the neuroses. The symptoms of these disorders consist either of a manifestation of anxiety as it is directly felt and expressed or of automatic efforts to control it by such defenses as conversion, dissociation, displacement, phobia formation, or repetitive thoughts and acts, Ordinarily repression, frequently aided by socially acceptable and useful reaction formations, enables the individual to deal comfortably with feelings and situations that tend to create anxiety. In the psychoneuroses, however, repression is never complete enough to prevent both the feeling and manifestation of anxiety and the formation of unconscious, repetitive techniques designed to control it. These feelings and manifestations of anxiety or the methods of adaptation (defenses) to it constitute the symptoms of the neurosis. The methods of adaptation utilized by those with a psychoneurosis, in addition to their repetitive and unchanging character, are considered to represent behavioral, affective, or psychological traits that proved satisfying at an earlier stage of development. In short they represent either a regression to an earlier, more gratifying type of behavior, or a failure to develop beyond a fixation at a developmental level that proves inappropriate and inadequate in the face of the responsibilities of later life. Neurotic adaptations are never fully satisfying, since secondarily they lead to feelings of inadequacy, shame, and guilt. In the psychoneuroses, therefore, the symptomatic clinical phenomena are usually not significant in and of themselves but merely indicate that anxiety-producing meaningful situations are perturbing to the individual. Although symptoms observed in the psychoneuroses are described in this chapter, these mental disorders should be studied from a functional rather than from a symptomatic standpoint. Many times, it is true, the symptom may afford a clue to the nature of the underlying problem, but the understanding of a neurosis depends on a recognition of the unconscious, neurotic purpose it serves.

The form of the neurosis is determined largely by the type of the defensive measure the patient employs to control anxiety. Relatively few patients confine themselves to a single type of measure. Many psychoneurotics, therefore, show mixed features. The patient's symptoms represent his defense reaction to an anxiety-producing situation that he finds unmanageable by other means. Regardless of the form that they may assume, it is now realized that the neurotic patient's symptoms are intelligible only in psychological, or rather psychobiological, terms. The relationship between his emotional conflicts and perturbing situations, on the one hand, and his disturbed personality functioning on the other is not recognized by the patient. For example, he may, without any apparent reason and without ideational content, develop an attack of anxiety, or without apparent reason develop a panic-like reaction in a crowd or in an open place. Again, without any recognition of its face-saving function, the patient may develop an invalidism that provides escape from a difficult situation. Another patient may experience the persistent recurrence of an appalling or disgusting thought, or feel an overpowering urge for the repeated, ritualistic-like performance of some act that serves to ward off anxiety. Aggressive, hostile wishes may become so threatening that the patient has to employ some neurotic mechanism for handling them. These defenses are often so ego-hampering that they are quite burdensome to the patient. Many persons presenting a variety of symptoms and known to the laity by such terms as "nervous invalids" are really suffering from psychoneurotic disorders. The term "nervous" is, of

course, a euphemistic and evasive term, since there is in fact no physiological disturbance of the nervous system. Each case is a problem of emotional dynamics.

Psychoneuroses Versus Psychoses

For a long time psychiatrists have placed much emphasis on a supposed distinction between psychoses and psychoneuroses. Countless hours have been spent at clinical conferences in discussions as to whether the diagnosis in a particular case should be psychosis or psychoneurosis. If, for purposes of the present discussion, one disregards those mental disorders caused by or associated with impairment of brain tissue function, then the remaining ones are regarded as disorders of psychogenic origin (or without clearly defined physical cause or structural change in the brain). It is increasingly accepted that not only do such disorders as the psychoneuroses but also schizophrenia, manic–depressive psychosis, involutional psychosis, and the various paranoid states belong among those in which psychodynamic factors are largely or solely operative. To a constantly greater extent it is felt by psychiatrists that there are no such differences in the fundamental nature of psychogenic disorders as to warrant the present rigid and meticulous distinction between psychoses and psychoneuroses. Many agree with Bowman[*] that the distinction is without scientific proof and has been based on rough descriptive differences in symptomatology, also that precise and universally accepted definitions of the two terms have never been established. There is an unbroken line of continuity from the "normal" through the neurosis to the psychosis.

Although it is doubtful if there is any scientific basis for the distinction between "psychoses" and "psychoneuroses," classifications of symptom-complexes that have become so well established must contain some value. The value in this distinction has been largely legal, social,

* Bowman, K. M., and Rose, M.: A criticism of the terms "psychosis," "psychoneurosis," and "neurosis." Am. J. Psychiat., 108:161–166, 1951.

and administrative and is based arbitrarily on symptomatology. Since differences in symptomatology readily conduce to the establishment of diagnostic categories, the distinction has also been of value as a teaching aid. The matter of classification, too, may be of importance in selecting the type of therapy.

Many criteria have been suggested to differentiate between psychoses and psychoneuroses. The great variations in those proposed suggest, as Bowman points out, that the distinction is not basic but superficial. Some psychiatrists have designated the psychoses as "major reactions" and the psychoneuroses as "minor reactions," the distinction being made on the extent of the involvement of the personality. Other psychiatrists look upon psychoneurosis and psychosis as successive stages in the same mental process.

Although it must probably be conceded that there is very little scientific basis for the distinction between the psychoneuroses and other psychogenic mental disorders, there is nevertheless a sufficient difference in their clinical nature to justify the distinction on pragmatic grounds. In general, the diagnosis of psychosis implies a greater severity of personality disturbance than occurs in psychoneurosis. The psychoneurotic's defenses against anxiety are largely substitutive or symbolic; the psychotic's defenses are more extreme, regressive, and disregardful of reality. In many instances, there is a difference in their outcome as regards the integrity of the personality. In the psychoses, the distortion or disorganization of personality is often great, and its social functioning is greatly disturbed, whereas in the psychoneuroses the personality usually remains socially organized. In the psychoneuroses, inner experiences do not upset external behavior to the extent or in the abnormal manner that occurs in the psychoses. In the psychotic individual, the capacity for discriminating between subjective experiences and reality may be greatly impaired. In the psychoneurotic individual, there is no grave interference with reality-testing; that part of the personality that the analysts speak of as the ego remains sound. Any evasion of reality is partial and at comparatively little expense to the personality. "Neurosis does not deny the existence of reality, it merely tries to ignore it; psychosis denies it and tries to substitute something else for it."[†]

The psychotic creates a new environment to which he imputes the forces and properties of reality. He may distort or falsify reality in the form of delusions or hallucinations. The environment of the psychoneurotic remains unchanged, although certain elements may be invested with abnormal affective values. The thinking of the psychotic may be dereistic, a type of thinking not occurring in the psychoneurotic. The content of thought in the psychoneurotic may be temporarily restricted by overvalued ideas, yet true delusional formation does not occur. Associations are frequently disturbed in the psychotic but remain unimpaired in the psychoneurotic. Desires and motives are often projected in the psychotic, but they are never so externalized in the psychoneurotic, at least not to the extent of producing delusions. In the psychotic, repression may be destroyed, the ego being so changed that it will tolerate repressed impulses or fantasies uncritically, or will fail to recognize that they arise from itself. In the psychoneuroses, repression appears to be maintained, but nevertheless the repressed material returns, although in such a distorted form that it is acceptable to the ego. Conation may be profoundly disturbed in the psychotic, but only to a slight degree does it suffer in the psychoneuroses. In the psychotic the changes in affect may be great, and affective lability is often decreased, while the psychoneurotic affective changes are slight and lability is maintained. Any depression in the psychoneuroses is determined more by evident environmental factors than is the case in psychoses and is accompanied by a greater degree of insight and by an absence of retardation. The psychoneu-

[†] Freud, S.: The Loss of Reality in Neurosis and Psychosis. Collected Papers, II, p. 278. New York, Psychoanalytical Press, 1924.

rotic usually retains well his interest in
the outer world and he remains sensitive
to changes in the social atmosphere;
the interest of the psychotic may be
lost. The psychoneurotic conforms more
nearly to the social norm in his relationships, while the regression of the
psychotic may be extreme, but it is not
an important mechanism in the psychoneurotic who never, if consciousness
is clear, degresses to an infantile level
with its excretory soiling. Generally
speaking, the psychotic does not recognize that he is ill and therefore has no
desire for change in his subjective status.
The psychoneurotic, on the contrary,
usually feels keenly his subjective suffering and consciously wants to get well,
although it is known that his more powerful unconscious desire is to the contrary.
The psychoneurotic, especially the hysteric, often exploits his symptom for secondary gain, whereas the psychotic patient
acquires no secondary gain from his illness. Finally, as already stressed, there is
no sharp line between the psychoneuroses
and the major psychoses. They merge one
into the other by intermediate, scarcely
perceptible stages. The differences are
largely descriptive and ones of degree.
Given psychogenic factors may in one
individual lead to defenses and reactions
characterized as psychoneurotic and in
another person to those classified as psychotic. Frequently a reaction that would
be classified as neurotic will later assume
a form descriptively classified as psychotic. This does not mean that one type
of mental illness is being superseded by
another form fundamentally different in
nature. It is, in fact, the opinion of some
psychiatrists that if the life history of a
patient suffering from a psychosis not
associated with toxic or organic factors
is fully known, evidence will always be
found of an untreated or inadequately
treated pre-existing neurotic-like syndrome out of which the psychosis grew.
In the so-called borderline cases, both
neurotic and psychotic mechanisms may
be noted.

Classification of Psychoneurotic Disorders

The Standard Nomenclature adopted
by the American Psychiatric Association
classifies the psychoneurotic disorders as
follows:

1. Anxiety reaction
2. Dissociative reaction
3. Conversion reaction
4. Phobic reaction
5. Obsessive compulsive reaction
6. Depressive reaction

The so-called "types" are not disease
entities in genesis, mechanisms, or manifestations. Rather should the psychoneuroses be regarded as a series of varying
types of reaction brought about by multiple causative factors that vary from case
to case. The more carefully the reactions
of the neurotic are examined, the more
frequently it will be found that there are
no sharply defined lines among the various types of neuroses. It is rare, for example, to find a "pure" hysteria or "pure"
obsessional neurosis. Frequently the neurotic will, in varying degrees, show hysterical, obsessional, anxiety, and even
psychosomatic manifestations. Thus its
definite assignment to a certain type may
be difficult or arbitrary. Overt anxiety,
for example, although the most conspicuous and characteristic symptom in anxiety
states, is frequently an important picture
in other forms. Also, just as there is no
sharply defined distinction between the
psychoneuroses and the psychoses, so
there is none between the psychoneuroses
and many character traits of the so-called
"normal" person. Far more frequently
than is realized, outstanding character
traits are really neurotic reaction formations that serve as defenses. Neurotic
syndromes fit into the personality pattern
of the individual and are allied to the
techniques he has employed all his life
in handling situations. As will be pointed
out in the following paragraph, there is
an increasing tendency, not to classify the
psychoneurotic states into distinct and
definite types, but to divide them clinically according to the nature of the principal mechanism the patient employs as
a means of defense or compromise. In
conversion reaction (conversion hysteria),
for example, the repressed impulse pro-

ducing the anxiety is "converted" into functional symptoms involving voluntary musculature or special sense organs. In phobic reactions (phobia), the anxiety is handled by detaching it from some specific idea or situation and displacing it in the form of a neurotic fear of some object or situation that serves as a symbol of the idea or situation from which the anxiety originally arose. The various forms or mechanisms of anxiety-relieving devices are discussed as different psychoneurotic reactions are described.

Causes

When we seek for the causes of the psychoneuroses, we must conclude that emotional, meaningful factors play a predominant and, in a broad sense, perhaps an exclusive role. Usually from early life the psychoneurotic has shown personality traits that are so deeply rooted in the make-up of the individual that some psychiatrists refer to them as constitutional. Probably, however, these traits are not inherited but are acquired during impressionable years through close association with and dependence upon various members of the family. There is an increasing belief that most major neurotic patterns are basically dependent on conflicts and feeling-attitudes that arose in childhood and that, in order to understand a patient's neurosis, an attempt should be made to connect the patient's present symptoms with some unliquidated childhood situation. One will therefore agree with Freud's statement that the analyst deals more with scars than with bleeding wounds. Presumably this is not always true, yet often the childhood of the psychoneurotic was characterized by such disturbances as sleep walking, crying out in sleep, enuresis, disturbances of speech, food idiosyncrasies, delirium accompanying slight rises in temperature, destructiveness, emotional excitability, temper tantrums, phobias, compulsions, shyness, nail-biting, and other disguises looked upon as constituting personality and behavior problems. Probably these manifestations should be regarded as evidence that spe-

cific conflicts and situational factors have always produced anxiety and led to neurotic symptoms or character traits. It is necessary, however, not only to examine the childhood background for scars that the special circumstances of early life have left, but to be alert for feelings of guilt, conflicts over unconscious needs, meaningful life-events, recurrent, cumulative stresses and tensions of interpersonal relationship difficulties, and the everyday stresses of family living, including marital or sexual problems. It is also important not to consider immediate reality factors as always being fundamental etiological ones rather than precipitating causes. Often it will be found that an apparently smooth adjustment has been a cover for stormy problems that have long existed beneath the surface.

Whatever determined their personalities, there seem to be individuals who are unusually sensitive to tension and conflicts of life, persons who have never really faced its problems and are especially prone to deal with its tensions, wishes, and conflicts by the faulty reactions designated as neurotic. Although the efficiency of most persons is impaired by psychoneurotic tendencies, much of the best work of the world is done as an expression of neurotic disorder. This has been particularly true in the case of art and literature.

Of the immediate causes for the development of the psychoneurosis, it may be said they are frequently to be found in the necessity to repress, distort, or displace emotions of hostility or rage, or the drives of sexuality and dependency as they emerge and conflict with order and peace in the patient's personality. These and similar factors, often of a conflict-producing nature, create *anxiety*, which is the commonest and most important source of psychoneurotic disorders. Anxiety, engendered by a too severe and exacting superego but perhaps stimulated by an external situation, mobilizes the defenses of the personality. As already indicated, the manner in which the patient adapts to this anxiety, which is sometimes characterized as the most unpleasant of subjective emotional states, and tries to mobilize the defenses of the personality against it, determines the type of the psychoneurotic reaction. If the anxiety is felt and expressed directly, is "free floating" and is not confined to definite situations or objects, the neurosis is spoken of as an anxiety state or anxiety neurosis. If the repressed wish or impulse causing the anxiety is "converted" into functional symptoms in organs or parts of the body, the clinical picture is that of conversion hysteria. If the anxiety overwhelms and temporarily controls the individual, the clinical picture is that of hysterical dissociation as in hysterical stupor, fugue, or amnesia. In compulsion neurosis, the patient controls his anxiety by a repetitive activity. This activity or ritual protects the patient against the threat of repressed impulses. In phobias, anxiety is controlled by detaching it from some idea or situation and, by displacement, attaching the fear to some specific object or situation that serves as a symbol.

The psychoneuroses are more frequent in women than in men, partly because of the fact that a more rigid repression of basic biological needs and instincts is required of women, with the result that anxiety defenses in the form of neurotic symptoms are more frequently required than in men. The psychosexual life, with its many taboos and social restrictions, is by no means, however, the only factor, since any fundamental urge or desire against the expression of which a defensive barrier must be constructed, or the gratification of which must be vicarious, may give rise to neurotic symptoms. Feelings of guilt, social situations, or irritating relationships that strain the ability to adjust, or marriage with its new responsibilities are examples of the many factors that may contribute to a neurosis. In a married woman, a chronic marital dissatisfaction and disappointment may contribute to the development of a psychoneurosis. The husband may not have proved to be the ideal mate that was expected, desired demonstrations of affection may have been lacking, or marriage may have failed to be the sustained romance that the wife had dreamed it would be. She may deny any dissatisfaction that may be consciously acknowledged only if she frankly faces her feelings. Other women, interested in a business or professional career, or hesitant to exhibit any interest in, or behavior toward, the opposite sex that would lead to marriage, may put it off until they reach an age when opportunities for marriage are infrequent. The sense of frustration and of a certain emptiness of life may lead to a neurotic reaction. Again, the involutional period, with its reluctantly acknowledged psychological implications, may be accompanied by anxiety, depression, or irritability that is readily converted into functional symptoms.

At times a psychoneurosis may develop as an indirect result of long-continued physical illness. In such a case, the prolonged and perhaps severe illness may threaten the patient's sense of security, compel him to give up activities and interests that have been highly prized, or jeopardize his ability to function at his previous level. Such factors may stimulate an anxiety that had previously been handled without difficulty.

Most neuroses of adults develop between late adolescence and 35 years of age. This is the period when the individual becomes confronted with the problems of adult adjustments and responsibilities. It is the period when satisfying social, economic, and sexual situations should be established. Frustrations in these critically important fields may lead to conflict and anxiety that can be met only by neurotic mechanisms.

Elaborate disguises, including fears, which have no obvious connections with immediate realities and make the neurotic's behavior more or less incomprehensible both to himself and others, are among the conspicuous features of neurotic behavior. A rational explanation for the apparently unintelligible behavior will be found, however, when its psychodynamics is studied. It will be observed, too, that neurotic syndromes tend to fit into the established personality pattern of the individual and are allied to the techniques he has employed all his life in handling difficult situations.

In some psychoneurotic reactions, particularly in anxiety states, the patient often fears the existence of some serious physical disease, whereas the causes of the symptoms are in fact purely psychogenic. In such cases, the patient will usually not accept the psychiatrist's assurance of good physical health unless the physician has first made such a painstaking physical examination and has shown such open-mindedness and true interest concerning the possible existence of physical disease as will make the patient willing to accept the physician's statement that he has no organic basis for the symptoms. It should be emphasized, however, that a diagnosis of psychoneurosis cannot be made merely by the exclusion of organic factors. It can be made only on the discovery of positive factors in the psychological sphere sufficiently pertinent to offer a logical explanation for the symptoms. This evidence is to be found in a study of the patient's personality aimed both at an analysis of the present picture and at a reconstruction of the sequences of psychological experiences that have influenced personality development and structure. It will frequently be found that as time passes a neurosis becomes more complex and irradiates into more aspects of life.

ANXIETY REACTIONS

As previously indicated, anxiety may be described as a painful uneasiness of mind, a state of heightened tension accompanied by an inexpressible dread, a feeling of apprehensive expectation. It may arise under any situation that constitutes a threat to the personality. The emergence of repressed material is particularly apt to be anxiety-producing. Anxiety may arise, for example, when self-requirements and the security of the personality are threatened through the fact that the repression of forbidden sexual desires or dependency strivings to ward off loneliness or of unconscious hostile and aggressive feelings is in danger of giving way. Again, anxiety with its obsessive apprehensiveness may arise in association with frustrations or dilemmas occurring in some major life problem related to such topics as vocational, sexual, or marital adjustment.

In the other psychoneurotic reactions, some specific, auxiliary form of psychological defense mechanism is devised to control anxiety. In anxiety reactions, however, there is no such specific method of defense. Repression alone is insufficient to control the anxiety. As a result the anxiety, not being displaced as in phobic reactions, not being "converted" into functional symptoms as in hysteria, not being discharged by some gross personality disorganization such as dissociation, fugue, or amnesia, and not being automatically controlled by some repetitive thought or act, remains diffuse and uncontrolled, with the result that the patient is in a state of constant anxious expectation. Anxiety reaction is therefore sometimes spoken of as the simplest form of neurosis.

If the diffuse anxiety is not too painful, it may be expressed or controlled through certain personality traits. Individuals who are constantly beset by pervading anxiety are characteristically tense, timid, apprehensive, sensitive to the opinions of others, easily embarrassed, and tend to worry. Many persons with such a constant sense of anxiety are self-distant, given to inferiority feelings, experience difficulty in making decisions, and are afraid of making mistakes. Usually they are scrupulous, overconscientious, ambitious, and feel that they must live up to self-imposed high standards. Although such a person suffers moderate distress through apprehension and other tendencies previously noted, the tension is not usually intolerable. If, however, the anxiety becomes more disturbing, it may be expressed in such symptoms as depression, sleeplessness, irritability, restlessness, a paralyzing indecision, psychosomatic disturbances, outbursts of aggressiveness, attacks of weeping, and feelings of inadequacy and inferiority accompanied, perhaps, by a paranoid attitude. Usually the patient with an anxiety reaction feels chronically fatigued and complains of inability to concentrate. Some express the fear that they are "becoming insane."

Anxiety Attacks

In addition to a chronic state of tension and mild anxiety, the patient with anxiety neurosis may be subject to acute, terrifying, panic-like exacerbations lasting from a few moments to an hour. The patient suffers therefore from rapid heart, palpitation, precordial discomfort, nausea, diarrhea, desire to urinate, dyspnea, and a feeling of choking or suffocation. The pupils are dilated, the face is flushed, the skin perspires, the patient suffers from paresthesias and tremulousness, feels dizzy or faint, and often has a sense of weakness and of impending death. Restlessness is acute, and the patient may express beseeching and apprehensive appeals. In chapter 27 the psychophysiological mechanism of hyperventilation is described; this is the mechanism that causes these symptoms in perhaps the majority of acute anxiety attacks. Other physiological expressions of acute anxiety perhaps occur through activation of various segments of the autonomic nervous system and the adrenal medulla and its secretions. In an acute reactive anxiety attack, the clinical picture may be colored by a traumatic situation. This is well illustrated in the anxiety attacks of combat neurosis.

The patient who is subject to acute anxiety attacks usually suffers also from a chronic anxiety state. He experiences difficulty in falling asleep, is disturbed by fearful dreams, suffers from coarse tremors or "trembling," and complains of a "band around the head" or of a "quivering in the stomach." He is absent-minded and seems worried without knowing about what or why. He complains that his mind is in a constant daze and that he is unable to control his thoughts. He is apprehensive and is afraid to be alone, yet he does not desire conversation. He feels too tired to attempt anything constructive and continually seeks a physical explanation for his distressing mental state.

Physicians lacking an appreciation of psychological factors in the production of symptoms have at times erred in failing to recognize that anxiety attacks are psychological, not physiological, disturbances and have diagnosed them as heart disease, thyrotoxicosis, hyperinsulinism, or dysinsulinism.

Treatment

Two phases of an anxiety reaction require attention—one, the acute anxiety attack, the other, the anxiety neurosis. During the attack, the rapid pulse and pounding heart lead the patient to believe that only a heart attack could have produced his distress. After an examination of the heart and other organs has been made and no physical disorder discovered, the patient should be confidently assured that he has no heart disease. Frequently the cause of the symptoms may be demonstrated easily by the simple medium of requesting the patient to overbreathe for a period of two minutes, as described in Chapter 27 under the hyperventilation syndrome. Further somatic complaints should be disregarded and the examination of the heart should not be repeated. The patient should not, through the use of drugs, be led to believe that his pathologic condition is physical rather than emotional, and rest should not be advised, nor should personal reassurance be repeated to a degree that the patient constantly feels the need for it.

Treatment of the basic neurosis is psychotherapeutic and requires that attention be directed to an uncovering of the unrecognized sources of anxiety, to the action of psychodynamic factors, to their adjustment, and to re-education. Less attention should be paid to the anxiety attacks than to a study of the patient's personality and to attitudes and situations that cause frustration and tension. Although a more formal analysis is desirable in severe anxiety neuroses, many patients with milder cases can be helped by a psychotherapy on the conscious level and by a face-to-face discussion. Consideration should be given to the meaning of symptoms, the role of emotions, the stress of present circumstances, and the effect of well-remembered past experience in molding present attitudes and habits of thinking and feeling. The demonstration of a correlation between the time when anxiety appeared and certain preceding events in the patient's life history may give insight sufficient to produce considerable relief. A desire to violate self-imposed rigid standards may at times be discovered. Troublesome sex problems, including any arising from faulty contraceptive technique, should be adjusted. The patient should be encouraged to continue physical exercise and recreation. If chronic tension states and associated muscular pains occur in neck and shoulders, physiotherapy is helpful. Meprobamate, the various phenothiazines, and the barbiturates may be used to provide symptomatic relief from the chronic symptoms of anxiety. Prolonged and permanently disabling anxiety states have been benefited by prefrontal lobotomy when all other measures have failed.

The anxiety reactions are most frequently associated with phobic defenses that are often overlooked in originally describing the anxiety neuroses. Untreated, the phobic anxiety state may extend with either the development of obsessive ideation and disappearance of the acute anxiety reactions or progressive withdrawal associated with phobic diffusion that leads to a state of helpless isolation simulating a psychotic regression.

A 27-year-old woman entered the hospital complaining of multiple fears. She was too frightened to get on streetcars or buses, to go to the movies, and to go out to supper. She was also afraid that she would not live up to the expectations of her mother, was dubious about her own capabilities, and indicated that her marriage was in difficult straits and that she had previously been separated from her husband for a period of 18 months. She stated that their only son was a bed wetter. In addition, she presented the symptoms of acute anxiety with palpitation, perspiration, dizziness, and shortness of breath caused by the hyperventilation syndrome.

Brief questioning elicited the information that her mother had been a nagging, sadistic person, who unmercifully switched the patient and her brother whenever they failed to obey her command. The father, a mild, subservient individual, had seldom been at home. The patient was a quiet and obedient, though fearful, child, usually timid and retiring, who felt that she must always acquiesce to the wishes of others or be subject to their criticism and withdrawal of affection.

The diagnosis in this case was long-standing anxiety neurosis, associated with the hyperventilation syndrome and a phobic state. The anxiety attacks occurred regularly in situations in which the patient's husband or mother or even the doctor did something or said something to arouse her anger. She could not allow herself to express her anger, as she feared that this would lead to further criticism and rejections. Although the majority of anxiety attacks were relieved after several months of psychiatric treatment, she was not entirely free of her symptoms of dizziness and palpitation and of her phobias until a year of regular visits had elapsed.

Freud delineated in detail the physical symptoms of anxiety and their intimate association with phobias. Since anxiety and phobic reactions are so frequently associated, the latter are brought to discussion for clinical reasons at this point.

PHOBIC REACTION

A phobic reaction is a defensive one in which the patient attempts to deal with his anxiety by detaching it from a specific idea, object, or situation in his daily life and displacing it to some symbolic idea, object, or situation in the form of a specific neurotic fear. Although the patient consciously recognizes that no actual danger exists, yet if exposed to the specific phobia-stimulating, symbolic object or situation, he is powerless to prevent experiencing an intense sense of fear. The intensely distressing sense of apprehension associated with the consciously feared object or situation is actually derived from other sources—sources of which the patient is unaware. A defense against the anxiety arising from his unrecognized source is provided through the mechanisms of displacement and symbolization. By these means, the anxiety is detached from its real source—unconscious, forbidden tendencies and impulses, for example—and displaced to some situation or object that is usually symbolic of the threatening tendency or wish. A great variety of phobias has been described. Among them are fear of dirt, of bacteria, of certain animals, of travel by a certain type of vehicle. Many of them have Greek names attached to them, as agoraphobia, a fear of open places or claustrophobia, a fear of confined spaces. A claustrophobia might, for example, prevent the occupancy of a Pullman berth. When exposed to the specific situation that evokes his fear, the phobic experiences faintness, fatigue, palpitation, perspiration, nausea, and tremor. He may be unable to continue with the duty at hand and be overwhelmed with panic. He can control his anxiety if he avoids the phobic object or situation. If the patient were to carry out a phobic activity, it would unconsciously mean to him that he was performing the forbidden activity that arouses the dreaded anxiety. He also constantly punishes himself for his unconscious tendencies and impulses by the distressing restrictions and sufferings imposed by his phobia. Phobias are twice as common among women as among men.

The phobic sufferer oftentimes comes from a family in which the mother is fearful of her aggression, is herself phobic, and is unable to exact conforming behavior except through nagging insistence from the children and even the father. If the father overtly complies with the mother's phobic insistence, even though he appears firm, some of the children may become phobic as well, as this becomes the dominant adaptation for control.

DISSOCIATIVE REACTION

At times anxiety may so overwhelm and disorganize the personality that certain aspects or functions of it become dissociated from each other. In some instances, the personality may be so disorganized that defense mechanisms govern consciousness, memory, and temporarily even the total individual, with little or no participation on the part of the conscious

personality. In such a case the patient may at times appear psychotic. Formerly the dissociative reactions were classified as a type of conversion hysteria.

One of the commonest anxiety-stimulated and defensive dissociative reactions is *amnesia*. Forgetting is a simple expedient. It is therefore not surprising that amnesias obliterate recollections, particularly for definitely circumscribed periods of time. Dissociative amnesia is, however, not a mere forgetting. It is an active process, a blotting out of awareness of unpleasant features. Periods of stupor or of twilight state may precede such an amnesia, which then tends to become selective and limited to the particular element or experience that evoked it. Among experiences that suspend the ability to bring pertinent factual data to consciousness are those involving great terror, as in war, or covering periods and behavior with which shame, guilt, or other intense feeling-tone is connected. How satisfactorily an amnesia exercises its protective and escape purpose is shown by the unperturbed manner in which the patient accepts his loss of memory. Although most dissociative amnesias are of brief duration, they sometimes blot out long periods, sometimes even the patient's entire previous life. In some instances, there is a reversion to an earlier period of the patient's life, with retrograde amnesia for events subsequent to that period. In differentiating between an organic and a dissociative amnesia, it will be found that a sudden return of memory is indicative of its dissociative loss. The onset, also, of the dissociative amnesia will have been sudden.

Dissociative reactions are at times characterized by mental symptoms involving *disturbances of consciousness*. These may be in the form of stupor or of various forms of "twilight state." Frequently the latter suggests delirium. Such psychogenic delirious states are usually preceded by marked emotional experiences or displays and consist of dream states accompanied by more or less confusion, dramatic posturings and activities, and an excessive flow of speech appearing nonsensical, but in which occur references to strongly affective experiences. Dissociative delirium often represents the dream-like realization of a wish or the dramatic re-living in fantasy of an affectively traumatic experience. Its clouding of consciousness and the presence of illusions and hallucinations may exclude the reality of the outside world and falsify it in accordance with deep-seated motives and unsatisfied wishes. Occasionally the patient spins fantastic stories. Such instances usually represent an effort to supply romance and drama to a life devoid of emotional satisfactions.

At times a psychic escape may be in the form of a dissociative *fugue*. In this there is a sudden change in state of consciousness, during which the patient may be impelled by unconscious forces to perform complicated activities, perhaps involving travel over long distances. Throughout this period, the patient may appear quite normal to the casual observer. In some instances there is a loss of personal identity. In the fugue the patient indulges in acts of fantasies that are in conflict with his superego, and the function of the fugue is to permit the carrying out of these acts or fantasies. A further defense mechanism becomes necessary, however, and so the patient attempts to protect his ego by forgetting his name and past history, that is, by losing his identity. In other instances there is not a loss but a change in personal identity. In such a case the patient assumes a false name and identifies himself with the person whose name he takes. The assumption of the false name is associated with the unconscious fantasies responsible for the genesis of the fugue. O. Henry has presented a delightful picture of a dissociative fugue in his misnamed short story, "A Case of Aphasia." As Fisher** points out, the psychological formula is as if the patient says, "I did not commit this crime, because I am not I; I am somebody else."

After the termination of the fugue, the

** Fisher, C.: Amnesic states in war neuroses. The psychogenesis of fugues. Psychoanalytic Quart., 14:460, 1945.

patient may have a complete amnesia for his journey until the memory of it is restored by hypnosis or other psychic means. Examination of the patient either by sodium amytal narcosis or by other means of ascertaining subconscious mental content usually reveals the personal, emotional factors that prompted an escape mechanism in the form of an automatic, unconscious, uncontrollable withdrawal. In certain recent studies, it has been found that the fugue state is preceded by depression and may be regarded as an attempt to ward off this affect. The model for a number of fugue states apparently has been supplied by a previous head injury with a resulting amnesia, or amnesic states induced through alcohol, or identification with others who suffered dissociative reactions.

Ganser Syndrome

The Ganser syndrome, with its combination of instinctive, rational, purposeful, and deceptive elements and theatrical behavior, is an alteration of consciousness allied both to simulation and to dissociative dream states. In this syndrome, occurring largely among prisoners under detention while awaiting trial, the patient, being in a situation that would be solved or mitigated by irresponsibility, desires, although not consciously so acknowledged, to appear irresponsible, and accordingly, without being aware of it, actually does develop mental disturbance. The conspicuous features of this disorder consist of a childish, ludicrous performance of simple acts, the correct procedure for which is fully known by the patient. The patient's responses to questions are wrong but are not far wrong and bear an obvious relation to the question. His replies show that he understood the meaning of the questions, but they are beside the point and are in the nature of approximate answers—a phenomenon known as paralogia, or "Vorbeireden." The purpose of the patient's behavior is so obviously to appear irresponsible that he may seem to be malingering. Since the circumstances under which the Ganser syndrome occurs are such that the advantages to be gained by a mental disability are greater than those obtained by physical disorders, the reaction takes place in terms of the former rather than of conversion hysteria. As in other dissociative reactions, the protection from a full realization of his situation affords the patient a relative freedom from the anxiety that might otherwise be intolerable.

At times dissociation may suggest a schizophrenic reaction. Usually a dissociative reaction is of more sudden onset and is preceded by more conscious or felt anxiety. The pre-illness types of personality are not similar.

CONVERSION REACTIONS

The term "conversion reaction" is synonymous with "conversion hysteria," the name by which it is better known. Because of the striking and dramatic manifestations that may accompany this reaction, it was the first of the psychoneuroses to receive attention. In a conversion reaction, anxiety, instead of being consciously experienced, either diffusely as in anxiety reactions, or displaced as in phobias, is "converted" into functional symptoms in organs or parts of the body innervated by the sensory-motor nervous system. The conversion symptoms serve to prevent or lessen any conscious, felt anxiety and usually symbolize the underlying mental conflict that is productive of anxiety. The reaction usually meets some need of the patient and therefore not merely serves as a defense against anxiety but also provides some more or less obvious "secondary gain," a phenomenon discussed in this chapter. Viewed a little differently, the hysterical symptoms may be regarded as expressing a conflict or an idea in symbolic form. It may, for example, "convert" a mental concept into a significant body symptom, as when hysterical paralysis of an arm expresses a wish to do a forbidden act, yet ambivalently prevents its accomplishment. The form of the conversion symptom is de-termined by some feature of the situation it was designed to meet.

If a person were consciously to counterfeit some physical sign or symptom or some mental disturbance for the purpose of attaining a particular objective, we would say that he was *malingering*. Conscious recognition of its intent is not necessary, however, in order that behavior may be purposive. In conversion hysteria, the symptoms, without awareness on part of the patient, provide some form and extent of solution for his problems and afford him a certain relief from the anxiety involved in the perturbing situation. Nature's methods are not of a sharply defined and delimited character but form imperceptibly graded series, so that there are found all degrees of awareness and many types of reaction between simulation, consciously adopted to solve some clearly defined external difficulty of which the individual is clearly aware, and hysteria, in which to satisfy unrecognized inner needs similar reactions take place without conscious participation. Some hysterical phenomena are on the borderline between psychoneurotic reactions and simulation and therefore come close to malingering. Just where, as to awareness, the line between simulation and hysteria should be drawn is therefore arbitrary. In both there is a subtle interweaving of conscious factors. Both are related to some definite purpose, usually protective or wish-fulfilling in nature. It is not surprising that the difference in the hysteric's mind between reality and fantasy is often vague.

Causes

The immediate factor in the production of hysteria is some anxiety-producing situation. With the frequent exception of the traumatic hysterias, we find that the hysterias of civil life tend to develop on a certain personality background characterized by immaturity in the psychosexual and emotional fields. Puberty is a favorite period for the appearance of hysteria. What may be called the normal psychic characteristics of that period are often found to persist in the mental life of the adult hysteric. Maturing drives, for example, may remain in an arrested or infantile state of development, a state to which a failure to attain an emotional independence from a parent sometimes contributes. Impulses, sentiments, and other bases of the personality are not integrated into a harmonious system. Some hysterics, with their immature personality development, are basically hostile and aggressive persons.

Kretschmer divides persons of the infantile, psychobiologically inhibited, hysterical character into two groups. In the first group he places persons of normal intellectual development but whose other psychic characteristics, particularly the emotional ones, are of an immature, pubertal type. They are childishly egocentric, selfish, vain, like to be the center of attention, take pleasure in exhibiting their virtues, are oversensitive, irritable, petulant, exhibit emotional capriciousness, moodiness, histrionic poses and pathos, and fleeting enthusiasms that often represent identifications.

In the second group of persons of hysterical personality, Kretschmer places those whom he characterizes as having a stunted psyche. These persons are immature, emotionally indifferent, shy, fearful, excitable, of rather inferior intelligence, and, because of their primitive and impulsive reactions, they may become social defectives, criminals, and prostitutes. The grosser varieties of hysteria are more common in these persons of inferior make-up than in those of better endowment.

Kretschmer's suggestion as to the genesis of hysterical symptoms is of theoretical interest. After the initial formation of symptoms, there is, in his belief, a period when conscious volition and interference could be effective, but after that, deeper lying automatic mechanisms take over. These become unconscious and put the process of symptom formation beyond the range of volition of the patient.

In ordinary civil life, wishes, struggles, and disappointments associated with the sex life form, especially in women, one of the most important groups of experiences that produce the major forms of hysteria. The sexual impulse, although often active, may fail to develop toward a natural goal and is gratified in fantasy and auto-erotic habits. A confused admixture of sexual desire and aversion, of erotic feelings and prudish attitudes often exists. Erotic fantasies often contrast with conscious expressions of fear and disgust in regard to sexuality. Among the problems that in women may give rise to hysteria are an unsuccessful love affair; jealousy, perhaps arising from the marriage of a sister; an undesired marriage; fear of pregnancy; difficulties in intercourse; or an unhappy marriage. Many such women are sexually frigid.

The developmental histories of such women make evident the sources for the disordered psychosexuality. In contrast to the earlier concept that the disorder resulted from disturbances in the Oedipal period, it often commences in the initial maternal relationship. In many instances the mother, hysterical herself, has been rejecting, arousing in the child retaliatory fantasies that have been repressed. The mother often has been recognized as hypocritical about sex, dependent herself, and subtly clinging to the child for whom she has special ambitions. The father of such patients is inadequate, repressing this through either alcoholism or passivity and usually derogated by the mother. This family situation forces the child to perceive her mother ambivalently —as "good" or "bad"—often "good" in the sense of offering concern during illness and as setting idealistic standards for repression of sexual and aggressive activity. She, however, is "bad" in lacking in tenderness, and her interest, even though denied, in the father and other siblings exaggerates feelings of jealous rivalry in the child. The latter, rejected herself, envies the father or male siblings, whom she considers receive preferential treatment from the mother. Fixed to the mother, yet envying the father and brothers, she displays early tomboyishness, enuresis, difficulty with menstruation, and later difficulty in acceptance of the feminine role, which is shown in frigidity, vomiting in pregnancy, or hostile seductiveness with men. In all these reactions, the hysterical symptoms symbolically express her conflicts and confusion in regard to her sexual identification.

In men, threats to self-esteem, to economic success, or to self-preservation more frequently present situations from which escape is sought through the hysterical symptoms. Many men are of immature personality with a strong, dependent attachment to a mother. Striking forms of hysterical reactions, such as functional incapacities and symptoms with histrionic features, occur largely among young people. Such hysterical states rarely occur during or after middle age, by which time more permanent and less dramatic protective mechanisms have been established.

Frequently the factor or event that precipitated a conversion reaction may have been trivial but had some special meaning to the patient. Sometimes the precipitating situation may have some special similarity to a previous occurrence. It is therefore well to ascertain what the setting was at the time of appearance of the conversion reaction and also what the patient's emotional state was at the time. The nature of the earlier experiences that give special meaning to the precipitating event and the patient's predisposition to respond with a selective conversion mechanism may usually only be determined by psychoanalysis, although much recall may emerge in hypnotic or narcosynthetic states.

Painful complaints today are among the most commonly encountered conversion symptons. Their determination appears to rest on any one of the following parent–child interactions.

Oversolicitude by the mother following minor painful experience may establish the predisposition to obtain gratification, in the face of conflict, by means of painful complaining in later life. Envious observation of the attention given to another sibling or home member sometimes arouses fantasies of suffering that are repressed until the later conflictful period

and are then aroused as a substitute means of allaying anxiety. Of greatest importance are the childhood experiences of pain that lead to masochistic suffering in order to obtain gratifying affectional responses. In some instances, parents suffer guilt on punishing the child for misdeeds and then lavish affection following punishment as a means of assuaging their own anxiety. If this is the means by which the patient as a child repetitively obtained emotional satisfaction, a pattern for later masochistic pain and suffering is established. Another method, described by Freud, has to do with the guilt suffered by a child after secretly enjoying the punishment offered an envied brother or sister. To assuage this guilt, he must then suffer some distress. In all these instances, the basic issue is the wish for the affection and acceptance by the parent or parental substitute. With the masochistic expression, pain or distress must be expressed in order to obtain the wished-for affection and acceptance denied in reality.

Symptoms

Although reference has already been made to the type of individual who seems predisposed to hysteria, further mention may be made of some of the personality characteristics frequently observed in the hysteric. It will often be found that evasions and mechanisms of retreat have been habitual since early life. The narcissism that tends to characterize her arrested personality development gives her a proneness to self-display that is often expressed in childish and dramatic ways. Persons of the hysterical type of personality desire an immediate gratification of their wishes but avoid effort to gain their goal. They are self-engrossed, offended by trifles, and dependent in attitude; they bid for sympathy and attention and are given to suicidal "gestures." Such acts are without intent to die. The threat or shock of the apparent attempt is used by the hysteric to control her environment, to gain attention, to arouse sympathy, or to frighten others into submission. Many seek to rule their environment by being sick, pitiful, and appealing. Such persons exaggerate any existing physical symptoms and even precipitately develop those of a critical or unique nature. Attention-getting, secondary-gain complaints are common. Craig called attention to the fact that hysterics, with their immature personalities, rarely react with awe, reverence, wonder, or pity; they may exhibit self-depreciation, remorse, or grief, but if so, it is because those emotions are the ones that gain them the greatest attention or best obtain a desired domination over their environment. Her childish egocentricity and inner fantasy poorly fit the hysteric for adult reality.

Hysterical patients are notoriously suggestible, and their symptoms tend to follow the fashion of their particular period. One now rarely sees the dramatic posturings that were common in Charcot's clinic or the astasia–abasia of Victorian women. They are frequently, however, imitations of actions or disabilities either seen or read about. If a hysterical patient, confronted with some difficult and unpleasant situation, observes the successful evasion of a similar situation by another person, he may develop the same symptoms as a means of escape. Such imitations of symptoms were so frequent in World Wars I and II that attempts were made to isolate from the observation of his associates the soldier who had escaped combat service through his hysterical disability.

The nature of the hysterical symptoms is often determined by some need or feature of the situation that produced them and by the type of disability that will be most useful in satisfying the subconscious purpose they are designed to meet. As a rule, the more turbulent the emotional undercurrents and the greater the disturbance of strong impulsive strivings, the more acute and striking the manifestations and the greater the evidence of anxiety.

Physical Disturbances

Physical symptoms may be sensory or motor. The *motor disturbances* in hysteria are various. In all of them, function is disturbed without demonstrable physiological or anatomical change. Paralyses may be in the form of monoplegia, hemiplegia, or paraplegia and may be either flaccid or spastic. The deep reflexes are not lost in flaccid forms; they may be exaggerated in the spastic forms, but there are no true clonus and no Babinski reaction. In hemiplegia the paralysis of the proximal muscles is greater than of the peripheral, being in this respect the contrary of that existing in organic hemiplegia. The forearm is extended instead of being somewhat flexed, as in organic hemiplegia; the leg is dragged instead of being swung in circumduction. There is no appreciable wasting of the paralyzed extremities. The maintenance of normal electrical reactions in flaccid paralysis is diagnostic, as is an absence of bladder symptoms or of tendency to bedsores in paraplegia. Contractures are not uncommon. A fairly frequent form is that of a tightly clenched fist. In hysterical paralyses, the muscles in question may be used in one voluntary movement and not in another. An attempt to exercise the paralyzed function is accompanied by a display of excessive effort.

Tics, tremors, usually coarse in nature, and choreiform and clonic movements occur. Aphonia, in which the patient cannot phonate speech but continues to cough as formerly, is not rare. Whereas in aphonia the patient finds no difficulty in communicating in whispers, the patient with hysterical mutism can utter no word, although he communicates freely and correctly in writing—a point of differentiation from aphasia. One patient who developed hysterical mutism in prison dreamed that the institution for mental diseases to which he had been transferred was on fire, whereupon he screamed and thereafter talked normally.

The occupational neuroses, such as writer's cramp, usually belong among hysterical reactions. The hysterical tic consists of a spasmodic, co-ordinated twitching movement of a small group of functionally related muscles. It may take the form of twitching of the facial muscles, blinking of the lids, sudden turning of the head, or a gesturelike movement of the hands. Such tics may represent dramatization of psychic experiences. Because of the suggestion of defense that they manifest, they may appear purposive. Care must be taken not to confuse hysterical tics with the more complex, co-ordinated tic-like movements observed after epidemic encephalitis and certain other organic diseases of the brain.

Sensory symptoms, like other physical disturbances, are usually those of functional incapacity. Among the more frequent ones are anesthesias, paresthesias, and disturbance of special sense organs, such as blindness or deafness. Hysterical anesthesia does not follow the distribution of a nerve but involves an extremity up to a sharply defined line above which sensation is normal. It follows what the patient believes to be the distribution of the nerve, which is represented in the patient's mind as a functional unit. One-half of the body may be anesthetic, in which case the special senses—hearing, smell, taste, and sight—may be lost on the same side. Hysterical anesthesia may be extended in area by the suggestive and repetitious procedure of the physician in examination. Anesthesia probably cannot be produced *de novo* by the physician's examination, although this was believed by Babinski. The area and degree of the anesthesia may vary from one examination to another. Hysterical disturbances of vision are of various forms, the most frequent ones being blindness and narrowing of the visual fields. Hysterical blindness usually has a sudden onset. The pupils continue to react to light, and usually, but not always, the patient avoids objects that would injure him if he came into collision with them. The onset is usually either closely related to some distressing visual experience or has a fairly obvious symbolic relation and significance.

Painful complaints are often hysterical in nature and may sometimes be hallucinatory. This conversion symptom is perhaps the commonest expression of the illness at the current time and is frequently misdiagnosed and mistreated. As with other hysterical symptoms, the patient presents a bizarre or unusual account of the symptoms that is not easily recognizable as a result of the usual physical illnesses, or he may exaggerate the pain of a relatively minor physical disturbance. In spite of his insistence on the severity and disabling nature of the symptom and his demands for medication and care, he may be observed frequently to appear indifferent and undisturbed by the symptom. Placebos may relieve the symptom. There is often an intermittent history of its occurrence, and exacerbations may be found related to incidents arousing emotional conflict. In taking the history, the examiner may induce many hysterical patients, apparently indifferent to the symptom, to complain at the point where the psychiatrist touches upon the emotionally disturbing relationship or incidents in his life. If the psychiatrist is easily dissuaded from the task of history taking in an effort to provide immediate relief of a sudden complaint of pain offered by the patient during the interview, a valuable opportunity and a significant clue pertaining to the emotional connotation of the symptom are missed. Reintroduction of the anxiety-ridden topics or associated themes often gives rise again to painful complaining. The arousal of painful complaining may be regarded as perhaps hallucinatory. It may occur in the course of psychoanalysis when the patient associates pertinent information symbolizing the conflicting needs that underlie the symptom.

Organic Factors and Conversion Reactions

The existence of organic symptoms does not exclude the presence of conversion ones also. Symptoms of organic disease that still exist may be exaggerated, or symptoms may persist after the organic basis for them no longer continues. In such cases, the symptoms produced by the disease were found to serve some psychological purpose, to be of value in themselves. Because of their usefulness in providing protection, escape, or advantage, they are unconsciously exaggerated or prolonged. Hysterical symptoms of this nature occur particularly in industrial, insurance, and traumatic neuroses, but they are by no means confined to them, since there are many situations in which physical symptoms may serve some useful function. At times the organic disease may impose sufficient additional stress so that emotional problems can no longer be dealt with in a realistic manner. Exhaustion, whether a result of fatigue or of anxiety resulting from prolonged indecision or from emotional conflict, may predispose to a hysterical retreat from a situation that would otherwise have been met with ease. The person already having some organic disease will often, if his situation does not demand some other special symptom, select one related to the organic disorder with which he is already familiar. The organic symptoms may merge imperceptibly into the hysterical one.

Psychopathology of Conversion Reactions

It is not surprising that theories formulated to account for the etiology and nature of a personality disturbance that may manifest itself in symptoms apparently purely physical in nature should be various. As would be expected, these theories have been influenced by the concepts that have prevailed during different periods relative to natural phenomena in general, and human behavior in particular. Among these theories are the teaching of Hippocrates that hysteria is caused by the wandering of the uterus through the body in search of humidity, the belief of the 17th century that its striking manifestations seen in that period were a result of witchcraft or demoniacal possession, and the conviction now generally accepted that it is an adjustmental technique to which the personality may resort.

Among those who have contributed most to our understanding of conversion and of dissociative reactions are Charcot, Janet, Bernheim, Babinski, Morton Prince, and Freud. Although his point of view was entirely neurological, Charcot was the first to demonstrate that the dramatic manifestations of hysteria could be produced and allayed by hypnotic suggestion. He thus demonstrated that psychological influences could affect bodily mechanisms, although, with his lack of aptitude for psychological investigation, he assumed that a hereditary degeneration was an essential prerequisite for hypnotic or hysterical phenomena. His discovery did, however, lay the foundation for investigative work by others.

Janet, a pupil of Charcot, in an attempt to account for the phenomena of hysteria, developed the concepts of dissociation, the subconscious, and psychological tension. Janet, it will be remembered, believed that the integration of the organism, whether considered from the standpoint of consciousness or of function, depends upon an energy that he called psychic tension. If this hypothetical psychic tension is adequate, there is a unity of the personality with a synthesis of consciousness and of functional processes. If, however, there is a weakness in this tension or energy, caused particularly, Janet believed, by emotional shocks and traumatic memories, there is a lowering in the level of psychological performance, and certain mental processes go on in the subconscious independently of (dissociated from) the main stream of consciousness. According to this view, hysteria would be considered a defect, a negative process, rather than a dynamic, purposeful one.

Bernheim emphasized the importance of suggestion and expressed the opinion that all hysterical symptoms are the result of suggestion. Babinski also believed that in the hysteric there is a particular susceptibility to stimuli that therefore are peculiarly potent in inhibiting or dissociating mental processes. He added the opinion that not only could all hysterical phenomena be produced by suggestion but they could be removed by persuasion.

It is now universally agreed that conversion hysteria and dissociative reactions are of psychogenic origin. The greatest influence in creating this point of view is to be found in the contributions of Freud. Most psychogenic theories as to the nature of conversion hysteria go back to the concepts of conflict and of repres-

sion. According to Freud, the wish or
other repressed material, although not
permitted frank expression, obtains release
in disguised form through the mechanism
of conversion, by which the psychic conflict is transformed into a physical or mental symptom. Freud explained the hysterical symptoms as caused by a conflict between the superego and some wish that
because of its consciously objectionable
nature, is repressed by the superego. This
repression is not, however, entirely successful, and the wish therefore obtains
disguised expression by its "conversion"
or transformation into the symptom. The
nature and localization of the symptom
thus produced are such as will symbolize
or provide disguised expression of the repressed wish and at the same time provide some degree of its fulfillment or of
relief from the emotional conflict. Many
psychiatrists who accept the role of repression in the production of the hysterical symptom hesitate to accept Freud's
belief that a repressed Oedipus complex
is an essential condition for the development of hysteria.

At the present time, the most widely
accepted explanation of the mechanism
known as conversion is that impulses and
unadjusted, repressed elements in the
personality, highly charged with emotion,
are productive of anxiety. The anxiety
is then mitigated or dispelled by being
"converted" into functional symptoms
manifested in the voluntary musculature
or in special sense-organ systems. The
exact process involved in this "conversion" is uncertain.

In conversion hysteria, we find an excellent illustration of both primary or
neurotic gain and of secondary gain. The
conversion mechanism yields a primary
or neurotic gain through its anxiety-de-
fense function. It also yields a secondary
gain by producing something to the advantage of the patient. A hysterical paralysis, for example, may enable one to
evade some situation that he feels incapable of mastering.

The manner in which conversion, or
the transformation of an anxiety-producing emotional conflict into a specific

symptom, alleviated the anxiety caused
by the patient's conflicting desires, and
at the same time yielded a secondary gain
that enabled the patient to escape from
an extremely unpleasant situation, is
illustrated by the following case.

M., a young man who had been a dancer and
an acrobat in a circus, enlisted in the army long
after World War I. Here he found the discipline
rigid, his duties irksome, and his experiences
monotonous. He longed for travel, excitement,
attention, and the opportunity for exhibition enjoyed in his former life. The situation became
quite intolerable, but to leave meant that he would
be treated as a deserter. A hysterical conversion
reaction, induced by two conflicting motives, the
one to conform to the requirements of military
life, the other to secure escape from a hated situation, provided a solution that permitted him to
gain his own end, i.e., to obtain immunity from
unpleasant experiences and tasks, and at the same
time alleviated his anxiety and enabled him to
maintain his self-respect. On arrival at the mental
hospital to which he was transferred, he could
neither walk nor stand, and his legs were anesthetic to even vigorous prickings by a pin. At the
same time, he displayed a significant attitude of
unconcern (*la belle indifférence*) as to his disabilities, although, as far as he was consciously aware,
they were complete and incurable. His absence of
concern is to be explained by the fact that the
penalty was less than the gain, although one must
not conclude that this weighing of advantages and
disadvantages was at all a matter of conscious
reflection. A few months later, the man was discharged from the army on a surgeon's certificate of
disability. Soon the suspended motor and sensory
functions began to return. Persistent efforts to
walk met gradually with success, and in another
three months he left the hospital practically well.

In the case of this soldier, it can be
seen how a psychological mechanism
"converted" the anxiety stemming from
his repressed hostile drives against those
in authority and his wish for release from
military service into an overt and incapacitating symptom that, however,
yielded a definite secondary gain.

The hysterical conversion reaction may
provide the patient with a defense against
anxiety, enable him to maintain his self-
respect, and at the same time accomplish
some purpose, the achievement of which
respect for self would otherwise have been
forbidden. It may make possible an escape
from an intolerable situation; it may afford an exoneration for oneself, an excuse

for one's failures, serve as an attention-getting device, or enable one to evade some duty, shun a responsibility, express some spite, or realize some purpose that would not bear the scrutiny of consciousness.

Hysteria has its analogue in many acts of everyday life, when many psychological processes considered normal take place without full consciousness of their methods and motives, particularly if there is some reason for hiding the truth from oneself. The hysteric is always desirous never to disclose to himself the real nature of his illness, an effort that is successful, since the conscious personality has no access to the cause of the illness. Universal, too, is the tendency to project one's difficulties upon something tangible. Similarly, any physical basis for an explanation of the symptom is welcomed and assigned an important place.

In connection with conversion reactions such as the one cited, it should be kept in mind that several factors usually play a role in determining the specific nature of the neurotic reaction. This concurrence and integration of adaptive functions unconsciously served by the symptoms is known as *overdetermination*. Through this process, a single symptom or neurotic reaction may be a complex compromise formation, to the production of which several needs have simultaneously and unconsciously contributed. If an overdeterminative process is analyzed, it will be found that in many neuroses there are anxiety-relieving values that have been produced by the symptom, together with further advantages that the patient secondarily derives from his illness once it is established. Two or more birds are killed with one stone, so to speak.

As already indicated, these two sets of values derived from the neurosis are the primary and the secondary ones. The primary gain is the defense against anxiety supplied by the symptom. The secondary gain is a material advantage that is contributed by the symptom. In the case of the soldier just mentioned, the conversion symptom (hysterical paralysis) relieved him from the anxiety incident to his ambivalent wishes. It also afforded what was to him a very important secondary gain: it rendered him unable to perform military services and therefore made his discharge necessary. Conversion reactions usually meet some immediate need of the patient and are therefore associated with more less obvious "secondary gain." The secondary gain is not always material but may be emotional or social, e.g., the extraction of love, sympathy, or consideration from other people. Usually the element of "secondary gain" secured from the disturbing conversion symptoms seen daily in the general practice of medicine is less apparent than in the case of the soldier. Frequently, in fact, when symptoms of anxiety are also present, the element of secondary gain may be slight.

In the case of the soldier, comment was made concerning the attitude of unconcern manifested toward his disability. This satisfied indifference and pathological tranquility, characterized by Janet as *la belle indifférence*, is of diagnostic significance in a conversion reaction, representing as it does the characteristic use of denial as a means of defense. The conflict having been solved and anxiety having been relieved through conversion of the repressed impulses and wishes into a functional symptom, an outward calm follows, even though the symptom produced is so disabling that it would presumably be a source of great concern.

Accident or Compensation Neurosis

Industrial accidents, in which a question of indemnification for a real or presumed disability may arise, are frequently followed by a definite psychoneurotic reaction. The presenting features of these reactions may be those of anxiety, hypochondriasis, conversion, or mixed types. Frequently the conversion symptoms are sufficiently prominent so that compensation neuroses are often classified among the hysterias. It was formerly considered that a desire for what the patient considered adequate compensation was the principal, if not exclusive, factor in the production of neuroses following industrial accidents. In recent years, closer studies of the patient's personality have shown that other factors also are usually dynamically important.

Persons of a paranoid tendency, those who are insecure, and those who crave sympathy and attention are predisposed to compensation neurosis. The same is true of the individual who finds himself in an employment situation that is becoming progressively more unbearable. The necessity, because of financial obligations, for continuing work beyond mental or physical capacity, or the failure to derive satisfaction from one's work may predispose to a traumatic or compensation neurosis. Some incidental gain resulting from an injury, such as escape from dreary or wearisome conditions of employment, may be important contributing factors.

Oversolicitude on part of the patient's family or an injudicious remark by the physician in the first days or weeks after an injury concerning its severity may create fear in the mind of the patient and predispose to the development of a neurosis. Experience connected with bodily helplessness, disturbance of business resulting from the accident, or worry about cure may conduce to its development. Not only a desire for financial gain but the conviction on the part of the patient that he has the right to expect indemnification may be motivating factors. Social custom and public opinion tend to encourage the development of accident neuroses by their attitude toward the question of responsibility.

The probability of developing a compensation neurosis following a relatively slight injury is greater than if the injury is so disabling as to be obviously compensative. Mild traumatic residuals may become heavily overlaid with hysterical elaborations. The traumatic or accident neuroses rarely occur when the victim of the injury must bear the brunt of the financial responsibility for the accident, as in the case of injuries sustained in sports. There is usually an incubation period between the injury and the appearance of the mentally determined symptoms. This interval before the development of the chronic disabilities is of value in excluding an organic source. It is usually occupied with vague ruminations that tend to be of an imaginative, affective, resentful, wish-determined, and suggestive nature.

SYMPTOMS. The symptoms of the accident neuroses are various, but these neuroses differ in no essential feature from others except in the matter of compensation. Frequently the symptoms include irritability, stubbornness, argumentativeness, crying spells, anxiety, depression, sleeplessness, headache, and dizziness. The patient is garrulous in describing his feelings and may complain of poor memory and inability to concentrate. If the foreman, "company doctor," or insurance adjuster questions the genuineness of his symptoms or the validity of his claim that the injury was sustained while at work, the patient frequently reacts with an indignation and resentment that aggravates and prolongs his symptoms. The fact that a hysterical reaction may be superimposed on an organic injury that has escaped attention should not be forgotten. Sometimes the neurotic symptoms do not become seriously troublesome until after the patient has returned to his employment, when they become so aggravated that he gives up work.

Tremors, paralyses, and other motor and sensory conversion symptoms occur. At times the necessary form of treatment for the original injury may be instrumental in suggesting a disability in a person of a hysterical type. Immobilization by splints of an injured extremity, for example, may be followed by its paralysis. As in other psychoneuroses, symptoms may be firmly fixed by over-examination or by over-treatment based on wrong premises. The development of symptoms through suggestion is, of course, in no way limited to accident neuroses involving the matter of compensation. A repetition of physical examinations may aggravate symptoms when organic disease exists and produce them when no disease exists. The fact that the physician's words and acts may have a suggestive effect upon the patient imposes a special responsibility upon him. In those cases in which indemnification is a participating motive, the patient remains unaware of such an influence and denies that he desires compensation, declaring that he would gladly forego any financial satisfaction could he be restored to health. He complains of his symptoms, but he rarely asks how he may get rid of them. Underlying feelings of guilt may be over-compensated and experienced as self-pity.

Workmen's compensation acts and industrial accident insurance have greatly increased the incidence of compensation neuroses. The effect on the worker of the general practice of awarding compensation for injury is to create a receptive mental state so that, when injury occurs, there follows an unconscious wishing for compensation. This does not at all mean that a worker who, following an industrial accident, complains of symptoms without organic basis is a malingerer or that compensation is not merited. The disability, it is true, would not have occurred had the results of the injury not possessed potential benefits in some form. The misfortune is that the injury in the "damage-suit" hysteria occurred in a person who was psychologically predisposed to a neurotic reaction. The existence of litigation tends to maintain the patient's focus on his injury, particularly if legal processes are prolonged. Contrary, however, to a frequent belief, the end of litigation does not always terminate the symptoms promptly. A termination does usually, however, have a salutary effect on the symptoms by removing one factor that has tended to keep the patient's attention focused on himself.

Mention should be made of the *occupation neuroses*, a large proportion of which, particularly those characterized by spasms, are to be looked upon as hysterical. In these neuroses, the patient, on attempting to execute some specialized movement in an occupation requiring the co-ordination of groups of muscles, suffers from a spasm of the muscles involved

in this act. Their function remains unimpaired when an attempt is made to employ the same muscles for the performance of some other act.

Diagnosis of Conversion Reactions

In addition to differentiation from the other neurotic reactions, features of which it often shares, hysteria is to be differentiated from organic disorders, malingering, schizophrenia, and the psychophysiological reactions. A conversion reaction may simulate an astonishing variety of organic symptoms, in making a differentiation from which certain principles should be held in mind. One should, of course, ascertain if sensory and motor disturbances are consistent with known anatomical facts. Conversion symptoms often change from time to time and with suggestion. Reflex and trophic disturbances do not accompany hysterical disturbances aside from the changes that may come from chronic disuse following a paralysis. Before deciding that a physical sign or somatically expressed symptom is of psychogenic origin, one should carefully attempt to ascertain if a setting of affective dissatisfaction existed before the appearance of the sign or symptom.

The patient's attitude of satisfied indifference toward his disability and the circumstances under which the disorder arose are often significant. The coincidence or immediate sequence of an acute emotional state and the appearance of physical phenomena are suggestive, especially if the connection between the psychological event and the sign is unrecognized by the patient. In actual physical disease, the patient readily accepts or even suggests the statement that his disability is of mental origin. On the other hand, the patient whose disability is psychogenic eagerly seeks for a physical basis. Both patients, of course, are really attempting to avoid the truth. It is always well for the physician to ask himself if the signs and symptoms serve a purpose in the life of the patient (secondary gain) and not let the apparent loss or suffering exclude hysteria from consideration. In making the diagnosis of conversion hysteria, too, one should not rely solely on the presence of conversion symptoms but should also consider whether the patient is an emotionally immature type of person. It must be remembered, too, that organic disability and a conversion reaction are not mutually exclusive. Organic neurological disabilities are not rarely complicated by superimposed conversion phenomena.

The confusion of a conversion reaction with malingering is most apt to be made by persons who consider all hysterics as malingerers and mistakenly believe that the hysteric could control his symptom if he wanted to. Discrepancies, contradictions, and exaggerations of symptoms are more frequent in malingering; also, the malingerer usually expresses much concern about his symptoms. In the classical form of major conversion hysteria, the patient manifests little concern about them. Because, however, of the considerable component of anxiety often accompanying a recently established conversion reaction, the patient may show signs of concern. Surprise examinations or observation of which the patient is unaware may reveal the deception in malingering. Conversion reactions and malingering have much in common. The difference is largely one of the relative degree in which consciousness participates in the reaction. In malingering there is a subtle interweaving of conscious and unconscious factors.

Since there may be reactions in schizophrenia strongly resembling hysteria, the diagnosis is not always easy. The native temperament of the patient may be somewhat indicative, that of the hysteric person having been characterized by more easily shifting emotions. In hysteria a dominant affect usually exists, there are no inconsistencies in symptoms and no disturbance of associations, there is a greater response to any emotional reaction on the part of nurse or relative, and there is no deterioration in habits of dress or cleanliness. In hysteria there is an apparent desire to be the center of attention, and it will usually be found that either parent or mate has been accustomed to exhibit a sympathetic and exaggerated emotional reaction to any illness on the part of the patient. Here the aid of the clinical psychologist may be most helpful, particularly as the usual diagnostic interviewing with the hysterical patient is distorted through his unwitting use of denial and the force of repression.

Attention was called in Chapter 27 to the fact that conversion reactions should be distinguished from psychophysiological reactions, in which tension and anxiety arising from psychological conflicts and emotional stresses are allayed, not by channelizing them through voluntary muscular and special sense systems (conversion), but through the vegetative nervous system into visceral organ symptoms and complaints. Yet many patients show combinations of both varieties of reaction.

Prognosis

The degree to which conversion mechanisms can be eliminated depends to a considerable degree on the extent to which evasions become habitual in early life and on the maturity and independence of the personality pattern. The prognosis depends, too, upon the strength or weakness of the patient's personality resources in relation to the environmental demands and to the other stresses that he will be called upon to face. If the patient's capacity for social adaptation has been limited, if it has been his habit to deal with minor difficulties by evasive methods, or if he has led an aimless existence without drive or ambition, it is probable that further conversion defenses will be employed. Symptomatology alone is a poor guide as to the future. If the patient was formerly well adjusted and the conversion reaction was brought on by unusual stress, the prognosis is favorable, provided return to the precipitating situation is not required.

The patient who has consciously thought how his difficulties would be solved by the chance appearance of disabling illness may easily and unconsciously permit the thought to become a reality. The presence of felt anxiety, with its indication that the conversion reaction is not providing an adequate defense, makes the prognosis less favorable. The childish egocentric patient who becomes increasingly dependent on his conversion symptoms has a poor prognosis. His conversion reaction becomes a more or less permanent mode of life, and he grows increasingly dependent on his symptoms.

The conversion reaction, in many instances, is engrafted upon a basically schizoid personality structure. With such persons, the psychotic reaction eventually becomes apparent. This is particularly so in groups of patients diagnosed as hysterical and followed for years after their initial admission to a mental hospital. On the other hand, similar follow-up studies over a period of a decade on patients who presented in a general hospital or outpatient clinic a monosymptomatic conversion make it clear that, even with treatment by measures designed only to modify the symptoms without restructuring the personality, the majority remained well and made excellent social adjustments. The outlook is best in the monosymptomatic hysteria that occurs in adult life rather than adolescence. Presumably here the response takes place in the face of a severe stress.

Treatment

In the treatment of a conversion reaction, the psychiatrist attempts to ascertain the purpose of the symptom and to discover the factors causing anxiety so great that it could be handled only through the mechanism of conversion with functional physical symptoms. Since the patient's disorder arose through mental causes and through the operation of mental mechanisms, the treatment should basically be that of psychotherapy.

The nature and energy of the dynamic factors that have led to the patient's symptoms are concealed from his recognition, and any explanation of the underlying mechanism is often received with resistance and protest. The patient's conversion reaction may, too, appear so remote from his emotional problem that only a searching analysis can uncover the relationship between the two.

Before beginning psychotherapy, the physician should first make a thorough physical examination. If no evidence is found that there is physical disease, no more physical examinations should be made, even though new symptoms occur. Continued examinations and long hospitalization may cause new symptoms to appear and old ones to become fixed.

The psychiatrist should remember that he must deal with two distinct although related problems: one, the removal of the symptom, the other, that of enabling the patient to apprehend the source of his anxiety and the significance of his symptom in order that he may form a more constructive method of action for the future. It is much easier to dispel a conversion than to help the patient to achieve further emotional growth. The principal attention, too, should be directed to a discovery of the psychogenic factors and their adjustment. If this objective is attained, the symptom will, of itself, disappear. It is important to make a correct estimate of the patient's personality stability and maturity and of his intellectual resources. If the personality limitations are relatively minimal, the treatment may be psychotherapeutic and based on analytical principles, with an investigation of the dynamic factors of repression. In a majority of cases, however, an extensive investigation of the whole personality and its development is not essential. In the person of low intelligence and in the unstable individual who develops a conversion reaction in a relatively uncomplicated situation, the principal therapy will probably have to be limited to suggestion, hypnosis, and re-education. In no case must the patient be accused of dishonesty or of a lack of desire to get well.

When the conversion symptom presents as a major disability incompatible with return to social and vocational activities, consideration must be given to its rapid reduction by the methods just described. In making this clinical judgment, the psychiatrist keeps in mind the defensive nature of the symptom and should evolve a concept of what the symptom defends against. With its rapid removal, he is aware that there will occur either overt anxiety or substitution by another symptom with equivalent symbolic significance. Either of these alternatives may be more suitable than major paralytic symptoms, blindness, choreiform states, or astasia–abasia. However, in those instances in which rapid symptom removal is likely to induce serious disruptions of self-esteem with anxiety, shame, and guilt, associated with regressive phenomena, this judgment is avoided. Such serious regressions are likely in those in whom the personality is essentially schizoid or there exist other symptoms indicative of an underlying schizophrenic reaction. Narcosynthesis, persuasion, or hypnosis, as described in Chapter 32 are the therapeutic measures of choice for rapid removal of symptoms. Once the acute symptomatic disability is modified, the psychiatrist will then determine the potential for character change through the use of a dynamic psychotherapy. If this potential is considered to exist, psychoanalytic psychotherapy is recommended as a means of avoiding further symptomatic recurrences. These methods of treatment are described also in Chapter 32.

Evidence for the presence of a schizophrenic disturbance may be gained by careful assessment of the developmental history. Family history of psychotic disturbance or pre-existing information of a dependent, withdrawn, and isolated life with resort to fantasy or other disordered behavioral traits should arouse suspicion. Often, because of denial by the hysteric in presenting his life history initially, valid information is not obtained. Many consider that the aid of psychological tests, particularly the projective methods, should always be sought in such instances before treatment goals are determined and therapy is initiated. Such tests may provide clues as to the potentiality of

severe regressions that will require hospital treatment if sudden removal of symptoms appears to be the method of choice. One of the authors has been impressed with the frequency of such regressions in patients who present numerous pure color reactions in their Rorschach responses.

In the treatment of *accident neuroses* there are certain factors that require special attention. In case of injury any suggestion that it is serious should be carefully avoided. If possible, the injured person should be kept at work, and if his condition does not permit this, he should return as promptly as possible. Care should be exercised that the treatment of any physical complication is not prolonged. The attitude of the physician toward a patient suffering from a traumatic neurosis should never be one of suspicion or antagonism. If he approaches the patient in a biased, skeptical attitude, disregards his complaints, and makes but a superficial examination, he destroys the possibility of any therapeutic rapport and may even contribute to further psychological elaboration.

A hope for indemnification on the part of the injured employee makes it impossible for him to disregard unpleasant sensations or unpleasant subjective experiences or to adjust himself to them. In contrast to an athlete similarly injured, the workman, doubtless unwittingly, is prompted to magnify rather than ignore the discomforts resulting from his injury. The harshness and disregard of complaints by representatives of insurance companies, a ready assumption of intent to swindle, and the delays and technicalities of court procedure tend to stimulate unwholesome patterns of reaction. Such attitudes engender resentment and discouragement and may force the injured person to resort to a primitive (conversion) mode of response. Whether a compensation award granted to the workman suffering from a traumatic neurosis is paid in a single sum or extended through a number of installments makes little difference so far as the neurosis is concerned. It is important, however, that a settlement be made promptly and that any litigation be terminated.

OBSESSIVE–COMPULSIVE REACTION

In the obsessive–compulsive reaction, the patient's anxiety is automatically controlled by associating it with persistently repetitive thoughts and acts. The patient recognizes that his unwanted thoughts and ritualistic acts are unreasonable, but he is unable to control them. The obsessive–compulsive reaction may be expressed in three clinical forms: (1) the persistent recurrence of an unwelcome and often distressing thought; (2) a morbid and often irresistible urge to perform a certain repetitive, stereotyped act; and (3) an obsessively recurring thought accompanied by a compulsion to perform a repetitive act. Obsessive ideation may be concerned with various topics. Frequently the patient must fight against thoughts that are repugnant to his conscious moral and esthetic feelings, such as thoughts of a blasphemous nature or fantasies of killing a beloved member of his family. Although horrified that he should entertain such thoughts the patient is unable to rid himself of them. The intruding and constantly recurring thought may be pointless and absurd, such as the case described by Ireland, whose well-educated patient persistently wondered why a chair had four legs instead of one leg, or a ruminative preoccupation and speculation on such topics as creation, infinity, or other philosophical or religious questions. The condition of being obsessively preoccupied with an apparently indifferent topic, with marked exclusion of other interests, is sometimes known as an obsessive–ruminative state. At times, considerable overt anxiety may be associated with such states. The greater the effort to dispel obsessive thoughts, the more stubbornly they return. Ritualistic activities may be performed in an effort to dispel or counteract the thoughts. Practically never do such patients carry out any recurring thoughts suggesting an immoral or violent act, although they may become very apprehensive lest they do so. The inability of the patient to free himself from the distressing thought may rarely lead him to suicide.

Types of Obsessive–Compulsion

FOLIE DU DOUTE. Some obsessive thinking assumes the form of *folie du doute* characterized by persistent doubting, vacillation, and indecision, usually with compulsive ruminations that lead to repetitive acts aimed to dispel the irrational doubts. Because of them, the patient must check and recheck even the simplest acts. He may, for example, lock the front door at night, but no sooner has he reached his bed than he is in doubt about the security of the door. He must therefore return and try the lock. Even then his doubts may recur after he is again in bed and require further visits to verify that the door is locked. Obsessive doubts and indecisions not rarely arise in case of conflict between desire and counterdesire.

Insistent, obsessive thoughts are defensive in purpose. The persistent idea is not to be taken at face value, so to speak. It is a substitute for another idea and thereby serves an anxiety-preventing function. Other affects are concealed behind the apparent content. The real sources may be any impulse, tendency, or wish that would be consciously intolerable to the patient. A hidden feeling of guilt is not an uncommon source. The manifest and recurring idea is the result of an effort to keep something else out of the mind and is formed by the mechanisms of displacement, symbolization, and condensation. The process is much the same as that occurring in a dream, where the latent or true content is concealed by these mechanisms so that the idea, wish, or impulse appears in the conscious dream in distorted and symbolized form.

COMPULSIVE ACTS. A second clinical type of obsessive–compulsive reaction is that of compulsive acts. In this there is the obligatory repetition of a certain act. The forces that produce the compulsive act are, of course, unconscious. Since the symbolic act cannot adequately satisfy the forces that produced it, the act is stereotyped and repetitive. When the patient is asked the reason for his behavior, he may either offer some explanation that he knows has no rational basis or he may admit that it is absurd and purposeless. Usually the patient consciously experiences some rejection and resistance to the carrying out of his defensive, compulsive act, but tension and anxiety mount until the urge to repeat becomes irresistible. If the patient is prevented from carrying out his compulsive ritual, overt anxiety appears. One of the most frequent forms of obsessive–compulsive rituals is that of handwashing, which has for its purpose the warding off of anxiety.

Most obsessive–compulsive acts consist merely of such simple, useless acts as touching or counting, or excessive ones, such as repeated handwashing. Some, however, become elaborate rituals or ceremonials. They superficially appear as meaningless formalities and are only recognized as neurotic ceremonials when a necessity for renouncing them is accompanied by discomfort and anxiety.

The ritualistic ceremonial described by Freud in one of his earliest papers (1896), entitled "The Defense Neuropsychoses," is often quoted and is an excellent illustration of the complexity that may be assumed by these compulsive devices designed to protect against anxiety:

"An 11-year-old boy had instituted the following obsessive ceremonial before going to bed. He did not sleep until he had told his mother in the minutest detail all the events of the day; there must be no scraps of paper or other rubbish on the carpet of the bedroom; the bed must be pushed right to the wall; three chairs must stand by it and the pillows must lie in a particular way. In order to get to sleep he must first kick out a certain number of times with both legs and then lie on his side."

The function of compulsive acts also is to allay or bind anxiety. The compulsive act that the patient performs has, it will be found, a symbolic significance. This symbolic act serves as a sort of magic ritual by which he undoes or annuls the possible effect of his unrecognized impulses and achieves a distorted satisfaction, self-punishment, and atonement. The compulsive act serves as a sort of magic ritual that temporarily dispels the dangerous situation; as long as it can be carried out, the intensity of the anxiety is reduced. If the performance of the ritualistic substitutive act is resisted or impossible, the effectiveness of the protective obsessive–compulsive defense is eliminated, and the forbidden wishes and impulses arouse anxiety. The need for ritualized behavior increases, since the unconscious striving threatens to erupt into consciousness; more and more symptoms must be constructed to provide defenses against the forbidden tendencies. In many respects, the defensive patterns of the compulsions resemble penances, atonements, and punishments, or serve as precautions, prohibitions, and restrictions. In many ways, they are closely allied psychologically to the ceremonies and taboos that primitive people devise as protections against demonological and other supernatural forces.

Compulsive acts are not uncommon in children and adolescents, in whom they originate as expiatory ceremonials or as means whereby, through attributing a certain magic-like power to an act, a particularly desired wish may be attained. The acts then become established through habit, but they normally disappear as repressed tensions subside and more adequate social adjustments are established.

PHOBIA WITH COMPULSION. The third type of obsessive–compulsive reaction is that in which a phobia or obsessively recurring idea is associated with a compulsion to perform a repetitious act. This association occurs when there exists an overpowering fear of intolerable impulses. Usually considerable anxiety is observable. One of the commonest examples of this type of reaction is a repetitive handwashing, the result of an obsessive fear of dirt or uncleanliness. Whatever object the patient touches has, he is confident, left his hands contaminated. Since he can scarcely avoid touching objects, he must repeatedly wash his hands. As every object is a possible source of contamination, the patient may resort to complicated and troublesome means of avoiding the touching of objects. He may open doors with his elbows or handle articles with gloves or other coverings. One patient washed each Saturday the church pew she expected to occupy the following day. Because of this tension, preoccupation, and irresistible handwashing, the capacity for gainful employment may be destroyed.

Here, too, are found the same mechanisms of displacement and undoing. The real fear is, of course, not of dirt but of intolerable impulses or guilt-laden strivings that have been displaced and symbolized by constant preoccupation with fear of dirt. The anxiety to which they have given rise is temporarily alleviated by the compulsive washing, with its symbolically cleansing significance.

Adolf Meyer described a group of persons characterized by difficulty with decisions, by doubts, rituals, and fears, and with anticipation of panic should fulfillment fail to be achieved. Anxiety and depression are common accompaniments. He designated these reactions as "obsessive–ruminative tension states."

Psychogenetically, the origin of obsessive–compulsive behavior is believed to rest in the early struggle of the growing child between his drives for omnipotent self-assertion and the necessity to conform to the demands of his parents in order to maintain their love and respect. The early period of toilet training initiates the conflict. Often the later obsessive–compulsive individual is one brought up by a rigid compulsive mother, who insistently demands compliance and threatens both loss of love and various forms of punishment for failure to behave properly. The growing child is then exposed to repeated arousal of rage through the insistent requirements for cleanliness and compliance but must repress them in order to retain his relationship with the parent. Very early he

learns to regard his underlying thoughts of hostile reprisal to be taboo, and therefore, subject to punishment and requiring penance. He may learn, by observing the parents, that his defiant behavior provides gratification in the attentions of the parent, yet at the same time he must then atone both by carrying out the parental desire as well as an associated expiatory act. This train of behavioral responses, derived from the long-continued relationship with such parental figures, becomes internalized and unconscious so that each thought reflecting rage or hostility sets in action the psychodynamic train of ambivalently balanced action and counteraction symbolizing rage, gratification, compliance, and expiation.

The following case illustrates many of the features of a mixed phobic and compulsive reaction.

S. K. was admitted to a mental hospital at the age of 29. The family history revealed no significant history. During the second and third grades of school "he was a problem to the nuns because of his stuttering. They would ask him to read a paragraph over two or three times." For a considerable period at this age "he felt he had to bless himself a certain number of times in the evening." When in the fourth grade and after an illness "he was afraid to go to sleep at night for fear he might die. He would call his mother two or three times before going to sleep. He would not go to sleep unless she reassured him that he would not die. This lasted for two or three months." He bit his nails until he was 16 years of age.

At the time of his admission, the patient's mother and wife were requested to describe his adult personality characteristics. He was, they reported, a quiet, serious, honest, thrifty, saving, stubborn, and somewhat worrisome person. "He was ambitious. He wanted to go through college and be more than an ordinary working man. In college he studied very, very hard, and was an honor student." When 18 years of age the patient drank excessively for a period of several months. He then suddenly stopped and became so opposed to liquor that, to quote his wife, "He wouldn't touch a drop, and I remember once when we were both young he walked out of a home where liquor was being served because he was so opposed to it."

He enlisted in the Marine Corps. When, after his admission to the hospital, he was asked what prompted him to volunteer, he replied, "Well, I felt uneasy a little bit with my scrupulosity. I wasn't too uneasy, but I thought somehow the service would take it away." Asked what he meant by 'scrupulosity,' he said "I was doubtful about my confessions." Asked if he was doubtful that he didn't confess enough, his answer was, "That's right; I didn't have enough sorrow for my sins." When the admitting physician asked the patient about his duties in the military service, he replied, "I had a job cleaning urinals. I probably was very good. I tried to do a thorough job. I saw cigarettes, but I always kept on cleaning all the time. It could have been done in 2 or 3 hours, but I worked 8 or 9 hours. I volunteered for the job." Two years later he wrote his fiancée that he wished to break his engagement as he was going to study for the priesthood after discharge from service. Six months later he wrote again, saying he had decided not to become a priest and asked that their engagement be renewed. Twenty-four months later he was married but had no sexual relations with his wife until 17 months later.

After his discharge from military service two years later, the patient entered college, from which he was graduated, although several months before, his neurotic reaction had become so disabling that he was unable to continue his studies for the final two months of his senior year.

Soon after the patient's admission to the hospital, his wife was asked to give a history of the patient's illness. She reported that he had exhibited a compulsive handwashing for several months but that it became more serious. "He used to wash his hands and keep the water running for 15 minutes at a time. After he had washed them, he would turn off the spigot with his elbow. He had to count and wash and rinse his hands a certain number of times. If he had touched the door or door knob, he would go back and wash his hands again. One time he began to wash his hands at 1 o'clock in the morning. After we moved into our own house, he refused to use the front door or to turn the knob on the door for fear there might be germs. He used to go to the back window and call me to go to the front door and open it for him. He reached the point where he would climb in and out of windows so that he wouldn't have to enter the doors at all." The wife described also the following compulsion: "He also had the idea that when he walked there was something under his shoe. He would stop and look on the sole of his shoe, but there would be nothing there. He also worried as to whether or not his shoe laces were tied. He would pick up his foot and look to make sure. He had to do that a certain number of times before he was absolutely sure they were tied. When he walked down a street, if he kicked a stone he felt that he should put it back in the same place. If he walked on a line, then he would have to walk on all the cracks in the sidewalk."

On arrival at the hospital, the patient stated to the admitting physician, "I like to wash my hands many times a day in order to get them good and clean." While talking to the physician, he stood with his arms folded in order to avoid touching anything. He readily acknowledged that he was worried about touching objects lest he give others disease. As he seemed somewhat depressed, he was asked about suicidal thoughts. He replied that he felt he would be better off dead than to be thinking of the things he did but added that he would "not really" commit suicide. He then added, "When I say things, they have to be said a certain way. If I don't say them properly, I must apologize. I do this all the time. This irritated my wife and was another reason why she couldn't live with me. I would leave my books to apologize to her. It was the apologizing that was bothering her—not being at peace. I thought if I rubbed my hands 88 times, shut the water off, and then went back again, it would be all right. Then I thought maybe it hadn't been 88 times."

A month after the patient's admission, his ward physician entered the following note in the clinical record: "This patient has become extremely disturbed over his obsessive–compulsive ideation during recent days. He stops his physician at every opportunity and repeatedly asks the same questions, which include the following: "Should I wash my hands after I go to the bathroom and just do number one? Should I wash my hands when I go to the bathroom and have a bowel movement? My penis touches the toilet seat. Do you think I should wash it off with soap and water so there won't be a spread of disease? I wouldn't want anyone to get this disease. There's a rash there. Do you want to look at it? I think it is some sort of a disease. I'm afraid everybody will get it. I don't know, doctor, I'm afraid something is going to happen. I have a feeling that I might go crazy or something. Someone asked me if I thought these things were silly and I said, 'Yes,' but now that I think of it, they don't seem silly. I just can't quite explain them. They must not really seem silly to me or I wouldn't have to do them like I do." The patient manifested an interesting inability to make any definite statement or to take any decisive action. When discussing a point he would say such things as the following: "Well, doctor, it's just like this. Well, no, it isn't exactly like that. I should say rather that's a little on the order of—well, that isn't quite right either. Perhaps I should put it this way. It's more of—uh—well, no, that isn't it."

Under therapy, the patient gradually improved. Two years after his admission he left the hospital for employment in a brick plant. A report received a year later stated that, although not entirely well, he was successfully employed.

Prognosis

In adults the prognosis in obsessive–compulsive neuroses is not good, although a recent study has shown that a large percentage of individuals with this condition suffer episodic attacks and are able to adapt socially. The patient's compulsive needs frequently interfere seriously with his comfort and efficiency. In extreme cases his constant preoccupation with his protective rituals renders him socially impossible. Some psychiatrists characterize the obsessive neuroses as intermediate between neuroses and psychoses. The obsessive–compulsive states of children usually disappear with time if not taken seriously in the presence of the child. Such compulsions grow out of childhood anxiety, often a single one. The prognosis is much more serious if the onset is during adolescence or early adult life.

Diagnosis

In all the neuroses, there are fine gradations between what at one extreme are usually looked upon merely as personality traits to incapacitating distress at the other extreme. One, therefore, may well be in doubt at times whether a given person should be considered within the limits of normality or whether he should be looked upon as a compulsive neurotic. In the fully developed cases, with their well-marked obsessive thinking, fears, or compulsive acts, there is, of course, no question. Since, however, we all have defensive character traits, the decision must often be arbitrary. Perhaps the criterion should be whether there are repressions that require such drastic supporting measures that these defenses seriously disturb the subjective life of the individual. Ordinarily, the exaggerated traits of character, such as stern conscientiousness or over-moral and over-ascetic scruples, are not included, although, like the frankly neurotic symptoms, they are defensive in purpose.

A diagnosis between early schizophrenia and the obsessive–compulsive neuroses is at times exceedingly difficult. The obsessive thinking of the psychoneurotic may not be unlike the subjective rumination of the schizophrenic, although the compulsive ritual of the former may suggest the mannerisms of the latter. The symbolisms seen in the compulsive acts of the neurotic individual, as well as the substitutive nature of the phobias, are close both in resemblance and in relationship to the symbols seen in schizophrenia. It not infrequently happens that what is first thought to be the ruminative and obsessive tension state of a neurotic subsequently becomes an obvious schizophrenic reaction, usually of the paranoid type. In general, it may be said that the greater the rumination and the less the tension, the nearer does the reaction approach that of the schizophrenic. A failure on the part of the patient to regard his phobias and compulsions as absurd and particularly to refer them to external influences indicates a malignant, schizophrenic origin. The compulsive neurotic never loses the capacity for discrimination between subjective experiences and reality, as is the case in schizophrenia. Finally, as Bleuler points out, the compulsive neurotic struggles *against* his obsession, whereas the delusional patient struggles *with* his idea.

At times the genuine depressions of manic–depressive psychosis may be accompanied by obsessive ideas. In differentiating such cases from compulsive states, one will inquire which appeared first, the depression or the obsessive idea.

Treatment

Fully developed obsessional and compulsive reactions are even more refractory to treatment than the milder psychoses. It is therefore important that treatment be early. The obsessive–compulsive neuroses usually develop in individuals who have been characterized by compulsive personality traits. The neurosis is in many ways an exaggeration and caricature of that pattern. Effort is made, therefore, to discover the factors that, through their dynamic action, led first to the personality make-up and then to the neurosis. Treatment, then, should be psychotherapeutic and either consists of a formal psychoanalysis or is based on analytical principles. Guided by the therapist, the patient's unconscious is explored and his apparently irrational fears and compulsions take on new meaning when understood in terms of chronologically earlier experiences and early life dynamics. In all cases, but particularly in rigid personalities and in those of limited intellectual development, re-educational measures should be employed. The patient should be encouraged to evaluate the relative importance of matters and to learn that indecision and perfectionism should be curbed, even at the cost of errors and mediocrity. Such attitudes as excessive guilt and overconscientiousness should be discussed. Cultivation of latent interests may help to reduce the ruminative thinking to which these patients are often addicted. Self-preoccupation and self-analysis are to be discouraged. Prefrontal leukotomy has at times been followed by improvement. It should, however, be confined to cases so severe that the patient is practically confined to his home and incapacitated for any useful activity because of his compulsions. Results are better when there is evidence of persistence and drive and when the obsessional symptoms are accompanied by considerable anxiety.

Although not included in the present official classification of psychiatric disorders, the term *hypochondria*, or hypochondriacal reaction, is one that was long applied to a group of psychoneurotic symptoms. Patients presenting these symptoms are now usually included in the obsessive–compulsive reaction group. The reaction is characterized by an obsessive preoccupation and concern of the individual about the state of his health or the conditions of his organs. Often he expresses a multiplicity of complaints about different organs or body systems, which, the patient reiterates, must be incurably diseased. The hypochondriac is not only aware of various sensations that most persons disregard, but he also magnifies the intensity of normal sensations of fatigue, et cetera. In many cases, the hypochondriasis seems to be a displacement of anxiety onto the body, with the resulting somatic complaints. Some hypochondriacal reactions may become excessively and persistently obsessional, and associated compulsions may develop.

GROSS STRESS REACTIONS

Following severe threat to life, whether as the consequence of stress in civilian life in the form of catastrophies experienced in accidents, floods, tornadoes, or volcanic eruptions, or as the stress of warfare and combat, a well-defined personality disorder frequently results. This condition, known much earlier in the German literature as fright (*schreck*) neurosis, in the English as a traumatic neurosis, may occur as an isolated disturbance or may complicate pre-existing personality disorders. In the United States, it probably occurs most commonly, and is most frequently unrecognized, after automobile accidents. Adler differentiates two types of post-traumatic states: those with immediate, and those with delayed, onset. In the current nomenclature of the American Psychiatric Association, this syndrome is not listed under the neuroses but under the Transient Situational Personality Disturbances as "gross stress reaction." The more profound reactions to catastrophic stress produce long-continuing disruption of personality functioning both in previously healthy and in neurotic persons. For this reason they are discussed here as a neurosis. Since the combat neuroses have been most thoroughly studied, they are given extended comment.

Combat Neuroses

Presumably combat neuroses have long been associated with warfare, although their real nature and psychopathology were not recognized until relatively recently. During the Civil War, DaCosta described the "Irritable Heart of Soldiers." This was undoubtedly a neurosis induced by the stress and anxiety of combat and closely resembled the "Disordered Action of the Heart," 80,000 cases of which, it is said, occurred among British soldiers during World War I. It is of interest that this high incidence was not reported in World War II, presumably because its nature had become recognized so much more fully and it was designated as a neurosis.

In World War I, artillery fire reached a new intensity, with a fear-producing potentiality probably never before attained by weapons of warfare. It was noticed that with this terrifying shell-fire, often combined with fear-inspiring air attacks, there appeared a striking variety of symptoms, including paralysis, gross tremors, mutism, blindness, confusion, or intense anxiety. In apparent absence of other etiological factors, it was at first concluded that the brain must in some undetermined manner sustain damage by a blast concussion attending the nearby explosion of a shell. Soldiers readily accepted the opinion of their physicians that their mental disabilities were of an irreparable nature as a result of brain injury. The term "shell shock" was therefore applied to these psychiatric casualties and prolonged hospitalization was prescribed for their treatment. Gradually it was recognized that "shell shock" was primarily a psychological problem and that the effect of air blast could not explain the immediate symptoms and subsequent persistent illness. Late in the war it became apparent, too, that prolonged hospitalization merely fostered and fixated the mental symptoms, which, because they prevented return to combat and even brought a compensation pension, provided a considerable secondary gain.

Before the end of World War II, it was recognized that recovery was much more prompt and lasting if the patient with an acute, battle-induced neurosis was treated near the front lines and returned to duty as soon as possible. It was also noted that the percentage of recoveries was greater if the attitude of the psychiatrist indicated that no organic damage had been sustained and if the name by which the neurosis was known to the soldier implied that the disability was temporary and recoverable and that no actual physical or mental illness existed. In the opinion of many psychiatrists, the term "shell shock" used during World War I probably set off more neurotic reactions through its injudicious use than did battle. In 1943, therefore,

the United States Army adopted the term "combat exhaustion" for the labeling of nearly all types of psychiatric casualties appearing in the forward areas. This term was adopted advisedly because of its implication that the disability is of a temporary and honorable nature, that it is the logical result of combat, and that rest and recuperation lead to recovery.

Extreme and repeated battle fear, with a constant threat of death plus intense fatigue, are the precipitating factors in the production of combat neurosis. Physical exhaustion alone is not sufficient to produce the neurosis, but it does serve to lessen resistance so that psychodynamic forces are more easily released. The greater, however, the element of decreased physical efficiency resulting from fatigue, lack of food and sleep, or intercurrent illness, the more easily does emotional breakdown occur and the greater is the possibility of not returning the soldier to active duty.

Although, as has been indicated, exhaustion, hardship, and fear are the most important and the precipitating factors in the development of war neuroses, other factors are often of significant influence in preparing the soil, so to speak, for the mental breakdown in battle. It is not easy to select the man who will maintain emotional equilibrium in combat and eliminate the one who will prove inadequate for the stress. It is not always the unstable and neurotic man who, as might be supposed, lacks resistance to the terror that accompanies long and intense combat. In general, it is the timid and passive person who cannot mobilize and externalize his anger and react aggressively toward the enemy and thus discharge his tension who is prone to develop a combat neurosis.

Most men, although wishing to meet the demands of their country, are inducted into the armed forces without strong, conscious desire for military life or for combat experience. Many at the time of induction are still emotionally dependent on their families, perhaps overprotected by their mothers, and intimidated by cruel fathers. It has been found, too, that an unduly large number of combat neuroses occurred in individuals from broken or distorted homes unfavorable for the development of a well-integrated and mature personality. Induction into military service is accompanied by the abrupt loss of emotional support provided by family and friends, the deprivation of female companionship, and the loss of individuality and privacy. Frequently, too, the unseasoned soldier has a feeling that he is not appreciated and nurses resentment resulting from the change from the relatively flexible and permissive civilian pattern of living to one of subjection to strict discipline, regimentation, and subordination.

The stresses and conflicts to which the soldier is exposed during his training period are relatively mild and are handled by most trainees without the development of protest symptoms in the form of neurotic or psychotic syndromes. Even though the period of training is not accompanied by the hazards of combat, normal gratifications are renounced and destructive goals are substituted for the constructive ones of previous civil life. New relationships that would meet the soldier's emotional needs in the strange and abnormal state of affairs have to be established. Under these circumstances, the most constructive relationship is the soldier's identification of himself as an integral part of his unit, and his unit as a part of himself. He should have confidence in his unit and in the character, capability, and bravery of his leader. With the formation of deep emotional relationship with his leader and his buddies, the soldier's feelings of security and power are increased and his morale, or those attitudes, feelings, and beliefs that promote participation in a united effort, is promoted.

In World Wars I and II and in the Korean campaign, the American soldier, following a period of overseas training and waiting with its boredom, suspense, and inactivity, moved forward to the field of combat warfare. Arrived there, he was precipitated, often without sufficient time for rest, into a situation fraught with constant danger and hardship and intense emotional and physical stress. The particular combat experiences of the soldier depend upon the branch of military service to which he is assigned, but in nearly all instances there is the continued threat of injury and death, accompanied by feelings of great intensity and wide variety. Common to all experiences is the emotional reaction of fear, the most potent source of emotional tension in combat.

Fear, it will be remembered, is an emotion experienced in response to a stimulus having actual reality, one that either constitutes a present threat to the individual or portends real danger. Anxiety, on the other hand, is an expectation of danger, an emotional state of apprehensiveness, uncertainty, and insecurity, that may be produced either from situations symbolic of external danger or from internal conflicts and tensions present in the unconscious. Frequently it springs from the threats of repressed hostility, aggression, or resentment. Although this distinction between fear and anxiety can be made, yet in war situations they operate jointly. Their feeling-tones and their accompanying physiological expressions are the same. Although anxiety really arises from internal threats, it is attributed to (projected upon) some real external source. In the war neuroses, this projection is upon a dangerous external situation that is also provocative of fear. Both fear and the feeling of apprehension and insecurity characteristic of anxiety may therefore seem to have a common source. To draw the line between the two is not always possible. In the battle situation, fear and other powerful external and emotional forces play upon the internal tensions and threats, upon the unconscious sources of anxiety. Of these sources of emotional stress in combat, fear is the most potent, its somatic and physiological effects being a source of great strain. Under combat circumstances, the various external and internal stresses conspire to produce a conflict that may become intolerable. The psychological defenses hitherto effective collapse, with a consequent rise of anxiety and the production of the neurotic symptom. Anxiety and its management constitute, therefore, one of the basic problems in war neuroses.

FACTORS CONTRIBUTING TO WAR NEUROSES. As already indicated, fear and an impairment of the ability to repress fear reactions are highly provocative of anxiety. A breakdown of group morale or an attitude of defeatism within the combat unit greatly increases the psychological strain. Such a loss of morale is particularly prone to exist in case of lack of faith in commanding officers, in the absence of identification with one's unit, or during a retreat. The quality of leadership is one of the most important factors in the incidence of neurotic breakdown in any given unit. Prolonged periods of enforced inactivity during which men are exposed to danger predispose to an anxiety reaction. So does the loneliness of foxhole fighting with the usual inability to communicate with comrades. Repeated narrow escapes, high combat losses, and repeated exposure to the mutilation and death of close friends increase apprehension and stimulate guilt and anxiety. Fear of being a coward or of losing one's self-control, a realization of the responsibility for the lives of others, and an insufficient understanding of war or a lack of conviction of the need to fight. A sense of guilt over expression of hostility is at times a psychogenetic factor. The regimentation and frustration of service life, separation from home and the existence of domestic difficulties are often of much greater significance than more dramatic events.

The necessity that the man "sweat it out" in a continuously hostile environment results almost inevitably in at least some degree of anxiety; there are also certain internal as well as external factors that tend to increase anxiety. One of these internal problems is the soldier's handling of his hostilities. During his civilian life he was called upon to inhibit any hostile or aggressive drives. Whereas he formerly had the value of human life constantly impressed upon him, the soldier is expected to kill as many men as possible. His hostility, which through long inhibition had become well repressed, is now to be released to kill men like himself. This release of hostile and aggressive drives in most destructive expression evokes anxiety. The problem of control of aggressive impulses is probably one of the soldier's heaviest psychological burdens. The combat situation demands release of hostility. Whatever their origin, any anxieties and tensions that add to the burden of the ego weaken its defensive functions and increase the possibility of a neurosis. Frustrations, such as unfair treatment in regard to promotions, citations, or leaves of absence, also bring to the fore resentment, hostility, and anxiety.

Feelings of guilt provoke anxiety as well. Such feelings may arise from the soldier's thought that he has been responsible for the death of someone else, perhaps of civilians as well as an enemy. Again, the death of a comrade toward whom the patient entertained ambivalent feelings or whom he had identified with a sibling rival may create feelings of guilt with anxiety or depression. An unconscious hostility may lead to a conviction on the part of the patient that he has actually caused the death of a comrade. At times, following the death of a buddy, a man develops a feeling of guilt through a belief that he failed to take care of his friend. Frequently the loss of a buddy or of a respected officer, by creating the feeling that one is being left alone, helpless, and deserted, deprives the soldier of emotional support and leads to an unendurable anxiety.

One important factor, then, in the production of combat neurosis is the excessive mobilization of emotions that have always been important in the personality but have not previously strained or overwhelmed the forces of control. Neurotic anxiety in battle may be rooted in passivity, hostility, or aggressiveness, and in the character of the personality defenses constructed against them in early life.

NEUROSIS-PREVENTING FACTORS. One of the most important mechanisms in strengthening the ego against factors productive of anxiety and other neurotic reactions is the soldier's identification with his unit. By this mechanism, he transfers a considerable share of his personal self-love to affection and pride in his outfit. His feelings of obligation and loyalty, having their source in this mechanism, overrule selfish, personal interests and provide one of the strongest motivations for combat and most effective protections against any expression of his conflicts. The group relationship and its emotional bonds are among the most constructive and integrative forces for the individual. Similarly, an intense loyalty to each other on the part of the fighting men and their immediate leaders promotes morale and raises the threshold against anxiety. A resolute personal motivation, good morale, sustained by pride in one's organization, good leadership, respect for officers and fellow soldiers, confidence in equipment, the feeling of being properly trained, high quality of food together with adequate recreational outlets are of great importance in preventing war neuroses. Other factors that aid in warding off anxiety are the desire to avoid loss of the esteem of the group by any failure in courage or in other demands of military tradition and also the habit of obedience and of disciplined behavior established by military training.

An additional factor that doubtless assists as an aid in the prevention of war neuroses is education through a series of lectures concerning the nature of fear. These lectures may be given to the soldier during his training period. He is told that fear is a normal emotion of battle and to experience it should not be considered as occasion for censure or self-depreciation. The soldier is given simple information concerning its physiological manifestations and the nature of the nervous reactions it produces. His recognition of fear and his effort to deal with it on a conscious level tend to minimize its anxiety-stimulating influence.

NORMAL BATTLE REACTION. To protect itself from an overwhelming threat to its existence, the organism becomes completely and continuously alert. This leads to severe and continuous emotional tension. In spite of the various factors that aid in the prevention of combat neuroses, such stresses as exhaustion, excitement, and mortal terror inevitably produce reactions that would be considered abnormal in a civilian setting, yet are not so incapacitating as to demand removal from combat. Unless extreme, such reactions must under the circumstances be considered within the range of normal. Many of the reactions represent psychosomatic responses to stress and fear. Among them are sensations of pulling or pressure over the back of the head and neck, muscular tension, shaking and tremor. In some cases, the soldier may be transitorily immobilized. Excessive perspiration is common, and some soldiers experience anorexia, nausea, vague abdominal distress, mild diarrhea, and urinary frequency. Tachycardia, palpitation, breathlessness, and a sense of thoracic oppression and of faintness together with generalized muscular weakness and lassitude often exist. Many soldiers experience difficulty in sleeping and have repetitive nightmares of battle and "startle" reactions to threatening noises. Irritability is normal in the soldier subjected to long-continued battle, and resentment is common among those who have lost friends and withstood privations and dangers.

An 18-year-old Navy radioman was admitted to a hospital with symptoms of anxiety and depression.

The patient was the youngest son in a happy family of four children. He was the favored child and throughout his early life gave no indication of instability. At school he was an average student and later was president of his high school class and an outstanding football player. At the outbreak of the war, he enlisted in the naval service with the consent of his parents, and immediately after completing his recruit training was detailed aboard a destroyer, where the morale was high. He made many close friends, and with the personal assistance of the communications officer, who helped him with the radio work, made a rapid advancement in rate.

The destroyer was part of the screen of an aircraft carrier engaged in the Coral Sea Battle, the raid on the Gilbert and Marshall Islands, and later the Battle of Midway. At the onset of each engagement, the patient felt apprehensive, but once firing commenced, he became entirely composed and attentive to his duties. While the destroyer was lying alongside a stricken aircraft carrier following a bombing attack during the Battle of Midway, the patient saw "torpedo wakes" approaching the ship; he resumed his post, until suddenly he was thrown out of his seat when the torpedo exploded beneath him. He plunged overboard, reached a nearby raft, and was later taken aboard another destroyer. He was then cognizant that his best friend, his immediate chief, and the communications officer, had all been killed. On being taken aboard the ship, he collapsed. Following his return to the naval base, it was learned that he had suffered blast injury to the chest and abdomen that eventually necessitated intestinal resection. During convalescence from this operation, he first had terrifying nightmares in which various scenes related to the sinking of the destroyer were continually repeated, and during which he awoke in a state of anxiety. Sudden noises also produced unusual apprehension.

There was no evidence of physical disease, but insomnia, anorexia, constipation, and fatigue were observed and psychiatric study was requested. The patient was listless, dejected, and emotionally labile. Discussion of his battle experiences was distressing to him, and he described in detail his sensitivity to sounds and various combat scenes in motion pictures. The latter stimulus invariably led to anxiety. After one month of treatment on the psychiatric service, he became more energetic and content, slept well, commenced to eat, gained some weight, and again desired to return to duty. Nightmares were infrequent and sounds were less disturbing to him.

NEUROTIC REACTION. As indicated, such symptoms as those described should, if of moderate degree, be considered as a gross stress reaction and as the base line from which pathological reactions should be evaluated. The combat neurosis consists therefore of pathological degrees of the reactions mentioned.

The most frequent form of combat neurosis is the *anxiety state*. This constitutes over 75 per cent of acute war neuroses. In moderate or mild anxiety states, the patient shows tension, tremor, apprehension, weeping, depression, feelings of guilt, dizziness, tinnitus, urinary frequency, insomnia, and battle dreams. Less frequently than in World War I, and usually in men of poor integration, the neurosis may consist of a *conversion reaction* with paralyses, sensory losses, aphonia, deafness, partial or total blindness, speech defects, astasia–abasia, a

fixed stooping posture known as camptocormia, and occasionally a persistent amnesia. Such patients exhibit little visible anxiety and may manifest "la belle indifférence." In the most severe reactions, the onset is acute and sudden. A coarse tremor is not uncommon. It may be difficult or impossible to establish contact with the patient. Even though no longer under fire, he may believe himself still in battle and behave accordingly. He may, with expressions of terror, call to his friends to look out for the shells. Some show highly dramatic reactions and excessive startle patterns in response to slight stimuli. In extreme cases, the soldier's behavior is one of panic reaction, in which there is apparently a complete disruption of personality organization. His uncontrolled, catastrophic reaction may vary from wild, impulsive flights to "freezing," or primitive protective withdrawal, with stupor, catatonia, or mutism.

Some cases of combat neurosis assume the form of *depression*, usually preceded by anxiety. The depression may not be particularly obvious until after the effort to control anxiety has failed. The depression is frequently precipitated by the death of a comrade to whose loss the soldier was unable to reconcile himself. The conscious mental content is dominated by ideas of failure, guilt, and self-condemnation. The patient is convinced that he has let his buddies down or that in some way he has been responsible for their deaths. Frequently such depressions arise in cases in which the patient has had ambivalent feelings directed toward a comrade. Upon the death of his buddy, the unconscious hostility that existed in these feelings stimulates the conviction that he actually caused the death of his comrade. This evokes guilt, depression, and self-punishment. The clinical symptoms are characterized by a rigid, mask-like face, by paucity of movement, and by ideas of self-accusation and self-depreciation.

A 17-year-old seaman had seven months' active duty prior to admission to the hospital with a tentative diagnosis of intracranial injury.

He was the third of four boys in a family of six. His father was a "shell-shocked" veteran of World War I, now alcoholic and a chronic complainer. The mother was migrainous. The home was kept discordant by parental quarrels; nevertheless, the patient, though of retiring and quiet nature, adjusted well at school, was accepted by his classmates, and was not considered temperamentally unstable.

Following his enlistment in the naval service, he received three weeks of basic training and was detailed aboard a transport for drill in amphibious operations. The patient had hoped for duty aboard a combat ship of the line. Three weeks prior to the departure of the convoys for the North African engagement, he was transferred to another ship. There he was barely acquainted with his new shipmates when the engagement opened. His immediate chief was regarded by him with little respect as an "old man." The seaman was extremely apprehensive as his landing boat approached the beach during the opening operations, but he quickly regained composure when not exposed to fire. The following day he was frightened to the point of believing his legs were paralyzed when an enemy plane strafed the ship and he threw himself on the deck. The fourth day the ship was suddenly torpedoed. He was blown against the bulkhead and struck his head but was not injured and quickly climbed down a net into a tank lighter below. While throwing out lines to men struggling in the water, he was fascinated by their cries and amazed to see some cast aside their life jackets. After helping one man aboard, the patient felt so weak that he lay upon the deck and later had to be assisted ashore. The following day a plane killed a French woman in town, and he morbidly examined her body and the leg wounds of a sailor wounded in the same raid.

He then realized how tense and anxious he felt, and in the following weeks had difficulty in sleeping, being repeatedly awakened by dreams in which his ship was torpedoed or he was shot in the leg. While aboard the transport returning home, he and the men in his division were quartered in a forward compartment. During a prolonged storm, the group repeatedly rushed to the boat deck in panic when a loose hatch cover slammed above them. He was given a 30-day leave after arriving in this country, but the change in his personality was so conspicuous to his family that his mother shortly sought medical advice concerning his symptoms.

On return to duty, the patient complained of headaches and dizziness and was transferred to the hospital for study. As there was no evidence of organic disease, psychiatric examination was requested. His extreme restlessness, amounting to agitation, and his inattentiveness and irritability were immediately apparent. He was unable to concentrate, expressed death fears, and presented the history of nightmares and sensitivity to sounds reminiscent of combat. His sleep was broken almost nightly by terrifying dreams. With sedation and psychotherapy there was some diminution in the restlessness, the insomnia, and his response to startle. He put on weight but continued to complain and insisted upon his inability to return to duty. It was evident that he would not again adjust in the service and, accordingly, he was recommended for discharge.

This youthful seaman, who was reared in a discordant home by a neurotic, alcoholic father and a high-strung mother, presented no evidence of emotional instability prior to his traumatic combat experience. He then developed nightmares, a startle reaction, and a personality change marked by agitation, anxiety, and preoccupation, with the complaints of headaches and dizziness. The case study illustrates the importance in determining the neurotic reaction of a disturbed home life with the possibility of neurotic identification, and the contributing factors of inadequate training, indifference to leadership, and low morale. The repeated panics during the voyage home probably further served to deepen the patient's anxiety by the process of conditioning.

PSYCHOPHYSIOLOGIC SYMPTOMS. Physical symptoms often associated with anxiety constitute a frequent form of psychiatric disability in military service. Such symptoms may be referred to any part of the body and may appear in the soldier's training period or may be precipitated or aggravated by battle stress. Sometimes they are seen in areas of the body previously the loci of disease, wounds, or injuries. The soldier then suffers pain or other discomfort out of all proportion to physical signs. In other cases, the emotionally upset soldier reports "sick" with types of disability—rheumatic, asthenic, gastrointestinal—that are acceptable to his group as having originated through no fault of his own but providing, nevertheless, a relatively nonpunishing escape from a psychologically intolerable situation. The somatic manifestations discussed in this paragraph should be regarded as physical expressions of anxiety rather than as conversion phenomena. If such cases are subjected to prolonged study and treatment, the symptoms may become fixed, and the patient may become a permanent military loss.

PSEUDOPSYCHOTIC STATES. In some cases the soldier, in his anxiety and panic reaction to combat stress, is so out of contact with reality and so confused and dissociated and his behavior so bizarre that he appears psychotic. The onset is usually sudden, and the clinical picture suggests schizophrenia. Many patients are disoriented and fail to reply to simple questions. Some cases resemble catatonic stupor; others suggest a catatonic excitement. These psychotic-like pictures occur in individuals who have not been psychotic in their previous reactions or in their basic personality structures. Such short-lived "three-day" psychoses usually disappear when the patients are removed from the traumatic situations. Sometimes sedation or electroconvulsive treatment is advisable.

PROGNOSIS AND TREATMENT. The presentation of this feature of the combat neuroses is based upon the procedure prescribed by the Office of the Surgeon General, United States Department of the Army.*

In dealing with these neuroses in the Army, emphasis is placed on preservation of medical discipline, early and vigorous treatment, the shortening of the period of hospitalization, the avoidance of unnecessary hospital atmosphere, and the promotion in the patient of the expectation of return to full duty. In his treatment, care is exercised to preserve the patient's identification with the combat group, to minimize the secondary gain of neurotic illness, and to avoid any suggestion of illness and disability. It is a basic principle in the attainment of these objectives that treatment should be as far forward as possible. So far as practicable, soldiers who show symptoms of becoming psychiatric casualties on the battlefield receive what may be called psychiatric first aid from members of their own combat unit. Here company officers promote morale by counsel, reassurance, exhortation, and leadership. Soldiers with relatively minor complaints may frequently be prevented from entering medical channels where the dissolution of group ties and the factors of secondary gain and suggestion tend to fix their symptoms.

If his motivation has been reasonably

good, the combat exhaustion patient responds rather well to proper therapeutic handling. If formal medical treatment is required, the patient is evacuated to the battalion aid station. Here most patients are those suffering from mild to moderate anxiety states complicated by physical exhaustion and the effects of exposure. They are usually wet, cold, dirty, and physically worn out. If the anxiety state is no more than moderate, the patient is kept at the aid station for 24 hours, where he is cleaned up, dried, adequately fed, and given sedation in the form of $7\frac{1}{2}$ to 10 grains of sodium amytal orally. By his manner and remarks, the battalion surgeon indicates that he expects an early return to duty of the soldier after he is rested. Many of the patients evacuated to the battalion aid station are simply suffering from normal fear reactions, with the somatic and psychological manifestations of that state. The patient has usually become alarmed by these symptoms that he has interpreted as those of cardiac, gastrointestinal, or other physical disorder. A careful physical examination is made. If no organ involvement is found, the cause of the symptoms is carefully explained to the soldier, who is assured that there will be no lasting effects or disability. After 24 hours of rest and psychotherapy consisting of reassurance, support, and exhortation, many patients are so greatly improved that they may be returned directly to duty.

The more severe and the pseudo-psychotic reactions are unsuited for management in the battalion aid station and are therefore transferred to the division clearing station. These patients exhibit marked anxiety states, extreme agitation and tension, acute panic, hysterical manifestations, or symptoms of acute psychosis. Upon arrival at the division clearing station, active psychiatric treatment begins. Sedation is given at once to those who have not already received it, and they are placed in adequately heated tent wards, are provided with cots for sleeping, and are given an abundance of hot food.

The psychiatrist combines an attitude of respect and sympathy for the patient,

* Ranson, Lt. Col. S. W.: Psychiatric treatment in combat areas. United States Armed Forces Medical Journal, *1*: No. 12, Dec., 1950.

yet he is also firm, decisive and realistic. He permits no doubt to arise in the patient's mind that he will not return to full combat duty after a brief rest. If the patient is allowed to ventilate his fears, hopes, and resentments, prompt symptomatic relief often follows. Since loyalty and sense of duty to his comrades are among the most important supports of the soldier in combat, an effort is made to strengthen these forces. Motivations for rejoining his outfit and active duty are strengthened. An attempt is made to avoid any suggestion of illness in the organization and atmosphere of treatment stations and in the attitude and action of the psychiatrist. As much care is used to avoid suggestion of serious psychiatric illness as of physical disease.

Both at the battalion aid station and the division clearing station, in order to emphasize the precipitating role of physical exhaustion, to imply a rapid recovery after a brief rest, and to avoid giving the impression of incurable mental illness, the term *exhaustion* is used for psychiatric casualities.

At one period in World War II, intravenous barbiturate narcosis was extensively used in severe anxiety states and in hysterical conversion reactions. During the narcosis, strong suggestion was used, with resulting emotional release, during which the patient relived his battle experiences. Few patients treated by this method recover to a degree that permits return to combat duty. It is now used in selected cases only.

The earliest possible return to duty prevents progress of the neurotic symptoms, minimizes secondary gain from their existence, and has a desirable therapeutic value in lessening guilt over separation from the group.

Inasmuch as psychiatric patients in the combat area are easily convinced that they are seriously ill, either physically or psychiatrically, it is important that, after proper physical examination, they be assured that they have no serious physical illnesses, that the psychiatric disability is temporary, that it is a reaction to the situation in which the soldier has been placed, that it has no relationship to "insanity," and that there should be no permanent after-effects. It is explained to the soldier that his psychological and somatic symptoms are but a frequent and essentially normal result from battle fear.

Since a neurotic illness occurring in battle places the patient in a safe situation with possible permanent removal from combat, it is important that the element of secondary gain be avoided so far as possible. If it is determined that a patient will not be returned to combat duty, he is informed of this decision and given reason to believe that it is final. The tension and pressure accompanying the anticipation of possible return to combat is thus eliminated, together with a further unconscious striving for the secondary gains of the illness. Such a soldier should, however, be returned to some type of duty as soon as possible lest prolonged rest and inactivity in comfortable hospital surroundings provide opportunity for brooding, tend to fixate the neurosis, and lead to demoralization and invalidism. Such measures should help to prevent permanent neuroses, so many of which followed the combat neuroses occurring in World War I. It should be remembered that the burden of guilt that a soldier may assume if he is evacuated from combat for less than excellent reasons may in some arouse intolerable and persisting guilt, by which his personality may be influenced morbidly or from which neurosis results.

BIBLIOGRAPHY

Adler, A.: Two different types of post-traumatic neuroses. Am. J. Psychiat., *102*:237–240, 1945.

Allen, D. W., and Houston, M.: The management of hysteroid acting-out patients in a training clinic. Psychiatry, *22*:41–49, 1959.

Alexander, V. K.: A case study of a multiple personality. J. Abnorm. & Social Psychol., *52*:272–276, 1956.

Bartemeier, L., et al.: Combat exhaustion. J. Nerv. & Ment. Dis., *104*:358–389; 489–525, 1946.

Beard, G. M.: A Practical Treatise on Nervous Exhaustion. New York, Wm. Wood & Co., 1880.

Berrington, W.. P., Liddell, D. W., and Foulds, G. A.: A re-evaluation of the fugue. J. Ment. Sc., *102*:280–286, 1956.

Bowman, K. M.: Modern concept of the neuroses. J.A.M.A., *132*:555–557, 1946.

Breuer, J., and Freud, S.: Studies in Hysteria. Translated by Brill, A. A. Washington, D. C., Nervous and Mental Disease Pub. Co., 1937.

Brill, N. Q., and Beebe, G. W.: A follow-up study of war neuroses. Washington, D. C., V. A. Medical Monograph, Dept. Med. Surg., 1955.

Carter, A. B.: The prognosis of certain hysterical symptoms. Brit. M. J., *1*:1076–1079, 1949.

Cobb, S.: Emotions and Clinical Medicine. New York, W. W. Norton & Co., Inc., 1950.

Darmstadter, H. J.: The superiority attitude and rigidity of ideas. Arch. Neurol. & Psychiat., *61*: 621–643, 1949.

Engle, G. L.: Primary atypical facial neuralgia. Psychosom. Med., *13*:375–396, 1951.

English, O. S., and Pearson, G. H. S.: Common Neuroses of Children and Adults. New York, W. W. Norton & Co., Inc., 1937.

Fenichel, O.: The Psychoanalytic Theory of Neurosis. New York, W. W. Norton & Co., Inc., 1945.

Fitzgerald, O. W. S.: Love deprivation and the hysterical personality. J. Ment. Sc., *94*:701–717, 1948.

Freud, S.: Collected Papers (5 Vols.). London, Hogarth Press, 1924–1925.

Idem: The Ego and the Id. London, Hogarth Press, 1927.

Idem: The Basic Writings of Sigmund Freud. New York, Modern Library, 1938.

Idem: The Problem of Anxiety. New York, W. W. Norton & Co., Inc., 1936.

Glass, A. J.: Combat exhaustion. U. S. Armed Forces Med. J., *2*:1471–1478, 1951.

Idem: Current problems in military psychiatry. J.A.M.A., *150*:6–10, 1952.

Grinker, R. R.: Treatment of war neuroses. J.A.M.A., *126*:142–145, 1944.

Idem, and Spiegel, J. P.: Men under Stress. Philadelphia, The Blakiston Co., 1945.

Idem: War Neuroses. Ibid., 1945.

Huddleson, J. H.: Accidents, Neuroses and Compensation. Baltimore, Williams & Wilkins Co., 1932.

Ingram, I. M.: Obsessional illness in mental hospital patients. J. Ment. Sci., *107*:382–402, 1961.

Jackson, D. D.: The question of family homeostasis. Psych. Quart. Suppl., *31*:79–90, 1957.

Janet, Pierre: The Major Symptoms of Hysteria, 2nd ed., New York, The Macmillan Company, 1920.

Kamman, G. R.: Traumatic neurosis, compensation neurosis or attitudinal pathosis? Arch. Neurol. & Psychiat., *65*:593–603, 1951.

Kennedy, A.: Recent hysterical states and their treatment. J. Ment. Sc., *86*:988–1019, 1940.

Idem, and Neville, J.: Sudden loss of memory. Brit. M. J., *2*:428–433, 1957.

Kubie, L. S., and Margolin, S.: The therapeutic role of drugs in the process of repression, dissociation and synthesis. Psychosom. Med., *7*: 147–151, 1945.

Laughlin, H. P.: The Neuroses in Clinical Practice. Philadelphia, W. B. Saunders Company, 1956.

Ljungberg, L.: Hysteria: A clinical, prognostic and genetic study. Acta Psych. et Neur. Scand. Suppl., *112*:1–162, 1957.

Masserman, J. H.: The Practice of Dynamic Psychiatry. Philadelphia, W. B. Saunders Company, 1955.

Idem: Principles of Dynamic Psychiatry. 2d ed. Ibid., 1961.

Michael, R. P.: Treatment of a case of compulsive swearing. Brit. M. J., *1*:1506–1508, 1957.

Noble, D.: Hysterical manifestations in schizophrenic illness. Psychiatry, *14*:153–160, 1951.

Idem; Roudebush, M. E., and Price, D.: Studies of Korean war casualties. Am. J. Psychiat., *108*: 495–499, 1952.

Ossipov, V. P.: Malingering; a simulation of psychosis. Bull. Menninger Clin., 8:39–42, 1944.

Pollitt, J.: Natural history of obsessional states. Brit. M. J., *1*:194–198, 1957.

Prince, M.: Miss Beauchamp—the theory of the psychogeneses of multiple personality. J. Abnorm. Psychol., *15*:67–135, 1920.

Idem: The Dissociation of a Personality: A Biographical Study in Abnormal Psychology. New York, Longmans, Green & Co. 1906.

Purtell, J. J., Robins, E., and Cohen, M. E.: Observations on clinical aspects of hysteria. J.A.M.A., *146*:902–909, 1951.

Seitz, P. F. D.: Experiments in the substitution of symptoms by hypnosis. Psychosomatic Med., *15*:405–424, 1953.

Thigpen, C. H., and Cleckley, H. M.: The Three Faces of Eve. New York, McGraw-Hill Book Company, 1957.

Ulett, P. C., and Gildea, E. F.: Survey of surgical procedures in psychoneurotic women. J.A.M.A., *143*:960–963, 1950.

Ziegler, D. K., and Paul, N.: On the natural history of hysteria in women (a follow-up study twenty years after hospitalization). Dis. Nerv. System, *15*:301–306, 1954.

Ziegler, F. J., Imboden, J. B., and Meyer, E.: Contemporary conversion reactions: A clinical study. Am. J. Psychiat., *116*:901–910, 1960.

Chapter Twenty-nine

PERSONALITY DISORDERS

The group of personality disorders includes a wide range of cases in which malfunctioning is expressed in inflexible and limited patterns of behavior. At times these personality patterns and traits are compatible with social success and satisfaction in cases in which the particular features of the individual make-up are both accepted and rewarded by the culture and the special vocational opportunities that are available. In such instances the inflexibility of the personality or its special vulnerability to particular stresses remains unnoticed except perhaps in the form of some peculiarity or eccentricity until that individual is required to adapt to another environment or is exposed to some personal or environmental pressure that he has previously avoided or escaped. In other forms, difficulties in social and sexual adaptation are evident and occur repetitively throughout life, in spite of adequate intellectual capacity.

The personality disorders differ then in that the psychopathologic manifestations do not present themselves in the grossly regressive disturbances of the behavior, affect, or thought of the psychoses or in the exaggerated and fixed psychological defenses that characterize the psychoneurotic. Nor does the disorder present itself in the form of somatic symptoms due to an expression of anxiety or other affect through disruption of psychophysiologic functions.

The Standard Nomenclature of the American Psychiatric Association classifies the personality disorders as those of disturbance of personality pattern, of personality traits and sociopathic personalities. To many psychiatrists the differentiations of the groupings are regarded as much too precise in terms of available knowledge.

Those personality disorders listed as disturbances of pattern include the *cyclothymic, hypomanic, melancholic,* and *schizoid.* They are recognized as forms of personality organization that contain many features similar to those found in patients with the various types of affective and schizophrenic reactions, but in the individuals in whom these disorders are present ego functioning and reality testing remain intact and allow an effective social adaptation. Presumably those with the cyclothymic, hypomanic, or melancholic make-up form a reservoir of persons vulnerable to manic–depressive or involutional reactions when exposed to a sufficiently severe and appropriate loss or frustration, with concomitant stress and emotional arousal. Also from the reservoir of schizoid personalities derive those reactive schizophrenic and paranoid disorganizations that occur in the face of affective arousal beyond the capacity of containment by their ego adaptive and defensive development.

The trait disturbances, as presently described, contain the *compulsive* and *hysterical* personalities. Also grouped here are the large number of individuals characterized by inability to delay or control their drives and associated emotions or to establish a personal autonomy and independence. This ill-defined aggregation of cases are classified as *passive aggressive, emotionally unstable,* or *inadequate personalities.* For the most part, this latter group of disordered personalities and those classified in the sociopathic group come to medical or psychiatric attention through contact in or referral from social institutions such as the courts, prisons, military organizations, and special schools. They now constitute problems in civilian life for large organizations such as the various labor unions. Together they were formerly considered as "psychopaths."

It was formerly believed that the unmodifiable behavior patterns of such persons were matters of inborn disposition and were constitutionally influenced or directed. Not only has the assumption of a constitutional basis failed to yield any understanding of the behavior of such persons, but it is only logical that such behavior disturbances should be susceptible of explanation by theories that are analogous to those that have been so fruitful in rendering other reaction types intelligible.

Thus the pathologic behavior of the psychopath presumably has a psychogenetic origin. The major defect in the personality rests in establishing an identity with constructive and socially useful adaptations or to evolve those controls that allow the delay and repression of anger or the many forms of hostile attack and retaliation towards others. Loss or absence of parents and parental substitutes and limited contacts with other adults and

peers often deprives the growing child, who later presents psychopathic features, of the experiences necessary to establish an ego identity through the process of identification. In some instances his behavior may be the result of frustration in his efforts to achieve a satisfaction of such fundamental needs as love, security, recognition, respect, and success. The child who was rejected may react by becoming resentful, rebellious, and antisocial, and thus establish a "negative identity," which brings him some ego satisfactions. The origins of these personality disorders can best be regarded as the expression of an arrested or deviated development of personality. Whether this behavior represents the consequence of a development fault—an experiential lack in the process of emotional maturation through deficiency of interpersonal contact or a character neuroses—it denotes the continuing activity of psychopathological forces set in motion very early in life. The persisting drive to or reaction to aggressivity, passivity, frustration, failure of deviated sexuality gives a compulsive chronicity to the psychopathic behavior.

As the result of studies of children deprived of early parental care through loss, or placement in foundling or foster homes, as well as by the developmental studies of animals exposed to maternal or peer deprivations at certain critical periods in early development, there is reason to consider today that such experiential deprivation often leads to persisting defects in social and sexual behavior. Whether such behavioral pathology may be modified by substitutive experiences later in life remain uncertain. For the growing child, neither the critical periods for social experiencing nor their duration or intensity are established or fully defined. Here future research promises much to the understanding of the psychopathology of the personality disorders.

Since all but the sociopathic disturbances have been described in Chapter 5, Psychopathology, the remainder of this chapter is directed to consideration of the antisocial and dyssocial reactions and the sexual deviations.

THE ANTISOCIAL PERSONALITY

Formerly the majority of patients now classified as antisocial personality were designated "constitutional psychopathic state" or "psychopathic personality." The present term provides a more restrictive application and is referred to those chronically antisocial individuals without the capacity to form significant attachments or loyalties to others, to groups, or to codes of living. Thus they are callous and given to immediate pleasures, appear devoid of a sense of responsibility, and, in spite of repeated humiliations and punishments, fail to learn to modify their behavior. They lack in social judgment, yet frequently are capable of verbal rationalizations that often convince them their actions are reasonable and warranted.

The essential defect in the character structure rests in the failure to develop a socialized superego and ego ideals. If they exist, they are directed to personal self-aggrandizement, acquisition of money and material goods, and the control of others for immediate pleasures and satisfactions.

Etiology

The future antisocial personality is often that of a child born to parents who did not want him, and not infrequently he is of an illegitimate birth. The mother's own early life and development have been unhappy, and her departure from her parents has been motivated by a wish to escape from them. She has little resources to offer others and thus comes to term feeling herself deprived. Any suffering with the birth or failures to realize her fantasies in the child serve only to increase her negative attitude toward the infant. Even when the parents have married, their relationship usually terminates in desertion or divorce. Thus the child may have been passed frequently between others or institutionalized. If he remains with the parents, he has been exposed to violent tempers, abuse, and a variety of brutalities and sexual observations that occur in parents frequently addicted to alcohol and to promiscuity. In this type of family, authority goals for the child are not clearly established and never are based on a foundation of mutual affection, tenderness, and trust. The attempt by school and other authorities to establish some control for the acts of the child are treated indifferently, openly defied, and fought off by the parents. The child is deprived again of other sources for establishing healthy identifications with those accepting the social values of the community. Further, both the attitude of the parents to outside authority and the child's own resentments are often deepened and embedded.

Even in childhood, the future pathological personality usually shows signs of emotional maladjustment and unwholesome personality traits. Typically, he is characterized by an emotional immaturity reflected by his impulsive and instant response to his feelings. His personality seems to be dominated by primitive drives to the exclusion of rational behavior. Certain lines of conduct, particularly of a socialized nature, are never learned. Some of these children are sensitive, stubborn, and given to tantrums or to outbursts of rage; frequently these pre-adolescent psychopaths steal, run away, suffer from enuresis, are destructive, quarrelsome, sulky, deceitful, obstinate, defiant, boastful, shameless, and erratic. Antagonism or open rebellion against a dominating parent may be shown. The adolescent resists the ideals and mores of his family and tends to socialize at a lower level. With approaching maturity and the weakening of the restraining forces of the home and with the increase of responsibilities and of environmental contacts and demands, the earlier tendencies become outspoken manifestations. These are elaborated in some as they obtain gratifications through cupidity, deceit, or sadistic acts as the only few means learned in such family environments to respond to their own needs and desires.

Many psychopaths, although not intellectually deficient, seem emotionally such. They therefore lack keenness and delicacy of sentiment. The psychopath is typically affectionless, selfish, ungrateful, narcissistic, and exhibitionistic. He is egocentric, demanding much, and giving little. His excess of demand is, in fact, one of the outstanding characteristics. He has no critical awareness of his motives and is unable to judge his own behavior from another's standpoint. In spite of the fact that his conduct is so inadequate or so hostile from a social standpoint, the psychopath is satisfied with it. He shows few feelings of anxiety, guilt, or of remorse. He lacks definiteness of objective, and his usual state of restlessness may result from a search for the unattainable. Occupational application and efficiency are usually faulty; routine is intolerably irksome. He demands immediate and instant gratification of his desires, with no concern as to the feelings and interests of others, with whom he forms few emotional relationships or stable affectional ties. He does not, either, build up a sense of social values as normally should occur through the process of identification. As a result, such a sense is frequently distorted. The demands of instinct are not adjusted to the demands of society. He is often plausible and talkative but absolutely unreliable. Frequently the only environment to which he can adjust is the one that he can dominate. Surprising irregularities of ability and inconsistencies of behavior are constantly demonstrated. A certain number escape from a difficult situation by way of a psychotic episode, while others at the slightest stress resort to alcohol or drugs. Many psychopaths bear alcohol poorly and under its influence become noisy, quarrelsome, and destructive. The sociopathic personality projects his own insecurity by blaming others. His behavior prevents proper psychosocial adjustment and ranges from "queerness" to criminality, with a large intermediate group made up of cranks, extremists, eccentrics, habitual delinquents, and other social misfits.

Sometimes one sibling in a family may manifest the behavior and personality characteristic usually associated with the sociopathic personality, while other siblings may present mature and well-adjusted personalities. Presumably this difference in personality characteristics is because of the fact that the effect of a particular emotional experience or social influence in the family was highly specific to the individual. This type of psychopathic behavior probably develops more often in upper or middle class families than that previously described. The superego defect or lacunae, as it has been termed, may be limited to a single form of behavior—such as stealing, running away, or promiscuity.

In this respect, concurrent studies of children exhibiting antisocial activity and of their parents provide new insights both into the form of deviant behavior adopted by the child and its impulsion for gratification. Johnson and Szurek have found that the more important parent, usually the mother, has unconsciously encouraged the amoral or antisocial behavior in the child. Although the parent verbally protests such behavior both to the child and to others, yet it is accepted, either unconsciously or with a guilty permissiveness, by the parent. The permissiveness has appeared to gratify vicariously neurotic needs of the parent that derive from her own lack of current satisfactions or unmet needs of childhood, or both. Since the parent's permissiveness is uncertain and incomplete, the child, and later the adult, is inconsistent and confused. Healthy discipline is not administered by such a parent—discipline combining firm prohibition with reward for socially acceptable behavior. Through his own overt acts, inconsistencies, innuendoes in speech, or various non-verbal means of communication, the child has been found to recognize the partial permissiveness. But since the child is both partially gratified and encouraged in his action and partially frustrated by the parent, there are associated with the act feelings of hostility toward the parent and perhaps of guilt. In instances in which this variety of family interaction exists, the antisocial behavior is fixed unless the several participating persons can be brought to understand and modify their behavior or they are completely separated.

Psychopathology

These sociopathic individuals show a moral and ethical blunting, a lack of sympathy for their fellow men, and a behavior destructive to the welfare of the social order. As children they are often self-willed, play truant, commit petty thefts, are cruel and untruthful, and as they grow older they may be inaccessible, boorish, and without a sense of responsibility. Their emotional life is superficial and affectively cold. They seem incapable of mature emotional relationships. They cannot organize an acceptable, constructive expression of their aggressions. They lack ambition, application, seriousness of purpose, and foresight. They are irritable, arrogant, unyielding, characterized by a brutal egoism, and rarely feel remorse for their most serious offenses against person or property. Frequently they show a rebellious attitude toward authority and society. Changes in mood are sudden and often without apparent cause. They are cynical, devoid of a sense of honor or of shame, and are lacking in sympathy, affection, gratitude, and other social and esthetic sentiments. When frustrated, they may be dangerous to others. Their offenses may constitute the whole register of crime—theft, embezzlement, forgery, robbery, brutal sex attacks, and other acts of violence. Many take pleasure in their struggle with the law and feel pride in their accomplishments. They are unable to identify themselves with society and its laws. Punishments are considered as expressions of injustice and have no deterrent effect.

Merely to indicate the wide variety of behavior patterns that the antisocial personality may manifest, a description is given of a group formerly characterized as pathological liars and swindlers. In this group are egocentric individuals whose social maladaptation consists of extravagant, often apparently purposeless, lying, frequently combined with swindling. They exhibit a marked excitability of imagination combined with an instability of purpose. They are usually good-natured, of agreeable manners, optimistic, of a light-hearted geniality, and make social contacts easily. A glibness of tongue, an unusual aptitude for the use of language, a self-confident manner, a frequently assumed dignity, and a misleading appearance of knowledge readily enable them to convince the credulous as to their statements. They acquire a smattering of art, literature, or technical parlance, which they employ to their own profit and to the expense and humiliation of their victims. They spin remarkable tales concerning past experiences and paint their future with a careless disregard for reality.

Some are guilty of sex offenses and others obtain large sums of money under promise of marriage. When discovered in their delinquencies, they profess amnesia, and if charged with offense, they often stage an emotionally affected exhibition designed to impress observers and arouse sympathy. They are restless and unstable and are incapable of exertion or responsibility. They never learn to meet the struggle for existence with industry and perseverance but live in a world of imagination and seek to acquire the necessities of life by deceit and fraud. They are unable to accept the limitations of reality. Their theatrical imitation, their tendency to day-dream, to boast, to avoid realities, and to surround themselves with an imaginary world suggest a childish immaturity of personality, while their wish-fulfilling fabrications have much in common with the fantasy of childhood. Many times their flagrant lying is defensive in purpose. On a less conscious level is the extravagant and often apparently purposeless romancing known as *pseudologia phantastica*. This egregious disregard of the truth seems to result from a pressing need to indulge in extravagant castle-building in order to make up for a reality that appears to be too onerous or prosaic. Inasmuch as the content of the fantasy is generated by unconscious forces, the patient is not entirely aware that his statement is a fabrication. His unusually rich imagination, stirred into active expression by acute emotional needs, enables the patient to live in a dream world. Psychometric tests usually disclose a normal or superior intellectual capacity, but as with other psychopaths, intelligence has little regulating influence on behavior. At times it would appear that such personality characteristics grow out of a feeling of inferiority, envy, or jealousy.

DIFFERENTIAL DIAGNOSIS. All delinquents and criminals, even though guilty of repeated offenses, are not to be considered as antisocial personalities or psychopaths. In previous chapters mention has been made of criminal behavior as incidental manifestations of the neuroses, affective, and schizophrenic reactions and the mental deficiencies. However, the personality structure and its precursors in the constitutional and psychogenetic history differ from that of the psychopath.

But, in addition, it must be kept in mind that cultural, economic, and social forces also may determine antisocial behavior and in some instances release it, as for example, in times of war, when the ordinary standards of social interaction are overturned or reversed even for those with well-established social values. There exist in many societies subcultures that live through their adeptness in defying the usual social codes, the members of which constitute a separate criminal class. Persons in these groups differ from the psychopath or antisocial personality in their personality structure and presently are separated in the classification of the American Psychiatric Association under the rubric, *dyssocial reaction*. In contrast to the antisocial personalities, individuals of this group are capable of warm and strong loyalties to others and to their group. To Jenkins and others they represent a criminal occupational group motivated as other citizens to gain, but through illegal means and, as such, learn, plan, and adapt as others without significant personality disorder. The major differences rest in their group loyalties and the nature of the early development, which has fostered the capacities for interpersonal contact and trust but through continuing life in a delinquent or criminal subculture that has limited its expression to behavior acceptable to those groups. Certain of the antisocial adolescent gang activity, now widely reported but known for centuries, represents culturally determined antisocial behavior.

Particularly to be distinguished from the sociopathic group are the *character neuroses*. Here the neurotic conflict is resolved through asocial or antisocial behavior rather than through a symptom neurosis; the psychopathology is expressed in social behavior rather than in neurotic symptoms. In the character neurotic, his compulsive "acting out" relieves anxiety that would otherwise be distressing. Oftentimes the "acting out" is motivated by a pathological sense of guilt due to an abnormal superego. The "acting out" is performed for the purposes of relieving the guilt through apprehension and punishment. Intellectually such patients are aware of the potentialities for punishment and humiliation but are unconsciously impelled to the repetitive antisocial act in order to assuage the unconscious guilty anxiety and need for punishment. The neurotic character then differs from the antisocial personality in that he, as well as the dyssocial personality, have evolved the ego structure that allows for trust and attachment to others and has internalized social codes. Thus he has available superego structure, but this is distorted and forces persisting unconscious irrational senses of guilt, shame, or unworthiness.

A characteristic of all antisocial psychopathological behavior is the fact that the drive or motivation behind it is intense and forceful. The immediate urges are stronger than any rational considerations. The pathological personality who repeatedly commits some antisocial act appreciates intellectually that he will doubtless be caught, and if so, will face severe punishment. His need for his customary anxiety-relieving means impels, nevertheless, the compulsive continuance of his behavior. He may make a genuine effort to "go straight" and yet find his efforts futile in the face of strong, unconscious forces. At times this may be the result of a vicious circle. His dynamically motivated aggressiveness, for example, may generate anxiety, and his anxiety, in turn, may generate antisocial aggressiveness. Although from a psychopathological standpoint the sociopathic personality may be looked upon as not responsible for his conduct, from a legal point of view he is regarded in most American courts as accountable for any violations of the legal code. The projective psychological techniques may yield significant information concerning personality structure and underlying psychopathology as well as reveal the areas around which the patient's major problems revolve.

Treatment

One must not oversimplify the factors that have determined the behavior of the sociopathic personality. It should be borne in mind, too, that the dividing line between normal psychology and psychopathology is not at all definitely drawn. Here, as elsewhere in nature, there are no discontinuities. Frequently environmental factors as well as inner psychic pressures have been operative. Internal ones, too, are frequently multiple and interacting. Pernicious social and cultural influences may contribute to the creation of the sociopathic personality, although they do not serve as the basic genetic agents. Often there is an interplay between psychological and social factors. If environmental influences are contributory, either their modification or the patient's removal from them is desirable.

The rational treatment of the antisocial and dyssocial must differ from that of those neurotics who perform delinquent or criminal acts. Essential to any effective therapy is the placing of the individual in an accepting and warm human environment where he may find it possible to develop a therapeutic relationship with some member of the treatment group whom he perceives as having his interests at heart and to whom he can given some trust. In dealing with delinquency of late childhood and adolescence, it is often found that one of the most effective corrective measures is a warm, authoritative father figure with whom boys can identify.

With the older psychopaths, this initial step becomes increasingly difficult and often is impossible due to the inherent ego defect of basic distrust. Psychiatrists and others treating such patients must be highly motivated and endowed with a mature patience to effect the development of the therapeutic relationship.

When the treatment relationship is established, either through individual or group identification, pressure through personal and verbal behavior must be initiated toward certain goals and standards of social relationship. Usually such efforts must be made continuously and slowly, and infractions should be treated by withdrawal of privileges and their reinstitution on improved behavior. The treatment relationship, whether established through the medium of a single psychiatrist or a group, makes clear certain standards of behavior, and their abuse is managed by frustrating loss of satisfaction in other areas. A sense of authority is consistently and firmly maintained. This treatment regimen can be attained infrequently without some type of institutional care. It clearly differs from the continually permissive attitude necessary for the treatment of the neurotic child or adult. If the latter is adopted throughout, no focus will be established for superego growth, and, if anything, the permissiveness may aggravate the antisocial behavior.

When the antisocial behavior of a child or adolescent has its origins in the family interactions described by Johnson and Szurek, in order for treatment to succeed, in most instances the parent of the patient must be treated as well or, in the case of a child or young adult, separated during the course of psychotherapy. Such separations are resisted by parents, whose major gratification comes from their dependent relations with the "scapegoat" child. In some instances, separation of the patient from the parent or change in the behavior of the patient during treatment has led to serious behavior disturbance in the symbiotic parent.

Treatment for those with a character neurosis that has led to repetitive antisocial behavior should conform to the psychoanalytic model as described in a subsequent chapter. Here the hope of the therapist is to relate past conflicts that have led to the erection of a pathological sense of guilt and its expressive force in masochistic "acting out." Since the patient has already established a set of values, it is unnecessary to intervene by providing an environmental setting that prevents actions and denies or punishes for failure to comply.

Sometimes the patterned response to pathogenetic factors is so fixed that it is not modifiable. Again, the patient seems to lack capacity to experience anxiety with its resulting desire for relief. The hostility, too, often shown by the psychopath may generate hostility in others and hamper treatment. Sometimes a secondary gain from his neurotic-like symptom neutralizes any wish for a change in his behavior.

A prison environment is a handicap to therapy. If the sociopsychopath's behavior brings him before court, the judge may be aware that ideally the treatment of the prisoner's behavior is by psychotherapy, through which its psychogenesis may be traced and its pathology cured. Like the psychiatrist, he may realize that punishment without recognition of the prisoner's emotional problems may intensify his social maladjustment. On the other hand, a person cannot be sentenced to therapy.

Frequently the psychiatrist is confronted in the case of the sociopsychopath with the question of criminal responsibility. As a scientific psychiatrist, he should seek to ascertain if the criminal behavior is susceptible of psychopathological interpretation, but he should also remember that it is not easy to prove

or disprove such interpretations, that society cannot yet evaluate them, and that it cannot yet, and perhaps should not, establish them as criteria of responsibility. The matter of judgment of responsibility rests solely with the law. The psychiatrist's function only is to provide his opinion as to the motivating forces for the criminal act and their origins as determined from the personality study.

SITUATION PSYCHOSES

If, according to the view expressed, the maladaptation of the antisocial personality is fundamentally an attempted solution of the individual's problems rather than the result of unwholesome social influences, we should expect a higher incidence of psychotic reactions among these poorly integrated individuals than among well-adjusted persons. This assumption is found to be true. The great majority of such reactions are schizophrenic, affective, or paranoid but some, occurring under circumstances involving great emotional distress, represent attempts, through disorders of belief or of sensorium, to escape from the hard and uncompromising reality of some specific, difficult situation and are therefore called "situation psychoses." Frequently situation psychoses are in the nature of confused states, paranoid episodes, or periods of irritability, excitement, or depression.

Prison Psychoses

Since the most difficult situation into which the behavior of the antisocial usually leads him is confinement, which he bears poorly, the most important of the situation reactions are the prison psychoses. It must not be concluded that all psychoses developing among prisoners belong to this group; in fact, but a minority of them belong to the true prison psychoses. In them, delusional ideas tend to be ideas of persecution, innocence, or pardon. The majority of the psychotic reactions observed among prisoners are of the usual clinical types, especially schizophrenia and paranoid states, the stress of imprisonment acting merely as the releasing agent.

Prison psychoses that begin after the prisoner has received sentence are most likely to occur among long-term prisoners and comparatively early during the period for which they are sentenced. The forms assumed by the psychotic reactions are various. Occasional forms are sudden excitements manifested by intense emotion, violent rage, cursing, and destructive attacks on the environment. Such attacks, usually brief, may, psychologically, represent a protest against an intolerable situation. Episodes characterized by delusions of persecution, ideas of strange influences, olfactory hallucinations of gas, or anxiety, irritability, and uneasiness are not common. Manic–depressive reactions rarely develop among persons held under indictment or sentence, and some psychiatrists of extensive experience report that they have never seen this form of psychosis in the case of life prisoners.

There are two forms especially typical of prison psychoses. One, expressing a deep-seated dissatisfaction, is characterized by querulousness. Patients suffering from this form have numerous delusions of ill treatment. They constantly grumble and maintain that all sorts of obstacles are placed in their way and that attempts are being made to annoy them. Frequently their complaints sound plausible.

One of the most frequent forms of prison psychoses found among long-term prisoners is that characterized by delusions of innocence or of pardon. The patient may experience auditory hallucinations wherein he is told that he has been exonerated from his alleged crime and is now to be liberated. Other, but similar, wish-fulfilling ideas are heard. As the patient believes himself an innocent and unjustly persecuted individual, he becomes bitter toward those who fail to set him at liberty.

Most of those with the acute prison psychoses recover after transfer from the prison to the hospital, where the general attitude is treatment rather than the maintenance of fixed and rigid discipline.

Many life prisoners thus transferred fail to recover but gradually deteriorate mentally. One of the most important elements in the treatment of the prison psychoses is to render the patient's points of contact as little irritating as possible. Occupation, games, amusements, and a friendly, although necessarily firm, attitude are helpful.

GANSER SYNDROME. An interesting type of mental disorder sometimes occurring in the case of prisoners under detention and awaiting trial was described by Ganser. It develops only after commission of a crime and, therefore, tells nothing about the patient's mental state when he committed the offense. This syndrome is described in Chapter 28.

SEXUAL DEVIATION

Persons whose biological sex urges are directed toward a normal heterosexual goal but who, because they are segregated from those of the opposite sex, casually seek sexual satisfaction through various perversions are scarcely to be considered as sexual deviates.* In the true deviate, the offending sexual act is the surface symptom of a more profound personality disturbance.

Although some of the current psychiatric theories concerning homosexuality and other non-biologically directed sex drives are presented, it must be admitted that established facts concerning sexual psychopathy are few. Even though lawmakers and courts look to the psychiatrist for information as to its etiology and for guidance in its treatment, he cannot yet answer these questions to the full satisfaction either of these agencies or of himself. It is a subject now receiving both psychiatric and social research.

* "It is said that only a small proportion of males convicted of sex offenses have been involved in behavior which is materially different than that of most males in the population. This small group, which numbers in the neighborhood of 5 to 10 per cent, is that which engages our attention as psychiatrists. They are hereinafter designated as psychiatrically deviated sex offenders." Group for the Advancement of Psychiatry, Report No. 9: Psychiatrically Deviated Sex Offenders.

In the opinion of many psychiatrists, the term sexual psychopath, or deviate, should be limited to the individual whose sexual impulse, through defects in the step-by-step development of personality, has either remained immature or has undergone deviation in the course of its maturation. The arrest or deviation in development is not, of course, in the anatomy or physiology of sex organs but in the psychosexual, i.e., the emotional, dispositional aspect of sexual expression. Psychosexual maturation may lag behind biological maturation or be so blocked that mature heterosexual impulses are not established. The emotional and instinctive aspects of sex are not harmoniously integrated into the total personality. Satisfaction of the sex impulse is therefore sought through such expressions as voyeurism, exhibitionism, homosexuality, rape, pedophilia, masochism, sadism, and other means. It must not be assumed that the biologically and culturally undesirable behavior of the paraphiliac is a matter of being "oversexed." Very few psychiatrists, moreover, regard the deviant behavior of the sexual psychopath as "constitutional" in origin.

In Chapter 3, Personality Development and Structure, attention was called to the fact that there is a progressive, sequential maturation of the personality, including its psychosexual aspect. Certain instinctive sex expressions are therefore normal and to be expected in the earlier stages of the individual's development. Sometimes, instead of being successfully modified or repressed, these infantile or immature expressions may continue or re-emerge. It is normal, for example, for the small child at one stage of his development to secure pleasure in looking at or exhibiting sexual organs. If such infantile habits continue and are not inhibited with the maturation of adult heterosexual drive and expression, the individual remains or becomes a voyeur or exhibitionist. Again, these or other infantile sexual expressions may have been apparently repressed or outgrown, but in adolescence, as the physiological forces that normally establish sexual maturity begin to exert their influence, the infantile sexual expressions may be reactivated and overtly manifested. The individual is then regarded as a sex delinquent.

If the family and social environment are not favorable to a healthy, mature psychosexual development, the drive toward mature heterosexuality will be blocked or deviated. Thus a boy held closely by his mother through his growing years and deprived of close association with a father, through the latter's absence, indifference, or hostility, is likely to have homosexual relations as his preferred form of sexual gratification in adulthood. There is much evidence from both the clinic and the laboratory that effective heterosexual development in man and animals depends upon continuing contacts with members of both sexes throughout growth.

Homosexuality

From the Kinsey studies, it is clear that there is a wide range of homosexual behavior in both men and women. Whereas some live an exclusively homosexual life and receive all adult sexual gratification from a partner of the same sex, others are predominantly but not exclusively satisfied in this way. With a large number of adolescents and adults, the major sexual expression is heterosexual, yet occasionally or incidentally these individuals have homosexual contacts. Such incidental contacts may take place when the person is deprived of heterosexual contacts, after alcohol debauches or head injuries, or in situations of homosexual license.

The term homosexuality is often used in ways other than to indicate a personality disorder wherein the predominant mode of sexual expression is with a member of the same sex. "Latent homosexuality" refers to the existence of a personality make-up similar to that of the overt homosexual, and associated even in some cases with fantasy formation of homosexual activity, but without overt sexual activity. Unfortunately, homosexuality is now used frequently as a derogatory remark, and some neurotic patients designate themselves as homosexual due to their feelings of failure and inability to express and utilize successfully their aggressive drives to mastery.

Among the groups of men charged with homosexual behavior in courts, one finds the female impersonator, as well as the isolated and dull person who has not had a loving relationship in the past, the resentful antisocial, those generally compensated individuals who are apprehended after an overt act while drinking in later life, and those whose homosexual behavior is a single component in a more serious psychotic disorder, most frequently schizophrenic or mentally defective. There is a group of homosexuals whose personality development and ego functioning otherwise appear intact and who conduct themselves both effectively and constructively in society. Yet all these individuals exhibiting homosexual behavior do show certain common features in the personality. They have difficulty in reconciling dependent and assertive drives, an ambivalent maternal relationship, and a high frequency of rearing in a broken home.

Homosexual behavior is determined on the basis of defects in psychosexual maturation. While Kallmann found a large number of identical twins concordant to homosexuality, more recently a study of a number of identical twin pairs showed one to be heterosexual and the other homosexual. In such twin pairs the opportunity is optimum to examine the differing psychogenetic forces that relate to the several forms of sexual behavior, and the findings of these studies gives a strong support to earlier psychodynamic formulations.

For a healthy psychosexual development, the child should form an identification with the parent or a member of his own sex. The future homosexual male has an inordinate attachment to his mother, fostered by her and leading to identification with her. This attachment flowers in the absence or indifference of a father or when the child fears or hates this parent or derogates him as the mother often does. The homosexual identified with the mother as the dominant person seeks out males as sexual companions, either motivated through fear or incest or loss of the maternal relationship that is threatened in his contacts with women. Then there are underlying castration fears and resentments toward women derived from the repressed hostilities toward the mother. The homosexual relationship may express as well his hostility to men. In a few instances, male homosexuality arises when the child has been separated from women and reared by men throughout life. Here he is deprived of the experience of heterosexual contact and also fears women.

Pedophilia

Pedophilia, or a pathological sexual interest in children, is regarded as a variant of homosexuality in which homosexual strivings are directed toward children. It occurs largely in weak and impotent persons. The pedophil acts toward the child as he unconsciously wished his mother to behave toward himself. Another, and perhaps more logical, explanation of the pedophil's behavior is that he functions on an immature psychosexual level because of his fearfulness and doubt concerning himself. As a result of these feelings, he expects rejection and failure in adult, heterosexual advances. His sexual expression is therefore released toward children.

Fetishism

Fetishism is a perversion peculiar to men. The fetishist is unable to love a real person but becomes attached to some material object having a feminine association, such as a lock of hair or an undergarment. This object attains a highly exaggerated value and becomes a special source of erotic gratification, a reliever of both psychic and sexual tension, as contact with it leads to orgasm. The fetish always has a genital meaning; it serves the purpose of denying the anatomical difference between the two sexes, a discovery of which caused an overwhelming genital fear.

Fetishism has usually been considered

as a substitutive genital drive necessary as the consequence of fears of castration. Some psychoanalysts consider the fetishistic attachment an effort to gain an ego identification through contact with a substitutive satisfying object and point to the fetishistic attachment of little children to blankets, toys, or other objects as a means of satisfaction in the absence of the mother. Thus, the act may be seen as one satisfying a pregenital wish.

Transvestism

Another deviation is that of transvestism, a morbid impulse to dress in the clothing of the opposite sex. Formulations of the psychopathology of fetishism and of transvestism are still largely speculative. Transvestism occurs more frequently in the male than in the female. Usually the patient's mother wanted a girl and literally reared her son to be one.

Exhibitionism

In exhibitionism, one of the commonest sexual deviations, one usually finds that the offender is a son of a dominant, aggressive mother who resents her feminine role and tries to live her life through her children, especially the sons. The father is frequently a weak and ineffective person who has exerted but little influence in shaping the son's emotional development. Because of the mother's spoiling and showering the boy with unusual affection, he comes to identify himself with her and incestuous wishes develop as well. With a strong taboo against such insistent but consciously forbidden wishes, the boy must build compulsive but unconscious defenses. The symptom of exhibitionism with genital exposure to others functions to reassure him against castration.

Pathogenesis of Perversions

In some instances, the infantile components of the aggressive–destructive instinct, normal at an early stage of personality development, are not outgrown or sublimated but persist into adolescence and seem to become associated with the sex instinct, each reinforcing the other

and therefore productive of sadism, with the result that the individual's sexual behavior is not merely socially unacceptable or disgusting but even mutilative and murderous. Society is then confronted with a potentially dangerous, perhaps criminal, sex offender. In many instances, however, legal codes do not adequately distinguish between sex conduct that is socially distasteful and that which is socially dangerous.

A characteristic common to all forms of sexually psychopathic behavior or perversions is their repetitive, compulsive, patterned nature. Such behavior represents the expression of an uncontrollable urge, committed without logic or rationale and apparently for the purpose of securing relief from an unbearable tension. The satisfaction derived from the commission of the sexually deviated and compulsive act is symbolic and substitutive; it is therefore temporary and requires repetition. These characteristics constitute the criteria of the neuroses. There is, in fact, an increasing tendency to regard the true sexual perversions as basically psychoneurotic in their psychopathology and therefore as a kind of mental illness. As in the case of compulsive handwashing, the apparent motive is not the real, or at least not the only, motivating factor. The real motive is to satisfy aggressive or various other immature and deviated aspects of the psychosexual component of the personality.

A majority of serious sex offenders are unable to comprehend the reasons, the inner compulsion, for their actions. The sexual psychopath's behavior is not a substitute for normal heterosexual relations. It is a form of sexual activity that satisfies some very specific need ungratified by normal sexual activity. The added fact that the offender is usually unable to comprehend the reason for his actions, that their motivations are to a large extent unconscious, gives the psychopath's behavior a neurotic characteristic. In general, sexual psychopaths are people with deep-seated personality disorders of which sex deviation is but one manifestation.

Recent studies in the pathogenesis of

the sexual deviations make it appear that overt antisocial misbehavior may be caused by parental, often unwitting, seduction. In infancy, nudity, fondling, and virtual absence of privacy are appropriate and even necessary. If, however, such evidences of kindly parental affection persist until childhood or adolescence, they become pathological. Under the guise of "motherly" or "fatherly" affection, boys and girls may be bathed by parents, often of the opposite sex, until adolescence. Sleeping with children of the opposite sex may be prolonged into the teen-age period. Habitual undressing may occur in the presence of children. Sometimes legitimate parental embraces of affection extend into the sphere of frank bodily petting of adolescent children. Stimulated by parental behavior, the boy finds no outlet for his aroused sexual impulses. Eventually, mounting frustration and anger force him to follow one of two courses. One is regression to the safety of more infantile attitudes of sexual behavior. The other is sexual aggression toward women. Neither course resolves the rage or dissipates the overstimulated unconscious sexual drives. The result may therefore later be a direct, sexual, destructive acting-out of the conflict.

In contrast to the direct, hostile acting-out stemming from the repeated seduction and frustration incident to the child's intimate association with the parent of the opposite sex, such sexual aberrations as exhibitionism, voyeurism, and transvestism may be traceable to the unconscious tendencies of the parent. In such cases, the instinctual sexual development of the child seems to represent or constitute an acting-out of the unconscious wishes of the parent.

Treatment

If, as is increasingly believed by dynamically-minded psychiatrists, the psychopathologic condition that results in the behavior of the paraphiliac is basically related in motivation to that of the neuroses, the treatment of his deviations should be by methods comparable to those employed in the neuroses, i.e., by psychotherapy.

Before considering therapy, a word should perhaps be said concerning the prevention of sex deviation. This requires a knowledge of its origin, also a recognition and emotional acceptance by the public of the fact that true deviation, in contrast to methods of sexual gratification adopted in absence of opportunity for the satisfaction of a biologically normal heterosexual impulse, is a manifestation of a developmental fault in the mental life that had its beginning in the early formative years of childhood. Any progress in reducing sexually psychopathic behavior must remain exceeding slow. The most hopeful approach is doubtless through more and proper sex education in childhood, the establishment of identifications consonant with the child's sex, and assistance in a constructive sublimation of sexual and aggressive impulses that may be misdirected by the vicissitudes of childhood.

Although psychotherapy utilizing psychoanalytical principles is the rational treatment for the sex deviate, yet in few cases are the unconscious forces that have laid the foundation of the deviated impulses redirected thereby. Some sexual psychopaths have no conscious desire to be cured of their behavior. Ideal conditions for therapy exist when the deviate has not been guilty of offense against the person, has therefore not committed a serious social offense, and has voluntarily sought therapy. If his offense has been so serious that the community must be protected, the deviate must be confined. The prison environment and routine are not, however, conducive to successful therapy. The personality factors and emotional conflicts that led to the crime will not, of course, be worked through by simply spending a certain amount of time in prison. If the offender has not been guilty of violence, it is usually desirable that he be confined in a hospital atmosphere in which the therapist may supervise the surroundings in accordance with the needs of the patient as the therapy progresses. Through therapy and subsequent parole, some such offenders, if their desire for improvement is strong, may be enabled to channel their impulses into constructive activities. Since sex perversions are of psychic origin, their treatment by glandular injections or by castration is, of course, of no avail.

The Committee on Forensic Psychiatry of the Group for the Advancement of Psychiatry, to whose report reference has been made, gave thoughtful consideration both to the psychiatric aspects of sex deviation and to legislation to be recommended for dealing with sex offenders. It suggested that a psychiatric examination be made of any persons convicted of sexual offense and that if the psychiatrists report the offender suffers from a fundamental personality disorder, the judge, if he deems it wise, should, in lieu of sentence, commit him for an indefinite period to an institution equipped to give psychotherapy. Such a law would satisfy the aims of both community protection from the potentially dangerous offender and treatment under conditions favorable to restoration. "If the offender is curable he can be eventually released to society; if not, he should never be released. . . . The Committee is unreserved in its opinion that the committed sex offender should be actively treated in a non-penal institution. . . . The stigma of sex offenses officially attached to the sex offender committed to a penal institution creates a formidable obstacle to treatment. At best consistency demands that if we diagnose the sex offender as mentally disordered he should be treated as a mental case in a facility for that purpose."

Not all persons concerned with the disposition of sex offenders recommend treatment in state hospitals for mental diseases. They contend that such institutions lack facilities in both housing and personnel, that sex offenders do not mix well with others, that treatment is unsystematized and difficult, and that there are no criteria of recovery.

BIBLIOGRAPHY

Aichhorn, A.: Wayward Youth. New York, Viking Press, 1935.

Alexander, F.: The neurotic character. Internat. J. Psycho-Analysis, 11:292–311, 1930.

Bieber, I., et al.: Homosexuality. New York, Basic Books, Inc., 1962.

Bowman, K. M.: The problem of the sex offender. Am. J. Psychiat., 108:250–257, 1951.

Brancale, R., et al.: Psychiatric and psychological investigations of convicted sex offenders. Am. J. Psychiat., 109:17–21, 1952.

Bromberg, W.: Dynamic aspects of psychopathic personality. Psychoanalyt. Quart., 17:58–70, 1948.

Idem: Emotional immaturity and antisocial behavior. J. Clin. Psychopath., 8:423–452, 1947.

Cleckley, H. M.: The Mask of Sanity. St. Louis, C. V. Mosby Co., 1941.

Eissler, K. (Ed.): Searchlights on Delinquency. New York, International Universities Press, Inc.,1949.

Ford, C. S., and Beach, F. A.: Patterns of Sexual Behavior. New York, Paul B. Hoeber, 1951.

Gardner, G. E.: The community and the aggressive child: The expression of the aggressive-destructive impulses in juvenile-delinquent acts. Ment. Hyg., 33:537–550, 1949.

Idem: The community and the aggressive child: The aggressive-destructive impulses in the sex offender. Ment. Hyg., 34:44–63, 1950.

Glueck, E. T.: Identifying juvenile delinquents and neurotics. Ment. Hyg., 40:24–43, 1956.

Glueck, S., and Glueck, E. T.: Unraveling Juvenile Delinquency. New York, The Commonwealth Fund, 1950.

Group for Advancement of Psychiatry. Psychiatrically Deviated Sex Offenders, Report No. 9. Topeka, Kansas, 1949.

Guttmacher, M. S.: Sex Offenses: The Problem, Causes and Prevention. New York, W. W. Norton & Co., Inc., 1951.

Idem, and Weihofen, H.: Psychiatry and the Law. New York, W. W. Norton & Co., Inc., 1952.

Hooker, E.: A preliminary analysis of group behavior of homosexuals. J. Psychol., 42:217–225, 1956.

Jenkins, R. L.: The psychopathic or antisocial personality. J. Nerv. & Ment. Dis., 131:318–334, 1960.

Johnson, A. M., and Robinson, D. B.: The sexual deviant (sexual psychopath)—causes, treatment and prevention. J.A.M.A., 164:1559–1565, 1957.

Idem, and Szurek, S. A.: Etiology of antisocial behavior in delinquents and psychopaths. J.A.M.A., 154:814–817, 1954.

Karpman, B.: The sexual psychopath. J.A.M.A., 146:721–726, 1951.

Kennedy, A.: Psychopathic personality and social responsibility. J. Ment. Sc., 100:873–881, 1954.

Kinsey, A. C., et al.: Sexual Behavior in the

Human Male. Philadelphia, W. B. Saunders Company, 1948.

Idem: Sexual Behavior in the Human Female. Philadelphia, Ibid., 1953.

Kolb, L. C., and Johnson, A. M.: Etiology and therapy of overt homosexuality. Psychoanalyt. Quart., 24:506–515, 1955.

Lorand, S., and Balint, M. (Ed.): Perversions: Psychodynamics and Therapy. New York, Random House, 1956.

Peabody, G. A., Rowe, A. T., and Wall, J. H.: Fetishism and transvestitism. J. Nerv. & Ment. Dis., 118:339–350, 1953.

Rainer, J. D., Mesnikoff, A., Kolb, L. C., and Carr, A.: Homosexuality and heterosexuality in identical twins. Psychosom. Med., 22:251–259, 1960.

Redlich, F. C., et al.: Narcoanalysis and truth. Am. J. Psychiat., 107:586–593, 1951.

Rexford, E. N., Schleifer, M., and Van Amerongen, S. T.: A follow-up of a psychiatric study of 57 antisocial young children. Ment. Hyg., 40:196–214, 1956.

Scott, P. D.: Homosexuality, with special reference to classification. Proc. Royal Soc. Med., 50:655–660, 1957.

Whitman, R. M., Trosman, H., and Koenig, R.: Clinical assessment of passive–aggressive personality. Arch. Neurol. & Psychiat., 72:540–549, 1954.

Yalom, I. D.: Aggression and forbiddenness in voyeurism. Arch. Gen. Psychi., 3:305–319, 1960.

Chapter Thirty

DRUG ADDICTION

Drug addiction is usually symptomatic of a personality disorder. It might well have been included in the previous chapter. Since, however, it is so large a subject, a special chapter is devoted to it.

OPIATES AND THEIR SYNTHETIC EQUIVALENTS

The World Health Organization's Committee known as the "Expert Committee on Drugs Liable to Produce Addiction" has suggested the following definition of drug addiction: "Drug addiction is a state of periodic or chronic intoxication, detrimental to the individual and to society, produced by the repeated consumption of a drug (natural or synthetic). Its characteristics include: (1) an overpowering desire or need (compulsion) to continue taking the drug and to obtain it by any means, (2) a tendency to increase the dose and (3) a psychic (psychological) and sometimes a physical dependence on the effects of the drug."

Perhaps there should be further explanation of some of the terms contained in this definition as well as certain others relating to addiction. By *habituation,* or habit-formation, is meant a psychological dependence on the use of a drug because of the relief from tension and emotional discomfort that it affords. By *tolerance* is meant a declining effect of the same dose of a drug when it is administered repeatedly over a period of time. As a result, it is necessary to increase the dose in order to obtain the original degree of effect. *Physical dependence* refers to an altered physiological state brought about by repeated ingestion or administration of a drug in order to prevent the appearance of a characteristic illness called an *abstinence syndrome.* Dependence on analgesic drugs is characterized, on their withdrawal, by autonomic dysfunction, such as yawning, lacrimation, rhinorrhea, gooseflesh, and symptoms reflecting general irritability of the central nervous system, such as twitching of muscles, insomnia, hypertension, and fever. Dependence on hypnotics and alcohol is manifested chiefly by the development of convulsions and delirium following withdrawal. Physical dependence is a self-limited process. The symptoms appear in a definite time sequence following withdrawal of the drug, reach maximum intensity at a definite time, and decline at a definite rate. The symptoms that follow withdrawal of drugs with relatively short lengths of action, such as heroin and dilaudid, appear quickly, become intense in a short time, and decline rapidly. Symptoms that follow withdrawal of a drug with a long length of action, such as methadone, appear slowly, are never intense, and decline more slowly.

Etiology

Addiction to drugs and the extent of its occurrence result from a complex interaction of cultural and familial forces that determine the availability of the pharmacologic agent, the opportunities for initiation to its usage, and the individual predisposition to continue its usage. In China and other Asian countries where opiates have been readily available in the past, addiction was common. Where the drug traffic offers opportunity for large profits and its usage is pushed, as in those areas of the United States offering sites of entry and distribution, prevalence of narcotic addiction is higher. Here, again, the initiation to its use takes a daring and defiant attitude that appeals to the adolescent and the immature. In those Western European countries, such as England, where narcotic addiction is managed as a medical problem, drug traffic is less profitable, and the culture places little prestige on its use by over-emphasizing its significance, the number of narcotic addicts is much smaller.

Those who become addicted are for the most part antisocial personalities, but the neurotic and psychotic also are predisposed in view of their affective problems. The majority of the narcotic addicts are those with arrests in the ego and superego development and, for the most part, fixed to an ambivalent maternal figure. The latter is both possessive and rejecting—on the one hand encouraging the addicted child to give up the habit, and on the other often offering or smuggling the addicting agent to him.

As in other families where psychopaths are reared, there has been an absence of a strong and consistent father figure. The addict fails to develop internal controls, hopes for immediate gratifications of his needs, and yet is continually frustrated due to his exaggerated demands, his psychosexual immaturity, and his lack of ego capacity that might bring satisfaction by delay and insistent efforts toward his goals. Whereas the psychopath is deprived of pleasure and pained by his frequent failures socially, the neurotic and psychotic suffer from either anxiety or depression, or both. Narcotics particularly, and other drugs as well, offer to such individuals both immediate reduction in the painful affects and the provision of a sense of pleasure or euphoria that provides a striking contrast to the usual state of those with personality disorders. The drug gives pleasure, satisfaction, and a sense of power as well as immediate relief to the tensions of disturbing affects. The narcotic agents particularly reduce hunger, pain, and the frustration of threatening yet unrelieved sexual urge. The drug then substitutes for satisfaction of the basic biologic drives. As the drug effect wears away, anxiety depression or the customary feelings of loneliness or hopelessness recur, compounded with neurotic or psychotic sense of guilt. The drive to be relieved again becomes insurmountable, and additional doses are taken. The euphorizing effects of the narcotics tend to subside with their increasing use. Here, again, in an attempt to regain the longed for experience of pleasure and relief from distress, the dosage is gradually increased by the addicted. There is now physiologic evidence to suggest that, after a few doses of the narcotics, those intracellular processes underlying the state of physical dependence commence to operate.

Although there is no proved explanation for the phenomena of tolerance and of physical dependence, there are now two proffered theories. According to one theory, morphine has diphasic actions—excitation and depression. The excitant effects persist longer than do the depressant effects. For this reason, as doses of morphine are repeated, excitant effects are accumulated, requiring larger and larger doses in order to obtain a sufficient degree of depression to mask the excitant effects. This is the suggested explanation for tolerance. Following a withdrawal of the drug, its excitant effects are released, thus accounting for physical dependence.

A second theory advanced to explain the development of tolerance and physical dependence is that known as the theory of cellular adaptation. According to this hypothesis, the administration of opiates stimulates compensatory homeostatic mechanisms that oppose the depressant effects of the drug. These homeostatic responses become strengthened upon repeated administration of the substance. More and more drug is therefore required to induce the original degree of effect, and when the drug is withdrawn, the enhanced homeostatic mechanisms are released from the brake imposed upon them by the continued presence of morphine within the body, thus giving rise to physical dependence. This theory is based largely on the observation that manifestations of abstinence are always opposite in nature to those of the direct effects of opiates. Thus in the non-tolerant, non-addicted person, morphine constricts the pupils, lowers body temperature, reduces blood pressure, and causes sedation. Following withdrawal of morphine from the addict, there are noted dilation of the pupils, fever, a rise in blood pressure, and insomnia. Although the exact nature of the changes responsible for tolerance and physical dependence are not precisely known, they must be due to biochemical changes within the cells of the central nervous system.

Still another process takes place as the narcotic user receives his drug from a peddler, injects it, and responds with euphoria and relief of tensions. There is now good evidence as in the research of Olds (who demonstrated that animals with implanted electrodes in areas of the midbrain and certain midbrain nuclei repeatedly stimulate themselves electrically as though receiving pleasure or a reward) of the drive of the nervous system to reinforce activities that provide satisfactions. It may be assumed that a conditioning process now takes place as well. Such a process, with the possibility of establishing as unconditional stimuli the presence of another narcotic user, the offer of a drug or syringe may well explain the propensity to relapse even long after a formerly addicted person has recovered

from a state of physical dependence and perhaps has even been relieved of the painful affect that originally led to the pleasure in the drug.

Extent of Drug Addiction

When the Harrison Narcotic Act was passed in 1914, there were 175,000 narcotic addicts, mostly women, in the United States. Reports show that there are now approximately 60,000 addicts, most of whom are men. About 35,000 of these are known to the authorities. Although addiction does exist among underprivileged adolescents, it is not as frequent as articles in the public press would indicate.

The large group of addicts is composed of individuals with personality disorders who became addicted to drugs through contact and association with persons already addicted. The addict often seeks to recruit new addicts in order that through sales to them he may secure funds in order to obtain a supply for his own needs. Most members of this group are emotionally immature, hostile, aggressive persons who take drugs in order to secure relief from inner tension. They have few healthy resources or interests and are motivated by immature drives for immediate goals. The addict-to-be finds in the drug a release from tension felt as a restless need for pleasurable or exotic sensations, the satisfaction of a longing for artificial elation or peace. Conscious discomfort is eliminated, repressed drives may be released, and responsibility is evaded. Another group consists of frankly neurotic persons with anxiety and obsessive, compulsive, or psychophysiologic symptoms that are relieved by drugs. A third group consists of persons who, in the course of physical illness, have received drugs over an extended period and after the termination of the ailment have continued their use. However, probably all persons who acquire addiction in this manner have some fundamental emotional problem that caused them to continue the use of drugs beyond the period of medical need. Many addicts were intemperate in the use of alcohol before they became addicted to drugs. In practically all addicts, their previous adjustment to life was marginal or unsatisfactory.

Opiate Addiction

Morphine, its derivatives, and its synthetic pharmacological substitutes are so allied in their addictive qualities that they are considered together.

The amount of morphine taken by addicts varies greatly. A few do not take over 2 grains per day. DeQuincey states in his "Confessions of an Opium Eater" that at one period in the history of his drug addiction he took 500 ml. of laudanum, or approximately 72 grains of morphine, daily. Perhaps the average addict takes from 10 to 20 grains per day when the drug is available. Today, most addicts in the United States subsist on a much lower daily dosage. Many addicts tolerate, without unfavorable symptoms, several times the dose they are accustomed to receive. This tolerance is destroyed following disappearance of the withdrawal symptoms. Addicts usually do not realize how rapidly they lose their tolerance for opiates. Sometimes during the "cure" addicts have obtained access to an opiate and have taken, with fatal results, what was the usual dose before withdrawal was instituted.

After recourse to his drug, the addict feels a sense of relief and perhaps of exhilaration, together with an increase in efficiency. The alleviation and sense of well-being obtained by the addict through a dose of the drug is so great that, as its pleasant effect diminishes, the desire for the satisfaction that the drug affords can scarcely be resisted. Although the continued administration of small amounts of the drug will prevent the distressing withdrawal symptoms to be described, increasing amounts are necessary to obtain the desired exhilaration and sense of increased capacity. As a result, the quantity taken is gradually increased until enormous amounts are required.

The eventual effect of the habit is impairment of a higher ethical sense, that is, the ego ideals. This moral and social deterioration is not a result of the direct effects of narcotics, but rather, of social consequences of the life of addiction. When the narcotic is taken in large doses, ambition and physical energy are lessened, lethargy is produced, and the pleasurable feeling that all is well makes the addict contented. As a result, he pays less attention to work and becomes an idler. Those who depend upon an illegitimate source for their supply of drugs are sometimes unable to work because of discomfort and weakness resulting from inability to secure the usual dose. When such patients, after a short period of deprivation, secure a supply, they often take more than is necessary to keep them comfortable. As a result, they alternate between physical and mental instability and physical and mental lethargy.

Frequently addicts are compelled to associate with low moral characters in order to continue their addiction. Financial embarrassment resulting from idleness or the high price of peddled narcotics may impel the addict to beg money, to obtain it by subterfuge, or to steal. He suffers from lowered self-esteem through the public attitude of contempt and through constant fear of arrest or because of a term served in the penitentiary for having narcotics in his possession. This chain of events results in habit deterioration and in a demoralization of character. It converts those who might have been fairly useful citizens into outcasts, idlers, and dependents. Contrary to popular opinion, the prolonged use of morphine, heroin, and marihuana has comparatively little effect on the physical health of the addict. Morphine addiction rarely produces psychotic reactions.

DIAGNOSIS OF OPIATE ADDICTION. Frequently the individual admits that he is addicted to and needs drugs. If he denies the habit, the diagnosis can at times be made by needle marks, indurations, and the scars of abscesses. Miosis is suggestive but not definite evidence. Periods of restlessness, irritability, and anxiety, followed rather suddenly by ones of euphoria and apparent relief and contentment, should be suggestive of drug addiction.

At times the only method of diagnosis

may be isolation of the patient from a source of drugs followed by observation for signs of abstinence. The addict may be exceedingly clever in concealing a supply of his drugs. He may enter a hospital for the purpose of being cured of his addiction, yet at the same time have a supply craftily concealed in personal articles or even in body cavities.

Recently, a diagnostic test of considerable sensitivity has been developed that depends upon precipitating the abstinence syndrome by the parenteral injections of N-allylnormorphine (Nalline), a morphine antagonist. Before conducting such a test, it is advisable to obtain written permission of the patient or his guardian. This test is performed by injecting subcutaneously 3 mg. of N-allylnormorphine. In less than 20 minutes after injection, clear-cut signs of the abstinence syndrome will be noted in addicts using 60 mg. or more of morphine daily or equivalent amounts of heroin, dihydromorphinone, methadone, or Levo-Dromoran. Symptoms of the abstinence syndrome are described in the next section of this chapter. If the response to the first injection is negative or doubtful, a second dose of 5 mg. should be given 30 minutes after the first, and again a third 30 minutes after the second. At this time, if abstinence symptoms have not become apparent and if the signs of the direct effects of the injected drug have appeared, the test may be read as negative. N-allylnormorphine directly produces dizziness, pseudoptoses, mioses, and reduction in the respiratory rate, with a drunken experience. The absence of response to this test may occur in addicts who have been withdrawn from narcotics for as short as a week's period, or in addicts taking scattered doses. It is unreliable for meperidine (Demerol) addiction and contraindicated in the presence of serious organic disease.

WITHDRAWAL SYMPTOMS. Whenever opium or its habit-forming derivatives are abruptly withdrawn, a definite train of symptoms known as abstinence or withdrawal symptoms appear. If, within 12 to 14 hours after the administration of morphine, the dose is not repeated, the so-called withdrawal signs and symptoms begin to appear. Among the first are yawning, lacrimation, rhinorrhea, sneezing, and perspiration. These symptoms become more marked, and anorexia, dilated pupils, tremor, and gooseflesh are added. About 36 hours after the last dose, uncontrollable twitching of the muscles appears and cramps develop in the legs, abdomen, and back. The patient becomes intensely restless, is unable to sleep, and both pulse and blood pressure rise. Vomiting and diarrhea are frequent. These acute signs and symptoms reach their height about 48 hours after the last dose of morphine and remain at this height for 72 hours. They then gradually subside during the next five to ten days. As the withdrawal symptoms develop, the patient becomes restless, pessimistic, surly, fault-finding, and irritable and exhibits an unpleasant, increased psychomotor activity. He has a marked subjective feeling of weakness, and considerable prostration may occur. He may curse, cry, be impulsively destructive, and make suicidal gestures. To quite an extent, the intensity of withdrawal symptoms depends on the amount of drug the patient has been receiving. To some degree, the extent of the symptoms can be controlled by the patient himself. Any patient who appears comfortable during the period of withdrawal should be suspected of illicit possession of the drug.

PROGNOSIS. It should be remembered that narcotic addiction nearly always results from emotional problems, compounded frequently with a complex system of habit patterns that add to the difficulty of treatment. In general, these emotional problems are the same anxieties, conflicts, and neuroses as those with which other emotionally unstable persons are confronted. Although probably more addicts than is commonly realized are permanently cured, they constitute a minority. The United States Public Health Service Hospital, Lexington, Kentucky, an institution for the treatment of addicts, found that only two-tenths of 1 per cent of the patients who left the hospital in less than 30 days remained off the drug, whereas 24 per cent of those who remained for the recommended period were believed to have remained free from addiction.

Some habitués, pretending that they no longer have any desire for the drug, look eagerly forward to an opportunity to return to their habit and devise every imaginable pretext to hasten their release from the hospital. Even those who believe they wish to be cured return to the drug on the slightest pretext, the alleged occasion being actually but a rationalization of their emotional defects and their psychological need for obliterating reality and its problems. They feel lost without the narcotic and the sense of physical comfort it imparts. Many, too, feel that they are not understood, are in a constant state of mild dissatisfaction, and long to return to the accustomed companionship of other addicts, by whom they feel they are understood and with whom they feel a sense of security and comradeship.

Other addicts, sometimes for the sake of self-justification, sometimes because, as vendors of morphine, they see in their unhappy companion a potential customer, urge the recently "cured" patient to share the alleviating agent. The profits from this "cured" patient will replenish their own diminishing supply of the drug, of course.

TREATMENT. On a rational basis, the preferable mode of treatment of the drug addict should be directed at relief of the distressing affective state that originally predisposed him to respond positively to its original use. Such treatment would be directed to correction of the personality disorder or the psychoneurotic or psychotic state by the therapeutic process most applicable for the particular patient. Withdrawal of the drug then would not be undertaken until there had occurred the development of a firm dependent therapeutic relationship with a physician or other member of the therapeutic team. This relationship might sustain the patient through the period of abstinence and provide positive support to sustain withdrawal.

Unfortunately, therapeutic efforts today are directed largely to simple withdrawal of the drug, which must be undertaken in an institution where the activities of the patient and the sources of the drug can be controlled. The period of hospital treatment should be four to nine months. The patient must remain long enough to be relieved of any physical ailments, to have opportunity to develop habits of living and working without drugs, and to be helped in discovering the source of his emotional difficulty.

WITHDRAWAL. It is not humane and it may be even dangerous to withdraw morphine abruptly. It may be withdrawn rapidly over a period of 10 days, in which case 30 mg. may be given every six hours for two days, with continued reduction thereafter until withdrawal is complete by the end of 10 days. It is probably more desirable to begin with the withdrawal of morphine, then shift to methadone, which suppresses the withdrawal symptoms in persons addicted to morphine. In this method, one should first ascertain the least amount of morphine that will prevent the appearance of withdrawal symptoms. This is termed the stabilization dosage and can usually be determined in two or three days. Once the stabilization dosage is known, 1 mg. of methadone may be substituted for every 3 or 4 mg. of the patient's accustomed dose of morphine. As methadone is a cumulative, slow-acting drug, the patient should be given one-half of his accustomed dose of morphine and one-half of his calculated dose of methadone during the first day of substitution. During the second day, only methadone is given. After substitution of methadone has been effected, the calculated dosage should be maintained for two or three days. The total dosage can be adjusted upward or downward, depending on the patient's response. Thereafter, methadone should be withdrawn over the course of 7 to 10 days, depending on the patient's response. Although withdrawal symptoms should be expected near the end of treatment, severe manifestations of abstinence are never seen when this method of withdrawal is used. Chlorpromazine is also useful in the tension states occurring in the withdrawal of opium and other narcotics. Great caution should be exercised in withdrawal of drugs from patients with evidence of myocardial insufficiency.

Sometimes the patient, without knowledge of the physician, has also been taking barbiturates before his admission. In that case the patient may develop an abstinence syndrome resulting from barbiturate withdrawal, as well. This will usually be in the form of a severe convulsion in which fractures may occur. The prevention of this additional abstinence syndrome is the continued but gradually decreasing administration of a barbiturate.

An effort should be made to establish rapport and positive transference between the patient and physician during withdrawal. The patient usually has a resistence to gaining insight into the real causes of his addiction. Psychotherapy should, however, be directed toward his motivations, defenses, and adaptations. Group psychotherapy is not successful. The usual recognition of drug addiction as a crime rather than as a disease reacts unfavorably on success of therapy. The vocational and social discrimination experienced by the addict following his discharge tends to lead to relapse.

The discharged addict should be required to report regularly for a period of five years to a center staffed with internists, psychiatrists, and social workers who are specifically trained to help him meet his problems. If left to solve his problems unaided, he usually returns to the use of drugs. It is frequently helpful if he joins the organization known as Narcotics Anonymous.

Other Opium Derivatives

Heroin, taken both hypodermically and by snuffing, has great addiction ability. Many consider it the most difficult of all addictions to cure. *Codeine* has a definite, though low-grade, addiction liability. Both *Dilaudid* (dihydromorphinone hydrochloride) and *metopon* (methyldihydromorphinone) have high physical dependence and habituation liabilities. *Demerol* (meperidine hydrochloride) is a synthetic analgesic that is not chemically related to morphine but is nevertheless addicting. It possesses considerable habituation liability, and after prolonged administration its addicts develop physical dependence. Any differences in the addiction liability of the new analgesic drugs from that of morphine are differences in degree, not in kind. The general features of the morphine abstinence syndrome are also characteristic of these drugs.

Cocainism

For many years cocaine addiction constituted one of the major drug problems, but because of legislation, its use among addicts is much less prevalent than formerly. At the present time, nearly all its habitués have acquired the addiction through other addicts. Strictly speaking, cocaine is not a narcotic. It produces a marked stimulation, a sense of exhilaration, euphoria, and self-confidence, an increased flow of ideas, and a pressure of speech and of activity. During this period of stimulation and sense of competency, there may be an actual increase in capacity for work. As the stimulus of the drug wears off, the patient feels weak, depressed, restless, morose, and irritable. Other abstinence symptoms are digestive disturbances, tremors, palpitation, specks in front of the eyes, muscular weakness, slight confusion, and impotence.

Frankly psychotic symptoms are common among those who continue the use of large doses of cocaine over a prolonged period. Such addicts may experience terrifying visual hallucinations, become suspicious, and perhaps show much excitement. Delusions of jealousy and of persecution are common and may lead to violence. A rather characteristic phenomenon is the frequent existence of formicative paresthesias, associated with which there may be the delusion that there are actually insects beneath the skin, the presence of which the patient may attempt to demonstrate.

The moral deterioration in the cocaine

addict is even greater than in the morphine habitué. The prospects of any permanent cure of the habit are even less favorable than in the case of the morphine addict. Withdrawal of the drug is not accompanied by the painful experiences and tendency to collapse occurring in the withdrawal of opium derivatives.

Barbiturate Addiction

Any of the barbiturates, when given daily for periods of three to six months in amounts approximately eight or more times the usual effective dose, produce addiction. Upon withdrawal, all patients who have been ingesting as much as 0.8 gm. or more of pentobarbital daily suffer anxiety, weakness, and tremor. Many will develop a psychotic reaction resembling delirium tremens, and probably a larger number has one or more convulsions. The nature of the biochemical and physiological disturbances responsible for the withdrawal symptoms is not yet known.

TREATMENT. Even a gradual reduction of barbiturates carries a certain risk. Patients should therefore be under constant supervision and observation during withdrawal, which should be carried out in a hospital. As already indicated, the drug in barbiturate addiction must not be withdrawn abruptly. For the first two days the patient will receive just enough of the barbiturates to maintain a mild degree of intoxication. This will usually be from 0.2 gm. to 0.4 gm. of pentobarbital or an equivalent amount of another barbiturate. Thereafter the drug will be very slowly reduced, the total withdrawal period being extended over two to three weeks. If excessive anxiety, insomnia, or tremor appears during withdrawal, reduction of the drug should be stopped and the amount held constant until these symptoms disappear.

It is important to remember that acute barbiturate intoxication is frequently superimposed on barbiturate addiction. After patients who have been acutely poisoned with barbiturates have recovered from coma, it should be ascertained whether they have been taking the drug chronically. In such cases, barbiturate intake should be restored and gradual reduction begun. After withdrawal has been completed, there should be a long period of psychotherapy.

Many believe that addiction to barbiturates is more serious than morphine addiction. Abstinence from morphine is less dangerous than abstinence from barbiturates, and morphine addiction causes less mental and emotional disturbance.

Marihuana

Because of its frequent use, marihuana addiction should also be considered. The active principle of this drug is an oil. The flowering tops of the female plant are used, the action being the same as that of cannabis indica. The usual form of taking the drug is by smoking it in the form of cigarettes, often referred to as "reefers." Much misinformation concerning the action of marihuana has created an unjustified alarm relative to its addicts. Unlike opium derivatives, it does not give rise to a biological dependence accompanied by withdrawal symptoms, and its indulgence can be discontinued without great difficulty. It does not lead to any physical, mental, or moral degradation, even after prolonged use. Following inhalation, the subject has a sense of euphoria and shows increased volubility and psychomotor activity followed subjectively by a feeling of calm and pleasurable relaxation. The individual may sleep for one to six hours, and on awakening he no longer feels exhilarated. Marihuana is probably taken by users for the purpose of producing sensations comparable to those produced by alcohol. It is probable that marihuana may precipitate a psychotic reaction in persons of a poorly-organized personality. One of the most undesirable results of marihuana addiction is the more serious addiction to opiate-like drugs to which the use of the former drug often leads because of the degrading social contacts with which marihuana addiction seems to be particularly associated. It is a popular misconception that the use of marihuana leads to criminal habits. This opinion is not sustained by actual experience. Bowman has correctly pointed out that alcohol causes infinitely more murders, rapes, and crimes of violence than do morphine, heroin, cocaine, marihuana, and all other drugs combined.

BIBLIOGRAPHY

Allentuck, S., and Bowman, K. M.: The psychiatric aspects of marihuana intoxication. Am. J. Psychiat., 99:248–251, 1942.

Council on Mental Health: Report on narcotic addiction. J.A.M.A., 165:1707–1713, 1957.

Hoch, P. H., and Zubin, J. (Ed.): Problems of Addiction and Habituation. New York, Grune & Stratton, 1958.

Isbell, H.: Addiction to barbiturates and the barbiturate abstinence syndrome. Ann. Int. Med., 33:108–121, 1950.

Idem: Medical aspects of opiate addiction. Bull. New York Acad. Med., 31:886–901, 1955.

Idem, et al.: Chronic barbiturate intoxication. Arch. Neurol. & Psychiat., 64:1–28, 1950.

Kolb, L.: Drug Addiction: A Medical Problem. Springfield, Illinois, Charles C Thomas, 1962.

Maas, J. M.: Increasing promiscuity and abuse with the barbiturates. Am. J. Med. Sc., 222:121–128, 1951.

Mason, P.: The mother of the addict. Psychiat. Quart. Suppl., 32:189–199, 1958.

Nyswander, M.: The Drug Addict as a Patient. New York, Grune & Stratton, 1956.

Idem, et al.: The treatment of drug addicts as voluntary outpatients. Am. J. Orthpsychiat., 28:714–727, 1958.

Plum, F., and Swanson, A. G.: Barbiturate poisoning treated by physiologic methods. J.A.M.A., 163:827–835, 1957.

Rado, S.: Narcotic bondage: A general theory of the dependence on narcotic drugs. Am. J. Psychiat., 114:165–170, 1957.

Report of Subcommittee on Barbiturates, New York Academy of Medicine. Public Health Reports, 71:1144–1155, 1956.

Report on Drug Addiction. Bull. New York Acad. Med., 31:592–607, 1955.

Wikler, A.: Opiate Addiction: Psychological and Neurophysical Aspects in Relation to Clinical Problems. Springfield, Illinois, Charles C Thomas, 1953.

Idem, and Rasor, R. W.: Psychiatric aspects of drug addiction. Am. J. Med., 14:566–570, 1953.

Chapter Thirty-one

CHILD PSYCHIATRY

The first organized psychiatric study of childhood maladjustments was undertaken by Healy, in Chicago, in 1909. Interest in the subject increased slowly at first but moved forward with greater impetus after 1919, when the National Committee for Mental Hygiene, supported by the Commonwealth Fund, initiated the sponsorship of child guidance clinics and provided fellowships for study in child psychiatry.

The treatment of children's psychiatric disorders differs in many respects from that of adult psychiatric problems. In large measure this is because the child is living through the most active phase of the developmental process. His personality is less structured and formed, and from one stage of growth to another he shows rapid modifications in behavior. The psychiatrist who works in the field of child psychiatry must have a knowledge of the ever-changing patterns of healthy behavior at the various age levels as a means of evaluating the existence of disturbance. Again, the environmental pressures leading to disordered personality functioning in the child may usually be discovered in the present or recent past. They contribute a continuing influence in the life of the child. Since at this age the child is dependent upon his parents emotionally and in all aspects of his living, the psychiatrist must deal directly with the parents in the course of arranging the treatment and in determining future management. The child seldom comes to treatment on his own; he is brought in by the parents or referred by community agencies such as schools or courts.

Still another difference is evident in the practice of child psychiatry. This has to do with the means of obtaining information and evaluating the problem of the child. Of necessity, much of the history must be obtained from the parents and from others who are related to the child in his school environment or in other aspects of his training. Inferences in regard to his emotional reactions and relations with others, particularly in the younger age periods, are derived from psychological testing and from play therapy, wherein the child acts out his fantasies. Because of the necessity of obtaining information from parents and social agencies and through psychological examination of the intellectual and emotional life of the child, the work of the child psychiatrist must be actively supplemented by the skills of the clinical psychologist and psychiatric social worker. Furthermore, in prescribing treatment, consideration must be given to the significant persons in the child's environment as well as to the child. The outcome of a particular problem depends to a great extent upon the family structure from which the child comes. There are some symptoms that are fostered by the family. In such circumstances, efforts directed toward understanding and modifying the behavior of the child remain unsuccessful unless the significant family members also come into therapy.

Child psychiatry is concerned with behavior disturbances, difficulties in social adaptation, unsatisfactory character traits, psychogenic disturbances of physiological function, or, less commonly, the forms of psychoneurotic or psychotic reactions characteristic of older-age periods, as well as delirious reactions, epilepsy, juvenile paresis, and the consequences of organic brain disease. Since there is less fixity of the patterns of disturbed behavior because of the plastic personality of the child, there is less unanimity in regard to the diagnostic schemata for the disorders of childhood than for those of adulthood. Although in recent years the tendency has largely been to consider the majority of behavior disorders as emotionally determined, there is a growing recognition of the great extent of brain injury consequent to childbirth as contributing to many of these disturbances. The specific problems of brain-injured, epileptic, and mentally defective children have been discussed in foregoing chapters. Whatever the type of disturbance or its etiology, it should be recognized that troublesome trends in the child that make it difficult for him to get along comfortably with other people or for others to get along with him are problems of mental health. They should therefore not be dealt with from the standpoint of moralistic disapproval.

Causes of Psychiatric Problems

The child is a changing personality, and in order for his emotional growth to proceed in a natural and spontaneous way it is necessary that he receive affection, understanding, security, and discipline and be stimulated by achievement and social acceptance. It is necessary, too, that he feel satisfaction in his relation with his parents, that he develop a feeling that he is lovable, that his individuality be respected by his parents, and that he have confidence in his own strength and capacity as a person in his own right. The maladjustments of childhood sometimes originate from a single cause, but more frequently they arise from the combined action of several types, particularly emotional and situational ones; also, in some instances, they arise from intellectual and perhaps other constitutional causes. Although care must be exercised not to oversimplify the problem and explain it by one formula, it is perhaps reasonable to assume that in many maladjustments of childhood human relationships have, through their influence upon the developing personality, acted as a significant etiological factor. Of all these relationships, that of parent and child is the one in which the problem is most frequently rooted. There are many phases of the parent–child relationship that may be pathogenetic, and there are many forms of personality maladjustment that may result from them. These will be discussed in this chapter.

According to psychoanalytical theory, the production of the behavior disorders and neurotic traits in children is attributed to an attempt to adjust two opposing forces in the personality—the *id* desires and the *super-ego* prohibitions. The child's neurotic symptoms, increased anxiety, and other clinical signs arise because he has not relinquished his infantile instinctual cravings normally during the growing-up process. He has failed either adequately to channelize them into reality-adjusted and pleasurable functions of the ego or to adjust them to the requirements of reality and of society by repression, reaction formation, undoing, isolation, reversal, or other mental mechanisms.

Others ascribe these manifestations to disturbances and distortions in the normal personality growth process. As a result, there is an undeveloped phase in some aspect of the child's personality. The undeveloped phases may have arisen through such factors as the striving of the mother to hold her child as an undifferentiated part of herself. Thus the child does not obtain the natural love, guidance, and direction necessary for his development into an independent personality, with fulfillment of his individual potentialities and responsibilities. Again, the failure of the personality development, with resulting inadequate capacity of the child to deal efficiently and realistically with the business of living, may result from the fact that he struggled to protect his dependency status against the demands of growth, against giving up his infantile relationship to the mother, and against an independent organization of his own powers and capacities. According to this point of view, the child has been delayed or blocked in some aspect of his growth toward a normally functioning self and cannot handle his feelings in a way that permits those growing relationships with others that are essential for his development.

To return to a consideration of factors and experiences that may be of importance in the production of the behavior disorders of childhood, including those that are neurotic, a number of factors must be considered.

Age. Observation of infants seems to show that the need for mothering, sensory stimuli to skin and mucous surface, and instinctual emotional gratification is present from the time of birth, and that the lack of these may result in evident inhibition of personality development. Sudden weaning or attempts to establish toilet training at too early a stage of the child's development may indicate parental attitudes that pave the way for later emotional and behavior disorders. At about the beginning of the third year, the necessity for growing into relationships with other people and accepting their values becomes definitely greater. Confrontation with this problem may stimulate insecurity and anxiety that then create defense reactions in the form of feeding problems, destructiveness, or temper tantrums. Puberty, with its social and sexual problems and its urge to effect emancipation from the home, offers many possibilities for friction and inner conflict with resulting emotional and behavior maladjustments.

Environmental and Interpersonal Factors. It is generally agreed that the influence of the child's environment is the most important factor in the development of neurotic symptoms or behavior problems. To a large extent those environmental factors that are of greatest influence in molding the personality of the child are interpersonal ones, particularly those in the family. In fact, the determining influence of the family circle on the developing personality of the child is one of the cornerstones of child psychiatry. The healthy family is the ideal medium for fulfilling the basic emotional needs of the child. In the family may arise many, perhaps most, of the psychopathological processes that lead to neurotic reactions, personality difficulties, or behavior disorders. Here are such disturbing influences as parental dissensions, parental alcoholism, hostility, cruelty, neglect, overprotection, and excessive parental ambition for the child. Even though the mother be highly intellectual, she may be incapable of mature emotional relationships.

Other factors that may distort parent–child relationship and disturb personality development are neurosis, psychosis, or psychopathic, antisocial or aggressive tendencies on part of the parent. The psychological fate of the child is to a considerable extent determined by the emotional health of the parents and by the complex forces interacting within the family group. Many faulty parent–child relationships are related to the parents' own personality structure, their emotional conflicts, biases, and past experiences. To secure a clear picture of the influences to which the child is subjected, one should know how the parents feel unconsciously about the child, what conflicts disturb the parent–child relationship, even what conflicts have existed between the parents and their parents, and how these have affected the ability of the parents to relate themselves to the child. The emotional reaction of the parents to the behavior of the child should not be overlooked. Occasionally the behavior of the parents is a result of the child's behavior rather than the cause of it. Early institutional care or other interruptions in the continuity of parent–child relationship are harmful and lead to defects in personality development expressed as emotional apathy or inadequacy in forming relations with others, inability to accept obstructions, failures, and separations, as well as perceptual, intellectual, and language disturbances.

Relations to siblings may be the source of personality problems. Parental favoritism and a feeling of being supplanted by the birth of a younger sibling may arouse abnormal sibling rivalry and jealousy. It should be remembered that it is particularly difficult for some children to share an adult (especially a parent) with another child.

The broken home is a common source of personality difficulties. The prolonged deprivation of the young child of maternal care may have warping or inhibitive effects on his personality development. Frequently this gives rise to a sense of insecurity, a frequent cause of neurotic behavior. Parental instability with resulting shifts of attitude on the part of the child may prevent identification, one of the most important mechanisms in shaping character. Death of a parent, or more frequently desertion or divorce, preceded, usually, by a long period of domestic unhappiness, may be important in the production of personality disorders. Attitudes experienced by the stepchild or the foster child may create personality maladjustments. Many school experiences are important in giving rise to personality problems. Failure in school and the factors that contributed to the failure, such as mental retardation or unhappy home conditions, faulty handling by teachers or difficulties in relations with classmates, often are sources of personality difficulties. Sometimes poverty and privation operate to produce

neurotic traits or behavior disorders. In such a case, the deprivation has some special meaning to the child.

There are many situations and features in the child's environment that have a great influence upon the developing pattern of his personality. Anxiety, frustration, deprivation of love, overprotection, and lack of consideration of the individual factor and of personality needs unfavorably influence the developing personality. The emotional attitude of the environment, for example, may promote security or it may create anxiety that evokes various defensive behavior reactions. Hate, fear, worry, and rejection and critical, punitive, and other environmental attitudes may exercise distorting effects and prevent the development of a rounded and smoothly functioning personality. An environment that presents constant frustrations or deprivations stimulates resentment that later takes the forms of a persistent hostility and aggression, or again it may lead to a pattern of withdrawal. Much of the child's behavior is determined by the manner in which he deals with his aggression.

Belonging to a social group regarded as inferior or alien to the major environmental one with the resulting conflicts in identification with one's own family group in ideologies and in accepted culture may create many emotional problems. Difficulties in language and lack of social and educational privileges and experiences also contribute to the problems. The child who feels rejected is often insecure and anxious, as a result of which he is hyperactive, emotionally unstable, has difficulty in concentrating, feels resentment toward the person who denies him the love he wants, and expresses his hostile feelings by temper tantrums and disobedience. He may cover up his need for affection by an air of bravado and attack. Students of child delinquency report that generally the delinquent has had an unhappy childhood characterized by feelings of rejection, inadequacy, and guilt and by lack of affection.

It has already been indicated that the

parent–child relationship is one of the most determinative interpersonal relationships in respect to the child's mental health. The attitude of the parents toward the child is greatly influenced by the degree of satisfaction and contentment they have been able to achieve in their own lives. Frequently the mother carries over into her relationship with her child the unresolved conflicts that arose in her relationships with her own parents. Hostilities and resentments from such a source may enter into a disturbing relationship with her child that has a harmful effect on its social and emotional growth and development. Conflict over hostile feelings is common in parents, and much of the behavior expressed in troublesome parent–child relationships derives from that source.

Parental oversolicitude is much more frequent than neglect and is equally pernicious in its results. Such overprotection in every phase of the child's life, including dress, health, food, play, and association with other children prevents the development of independence, responsibility, and maturity of personality essential for successful adaptation. Such children, shielded from all the ordinary hazards of life, are rendered dependent, infantile, and frequently hostile. They lack the satisfying pleasures of childhood and are usually whining and deceitful. Oversolicitous parents, in their anxiety to protect the child against imaginary harm, usually nag, scold, and constantly admonish him. As he grows older, they continue to treat him as a child rather than as a responsible, or at least partially responsible, person.

Maternal overprotection is more frequent than is paternal oversolicitude. It may be manifested in the case of both the wanted and the unwanted child and for various reasons. In the unwanted child, the fact that the prospective arrival of the child was unwelcome may have made the mother feel guilty for having entertained such a thought. A smothering oversolicitude then represents the denial and disguise of a hostile rejection of the child—a device for the denial of hate. The defensive reaction to her unconscious hostility to the child may lead her to extravagant measures of protection resembling an obsessional neurosis. Perhaps her marriage proved frustrating and she finds in her child a solution of her own emotional needs. Overprotection may take the form of continuing such activities as feeding, bathing, nursing or dressing the child long past the usual time. It may be shown, too, by the mother's practice of sleeping with the child even in his teens, or by a desire to have the child constantly in her presence. Usually, also, there is oversolicitous protection against physical danger, illness, or the "bad influence" of other children.

Levy points out that in her training of the child, the overprotective mother is either indulgent or dominating. The child of the indulgently overprotective mother continues his infantile demands and expectations long after they should have been outgrown. He is often a disciplinary problem, and his behavior may be characterized by disobedience, impudence, tantrums, an aggressively demanding attitude, and varying degrees of tyrannical behavior. He may be selfish, conceited, and a show-off. His bossy and demanding attitude betrays the fact that maternal indulgence has stimulated the development of aggressive components of the child's personality. Feeding problems are common in the child of the indulgent, apprehensive mother. The problems of the dominatingly overprotective mother's child are largely of anxieties, fears, shyness, and submissive behavior. In both cases, the overprotection operates against outside influences that make for growth in social adaptation. The child may use neurotic symptoms to control the mother and retain the infantile advantages of the emotionally intertwined mother–child relation.

Levy has shown, too, that many instances of the overprotective relationship arise from the mother's insatiable hunger for love, a hunger based on a severe privation of love in her own childhood. To this impoverishment in the child of all those positive feelings implicit in parental love—recognition, security, affection and sympathy—Levy gives the term "affect hunger."

The emotional influences in a particular family are never identical for any two children. Probably, too, a mother's psychology is such that no two children can bear for her the same emotional meaning. Occasionally a mother may entertain a hostility toward a particular child, arising, perhaps, from a hatred that is directed primarily toward her husband and then transmitted to a child who resembles him. Again, disappointment concerning the sex of the child may create a maternal attitude that is traumatic to it.

The overstrict, punitive father may arouse disturbing tensions and such emotional reactions as fear, anxiety, resentment, and hostility, with consequent personality or behavior disorders. The tension of actively aggressive impulses evoked by the severity of a father who represents an object of frustration and fear may cause the boy to erect defenses against his aggression, perhaps in the form of an obsessional character or an obsessional neurosis.

In Chapter 3, Personality Development, attention was called to the mechanism of identification as one of the most important factors in affecting personality and in shaping character. Emotional deprivation makes it impossible for the child to identify with the parental figures and thereby utilize the constructive influence of that mechanism in personality development. Although identification is largely an unconscious process, it is based on a feeling of love, and without love, usually without a feeling of respect or admiration for someone or something, without a desire to be like some member of the environment, identification does not take place, the development of the super-ego is hindered, and behavior difficulties result. It should be remembered, too, that through daily association and identification the emotional difficulties of the parent may be transmitted to the child.

One must not forget the emotionally deprived child who appears to be retarded in every field of personality development,

including even intellectual functioning. Such children are most frequently found among those who were reared in institutions during infancy.

HANDICAPS AND OVERAMBITION. Although the majority of emotional and behavior disorders arise from situations, interpersonal relations, and environmental constellations that operate against personality development or produce conflicts, tensions, and anxieties, organic and other factors must not be disregarded. The child, for example, who is so retarded mentally that he cannot compete with his peers, the one who is small for his age but strives to compensate through his readiness to fight, the child who is deaf or who has suffered from a prolonged physical illness or from encephalitis may react with emotional or behavior disturbances. The brain-injured child must not be forgotten, either. Beneath this child's disturbed behavior there may be a rich and troubled inner life marked by anxiety, regression, and frustration. Neurological or orthopedic handicaps, obesity, or other physical abnormalities that attract attention require special consideration. Other factors that stimulate self-consciousness or an exaggerated feeling of difference in relation to those about the child also act as potentially pathogenic factors. Overambitious educational expectations sometimes evoke emotional and behavior reactions of a neurotic nature.

Forms of Psychiatric Problems

The anxieties of childhood are often expressed as transient symptomatic reactions related to some current situation or emotional conflict. Although the child may present a variety of manifestations of anxiety, one or another symptom is seen as most disturbing. When the child suffers from prolonged and definitive disturbances of the psychotic, neurotic, or defective type, these are to be discriminated from the forms of psychiatric problems classified under the Adjustment Reactions of Infancy or Childhood.

ADJUSTMENT REACTIONS OF INFANCY. Those transient disturbances in infancy, such as undue apathy, undue excitability, or the disturbances in feeding and sleeping, that take place on a psychogenic basis and are unassociated with physical disorder are usually classified under the nosological term mentioned. In most instances it will be found that as a result of the infant's interaction with the mother, or a mother surrogate, or because of a deprivation of such a relationship, these disturbances take place. An example of the types of disorders which one might classify as adjustment reaction to infancy are those symptomatic responses of the infant to separation from the mother. Disturbances of behavior due to isolation or maternal deprivation in children reared in institutional homes during the first two years of life have been known for the past three decades. Schlossman* coined the term "hospitalism" in 1926 to designate the condition. Levy† defined the genesis of the condition in his paper, "Primary Affect Hunger," in 1933, and Spitz has more recently studied experimentally the withdrawal of the infant, his apprehension on the approach of others, weepiness, sadness, loss of appetite and of weight, and insomnia, that take place in the periods between six and twelve months as a consequence of separation from the mothering one. The child may show a retardation of development, with inability to walk, delayed reaction to external stimuli, slowness of movement, and stupor if the separation is continued for a period of time. If the mother returns, there is a rapid disappearance of the evidence of disturbance and behavior. Illness, tension, or anxiety in the mother may also lead to similar, though usually less severe, disturbances in the behavior of the infant. Prolonged maternal deprivation is productive of severe personality maldevelopment, as described elsewhere in this chapter.

ADJUSTMENT REACTIONS OF CHILDHOOD. As mentioned, these reactions are

to be differentiated from the rare psychotic, psychoneurotic, or organic disturbances of childhood. They are usually subclassified according to the most prominent manifestations in the following ways.

Habit Disturbance

This is manifested in such simple repetitive activities as nail biting, thumb sucking, enuresis, masturbation, and temper tantrums. One group of these disorders concerns the manipulations of certain parts of the body. Here we find such conditions as thumb sucking, nail biting, nose picking, and tongue sucking. These conditions are generally differentiated from tics; they are felt to occur at a high level of awareness, are intermittently present, are variable in duration, intensity, and course, and the action in itself seems to be pleasurable. If they are interrupted at any stage of a single performance, they are recognized by the patient as actions for which he is responsible and that are subject to his control.

THUMB SUCKING. One of the earliest forms of body manipulation, this is usually either the consequence of deprivation in the early sucking activities of the infant or, in older children, a regressive act during periods of tension or fatigue. Levy, from his observations, concluded that in the majority of the infants thumb sucking is a result of insufficient lip movements or incompleteness of the sucking phases of the feeding act, regardless of the type of feeding. Thumb sucking results not only from difficulties in feeding the infant, expressions of anxiety in the mother, but also from faulty techniques of nursing. Probably of greater concern are those anxieties in the parents related to the presumed effects of thumb sucking. In the past, various statements were made to the effect that distortions of personality as well as malformations of the jaws and palate resulted from thumb sucking. The management of this adjustment reaction is to be directed to the parental attitude rather than to the thumb sucking of the infant.

NAIL BITING. This is probably the

---

* Schlossman, E. E.: Zur Frage des Hospitalismus in Sauglingsanstalten. Ztschr. f. Kinderheilkunde, 42:31–38, 1926.

† Levy, D. M.: Primary affect hunger. Am. J. Psychiat., 94:643–652, 1937.

commonest of the forms of habitual body manipulation occurring both in children and adults. It is usually first seen around the fifth year of life and increases in its occurrence up to the tenth or twelfth year, when children gradually relinquish the habit. Threatening efforts to prevent the child from carrying out this act are usually unsuccessful. The condition is now recognized as an expression of tension. Its removal may be attempted through understanding and relieving the source of the underlying anxiety.

MASTURBATION AND OTHER MANIPULATIONS. Masturbation, commonly practiced by children, requires treatment only if the parental or adult attitudes toward the act have instilled in the child anxieties and fears that affect his personality development adversely. More frequently the problems of masturbation in a child involve clarifying misconceptions of the ill effects of the procedure in the minds of the parents and preventing radical efforts to prevent the act.

The other varieties of body manipulation, aside from hair pulling (trichotillomania), are relatively of little importance. The latter calls for more careful attention and may be associated with serious problems within the family.

ENURESIS. This disturbance, the involuntary passage of urine, occurs commonly and is frequently referred to the child psychiatrist. In some psychiatric clinics, enuresis is the problem for which the majority of children are seen. At the age of two years, some 80 per cent of children have ceased to wet themselves. By the end of three years, the average child is usually able to keep his clothes and bed clean and dry. The condition occurs twice as frequently in boys as in girls, it is unrelated to intelligence, and in the majority of instances has been persistent. There is a group of children in whom the habit disappears only to recur at a later date during a period of tension. By far the most frequent variety of enuresis is the nocturnal type, although diurnal enuresis and combinations of both have been noticed.

In the majority of instances, no physical disturbances of the nervous system or genitourinary apparatus are found on examination. Enuresis may occur as a matter of inadequate training resulting either from parental attitudes or because of lack of opportunity for adequate training. In some infants, the mother is overprotective, and the child's continuing inability to maintain himself dry is accepted by her on the basis that he is too small or weak for training. The child is thus infantilized and retains an infantile lack of control. Lack of opportunity for training as a causative factor occurs only in children reared in rural homes or in crowded urban areas, where toilet facilities are inadequate and the child is not expected to visit the bathroom under conditions of cold or crowding. In other instances, enuresis occurs as an expression of revenge in which the child wets, a reaction to too rapid and punitive training.

A common type of enuresis is the regressive. In children suffering from this form of enuresis, wetting occurs as a means of again obtaining the gratification of maternal contact. Very frequently regressive enuresis may be seen as a consequence of the birth of a younger child, with the loss of the mother's attention. The child now wets in order to obtain the care and personal attention and affection he misses because of the mother's preoccupation with the newborn. In such instances, the proper parental reaction conducive to change is to allow the youngster more attention for a time in order that he may grow beyond his childish needs. Punishment seldom leads to modification of regressive enuresis. The series of studies by Margaret Gerard suggests that two-thirds of the enuretic children have failed to identify with the parent of the same sex. The failure of sexual identification seems to take place in families in which the parent of the opposite sex has a passive personality, while the parent of the same sex is feared as more strict and rigid. Enuretic boys consequently tend to be passive and unassertive youngsters who are unable to compete actively, while girls with the wetting problem are found to be tomboyish and aggressive.

Although enuresis occasionally is interrupted by simple suppressive measures, it is well to recognize that it is often symptomatic of anxiety-arousing problems in the family. On the other hand, the symptom is often severe, prolonged, and not easily modified by therapy. It leads, if continued, to many additional conflicts in the growing child, depending upon the attitudes of people with whom he is in contact. As a result of punishment and shaming, the enuretic child develops secondary feelings of inadequacy. Many suffer from sleeplessness in their attempts to control the bladder. These children have feelings of embarrassment and lack of self-confidence that restrict their capacity to form easy relationships with others, as well as feelings of helplessness resulting from their inability to control the habit. They are often told repeatedly that they suffer from "weak bladders" or "weak kidneys," their personal conviction of physical weakness and disability thus being deepened. Exposed to the consequences of teasing when sent to camp or to school with other children, their sense of social inadequacy is again magnified.

A 12½-year-old girl was brought to the pediatric psychiatric clinic by her mother, who complained that she wet her bed, was very nervous and restless, bit her nails, and screamed while playing with other children. The mother recounted that her daughter had been enuretic since infancy. Initially, she wet her bed every hour or so during the night; at this time, she wet it once or twice a week. The mother waked her up twice during the night. She stated that if the children got her daughter to laugh in the day time, she occasionally wet herself. The mother stated that the daughter had slept with her for two years in the same bed. Her daughter always liked exciting things and was admired by everyone around her, but she did not care for work about the house and wished to be a lady; nor did she wish to learn anything. When asked to help with the housework, she argued and became angry.

The daughter was the only child. The mother felt that the pregnancy was quite normal. The child was breast fed for 14 months and walked at one year but was slow in beginning to talk. Her dentition was completed at seven months, and bowel control, at three years. The mother continued to feed the girl until the age of 8, since she would not take a spoon in her own hand. Her mother bathed her until she was 11 years old and reported that her daughter had dressed herself only for the past six months. She first allowed her daughter to cross the street alone within the same period of time. The explanation for this was that the mother had seen another child run over some time before. The girl had had no unusual illnesses, but was sick with teething and vomited a great deal at that time. Her school work was good. She began school at six and a half and was regularly promoted with her class. On psychological testing, she was found to have an I. Q. of 113.

The mother described the father as a nervous man whose hand shook and who was pre-occupied with palpitation of the heart. He was seen as impatient and easily upset. The mother considered herself a fairly healthy person but nervous since an operation for appendicitis the previous year. She spoke of crying quite easily and complained about her marriage, stating it had not been happy in the early years as her husband was attached to his mother.

When the daughter was seen, she was found to be a tall, gangling, very talkative, "smart alecky" girl, rather restless, walking about uneasily. In discussing the problem of bed wetting, she stated that she used to have difficulty in sleeping because "I was afraid I couldn't wake up in time and then I couldn't get to sleep; then I would worry because I couldn't sleep and I wouldn't." She said she had slept better since her parents did not put her to bed so early. In discussing her parents, she said, "They have to love me, I'm the only one." She described her mother as "treating me like a baby. She won't let me go to the movies alone." She volunteered that she did not want to grow up but preferred to remain the same age as she is now. "It is more fun."

In subsequent treatment hours with the mother and child, it was learned that the daughter had been unwanted but always overprotected, the mother believing that some harm would come to her. Initially she was a shy child but later developed many friends, mostly among older children. Although she was at first distant with her father, she had become quite close to him since the mother became ill and was not available to do everything for her. She stated that her father was a mother to her. The child and her mother were seen only intermittently over the following three years, as they lived at a distance. She did better at school but continued to be enuretic, although with diminished frequency. After three years, the enuresis disappeared, but there was occasionally frequency of urination at night or during the day. In the meantime, the child worked out many of her conflicting feelings in regard to her dependent relationship with her mother and her ambivalent attitude toward her father.

Conduct Disorder

This difficulty includes those disturbances in behavior or social activity in the child that are of such concern that they are reported in the home, in the school, in the community, or in all three. Such conditions are noticed by parents, teachers, or members of social agencies. Among the common conduct disorders are disobedience, lying, stealing, destructiveness, fighting, firesetting, truancy, cruelty, running away, and various sexual activities. Occasionally such disturbances may be secondary to brain damage as a consequence of epilepsy or epidemic encephalitis or are caused by mental deficiency.

Usually the child with such disorders expresses little self-criticism or reproach, feels no guilt, and is unresponsive to punishment. He is frequently lacking in the capacity to relate himself emotionally to others or to receive affection. Many of these early behavior disorders represent transformations or reactions to aggression. Aggression may play a part in the very symptoms that at first sight seem to bear no relation to it. Frequently, in fact, the troublesome behavior of the child is not of such a nature as to suggest its real source. The conduct disorder may be an adaptation to submissiveness or may result from an effort to obtain substitute or compensatory satisfactions for those not received at home. Again, the conduct disturbance may represent an attempt to bolster up feelings of inadequacy or inferiority, an effort to make himself feel courageous and superior by overemphasizing his independence in the form of aggressive and disturbing behavior. Sometimes it serves as defiance of authority or as a means of controlling the mother or of tyrannizing the household. Some forms of conduct disorder represent efforts to escape from anxiety-ridden situations. In others, the behavior disorder arises as a consequence of a desire for punishment created in response to marked feelings of guilt.

In Chapter 29, Personality Disorders, the etiology suggested by Johnson and Szurek for such antisocial conduct disorders as firesetting, truancy, stealing, and unacceptable sexuality as it occurs in some children is discussed. Here the source for the antisocial behavior is believed to be in the parent's unwitting sanction or indirect encouragement of the child's behavior. In these instances, the child is healthy, not deprived emotionally or exposed to cultural patterns that encourage the pattern, but comes from an apparently "good" family. In such instances, the parent appears overtly to interdict the act that is the source of complaint. However, study of the parent–child interaction in the course of collaborative treatment has demonstrated that, through unconsciously driven behavior, the parent or both parents communicate their permissiveness to the child. The approval is often expressed in non-verbal forms by undue attention to the child's disturbing behavior, by the lack of consistent firmness, and in its management through unwitting and sometimes suggestive remarks, smirks, or encouragement. In such instances, change in behavior requires treatment of the permissive parent, who obtains a vicarious gratification from the child's misbehavior that acts out the parents' repressed impulses.

A 7-year-old boy was referred for psychiatric consultation from the Board of Education because of his inability to make a satisfactory adjustment in his class room. The teacher reported that he was constantly aggressive toward other children and that much of his behavior seemed bizarre. He had been discharged from a class the previous year because of similar disturbances of behavior. The mother reported that she had had difficulty in controlling him at home. To her he seemed very restless, blinked his eyes frequently, and masturbated constantly. She summed up her problem in one sentence, "I can't seem to get through to him." She dated the change in his behavior to the age of 2½, when he first was observed to be tense and seemed to joke about everything said to him. When the boy was examined, he was found to be pale, stocky, but well developed, and with a husky voice. He frequently asked what would happen to him when he would return to the class room. He seemed anxious concerning the possibility of bodily injury and became very apprehensive when feeling the cutting edges of carpentry tools in the play room. He did not talk spontaneously and was evasive in his replies. There was evidence of poor motor co-ordination and little patterning in what he did. Psychological tests showed him to be hesitant, suspicious, and interpretive of all remarks as hostile. He frequently evaded by apparent misunderstanding or not hearing what was said to him. It was felt the child needed assistance in a residential hospital setting.

In the discussion of the problem with the father, it was learned that on many occasions the father had beaten the boy severely. It seemed evident that the father was competing with his son in many ways, and he remarked in regard to games with him, "He can't lose, he wants to win the games we play. I usually win. It's hard for him to beat me. If he loses, he loses legitimately!" The father also indicated his resentment toward the son and spoke of his son's interest as silly. He expressed favoritism for a younger child. The mother was found to be an immature, dependent, and self-centered person, limited in her fantasy life and depressed in mood.

When the boy was brought to the hospital, he first expressed much concern about "who is boss" on the ward. He frequently insisted that he was "the boss" and often attempted to engage in power struggles with other children and the doctor. He remarked, "Well, if you are strong, how come you haven't killed me yet?" Frequently he talked of his own strength or expressed desires of being killed. In play sessions, he acted as the father and behaved in an impatient, angry, and cruel way to a doll. The game often ended with the doll killing all other little dolls and destroying the furniture and the parents. With continuing treatment, he became destructive and aggressive in the hospital. This behavior subsided when he was provided an interpretation that apparently it was his wish to provoke the psychiatrist to respond as would have happened at home. He then made efforts to seek closeness to the psychiatrist.

Additional history disclosed that the patient was a planned child, and his early development had been quite normal. The mother reported that bowel training had been difficult and that she had had a constant struggle with the child. She stated that she had beaten him if he failed to excrete properly and admitted being constantly frustrated and angry in caring for him.

In the course of the treatment of the child, it became apparent that the problem was one of a hateful struggle for control between the boy and his chronically distressed mother. His only conception of existence seemed to be in fighting and attaining the position of "the boss." The father contributed to the child's hostility through his competitive feelings and his hostile aggression toward the child. His behavior slowly but gradually improved in the protective milieu of the residential treatment center and with play therapy sessions in conjunction with special schooling. After 18 months he was discharged home. By then his parents had received some understanding of their problems through psychotherapeutic treatment.

Another common type of conduct disturbance occurs in children who have *learning disturbances* at school. As Levy has recently pointed out, the motivational explanation for the conduct disturbance is inappropriate in such instances. The motivational problem is secondary; the primary issue is the capacity of the child to learn. At the present time, approximately 12 per cent of all children in the United States fail to learn to read as well as the average. Although these children have better than normal intelligence and their social and vocabulary development is excellent, as well as their vision, they suffer from dyslexia, occasionally, but not always, associated with left-handedness and with difficulty in converting to right-handed writing. This disability manifests itself in a variety of ways, sometimes as confusion of one consonant with another, such as b's for d's, p's for q's, or t's for f's, or as a reversal of the syllables, words, or entire sentences as mere writing, with a complete failure to recognize words. Another group of children suffers from an inability to learn as a consequence of the newer methods of teaching reading. By these methods, children are taught to read whole words, phrases, and sentences, with an analysis of individual words into phonic sounds and letters undertaken only secondarily. Because of their particular perceptual capacity, some children are unable to learn to read or spell by this method of pedagogy. In such children the emotional expressions of fear and anxiety, caused by failure to meet the standards of the family or class and by hostility resulting from feelings of rivalry and jealousy, tend to imbue concepts of personal inferiority and encourage behavior disturbance.

Many conduct disabilities founded on such a basis disappear rapidly with improvement in the reading. The important element in treatment is recognition of the underlying incapacity to learn. Here the use of a remedial teacher is often the effective technique to bring about a satisfactory modification of the behavior disturbance. The following case illustrates this problem.

O. E. was an 8½-year-old boy referred for evaluation and for possible treatment of emotional problems involved in the patient's inability to read. The school teacher and psychologist felt the patient had an emotional block that prevented his learning to read. The child was restless and unruly in school and a difficult problem in management. Physical examination was negative except for confusion in handedness. Past history was free of gross emotional disturbances. He was well liked by his many friends and had many interests. His parents had high academic aspirations for him and were distressed by his poor scholastic performance. He was compared unfavorably with his very bright 10-year-old brother.

During the psychiatric interview he appeared friendly and co-operative and fully understood the reason for his being in the doctor's office. He said, "I can't read and it gets me worried." He handled a pencil very poorly in either hand, and in printing, reversed several letters and words. He could not read. Psychological tests revealed an average intelligence. He could not be tested in reading achievement since this was so defective. Bender gestalt designs were below his age level, but he showed difficulty in integration of the designs. A diagnosis of learning disability was made. It was felt that the problem of anxiety was secondary. A remedial reading teacher was engaged. Parents and teachers were encouraged to let him progress and learn at his own speed. He did well under special instruction, progressing slowly but quite satisfactorily in reading. His restlessness, tension, and disobedience subsided quickly.

Neurotic Traits

These qualities are closely related to habit disturbance, and the distinction between the two is often difficult. Here are classified tics, habit spasms, somnambulism, stammering, overactivity, and phobias. Tics occur as repetitious, involuntary but apparently purposeless, movement of interconnected muscles. They frequently involve the muscles of the eyelids, with blinking or squinting. Often, tics are first noticed in childhood; they then disappear, only to recur at a later date at the time of some conflict. Frequently it will be found that the tic was first noticed after a frightening experience leading to a fear of injury and that it represents a defensive muscular withdrawal response of small muscle groups appropriate to the expected trauma. Although initially the defensive muscular contraction may have involved many muscles, the tic represents a rudimentary response of small muscle groups. Because of the persistence of the response beyond the particular time of the injury, the tic-like movement becomes inappropriate and involuntary. The use of the small

muscle groups develops as a consequence of parental prohibition for the full movement. The tic then represents both the fear of injury and the attempt to maintain gratification by complying to parental wishes.

In addition to the tic, the child frequently is restless, self-conscious, sensitive, or spoiled, or may be overambitious and overconscientious. Frequently easy excitability and fatigability are observed. There are other children who are shy, seclusive, and embarrassed. The tics of psychogenic origin are to be differentiated from those that occur as a result of encephalitic disease affecting the basal ganglia. Treatment of the latter is often difficult.

A 6-year-old boy was brought to the clinic by his mother, who complained that he jerked his head and blinked his eyes frequently. She stated that he had begun this habit about four or five weeks previously. When the habit spasm began, she paid little heed to it, but later she slapped him in the face for it. At first she thought it might be caused by disease of his eyes. She became annoyed when he began to open his eyes with his fingers. The boy reported it was his feeling that his eyes were closing on him when the lids were heavy.

The mother went on to describe her son as restless, unable to sit in a chair, and very fidgety. She also reported that he had occasional headaches and had begun to suffer from asthma at 17 months of age. His last attack had taken place 12 months previously. Early in life he had played with younger children, but now he played only with those of his own age. The boy had been breast fed for six months and bottle fed until 1½ years. At five months of age, he had been able to sit alone and had stood up and taken some steps at 9 months. At the end of the first year, he had said a few words. She indicated that his bowel and bladder training had been completed in less than a year. The mother had dressed the boy until a year and a half ago and said that he wished her to dress him even now. It was only at this time that he had begun to wash himself. The story of his schooling showed that he had entered the first grade at 6, had done very well, and was advanced several classes. He was, at the time of examination, the youngest child in his class. It was the mother's impression that he felt uneasy. The father was described as a happy-go-lucky person who enjoyed his children. The mother thought of herself as being well. There were three children, the patient being the eldest. A sister is two and a half years younger and a baby was 18 months old.

When the boy was seen, he was found to blink, roll his eyes, and grimace about his mouth. He said that the trouble with his facial muscles came on after he had arrived home from school some weeks before and done his homework. He felt he could not stop the movements once they started. He also reported that he had been unable to sleep well and admitted some recent worries about masturbation. He saw himself as a sickly boy and described his fear of playing rough games with others. The matter of the boy's masturbation was discussed with the mother, who became overtly anxious in dealing with this subject. On returning home, she was able to talk to her son on the subject without threatening him. The mother discontinued bathing him and allowed him to go to bed later. During several additional hours, the matter of the sexual interests of the son was brought up for discussion by the mother. The physician worked with her and the boy, with gratifying results. The facial tics disappeared following a series of four visits. Treatment for the asthma was continued for several years.

STUTTERING. This disturbance customarily has its beginning in childhood and, when persistent, seriously impedes the child's social adaptation and development. It must be recognized that short periods of stuttering may take place between the second and fourth years, when the growing child's efforts at expression exceed his capacity to verbalize. Parents who have themselves been stutterers or have been related to a stutterer often become overly anxious and tend to emphasize the child's defect by their efforts at control through admonitions to speak more slowly and by their evident preoccupation with the speech difficulty.

The persistent stutterer is considered to have a conflict between passive and aggressive drives, which is reflected in his speech. Such a child often tends to show other compulsive and ambivalent traits. His speech expresses his obstinancy in his waiting for others to complete his efforts.

Treatment generally requires both the efforts of a psychotherapist and speech therapist, the latter to direct efforts at correction of established but poor patterns of speech.

PHOBIAS. These disorders, of a transient variety, are common in childhood, particularly those of heights, the dark, animals, and other frightening figures. To be considered pathological, the response to the feared object is grossly overdetermined and leads to gross disturbance of behavior, with anxiety or panic. Children who have been harmed by animals may be expected to have a generalized over-reaction to them. In these instances the reaction may be thought of as a conditioned response. In other children, however, the phobia represents a displacement of fear to some other object and derives from aggressive drives directed toward one or the other parental figure.

The *school phobias* are probably misnamed. In most instances, the anxiety reaction on going to school is due to response to separation from the mother —a form of separation anxiety. A therapeutic regimen that directs the prompt return of the child to school has a high chance of success, particularly with younger children. Older children with school phobia usually are found in families with highly disturbed parents who are incapable of mastering their own anxiety over aggressiveness and providing the firmness necessary to face the complaints of the child. Oftentimes parents of older children who have failed to enter school due to phobia are themselves severely neurotic or psychotic. Here therapy for the parent is necessary to effect change.

Psychological Tests

Psychological examinations often serve as an aid to the evaluation of the limitations and assets of the child referred for psychiatric study. This is especially true if there are questions involving learning difficulties, mental retardation, the possibility of brain injury, or the existence of a psychosis. They may, too, provide help in obtaining a general picture of the child's problem areas and intrapsychic dynamics. In deciding as to whether or not the child should be tested, consideration should be given not only to the amount of meaningful information that can probably be secured by his test performance, but also to the degree of emotional trauma the tests may cause him.

Three types of tests are generally used in children's clinics: intelligence tests, achievement tests, and projective tests. Although intelligence tests have a high degree of validity when used with children of school age or older, the reliability of those designed for infants and children of pre-school age is comparatively poor in and of themselves, exclusive of other studies of the child.

Achievement tests measure the benefits the child has derived from his educational endeavors. Often the lack of correlation between educational achievement and mental ability uncovers the nature of general learning problems or specific ones, such as in reading or arithmetic.

The Rorschach is the projective test most likely to reveal nuclear conflicts, basic anxieties, and the level of emotional maturation. The validity and meaningfulness of projective test results are dependent on the skill, experience, and the personality of the psychologist.

Therapeutic Measures

The treatment of personality difficulties of the child must vary with the individual and his problems. The principal emphasis, however, is on "the child's needs, strivings, and growth tendencies in a social and cultural background." The fundamental 'objective is a healthy reorganization of the personality and an improved emotional adjustment. Many of the child's behavior problems and neurotic difficulties arise from emotional handicaps sustained through earlier relationship experiences that were not conducive to healthy emotional growth. One seeks, therefore, to acquire an understanding of the forces that have been operating in the early life of the child. Although the child cannot, of course, develop beyond the limits of his constitutional potentialities, it is the aim of therapeutic measures to remove or reduce his persistent and crippling emotional difficulties and to aid him in reorganizing those emotional attitudes and patterns of reaction that have been governing his personality functioning. In this way, growth of the patient's personality toward new and more spontaneous and satisfying patterns is made possible. A growth-promoting relationship must be substituted for the previous ones that produced insecurity, abnormal aggression, or hostility, that reinforced infantilization and prevented growth in the direction of self-reliance and social maturity.

One element common, however, to all forms of therapy is the use of the *therapist–patient relationship*. Into this relationship the child brings the resentments, anxiety, fears, guilt, and the fantasies that have arisen from such feelings. The first essential is for the psychiatrist to establish a friendly, interesting, and satisfactory relationship between the child and himself. He accepts the child as an equal and as a person in his own right. He neither stresses nor ignores the difference in age and maturity but assumes it as a matter of course and does not assume an artificially childish language. In the therapist the child finds someone who can help him as he is. The therapeutic approach must be a gradual one. To hasten it may defeat the relationship and cause the child to withdraw into evasion, indifference, or falsification. Any early reference to behavior disorders may stimulate hostility or tension. Early discussions may therefore deal with the child's interests and activities and in direct questioning about neutral matters. With the therapist–child relationship satisfactorily established, the patient may, in this friendly atmosphere, verbalize his conscious conflicts, opinions, ideas, and feelings, which can then be discussed. In another way, too, the therapist–child relationship may be of value. Through this relationship, the child projects his anxiety and hostility onto the personality of the physician. By projection the child may make use of the therapist to symbolize an unacceptable part of himself as he moves toward freeing himself of the unacceptable aspect. The child may also project onto the therapist desirable qualities that he hopes to attain. The therapist will not be critical of the child's behavior and will take his ideas seriously and as worthy of attention and consideration. He will seek to feel and understand just what problems the child is trying to solve when by that very effort he is creating the problems that have brought him to the psychiatrist. His attitude will not be one of condescension. Within the security of the dependent relationship with the emotionally more mature therapist, whom he trusts and imitates, the child relives his emotional conflicts. The physician will aim to have the child feel that the therapist is a kindly adult, a helpful, protective father who understands his feelings and is helping him.

Occasionally with older children and adolescents, if the problem is a simple and largely environmental one, talks with the patient concerning situations that are troublesome may be not only a direct but also an important treatment. He may have reacted to a situation with confused apprehension and undesirable behavior because he did not understand the chain of circumstances that produced a given result. One must not, however, by merely attempting to have the child see what is wrong or undesirable about himself, expect him to relinquish his old ways or control them more effectively. Even with simple problems there must usually be a reorganization of emotional attitudes and patterns of reaction. To secure this the patient must not only have wholesome compensations and outlets but, through an acceptable and gratifying, and therefore therapeutic, realtionship with the psychiatrist, gain a stimulus toward new ways of feeling, i.e., to change, to grow.

The physician may wish to make use of *"environmental"* or *"manipulative"* therapy, consisting of clubs, camps, dancing classes, boarding schools, or other activities to enable the patient to make contacts with others and develop interests of his own. In some cases, separation for long periods of time from an overprotective mother may be desirable. In younger children, play techniques involving psychoanalytical principles are largely used.

Child–Parent Relationship

Since, as already indicated, the child's problem usually arises from the living relationship between himself and a parent and is interwoven with a parent's attitude, the parental attitudes form part of the examination. Frequently, therefore, it is not so much a symptom as the child–parent relationship that needs treatment. The psychiatric examination consists therefore of interviews with the parents and the examination of the child. Usually a series of interviews either with both parents or with the mother is desirable before the child is examined in order to discuss the problem that the latter presents. The physician, by giving the mother—but sometimes both parents—an opportunity to express and relieve her perturbation and anxiety, gains her confidence, often secures revealing information about personality characteristics of the parents, and assists the mother in seeing the child's trouble in a truer perspective. She may like to explain the child's behavior as a result of heredity, but the therapist will usually discover that the mother's neurotic conflict has entered the child's handling. Her expressions of guilt, accusations, hostility, anxiety, and excuses may betray the nature of interpersonal relations that have been a source of difficulty.

Inquiry should be made as to the onset of the child's difficulty, the mode and circumstances of its first appearance, and its development. The interview will presumably, too, assist the physician in securing desirable information concerning the child's cultural background, the family's ways of living, its intelligence, its beliefs and problems, the relationships between father and mother, and the child's group relations. Through a knowledge of the parents' past and present attitudes toward the child, the psychiatrist learns much as to what situations the child's behavior is an adjustment. As previously indicated, it will often be found that the mother is carrying over into her relationship with her child the unresolved emotional problems that arose in her relationships with her own parents. The aim is to uncover a dynamic picture of the experiences and emotions of the child in relation to those surrounding him.

The problem may have arisen from the father–child relationship, but more frequently it arises from that of mother–child. If, as is probable, the problem has arisen from the relationship between the child and the mother, both require therapy. They are not, however, interviewed together. In child guidance clinics, the psychiatric social worker will usually do case work with the mother at the same periods during which the psychiatrist treats the child. In other clinics or private practice, the problem of the mother may receive paramount attention from the psychiatrist while the child is seen by the social worker. The psychiatrist and social worker collaborate in helping parents and child to resolve difficulties that have arisen through living together. Through visits with the social worker, the mother acquires a new understanding of her relation to the child and a realization that she has a part in the child's therapy. The simultaneity of these appointments, usually held weekly and 45 minutes in duration, assists mother and child to realize that the problem requiring help does not exist solely in the child or in the mother but in the relationship between them. As previously indicated, the parents' psychological problems are usually one of the most serious obstacles to a resolution of the child's problem. It is the task of the psychiatrist or social worker to assist the mother to a better understanding and an emotional acceptance of herself in her relation to the child.

If the mother's feeling for her child is one of rejection, treatment of the latter's problems is often difficult. The mother, burdened with anxieties and fears, cannot emotionally accept or understand a direct interpretation of her unconscious feelings or her personality patterns. By indirect methods, therefore, the worker helps the mother to objectify the problem, to formulate her thinking, feeling, and behavior in relation to the child, and to allay her guilt and anxiety. She will assist the mother in establishing a normal and satisfying relationship with the child that will permit a progressive and wholesome growth of her personality. No attempt should be made to make the mother recognize that she is coming to the worker for treatment for herself as a patient. If a favorable rapport is established with the worker, the mother accepts her relationship with the worker as a search for causes for the child's difficulties, and in examining the family life, she may begin to examine herself. The mother's influence and behavior in relation to her child are partially dependent upon her own self-understanding. The worker may help the mother to see family members in their respective relationships and, knowing their life experiences, the parent may begin to find new meaning for their behavior. In this manner her understanding of, and her relation to, the problem child may become clearer. In addition to treatment with the parents, the social worker carries out any necessary manipulation of the environment.

Play Technique

It is well recognized that free association is a valuable technique in adults for the investigation of significant psychological material below the level of consciousness. In children, however, play is a more normal mode of expression than is one limited to verbal forms. Play technique consists of introducing a child to a group of toys and permitting him to use them freely while the observer looks on. The toys given him represent all the common interests of childhood—animals, building blocks, and other objects of a creative type. Dolls often represent members of the family. Play being the medium in which the child expresses himself most freely, the use which he makes of the toys reveals his fantasies, offers insight into his mental mechanisms, and gives clues regarding his unconscious. In the child, play may be regarded as the speech of the unconscious. He may use the imaginary characters of his play to express his own disturbed feelings. Being a projective technique, it may show human relations and problems arising out of them. It therefore sheds light on the family relationships as no other medium can. It illuminates both the relation of the child to his parents and of the parents to the child. Hiding behind the anonymity of a doll, he may tell of death wishes directed toward a parent or sibling. The child should be permitted to choose the toy and use it spontaneously, since he will select the medium of expression best suited to himself and therefore best adapted to express his immediate problem or situation.

In play, therefore, we find an excellent projective technique for the diagnosis of hidden aspects of the personality and for a study of the emotional life of children. We know that the child's emotional life revolves primarily around his mother, father, and siblings. Since play provides a feeling-projecting medium, we find in it a readily available means of investigating the child's emotional attitudes toward the family. These, it will be found, are often ambivalent. We have already seen that the child's problems often arise from the interpersonal relationships in the family. Play, therefore, is often used by the child as a spontaneous projective technique for expressing the nature of the relationship in which his problem is rooted. He brings into his play the reactions and feelings connected with this problem. Drawing and painting may also be used as projective techniques, not only for securing clues as to the child's problems and psychic dynamics, but also as therapeutic adjuncts. In his art sessions, the child may attribute various imaginary roles to parent or sibling and may use his products as a channel of release.

There are many interesting phenomena in play technique comparable to those observed in psychoanalysis. For example, the child may show an anxious care in excluding some toy from his play, or on approaching some aspect of the play that he seems to find unsafe, not permissible, or unsatisfactory to the point of discomfort, he becomes upset and is unable to go on playing in peace. This is strikingly similar to the signs of emotional disturbance present when, in free association, conflicts and anxieties push too near the surface. In this way, the psychiatrist may secure clues to the sources of the child's difficulties. To be able not only to interpret the disruptions or interruptions of play such as those just described, but also to interpret the symbolic gestures and words that the child constantly presents, is of great aid in ascertaining the source of his difficulties. To do so, however, requires experience, insight, and imaginative vision on the part of the psychiatrist.

Pharmacological Therapy

Pharmacological treatment with the phenothiazines, rauwolfia derivatives, and other agents is now attempted widely for a number of the disorders of childhood as a means of providing symptomatic relief and reduction in anxiety for both child and parent. The eventual place of such treatment in child psychiatry remains to be established. The use of these agents is described in Chapter 34.

BIBLIOGRAPHY

Allen, F. H.: Psychotherapy with Children. New York, W. W. Norton & Co., Inc., 1942.

Idem: Aggression in relation to emotional development, normal and pathological. Ment. Hyg., 34:353–363, 1950.

Idem: Psychopathic behavior—fact or projection. Am. J. Orthopsychiat., 20:236–240, 1950.

Baruch, D.: One Little Boy. New York, Julian Press, Inc., 1952.

Bender, L.: Psychological problems of children with organic brain disease. Am. J. Orthopsychiat., 19:404–415, 1949.

Idem, and Nichtern, S.: Chemotherapy in child psychiatry. New York State J. Med., 56:2791–2795, 1956.

Bornstein, B.: Emotional barriers in the understanding and treatment of young children. Am. J. Orthopsychiat., 18:691–697, 1948.

Bowlby, J.: Maternal Care and Mental Health. Geneva, World Health Organization Monograph Series No. 2, 1952.

Children's Bureau: Emotional Problems Associated with Handicapping Conditions in Children. Washington, Federal Security Agency, 1952.

Creak, M.: Psychoses in childhood. J. Ment. Sc., 97:545–554, 1951.

Despert, J. L.: Delusional and hallucinatory experiences in children. Am. J. Psychiat., 104:528–537, 1948.

Idem: Diagnostic criteria of schizophrenia in children. Am. J. Psychotherapy, 6:148–163, 1952.

Esman, A. H.; et al.: School experience in training

of the child psychiatrist. Dis. Nerv. System, *13:* 266–268, 1952.

Finch, S. M.: Psychosomatic problems in children. Nerv. Child, 9:261–269, 1952.

Idem: Fundamentals of Child Psychiatry. New York, W. W. Norton & Co., Inc., 1960.

Freud, A.: Introduction to the Technique of Child Analysis. Washington, D. C., Nerv. & Ment. Dis. Monographs, 1928.

Idem, et al.: The Psychoanalytic Study of the Child, II. New York, International Universities Press, 1947.

Gerard, M. W.: Enuresis: A study in etiology. Am. J. Orthopsychiat., 9:48–58, 1939.

Idem: The psychogenic tic in ego development. The Psychoanalytic Study of the Child, 2:133–162, 1946.

Greenwood, E. D.: The role of psychotherapy in residential treatment. Am. J. Orthopsychiat., 25:692–698, 1955.

Group for the Advancement of Psychiatry, Report No. 38: The Diagnostic Process in Child Psychiatry. New York, 1957.

Hoch, P., and Zubin, J. (Eds.): Psychopathology of Childhood. New York, Grune & Stratton, 1955.

Ingram, T. T. S.: A characteristic form of overactive behavior in brain damaged children. J. Ment. Sc., 102:550–558, 1956.

Johnson, A. M., and Szurek, S. A.: Etiology of antisocial behavior in delinquents and psychopaths. J.A.M.A., 154:814–817, 1954.

Josselyn, I. M.: The Happy Child. New York, Random House, 1955.

Kanner, L.: Child Psychiatry, 3rd ed. Springfield, Illinois, Charles C Thomas, 1957.

Idem: Problems of nosology and psychodynamics of early infantile autism. Am. J. Orthopsychiat., 19:416–426, 1949.

Klein, M.: The psychoanalytic play technique. Am. J. Orthopsychiat., 25:223–237, 1955.

Levy, D. M.: Maternal Overprotection. New York, Columbia University Press, 1943.

Idem: Critical evaluation of the present state of child psychiatry. Am. J. Psychiat., 108:481–494, 1952.

Idem: Capacity and motivation. Am. J. Orthopsychiat., 27:1 8, 1957.

Lewis, N. D. C., and Pacella, B. L. (Eds.): Modern Trends in Child Psychiatry. New York, International Universities Press, 1945.

Lippman, H. S.: Treatment of the Child in Emotional Conflict. New York, McGraw-Hill Book Co., 2nd ed., 1962.

Lorand, S.: The psychoanalytic contribution to the treatment of behavior problems in children. Am. J. Psychiat., 105:357–360, 1948.

Lowrey, L. G.: Therapeutic play technique; a symposium. Am. J. Orthopsychiat., 25:747–787, 1955.

Mahler, M. S., and Luke, J. A.: Outcome of the tic syndrome. J. Nerv. & Ment. Dis., 103:433–445, 1946.

Murphy, L. B.: Childhood Experience in relation to personality development. In Hunt, J. McV. (Ed.): Personality and the Behavior Disorders. New York, Ronald Press, 1944.

O'Neal, P., and Robins, L. N.: The relation of childhood behavior problems to adult psychiatric states. Am. J. Psychiat., 114:961–969, 1958.

Pasamanick, B., Rogers, M. E., and Lilienfeld, A. M.: Pregnancy experience and the development of behavior disorder in children. Am. J. Psychiat., 112:613–618, 1956.

Pearson, G. H. J.: Emotional Disorders of Children. New York, W. W. Norton & Co., Inc., 1949.

Redl, F., and Wineman, D.: Children Who Hate. Glencoe, Illinois, Free Press, 1951.

Idem: Controls from Within. Glencoe, Illinois, Free Press, 1952.

Rodriguez, A., Rodriguez, M., and Eisenberg, L.: The outcome of school phobia. A follow-up study based on 41 cases. Am. J. Psychiat., 116:540–544, 1959.

Spitz, R. A.: Anaclitic depression. The Psychoanalytic Study of the Child, 2:313–342, 1946.

Szurek, S. A.: Comments on the psychopathology of children with somatic illness. Am. J. Psychiat., 107:844–859, 1951.

Chapter Thirty-two

PSYCHOTHERAPY

Psychotherapy may be defined as the treatment of emotional and personality problems and disorders by psychological means. Although many different psychological techniques may be employed in an effort to relieve problems and disorders and make the patient a mature, satisfied, and independent person, an important therapeutic factor common to them all is the therapist–patient relationship, with its interpersonal experiences. Through this relationship, the patient comes to know that he can share his feelings, attitudes, and experiences with the physician and that the latter, with his warmth, understanding empathy, acceptance, and support, will not depreciate, censure, or judge him no matter what he may reveal, but will respect his dignity and worth. This desired, positive, patient–therapist relationship, with its psychotherapeutic value, is often known as transference.

Since the patient goes to the physician for help and the latter offers this to him, the patient usually brings a positive transference attitude to the therapeutic situation. This positive transference attitude is found in the vast majority of patient–physician relations that exist in medicine and psychiatry. It underlies the expectations for recovery and explains many magical cases of cure. Its psychogenesis

derives from man's long period of dependent development in which his early pains and fears were frequently and repeatedly alleviated and relieved by the attention, interest, and strength of his parents and those they brought to him for aid. This learned expectancy of help from the early support of parents is transferred to the physician as a professional and forms the fulcrum for all successful psychotherapeutic ventures.

It must be recognized that every patient does not bring to the therapeutic situation the hopeful expectancy that characterizes the positive transference. Pervasive attitudes of distrust, suspicion, and hatefulness may make it impossible for the patient either to come himself or to accept under pressure contact with the physician, whether he is in need of medical or psychological treatment. Patient attitudes of this kind, which prevent the early establishment of an effective psychotherapeutic relationship, usually are found in those deprived of parents in early life, frequently shifted from one institution or foster home to another, or brought up in a home situation limited in loving support and encouragement by too demanding or rejecting parents. For individuals whose development has taken place under these circumstances, the opportunity has been limited to learn and ingrain the important ego attitudes of hopefulness and trust. Thus those whose growth has taken place under conditions of severe deprivation of early healthy mothering may be expected to enter psychotherapy with an initial impediment in the central focus of the psychotherapeutic relationship—the hopeful and expectant contact between patient and physician. In such patients, the effort to overcome the initial distrust—the initial resistance—may consume many months of contact. There is theoretical reason to believe that some individuals have undergone such serious deprivations in mothering at critical periods during early infancy and childhood that the patient–physician relationship necessary for forms of individual psychotherapy may never be capable of establishment.

Types of Psychotherapy

Types of psychotherapy fall into two general groups. One may be described as genetic–dynamic, the other as supportive, suppressive, non-exploratory, or non-specific. In the former are included both psychoanalysis and the psychobiological therapy of Meyer. No single psychotherapeutic method, approach, or technique is desirable for all patients or for all kinds of emotional difficulties. The types of psychotherapy must be determined by such factors as nature of the patient's problems, dynamic diagnosis, age of patient, intelligence, emotional maturity, family and social situation, and the specialized training and skill of the therapist.

The therapist, regardless of the type of therapy he employs, must have certain qualities. He should have a liking for people, possess a warm capacity for projecting himself into the situations and feelings of others, and be able to understand human motivation. He should not possess too many personality characteristics that are defensive in nature. For psychotherapy to be successful, too, the patient must not only want to get well, but he must give genuine and whole-hearted co-operation to the therapist. Both therapist and patient must relate meaningfully each to the other.

GENETIC–DYNAMIC THERAPIES

Psychoanalysis and psychobiological therapy have in common the assumption that the patient's emotional or personality difficulty had its genesis in significant psychological experiences and developed in accordance with the dynamic processes that determine psychopathology. Both assume that the patient's present attitudes and modes of reaction to life experiences are largely governed by reactions and attitudes to experiences in the past. Yet these therapies vary significantly in their theoretical assumption and their technical application.

Since the theory and practice of psychoanalytic therapy has been most intensively studied and clearly defined, its assumptions and methods form a convenient model against which other treatment methods and variations in technique may be examined. For this reason, psychoanalytic treatment is described first.

Psychoanalysis

It should be borne in mind that the term psychoanalysis is used in two very different senses. Freud originally applied the word to a particular therapeutic method, but it is now employed also as the name of a system of theoretical psychology based on the assumption that there is a part of the mind of which one is not conscious. It is therefore a technique for both the investigation and the treatment of mental and emotional disorder.

Value and Indications

Some believe that the value of psychoanalysis, with its emphasis on the unconscious background of conscious phenomena and as a method of investigating the workings of the mind, has been greater than its value as a psychotherapeutic method. It has elucidated many aspects of human behavior that had baffled interpretation and has led to a deeper understanding of the factors that have been responsible for personality development and patterns. Through psychoanalysis it has been learned that phenomena in adult life that are seemingly unintelligible take on meaning when understood in terms of chronologically earlier experiences. It has, too, been of immense value in bringing into awareness the unconscious roots of the problem of the mentally ill.

The application of the increased knowledge of the mind secured through psychoanalysis has, moreover, been of great therapeutic value. As a system of psychotherapy, it aims to establish its methods on the general principles and knowledge of the dynamics of emotional life. Psychoanalysis makes possible a study of deeply-repressed psychological forces and attempts to demonstrate how certain inner situations and roles persist and result in attitudes and motivating mechanisms that lie behind consciousness but may determine the whole course of life. It emphasizes, more than other psychological theories, the role of infantile experience in determining adult behavior. Probably many psychoanalysts underestimate the influence of later experiences in life. Often these are of more precipitating significance.

It is an etiological, uncovering, or insight type of therapy in contrast to the supportive, non-exploratory types described in the following section. Doubtless the most important discoveries of Freud in relation to psychotherapy were those of free association as a means of exploration of the patient's mind, the study of resistance, and the analysis of the transference. Psychoanalysis should not be undertaken except by one who has had systematic training in its techniques. The goal of psychoanalytical therapy is the uncovering and modifying of unconscious psychological forces. Through the analysis, the patient should discover the influences of these unconscious forces upon the pattern of his daily life and upon his relationship to other persons.

Theoretically, psychoanalysis is the choice of psychotherapy if a thoroughgoing modification of the personality is sought. The analyst seeks to bring about changes in personality structure by undoing the unfavorable patterns established in earlier years. Psychoanalysis aims to explore the deeper layers of the patient's mind with the hope that thereby he may acquire a maximum of self-knowledge and effect an alteration in the structure of his personality by undoing and reorganizing the unfavorable patterns that were established in an earlier period.

PREPARATION OF THERAPIST. It is now generally agreed that an analytical psychotherapist should have a personal analysis as a basic preparation for analytical therapy. In this analysis, the prospective therapist undertakes a penetrating psychological study of himself. With the aid of his analyst, he is expected to explore thoroughly the unconscious realms of his mind, trace his personality development back to the formative experiences of his childhood, and arrive at a fuller knowledge and a more realistic appraisal of himself. Such an analysis helps the therapist to recognize his own impulses, wishes, anxieties, and defenses and reduces the danger that they interfere with the therapeutic relationship with the patient, or that the physician be rendered anxious by a hostile patient because of arousal of his own hostile or sadistic impulses. As in all patient–physician relationship types of psychotherapy, the therapist must avoid treating the patient as a projected part of himself. The personal analysis also enables the therapist to avoid many problems that may otherwise arise out of countertransference, discussed later. A personal analysis, too, is extremely helpful in acquainting one's self with the technique of an experienced analyst. The future therapist should also receive a long period of supervised clinical work before undertaking psychoanalytical therapy without the guidance of a trained therapist.

USE IN NEUROSES. Psychoanalysis finds its greatest therapeutic usefulness in the psychoneuroses, character disorders, and some cases of incipient schizophrenia. The greatest success obtained in these disorders is with what Freud designated the transference neuroses, in which he included hysteria, phobias, and obsessive neurosis. These neuroses are characterized by a greater potentiality for transference (a relationship discussed later) than exists in other neuroses, and are therefore more amenable to therapy. In the psychoses, the usefulness of psychonalysis is limited.

Even though the nature of his neurosis would indicate that a patient is a suitable subject for psychoanalysis, certain other elements may contraindicate any therapy of this nature. Unless the patient sincerely wishes for relief from the neurosis and is prepared to undertake the therapy seriously and resolutely, no attempt at psychoanalysis should be made. Since a person cannot profit by such therapy unless he has a well-developed capacity for introspective understanding, the analysis of a person of subnormal intelligence cannot be successfully undertaken.

Rarely can much be accomplished by the analysis of persons over 45 years of age, although more depends upon the plasticity and receptivity of one's personality pattern than upon chronological age. Psychoanalytic therapy is unlikely to be successful in the highly-dependent individual, those who demonstrate through their life history little evidence of self-reliance or efforts to gain a personal independence away from parents or parental substitutes. Where the life history shows that the patient has made efforts to give up their infantile attachments to the parents, even unevenly and irregularly, the potentiality for successful effort at analytic therapy is enhanced.

Principles and Technique

Psychoanalytical therapy involves, among other psychological principles, such important ones as *unconscious content, free association, resistance, transference, countertransference, interpretation,* and *analysis of dreams.* These are discussed briefly, but no attempt is made either to present them in detail or to examine the many problems that arise in the actual employment of the technique.

The analyst should be a graduate in medicine, have had considerable experience with both psychotic and neurotic patients, and be well acquainted with the principles of dynamic psychology. He should be relatively free from conflicts, anxieties, rigid convictions, and other personality defenses. Interviews are held five or six days per week for periods extending from 45 minutes to one hour. From one to three years are usually required for an analysis. It is generally considered desirable that the therapist and the patient should not have been previously acquainted, also that their relationship continue to be a strictly professional one, free from social association. In order that free association may be facilitated, the patient reclines during the interview, relaxed on a couch, while the analyst is seated a little behind and to one side of him. The analyst can observe the patient, but as the latter cannot see the analyst, he is not constantly looking for signs of the therapist's response. One of the basic steps in psychoanalytical procedure is an exploration of the unconscious.

Free Association

Although dream analysis and other techniques are employed as supplementary means, the principal method is that of free association. To obtain such consciously unguided associations, the therapist asks the patient to say whatever comes to his mind and warns him against changing the sequence of his undirected thoughts and against witholding anything because it seems irrelevant or distressing. There should be an uncensored, uninhibited verbalization of everything and anything that comes to mind.

The permissive atmosphere of the therapeutic relationship facilitates free association. Opinions and feelings are expressed with a minimum or no guidance by inquiry. As material through the free association process emerges, often in symbolic form, from the consciously inaccessible portion of the mind, it becomes conscious. That it may be used therapeutically, however, it is not only necessary that the patient's repressed material be made conscious but also that interrelations and implications of the material be recognized.

It is essential that the therapist be exceedingly guarded and discrete in pointing out connections among the material produced by free association or of suggesting interpretations of it. The meaning of the material, as pointed out elsewhere, must be largely discovered by the patient himself. Through the free association process, the patient explores early memories, recreates significant experiences and the feelings contingent on them, reactivates relations with parents, siblings, or other persons, and tries to bring into consciousness feelings and ideas about himself and his attitudes as they existed in childhood. The purpose of the analysis, however, is not in any way to secure a history but rather for the patient, through free association and his interpretation of its products, to discover the tendencies, motives, desires, and other influences that have led to his personality problems and his defenses against anxiety and have constituted dynamic forces in his life.

Gradually, as associations increase in number and in their richness of material from the unconscious, what has appeared irrelevant and meaningless to the patient begins to assume significance to him. As previously indicated, the therapist seldom provides interpretations of material replete with symbolic disguises, and the patient is advised to discover for himself the meaning of his associative products. This does not mean that comment or carefully restrained aid in interpreting these products is not permissible, but that the associations must be purely of an autogenous nature and that the patient must, insofar as possible, discover this significance for himself and come to appreciate that his symptoms bear a relation to some deep-seated personality problem. As is indicated more clearly else-

where, free association may be regarded as a method of recovering the history of a symptom and its defensive function. Because of the great degree of self-revelation that it makes possible, free association is perhaps the most valuable of all methods in disclosing psychodynamics.

Resistance

Free association does not, however, assure smooth and easy passage of all repressed memories and emotions into consciousness. Although the patient's trust in the analyst and the confidence that he is not being judged by the therapist aid him in facing emotional constellations with which he could not deal in the past, yet as certain repressed and forgotten experiences and emotions are about to be brought within the scope of immediate observation, an opposition to their complete awareness or an aversion to facing the unconscious basis of his motive, appears. This opposition, known technically as *resistance*, may be manifested by sudden silences, denials, blockings, forgettings, evasions, embarrassments, and strong emotional reactions. It derives from the patient's transference distortions of the therapist as a punitive, critical, or punishing replica of some significant person in his own past life experiences.

The dynamic significance of the repressed material may be estimated by the degree of resistance to its emergence, and by the severity of the defensive reaction. By noting the occasion and the topics that evoke the patient's defensive resistances, the analyst secures clues as to the nature of the repressed material. Usually the patient's inflection or sudden change of subject indicates that the nucleus of a conflict is being approached or that he is unwittingly attempting to avoid recognition of an unconscious motivation.

Again, the resistance represents an unconscious effort to evade memories or insight. The analyst seeks to detect and bring to the patient's attention a recognition of his deep-rooted and repressed feelings and drives. This tends, however, to lead to an unconscious resistance to therapy. The resistance serves, of course, as a defense mechanism against the anxiety that would be aroused by a threatening self-knowledge of repudiated feelings and impulses. Care is taken not to probe too deeply or too rapidly in the early stages of an analysis so as not to arouse too great anxiety.

Transference

What is perhaps regarded as the most significant concept in psychoanalytical therapy, and one of the most important discoveries of Freud, is the emotional reaction of the patient toward the analyst known as the *transference*. Transference is usually defined as a repetition in the patient's present life, and particularly in his relationship to the analyst, of unconscious emotional attitudes developed during childhood within the family group and especially toward the parents. It represents a carrying over, and attaching to the therapist, of the friendly, hostile, or ambivalent attitudes and feelings that the patient formerly entertained in relation to the parent or other meaningful person of the past who played a significant role in his life. The patient reacts toward the therapist as if the latter were this person.

The significance of the transfer is that it throws light upon the patient's relationship with the individual whom the therapist represents. The patient comes to react as if the therapist were actually the other person and therefore interprets the behavior of the analyst in conformance with his concept of the person toward whom he originally had the reaction. Important unconscious factors are therefore revealed, not only by free associations and dreams, but also by transference behavior. In the resulting reaction, often referred to as the transference neurosis, the original pathogenic conflicts of the early family relationships are repeated with lesser intensity in relationship to the analyst. This may lead to extreme anxiety, illogical hostility with paranoid implications, clinging affection, or serious acting out of impulses in order to invite the therapist's punishment.

The therapist must not be surprised or disturbed by a hostile or critical attitude of the patient toward him. Rather does he objectively study those feelings with the patient, point them out to him, and seek to trace them to their origin. An effort is made to make it clear to the patient how his feelings really arose out of earlier relationships. The patient's reliving of his original conflict in the transference situation is used by the therapist as an important therapeutic experience. By encouraging the patient to retrace his memories to early childhood, he may find the source of these feelings and make it possible to eliminate them or lessen their influence. The secret of the patient's illness may often be found in these transferred feelings. The discovery and understanding of the emotions originally felt toward other significant persons in the patient's past experience and transferred during therapy to the physician may have a definite therapeutic effect on him. This will be accomplished by the principle of interpretation, discussed elsewhere. One aspect of the transference situation that may arise is the tendency of the patient to repeat in relation to the therapist a pattern of dependent emotional relationship such as the one that hampered his emotional adjustment and personality development in the past.

Countertransference

A phenomenon that accounts for many mistakes and failures of psychotherapy is that known as *countertransference*. This consists of such negative attitudes of physician to patient as anger, impatience, or resentment. These and similar attitudes are almost certain to interfere with the therapeutic effectiveness of the physician. For the most part, the countertransference reactions arise in the therapist as a result of the patient's influence on the physician's unconscious feelings and have their origin in the latter's irrational projections and identifications. The therapist must not permit his own unconscious feelings and attitudes aroused during phases of treatment to intrude in his relations toward the patient. As a rule, the therapist himself should have received

psychotherapy in order that his own problems may not blind him to similar ones
in the patient.

It should be added, however, that just
as countertransference can account for
failure in therapy, so it can also in the
hands of a skillful therapist be put to
good use diagnostically and therapeutically. For instance, a patient, not in-
tending to do so, may nevertheless arouse
annoyance in the therapist. The latter
perceives this as an index of the patient's
hostility. The therapeutic task is then to
find out, first, why the patient is afraid
to express overt hostility, and second,
what the patient's hostility represents.

Interpretation

Another principle, especially important
in its relation to therapy, is *interpretation*.
This is the process whereby the therapist
helps the patient to understand the meaning of his mental phenomena and behavior—usually mental phenomena the
existence of which he is not even aware.
In order that the patient may acquire
an understanding insight into his difficulties and thereby improve his adjustment and reconstruct his personality to
a desirable extent, there are many phases
of his mental life of which he should
have an understanding knowledge—an
emotional, not merely an intellectual,
knowledge. The impairment of such an
understanding, however, is one of the
most difficult tasks of psychotherapy and
requires great skill and tact and discreet
timing.

The therapist attempts to penetrate
the patient's personality defenses and
bringing the anxiety and underlying conflicts into consciousness so that they may
be dealt with rationally. The acquiring
of an insightful understanding by the
patient is a slow process and must not
be hurried. Newly gained insights may
produce fright and terror. A premature
interpretation mobilizes anxiety and
alarms or antagonizes the patient. He
must not be expected to tolerate the
deeply-disturbing experience and painful
revelations that a self-knowledge of his
motivations may bring until preparatory

interpretations by the therapist have
brought about a necessary stage of readiness.

UNCONSCIOUS MENTAL CONTENT. An
interpretation of unconscious mental content as brought out by free association
is a necessary part of any exploratory
therapy. Before this is done, however,
there should have been sufficient interpretation of the patient's defenses so
that he is almost ready by himself to see
the implications of what is brought forth
through his free associations. A cautious
interpretation is necessary in order that
the patient may acquire an understanding
of the significance of transference phenomena. As is to be expected, the patient,
through his need for protection against
anxiety, will manifest a resistance to the
therapist's interpretations.

An added task for the therapist is
to assist the patient in interpreting his
resistance. As has already been indicated,
the therapist should never confront the
patient with a blunt interpretation of the
meaning of his symptoms. The more obvious their meaning, the more cautious
he should be in explaining them. It has
been correctly said that whenever the
patient cannot see the obvious it is because he needs his blindness. The therapist should not impose his own interpretations. The patient is likely to gain
more insight into his problems and behavior through making his own associations, or at least in being merely guided
and helped to draw his own conclusions
and fully assimilate his interpretations
into his psychology.

REPRESSION AND ANXIETY. The efforts
of the therapist and patient should lead
to an undoing of repression in order that
the repressed may be brought to consciousness and its critical judgments.
Thus a rational decision can be made if
all the facts are at hand instead of having only part of them available as was
previously the case when some were unconscious. One aim of analysis is to bring
about such a state that the conscious
ego, with its reason, logic, and critical
abilities, may assume control when it is
confronted with unrealistic, pleasure-

seeking, infantile demands that cannot be satisfied by reality. In other words, we can make a decision about our infantile demands when we see them and observe how inappropriate they are to present reality. Previously these infantile demands secured some gratification through neurotic symptoms.

In every neurotic individual there is overt anxiety when the repressed approaches consciousness. This anxiety then causes the ego to renew its efforts to secure expression, often through the aid of other defense mechanisms. In the analytical transference situation, the patient allows himself to experience the anxiety without renewed efforts at repression by the ego. This the patient can do, since he identifies himself with the analyst who is there to help him and will, he is confident, protect him from danger. Thus, over a period of time, there is a fractionizing of the anxiety, a gradual exposure of the repressed, until finally the reasonable, judging portion of the ego recognizes that what was repressed is not appropriate in the present life of the patient.

Dream Material

Another important method employed by psychoanalysis for rendering contents of the unconscious available for conscious scrutiny is the examination of *dream material*. The dream is no longer regarded as an accident of our psychic life but as a phenomenon directly connected with it. Since presumably it represents a product of the patient's thinking that lacks the directing and inhibiting forces exercised by awareness, the material it presents for examination discloses more clearly than does consciously directed thinking the underlying strivings of the personality. Tendencies that may not be expressed in the presence of clear consciousness work freely in dreams. They serve as a convenient disguise for the patient's unacceptable, rejected emotions. In them the analyst finds a symbolic expression of the patient's inner tensions and clues to his repressed thoughts, feelings, childhood memories, and experi-

ences. When a dream persists in memory or is repeated, it has special significance because it specifically fits and reveals something constant and basic in the forces that make the personality.

Freud divided the content of thought of dreams into two categories. One he called the *manifest content*—the content as it appears to and is recalled by the dreamer. The recollected or obvious content is not, however, the significant element that is contained in what is known as the *latent content*. The latent content, were it to appear in its naked form, would be too disturbing and painful and is therefore distorted and disguised so that its recollection will not disturb the dreamer. The disguise of mental material, the repression of which suffers nocturnal relaxation, is brought about by the mechanisms of displacement, condensation, symbolization, dramatization, and elaboration. The joint activity of these mechanisms is known as the *dream work*, a process by which the latent dream content is transformed into the manifest content. By condensation, two or more ideas, wishes, or persons are fused into one, emphasis on significant mental material is displaced, and the content is dramatized and filled out by a deceptive secondary elaboration.

As a result of the dream work, the manifest content may appear to be merely an irrelevant, confused product, yet it really represents the symbolic expression of inner tensions and of other important psychic material, the hidden meaning of which must be interpreted in terms of the total life situation of the individual. It will be noted that the mechanisms that in the dream work cause the latent content of the dream to assume the form presented in the manifest content are the same ones that are operative in producing many neurotic symptoms. Such symptoms are in their dynamics identical with dream processes. In both, one notes the operation of the psychological laws of the unconscious.

In psychoanalysis the dreamer is encouraged to report to the physician any recent or recurring dream. Starting from the manifest content of the dream, free associations are employed. The patient is requested to report all that comes into his mind in regard to the various objects, actions and affects revealed in the manifest dream content. The latent or underlying significance of the symbolic imagery in the manifest content is brought to light. There arises here, of course, the same problem of symbolization and interpretation as in free association, and the analyst must in the same way encourage the patient to discover the meaning concealed in the manifest content of the dream rather than impose the arbitrary acceptance of fixed symbols. It should be remembered, however, that the object in dream interpretation is not so much the translation of certain symbols as the discovery of the ideas and motives that are dynamic in determining the patient's reactions in his waking life. Jung speaks of the dream as essentially a rational and logical statement but one that appears illogical only because it is written in a language that cannot be understood without special study.

Personality Reorganization

To be successful, psychoanalysis should so thoroughly reveal to the patient his underlying strivings and problems that, with the assistance of the therapist, he can reorganize the forces of his personality, redirect his affective energy into constructive channels, and prevent its further dissipation in dissociation, substitution, and other evasive, neurotic ways. It aims to give the patient freedom from disabling fears, distress, and inhibitions and to enable him to achieve insight sufficient to handle ordinary conflicts and reasonable reality stress. In psychotic patients it is usually too difficult to overcome resistance or to establish transference to a degree that will permit successful analytic treatment.

Modified Psychoanalysis

Because of the time required for a standard Freudian analysis, and therefore the relatively few persons who can be treated thereby, attempts are being increasingly made to develop a brief interpretative psychotherapy based on psychoanalytical principles. Many psychiatrists combine selected features from psychobiological, supportive, and psychoanalytical therapies. Franz Alexander, although making use of psychoanalytical principles, sought to make psychoanalysis less time-consuming. He believed that prolonged, uninterrupted, daily interviews may favor the development of a too dependent relationship and consequently postpone recovery. He therefore reduced the contact with the patient as much as possible, gave the patient more independence, and discouraged regressive tendencies. Even in those modified psychoanalytic therapies, the therapist seeks to bring his patient to recognize the significance of his patterns of behavior and their relationship to early environmental and cultural influences or to interpersonal relationships and experiences.

Psychobiological Therapy

Although many other phases and differences characterize the techniques of the two therapies, it may be said that in psychoanalysis, problems and their genesis are ascertained by an exploration of the unconscious through free associations, and that in psychobiological therapy these problems are approached largely at a conscious level and discussed directly in the form of an ordinary conversation, with attention directed toward definite situations and the patient's reactions to them. Psychobiological therapy does not recognize nor does it systematically use the patient–physician relationship, the transference, to explore the genetic dynamics of the patient's behavior. In both forms, the therapist seeks to modify the unhealthy attitudes that have prevented the patient from carrying on his daily tasks without disturbing his relations with others or creating anxiety within himself. The therapist aims to assist the patient in establishing a more rational, more constructive, and therefore healthier pattern of living.

Distributive Analysis and Synthesis

Because of the principles involved, Adolf Meyer characterized as distributive analysis and synthesis the technique of psychotherapy often known as psychobiological therapy. Briefly, Meyer meant about as follows by this term: Guided by the therapist, the patient analyzes or critically examines one by one and in their relative importance the various factors and situations and his personality reactions thereto that in the light of his symptoms and complaints, may have been of dynamic importance in producing his emotional problem or pattern of behavior. Then by inductive reasoning and by discussion with the therapist, the patient, from the material secured through analysis, reconstructs his difficulties and formulates how the understanding acquired thereby may be used constructively to modify emotional reactions and established patterns of behavior and a wholesome integration of the personality be thereby achieved.

Some physicians, although adhering to the principles of distributive analysis and synthesis, believe there should be more emphasis on unconscious processes and therefore also use word association tests, Rorschach's ink blot test, dreams, and even Freudian free associations for securing material that may be used as topics for discussion. It is generally agreed that Meyer's psychobiological psychotherapy is more practical than orthodox psychoanalysis for the treatment of a majority of psychotic patients. If the patient has the intelligence and personality maturity to participate in analysis and synthesis, it is often helpful in psychoneuroses, affective disturbances that are of reactive origin, immaturity reactions, mild paranoid reactions, and psychosomatic or somatization reactions.

Recognition of Basis of Behavior

Included in the study of the personality are emotionally colored thoughts, desires, and strivings that may be only faintly recognized and not accepted by the patient. Occasionally the patient can be led to recognize that his behavior has been influenced by fear, resentment, hate, guilt, frustration, inferiority feeling, or anxiety. In such cases, a re-education of the abnormal attitude may be possible. In some cases, the patient–physician relationship helps the patient to acquire insight or to work through material that has been repressed. Since it is difficult for the patient to study himself objectively, the therapist must often give him direction and careful guidance.

Attention is directed more to actual situations and circumstances than to the discovery of unconscious attitudes and mechanisms. The therapist does not, as in psychoanalysis, attempt to have the patient relive early experiences but to have him understand the present meaning of them and his present attitude toward them. The physician's interested and receptive attitude and his noncritical acceptance of the patient's problems, feelings, and fears help him to recognize his own emotions and to understand himself better. In psychobiological therapy, as in psychoanalysis, one must be careful not to overwhelm the patient with interpretations and thereby cause him to build up his defenses and resistances.

The discussions aim to help the patient trace genetically the origin of his complaint in past experience, both in that of which he is aware and in that which has been excluded from memory. Such a biographical analysis includes a study of somatic factors, drives, and activities and a survey of the patient's psychosexual development. It emphasizes human relationships in general, including difficulties with others and social successes and failures. Not rarely, common factors are found to have been operative in the production of seemingly unrelated symptoms and reactions.

Only those factors are discussed that seem to the patient to be intelligible in terms of human experience, and with particular reference to those facts that appear, both to the patient and to the therapist, to have a meaningful place in the particular life experiences of the patient. The therapist asks questions frequently, not so much for the purpose of securing an answer as for promoting a study by the patient himself of his modes of reaction to life experiences. The patient is asked to analyze past experiences and to study them for factors involved. His conclusions are subject to a critical review and are made a topic for therapeutic discussion.

After various experiences, situations, and symptoms have been discussed and analyzed, the patient is asked to reformulate them into a dynamic life story with its motivations in order that thereby he may as nearly as possible reproduce the origin and development of his problem and understand the means whereby he attempted to meet it. Great care must be exercised lest any interpretations to which an effort is made to guide the patient be not made too early, without fact, or in terms not acceptable to him. Usually the psychological therapist makes use also of other appropriate measures, such as reassurance, guidance, persuasion, desensitization, and ventilation.

Word Association Tests

Reference was made in the previous paragraph to the use of word association tests. This is a method begun by Francis Galton but developed by Jung, having for its purpose the discovery of experiences and tendencies to which the patient is sensitive and therefore are of psychodynamic import. It is based on the observation that if a stimulus word arouses emotional conflict, the response is delayed, distorted, or inhibited.

In the use of this test, a list of 100 words designed to touch on all the common emotional problems is read to the patient and the latter is requested to respond after each word with the first thought that comes to him. Words that stimulate some sensitive topic are followed by a delay in answering, or they evolve unusual or apparently irrelevant response words. After the list has been called, the 100 words are repeated, with instructions to give after each word the same response as was first given. A failure to understand the word, or its repetition before giving a response, betrays the fact

that a sensitive problem has been touched. The topics and tendencies thus betrayed may be used as subjects of discussion. The unpleasant associations may also be used as starting points for psychoanalytic free associations.

OTHER PSYCHOTHERAPEUTIC TECHNIQUES

In addition to the genetic–dynamic therapies, in which group, psychobiological therapy and psychoanalysis may be included, there are various other psychotherapeutic techniques. These may be classified in numerous ways. The following classification seems, however, to be a logical one: (1) superficial expressive therapy; (2) suppressive therapy; and (3) supportive therapy. Although classical psychoanalytic techniques are not employed in these forms, the latter are often to some degree psychoanalytically oriented.

Superficial Expressive Therapy

In the discussion concerning psychoanalysis, attention was called to the fact that free association and an observation of its sequence of ideas, dreams, and the associations to them (transference phenomena and defensive reactions, such as resistances) served both as a means of exploration and of expression of unconscious material. In the superficial expressive therapies, various techniques, sometimes with associated adjunctive devices (such as drugs that alter the level of consciousness), are employed for the purpose of exploring and securing expression of the preconscious and other relatively superficial mental content. Among the superficial expressive therapies would be included narcosynthesis, ventilation, and abreaction.

Narcosynthesis

In this form of therapy, the patient is given an intravenous injection of pentothal sodium or sodium amytal to the point of thorough relaxation but not of sleep. In this state, censorship is less active and suppressed or repressed material emerges. Conscious control is obliterated and inhibitions removed. The patient's subconscious is revealed relatively rapidly and with the minimum of psychic trauma. Positive or negative feelings may be overtly expressed and trends disclosed.

The technique is of considerable value when the patient has recently been subjected to severe traumatic experiences that stirred impulses and anxiety to a degree that they could not be handled without repression and symptom formation. Under these circumstances, abreaction often contributes to the therapeutic process. The greatest usefulness of narcosynthesis is in acute anxiety states, early traumatic neuroses, conversion hysterias and the dissociative amnesias and fugues. It is not satisfactory in obsessive–compulsive states or in chronic neuroses. The technique not only breaks down inhibitions but favors the establishment of rapport, puts the patient in a suggestible frame of mind, and appeals to him because it uses a physical means of approach, which he usually accepts more readily. Resistance, or an unconscious effort to evade memories and insight, is reduced by the narcosis and interpretation is thereby facilitated.

Ventilation

Ventilation is an expressive type of therapy in which the patient's anxiety is relieved to a greater or lesser degree by his being given an opportunity in a tolerant, empathic setting frankly to "talk out" and discuss with the therapist personal problems and "worries" that he ordinarily would not discuss with others. The physician, with an attitude of understanding and encouragement, interrupts the patient as little as possible, although occasional questions may be necessary to keep the thread of the story in meaningful channels.

Among topics that may require ventilation may be doubts, impulses, conscious anxieties, family problems, and feelings of guilt. Some phases of the material expressed often represent confession of thoughts or actions considered intolerable and for which relief from guilt or shame is needed to alleviate anxiety. Others may consist largely of "blowing off steam" regarding resentments. Frequently a joint discussion of present conflicts and past life situations as they seem to relate to emotional or psychosomatic symptoms may bring relief to troublesome aspects of the patient's life. Perhaps in this way the patient may discover a linkage of events and feelings with present reactions and symptoms.

An occasional question may help the patient to find the meaning of his symptoms himself. A correction of misinformation regarding personal problems may result in some diminution of the patient's anxiety. The patient–physician relationship adds to the therapeutic effect of ventilation. Ventilation may at times be supplemented by a superficial psychotherapy based on a knowledge of psychodynamics.

Abreaction

There is a superficial expressive type of psychotherapy in which anxiety is lessened by an emotional reliving of the stress situation which produced the neurosis. A therapeutically beneficial discharge of damned-up emotions associated with the recall of a repressed memory occurs. The existence of a high degree of emotional tension is the basic indication for abreaction. It often tends to produce a desensitization, i.e., a reduction of emotional tension related to a repressed psychological conflict. The emotional reactions discharged are usually those of grief, rage, or fear. Sometimes the abreaction may include an expression of hostility toward the therapist.

Abreaction, with its beneficial effect in bringing about a reliving and possible working out of the emotional aspects of a stressful experience, may be spontaneous, suggested under hypnosis, or facilitated with barbiturates.

Suppressive Therapy

Suppressive psychotherapy aims to strengthen repression and other usual defenses or to lessen the intensity of a disabling symptom by such means as dogmatic assurance, persuasion, suggestion, and hypnosis. It makes no search for, or any effort to solve, the actual dynamic problem. If, therefore, it produces any relief, the problem still remains and may readily return under any stress or strain.

Persuasion

Persuasion as a form of psychotherapy is particularly associated with the name of Paul Dubois of Berne. This therapy is based upon the principle of intellectual explanations and moralizing discussions. It is explained to the patient how faulty intellectual and emotional attitudes on his part were reactions to certain difficulties; also how such tendencies led to undesirable habits and unhealthy emotional and mental conditions. According to Dubois, an important method of therapeutic approach is through self-criticism and through reasoning as to the nature of the symptoms and as to the false ideas and bad mental habits that led to the symptoms.

In persuasion the emphasis is on rationalism and on moral suasion, on an appeal to "reason" and to will rather than on an understanding of the personality and the dynamic factors in its formation. By means of persuasion, the therapist seeks to create, convert, or strengthen certain impulses and to remove or diminish others, to create or strengthen some inhibitions and to free the patient from enslaving ones. It is the aim of the physician, through reasoned argument, to implant in the patient's mind the conviction that his symptoms will disappear. Persuasion probably overestimates the potency of rational processes in any attack upon the products of emotional factors.

Suggestion

In suggestion the therapist seeks to aid the patient by subtly, often indirectly, implanting or inducing the idea or belief that unpleasant or disabling symptoms are being relieved. The successful use of suggestion requires that the physician manifest an attitude of assurance, professional authority, and sympathy. The patient, because of his respect for and confidence in the physician, tends to accept the idea presented. His critical ability is lessened and his mood is influenced. His attention becomes narrowed. In his state of expectancy, he comes to believe that the results predicted will actually take place.

The best results in suggestion therapy are secured when there is no deep-seated disturbance of the personality, as in hysterical conversion symptoms of recent and superficial origin, or in anxiety states following accidents. The employment of electricity, massage, or manipulation in conjunction with suggestion is not advisable, since the patient may attribute the recovery to external agencies. In such cases, the recovery is frequently not permanent and at best is only the disappearance of a symptom and not a cure. In the event of a probable recurrence, the same agencies must be employed in exactly the same manner and frequently by the same person.

Suggestion does not, of course, give the patient any understanding of the cause or dynamics of his disability, and in hysteria, it tends to fix even more firmly the usual propensity to receptivity so characteristic of that disorder. It tends to restrict rather than increase insight. Even though a symptom is relieved by suggestion, the problems and psychological needs that produced it remain unchanged and their evasion may soon be sought by some other symptom. For this reason, the use of suggestion should be accompanied by some kind of re-education.

INDICATIONS AND APPLICATION. In spite of the limitations of suggestion, its use may be considered permissible in children, in persons of limited intelligence and in immature, hysterical personalities.

Assuming, for example, that the symptom to be removed is a hysterical conversion symptom, such as a recent paralysis, the physician deals with it by direct suggestion accompanied by some explanation as to the nature of the paralysis. His attitude must be one of conviction, and certainty and the patient must have confidence in him. The physician demonstrates that the capacity for passive movement still exists. He informs the patient that no organic disability that can interfere with function is present. In referring to the patient's disability, the physician comments as to what a nuisance the former's disability must be to him. At the same time he instructs the patient to move the extremity naturally and without forced effort. The patient is apt to make the mistake of attempting the movement by a strenuous effort that leads also to an innervation of the antagonist group of muscles, resulting in a rigid immobility.

The interview with its atmosphere of conviction must continue until voluntary exercise of the function is restored, even though an hour or two be required. The physician, through the very full life story he has obtained from the patient and through a knowledge of the circumstances under which the disability occurred, must be able to convince the patient not only of the meaning and purpose of the symptom but also that the loss of function has persisted because he believed it to be a real loss. The restoration of function is not a matter of attempt to exercise it on the part of the patient, not a matter of "will," but a matter of belief that it is possible.

The physician must be careful both in word and manner not to create the impression that he considers the patient to be either feigning or exaggerating his inability. Anything that will tend to offend the patient's self-respect must be avoided. Ross emphasizes that the atmosphere of the interview during which the physician attempts removal of the symptom must be one of reasoned logic and of scrupulous avoidance of dramatic demonstration or of artful deception. The patient would prefer to believe that manipulation or some agency outside of himself removed the disability, but he must be made to see that no external interference was instrumental. The patient must be convinced that the disability disappeared because he recognized its purpose and unreality.

The loss of the sympton is at first accompanied by a feeling of relief and pleasure, but unless he fully recognizes the sequence and relation of events and feelings, the patient may suffer a relapse when again confronted with the same problem or unpleasant situation from which the symptom had unconsciously provided an escape. In that case, the sense of relief is followed by anxiety, sleeplessness, mild depression, physical distress, and perhaps by disability. A frank discussion of the situation with the patient may enable him to make an emotional adjustment to it; again, if the problem springs from the environment, a removal from the source of the difficulty may be wise. Unfortunately, the presenting symptom is often not an isolated affair but an expression of characterological tendencies that are apt to lead to difficulties of adjustment unless a thorough reconstruction of the personality occurs.

Hypnosis

Hypnosis has been defined as an induced state of dissociation produced through suggestion. Recent studies of the hypnotic state suggest it is more useful to consider it as a behavioral change understandable on the basis of the patient's preconceptions of hypnosis or the therapeutic interpersonal situation in which he finds himself, which leads to alteration of his perceptions of himself and his surroundings. Thus the psychiatrist who employs the method is perceived as an authority.

Through monotonous and repetitive verbal suggestions, the therapist diverts the patient's attention from all other stimuli and directs it to the therapeutic procedure. The patient's range of conscious perception narrows; he becomes increasingly drowsy and enters a trance-like sleep. By the psychiatrist's suggestions, the patient is motivated to carry out instructions and to accept the belief that in the hypnotic state he is capable of activities unusual for him otherwise. In this state of semiconscious suggestibility, inhibiting psychological defenses may be by-passed, at least temporarily. Suggestions given during hypnosis may be acted upon after its termination or even at a suggested period after its termination. These post-hypnotic suggestions have great therapeutic potential.

INDICATIONS AND VALUE. Although there is much prejudice against its use, hypnosis occupies an important and valuable place in the therapeutic armamentarium of the psychiatrist. Its greatest value is to modify conversion symptoms, recover amnesic defects, examine childhood behavior through suggestion of age regression, and as an anesthetic means in dentistry, obstetrics, and certain surgical conditions.

Although a symptom may often be made to disappear dramatically through hypnosis, yet the factors that produced it are merely repressed and the fundamental personality problem is unchanged. Another reason why hypnosis is not a measure that is permanently successful when used alone is because suggestions lose their effect after a time. It also has the disadvantage that, when the patient's symptoms are suggested away, he may become dependent on the hypnotist instead of developing an ability to solve his problems independently. For these reasons hypnosis, should be supplemented by an insight-producing and constructive form of psychotherapy. Any real cure requires a knowledge of the underlying factors that produced the symptoms.

Hypnosis may be of value when painful experiences have been repressed and have given rise to symptoms. The memory of the traumatic experience may be revived by hypnosis and the symptom made to disappear with an accompanying abreaction, in which the patient goes over and over the traumatic situation, crying and sobbing or showing other expression of pent-up emotions.

Mention has already been made of the fact that hypnosis may be used as a means of investigating aspects of the patient's mental life beneath full awareness. Under hypnosis, forgotten experiences may be revived, and the patient can discuss material about which he cannot or does not want to talk in the waking state. The use of intravenous barbiturates as a means of recovering repressed memories is more certain and requires less time than does hypnosis. It does not, moreover, involve the emotional dependence often prerequisite to successful hypnosis.

Supportive Psychotherapy

Support is particularly useful as a therapeutic technique in cases in which some immediate measures must be taken to relieve a patient, about whom little is known, with unmanageable anxiety. Thus it is an important technical procedure for management of acute peronality disturbances when time must be gained for further study and selection of more appropriate therapeutic approaches. For some patients in whom psychotic ego fragmentation is likely, it is often the only and most appropriate therapeutic method. Support may be regarded as a means of maintaining anxiety at a level at which the patient may successfully face his emotional problems.

TECHNIQUE. Through direct verbal statements of reassurance of the absence of danger and the ready availability of help and authoritative statements as to a plan for treatment, the hopeful expectations of the patient are enhanced. Sympathetic statements by the psychiatrist of his recognition of the patient's distress as he recounts his disturbing symptoms or experiences are helpful in fostering a sense of understanding and emotional relatedness, as sometimes do statements that reflect the physician's recognition of the patient's rationalizing defenses to protect him from anxiety. Verbal appreciation of the patient's constructive actions when he decries himself and his past actions form still another mode of bolstering the ego. As for other measures of support, the establishment of a regular system of therapeutic visits or other contacts by telephone or letter often forms the basis for a sense of constant reassurance.

Supportive psychotherapy is not based on genetic and dynamic considerations but aims to reduce the tensions of anxiety or of other incapacitating tensions by supportive techniques. Care must be taken, however, not to disturb important and acceptable personality defenses. The techniques employed are of a simple type, and the choice of selection will be determined by many factors, such as the personality characteristics, age, life situation, and the nature of the patient's emotional problem or illness. Among the measures employed will be reassurance, use of authority, permissive attitudes that relieve guilt, reasoning, encouragement, counseling, explanation, advice, and manipulation of environment, including, perhaps, an attempted alteration of attitudes of key persons in the patient's life situation. Little attempt is made to bring about an adjustive personality change but rather to help the patient to maintain or improve his ability to face and handle his reality at his best integrative level.

Although supportive therapy consists essentially of strengthening old, but socially acceptable, defenses and the cultivation of new but related ones, the therapist should usually not be satisfied with the exclusive use of such mechanisms, but as circumstances permit, he should try to work beyond the symptoms and aid the patient in acquiring at least some insight. In employing supportive therapy, the physician should bear in mind the danger that he may thereby encourage dependence and a regressive passivity in the patient. Support should be accompanied by efforts to promote maturity of personality. In both genetic–dynamic and in supportive therapy, only limited results can be expected if there are harsh environmental pressures from which the patient cannot escape.

Group Psychotherapy

Rationale

Following the utilization of a didactic discussion and inspirational group technique with tuberculous patients by J. Pratt in 1905, and later with psychosomatic disorders, the evolution of group psychotherapy into a useful psychiatric tool has been a gradual one to which many have contributed. It is now recognized as a valuable addition to our therapeutic armamentarium and is the object of continuing investigation, research, and application. The exigencies of World War II accelerated the wider use of group psychotherapy. Its rapid growth as a systematic treatment during recent years reflects the increased application in group therapy of the principles of dynamic psychiatry. In addition, the armed services initiated and pursued research projects that contributed to the recognition of group therapy as an effective and practical form of treatment. Although it was first used by Pratt and others for its effects upon the morale of physically ill patients whose activities were restricted, its scope has gradually been broadened through successive stages of experimentation and evolution to embrace both hospital and out-patient treatment of psychoses, psychoneuroses, emotional disorders of children, situational reactions, and behavior disorders. As a system of therapy, it has been born of three considerations: expediency, specific indications, and the sociodynamic nature of human maladjustment.

Its least recommending factor, perhaps, is that of expediency based on the fact that there are far more patients in need of therapy than there are therapists equipped to treat them on an individual basis. Although the latter is certainly true, the proponents of group psychotherapy maintain that this mode of managing psychiatric illnesses neither supplants individual psychotherapy nor necessarily offers itself as a substitutive treatment for those to whom other psychotherapeutic doors are closed. On the contrary, it is claimed that specific indications are found among patients for the use of group psychotherapy. Slavson notes that certain patients manifest aversion to the individual therapies because of fear, competitiveness, distrust, or antagonism toward all parental figures. Sometimes individual psychotherapy is too threatening and the patient finds in the group the acceptance and support necessary for the examination of his problems. For such persons, group psychotherapy alone may be successful, or it may serve as a preparation for individual treatment. Patients lacking sibling experiences, having antagonistic sibling attitudes, living in situations without opportunities for participation, experiencing destructive family relations, showing character disorders, presenting evidence of generalized social maladjustment, or those for whom the danger and fear of homosexual involvement with an individual therapist exist are often selected for group treatment. Patients with dull intelligence in peer groups may benefit more from group than from individual therapy. Generally, all children gain from group association, and it is believed that many children who need therapy are suitable candidates for the activity form of group treatment. Exclusive group treatment is frequently considered successful when feelings of inadequacy, sibling rivalry, and social maladjustments are the presenting problems in children. Analytical group psychotherapy is considered the treatment of choice for adolescent girls with confused sexual identifications.

Perhaps the most significant consideration giving rise to the concept of group interaction as a method of psychotherapy is the sociodynamic pattern of human maturation. The development of the infant from helplessness and dependency to tempered autonomy and acculturation is a social event. The need to adjust and the unprofitable systems for avoiding discomfort are created by group life. This consideration has given rise to the hypothesis that if maladjustments are caused to develop by inadequate or unwholesome group situations during the formative periods of life, it should be possible to undo and modify them by exposing the maladaptations to continuous, structured group action in a more adequate and more wholesome setting. Group psychotherapy provides an opportunity to relive and to correct in capsular form many traumatic experiences of earlier life, for example, destructive sibling rivalry, anxiety-provoking separation, premature liberation, spoiling, and loneliness. The psychotherapeutic group recommends itself through its employment of the following factors: acceptance of the selected individuals, avoidance of unnecessary restrictions, permissiveness toward uninhibited verbal expression, and critical evaluation of reactions to group interaction as opposed to platitudinous judgment.

In general, the constituency of the group is determined by the needs of the members, i.e., the group is structured to meet their needs. The approach in the case of schizophrenics is quite different from that in "psychopaths."

Some Dynamisms Relating to Therapeutic Groups

The group is virtually an amalgamation of individual needs. Experience with therapy groups has revealed that the principles of treatment employed in individual psychotherapy are applicable to groups. The relationship between each member and the therapist possesses the qualities of individual therapy, and in addition all the patient-members become, in a sense, auxiliary therapists, thus increasing the emotional interplay. The group setting is a continuous reality factor, which presents an ever-fresh stimulus and provocation to behavior that may be therapeutically directed. Although the group support diminishes individual anxiety, many group therapists feel that the amount and character of affective interactions may be increased and accelerated. The actual therapeutic benefits are realized by the participants rather than by the group as a whole.

A phenomenon of unmistakable significance is the factor of idea- and affectcontagion that permeates a group. Le Bon has likened the result with reference to group participants to the relationship between subject and hypnotist. The individual in a group behaves as though greatly influenced by a group will. Certain ego functions of integration, as well as of affective and conative censorship, are given over to the group and its leader. This factor makes group formation possible, but it also highlights the degree of immaturity of the members. The suggestibility and unreasoning obedience found in group participants demonstrate their dependency. This may be used as a criterion in determining therapeutic improvement, for as maturation progresses, some degree of individual independence develops and a more rational and more realistic relationship to the group ensues.

The group situation is such that mechanisms are mobilized for self-defense against real or imagined threat occasioned by the presence of others. In large part this is a result of *transference*, the avenue through which projections, displacements, and other mechanisms operate. While the entrance of this attitudinal force into the group work presents a barrier, it becomes the very focal point toward which therapeutic interpretations and insight formations are directed.

Aims and Goals

Although employing many of the skills, techniques and psychological mechanisms of individual psychotherapy, group psychotherapy is more complex because of the additional factors inherent in the group process. The complexity may impair to some extent the depth of insights that can be gained. Group goals represent a summation of the members' motivations and the leader's aims. Generally, group leaders aim to relieve emotional stress in their patients, resolve some of their conflicts, help them to a clearer realization of the reasons for their difficulties, and assist them in supplanting defensive reactions with more acceptable and satisfying modes of behavior.

When it is possible with some patients to make use of depth investigation and profound emotional experience, therapy may achieve a modification in super-ego qualities paralleled by an alteration in character structure.

Systems of Group Therapy

The large variety of conscious motivations entertained by patients usually gives way in the course of group work to the goal of insight formation. However, there are many people for whom the development of deep insight is impossible or even undesirable. Many therapists have experienced a progressive change in their methods of conducting groups. S. Hadden, an early leader in the development of group psychotherapy, who used this method without awareness that it had been concurrently innovated by others, and while working with psychosomatic patients in a general hospital, first used a directive, explanatory, reassuring, and inspirational approach. He later recognized the opportunity for the full use of the principles of dynamic psychiatry. Several schools of group treatment have therefore evolved, which range between extremes on a nondirective therapeutic scale. At one end of the scale are the analytical or free association therapies. At the other end are inspirational approches directed toward the suppression of symptomatic behavior. The following is not a comprehensive listing but sets forth a brief description of some representative group management systems. For the sake of psychiatric accuracy, all the methods listed cannot be called psychotherapy. There is much overlapping, and the classification scheme is entirely arbitrary. The number of systems of group organization does not reflect the psychotherapeutic validity of this mode of treatment but rather indicates the necessity for employing varying approaches to the manifold diagnostic categories group therapists undertake to treat.

I. Nondirective Methods (Psychoanalytical)

  1. *Analytical Group Psychotherapy and Group Analysis* (*Slavson, Wolf, Foulkes and others*)
    This system is applicable in psychoneurotic adults and adolescents. There may be

four to twelve participants. Some homogeneity in respect to age, sex, and type of problem is desirable. An analytically trained therapist is leader.

2. *Activity Group Psychotherapy (Slavson)*
This may be used with children from seven to fourteen years of age. There are usually seven to eight participants. It is especially indicated for children rejected by school and play companions. The atmosphere should be permissive and the therapist analytically trained.

3. *Activity-Interview Group Psychotherapy (Slavson)*
This is applicable in case of school-age children with serious problems or with deeply disturbed children who have need both to talk about their anxieties and to act out feelings. There may be eight to ten participants. The therapist should be analytically trained.

4. *Play Group Psychotherapy (Slavson)*
This is used for preschool-age children who are not mature enough to gain from acting out. Children are supplied with play materials. Hidden resentments, feelings of frustration, fears, and confusions are conveyed in play. An analytical therapist interprets the feelings expressed and the object in the family environment toward whom the feelings are directed. The number of participants varies from eight to sixteen.

5. *Group Interview Psychotherapy, Analytically Oriented (Wender, Hadden and others)*
This technique is applicable in most age groups and may be employed with psychoneurotic patients, psychophysiologic states, social maladjustments, and mild psychoses. Six to ten members are desirable. There is spontaneous verbal participation by the group. Group interaction with interpretation leading to mutual support and relative insights is desired. This method may be combined with a didactic approach.

II. Clinical Methods with Didactic (Educational and Directive) Orientation

1. *Group Interview Psychotherapy (Hinckley and others)*
This may be employed with most age groups and in a wide variety of psychiatric conditions. There may be eight to twenty members. The type of leadership depends on psychotherapeutic orientation.

2. *Interview-Inspirational Group Therapy (Pratt, Rhoads, and others)*
This technique may be followed with most age groups and diagnostic categories. There may be a variable number of participants. Spontaneous lectures are given by the leader, and free expression by participants is encouraged. Interpretations

may be analytically oriented or may be directed toward conscious dynamisms and social mechanisms.

3. *Social Relationship Groups (F. Redl)*
This method is followed with seriously disturbed and aggressive children who are usually denied other therapies. Camp activities, trips, tours, and group projects are employed. Leaders may aid rapport in traditional social ways, e.g., giving of gifts, treating, and group playing. Environmental manipulation is a part of the management.

III. Didactic Methods with Clinical Orientation

1. *Psychodrama (J. C. Moreno)*
There are two to six or more participants and the method may be employed in many conditions. A special stage is required. A spontaneous acting-out supplemented by discussion and interaction by audience ("auxiliary egos") is followed. A variation of this technique employs prepared scripts. Other therapeutic systems sometimes use the role-playing elements of psychodrama adjunctively.

2. *Group Orientative Therapy, "Affective Re-education" (Klapman)*
There may be a variable number of participants. Many conditions are treated. The leader plays an authoritative role. The following types are employed:
   a. Planned Program. A series of lectures is given by the leader. It may be used effectively with combat emotional casualties and veterans.
   b. Assigned Reading. A classroom method is followed.
   c. Call Method. This is often effective with groups having difficulty in developing group identity, e.g., seniles. Members are called upon by the leader.
   d. Rotation Method. A serial order of members agreed upon for recitation is established.
   e. Question System. In this method members submit problems or questions for group discussion or for leader-authority to answer.

IV. Nonclinical Group Management

(The nonclinical utilization of group therapies ranges from orthodox classroom techniques to so-called "brainwashing.")

1. Sociological Groups. Six to twelve members participate. Group tensions and group dynamics are observed, and interpretations are directed toward group development.

2. Social Group Work. Here there may be work and living project, recreational, or socialized occupation therapy groups.

3. Confessional-Inspirational Group Method (J. Pratt)
Inspirational talks are given by leader in

an attempt to stimulate admission of problems.

4. Counseling. In this, authoritative advice, guidance, and direction are employed. There may be changing leadership and variable membership.

5. Repressive-Inspirational Groups. (Anonymous organizations, e.g., Alcoholics Anonymous, Cure, Inc.)

There may be any number of participants, up to 500 or more. Group unification based upon group allegiance, mutual support, and the deep acceptance of cultural, moral, and religious values is developed. Appeals to reason and conscious elements of ambition are made. There may be changing leadership.

6. Revival Groups. There may be any number of participants. This well-known "religious conversion" experience may in its casual application convert some behavior problems into full-fledged obsessional neuroses. A reaction approaching revival may occur among groups led by amateur or unskilled "therapists."

Organization of Group

When possible, it is considered desirable to convene interview groups in round table formation in esthetically pleasant surroundings with an informal atmosphere predominating. Activity therapies may require work tables and a meeting room constructed of especially durable materials. Because of extra-therapeutic acting-out, which may limit group work or fragment the group, it is usually desirable to separate the sexes. Groups may meet at any time of day or evening on a rigidly scheduled basis. Except for the intensive therapies, the group convenes once a week for sixty-to-ninety-minute periods. More frequent meetings are necessary for groups having deep insight goals.

The proponents of the analytical psychotherapies urge that the group leaders have had personal intensive psychotherapy and further training in psychopathology. It is believed that group psychotherapists should have special training in the therapies, including a broad didactic educational background as well as a penchant for this form of treatment. The personality and motivations of the group leader are considered of importance, and it is felt that therapists who normally experience discomfort in groups should not undertake group therapeutic leadership. A competent therapist of either sex may be a group leader. When both group and individual therapy are required for a patient, the therapist must be the same person.

Many groups maintain "open" membership, allowing participants to terminate therapy when they wish to do so and permitting others to join at any time. As a rule, the deeper the insight goal, the less variable the group membership. Some groups set date limits, while others go on indefinitely for several years. Goals, number of participants, and systems of therapy vary according to whether the groups are composed of hospital or clinic patients. Group psychotherapy is used in mental hospitals, out-patient clinics, private practice, affiliate therapeutic agencies of educational institutions, family agencies, with relatives of hospitalized patients, and with children. Certain groups employ a totally permissive atmosphere without rules. Some groups employ agreed-upon taboos relative to group work. Many leaders, for example, regard it as desirable to inculcate ethical principles in the group relative to privileged communication and to forbid physical acting-out during meetings.

Group homogeneity and the number of participants are still debated subjects. Too much unification of interest may present the therapist with a symptom wall used as a rallying point for group resistance in the form of monothematic ruminations. On the other hand, too little homogeneity causes scattered interest. Extreme heterogeneity, e.g., alcoholic patients mingled with symptom-neurotic patients, or psychotic persons with transference-neurotic patients, may engender name-calling and mutual distrust. The groups should be large enough for an adequate amount of interaction, yet not so large that members are neglected. In formation of groups for psychotherapy, experienced group therapists suggest that the patients selected be: of the same sex, reasonably close to one another in intelligence, reasonably close in age, and fairly well balanced as to traits. Homogeneity of sex helps prevent acting-out. Similarity in intelligence is found to be important because misplaced retarded patients may delay group development. Closeness in age is significant because of the need for some uniformity in social values, outlook, and philosophical points of view. Group balance is needed in order to avoid overloading with a particular group of symptoms that may serve as a wall of resistance against the therapeutic effort. Generally, groups fare well when they are made up of multiples of a basic triad of patients: the activator, the mollifier, and the passive recipient.

The criteria for denying patients admission to therapeutic groups depend largely upon the orientation of the therapy involved. Most groups suffer from the inclusion of acute psychotic, aggressive paranoid, regressed schizophrenic, and manic patients. Patients with psychoses tending toward depression or those with potential or overt perversion, suicidal behavior, psychopathic personality, involutional states with compulsive and obsessional drives, or hallucinated thought-life are generally excluded from analytical groups. Such patients tend to disrupt, dominate, and exploit the group. They may also stimulate pathological processes in a deleterious way in other patients. In general, it is the feeling among group therapists that patients must have some capacity to participate in groups and at least a minimal amount of social hunger to gain from a therapy group.

The Group Process

Group psychotherapy possesses a characteristic that contrasts it with individual therapy in that it more closely resembles actual life situations and ordinary social intercourse, thus endowing the process with continuous reality meanings. Whereas in individual psychotherapeutic situations all attitudes, conditionings, and transferences are isolated in the patient and channelled into the one participant–observer, in group interaction there exists a multiplicity of targets and a dilution of transference. These have both positive and negative values. On the one hand, these factors reduce anxiety and fear activated by hostile and aggressive feelings toward figures of authority, and they allow for redirection or deflection of the hostilities and resentments toward fellow members. On the other hand, these factors may add an almost insuperable complexity to the production of insights. This is due to the multiplicity of possible emotional inter-relationships.

MECHANISMS. Probably all groups traverse phases of development roughly approximating three periods: (1) a stage of *group unification* with the emergence of group identity; (2) a stage of *group interaction* with the observation of dynamisms; and (3) a final stage of understanding and *resolution of dynamisms* with the production of insights.

Therapy takes place at different levels according to group goals. The factors of mutual support and reliance engendered by group sanction parallel the formation of group esprit and contribute toward the establishment of morale, which may be all that is desired for some groups. Simple ventilation through the phenomenon of emotional release may relieve tensions in given situations. Popular superstitions and ignorance may respond to educative group re-orientation, with the consequent lessening of fears and anxieties.

Analytically oriented group psychotherapies make use of the classical factors of catharsis, resistance, analysis of transference, interpretation, and insight formation. The leader plays an important role in interpretation when resistance must be overcome, also in the resolution of transference. The group setting offers opportunities for the manifestation of social mechanisms and dynamisms not ordinarily found in individual psychotherapy. In addition to those mentioned above, the following are a few commonly encountered.

Displacement. A variety of feelings toward the therapist, which the patient may be afraid to express, are displaced on less threatening group members or on persons not present.

Escape. This is achieved by selective silence or by a change of subject.

Deflection. This may be used for escape by re-directing attention to another group member.

Catalysis. This dynamism represents the manner in which each member activates all the others. Frequently it is valuable, especially in institutional group psychotherapy, to transplant a particularly alert or well-indoctrinated member as a nuclear cadreman, around whom new groups may be built. Such a catalyst accelerates early group work.

Identification. This primary mechanism in personality development is the insigne of civilization and enters importantly into the therapeutic process.

Universalization. This is the term given the dynamism occurring in patients when they discover that other people have problems similar to their own, that others entertain the same forbidden thoughts, or experience similar unacceptable impulses. This mechanism alone is considered by some to be therapeutic. It reduces guilt, heightens self-esteem, and diminishes emotional burdens.

ADVANTAGES. Frequently small groups not only have supportive value but permit the expression of hidden anxieties and conflicts. Also members, by seeing their unconscious motives in action in the ways the members feel toward each other and to the therapist, may gradually gain insight into their difficulties.

Since anxiety is reduced and transference modified in group psychotherapy, the depth of insight may be less than in intensive individual psychotherapy, although some therapists claim that a depth of insight comparable with that of individual psychoanalysis may be attained.

An important consideration of group therapy is the realization that in chronically aggressive children the very antagonisms and violent hostilities that constitute their antisocial tendencies are factors common to such groups and tend to promote unit formation, while the non-neurotic elements of the ego respond to the persevering interest and patience of the group leader.

The mobilization of certain defenses may be all that is desired in the treatment of many psychotic patients. The group process often encourages re-repression of unconscious fantasies that present themselves clinically as delusions. As the psychotic mechanisms are removed from consciousness, more normal ego elements resume their supremacy and the patient may become eligible for non-institutional life or individual psychotherapy.

Mention should be made of the ever-increasing senile segment of the population, with whom considerable group therapeutic work is now being done in some institutions. A significantly greater number of senile patients so treated is enabled to return to better levels of adjustment than is the case when group therapy is not employed. The group process appears to increase alertness, dispel confusion, bring affects toward nomal, and improve memory and orientation. Often the amount of incontinence is found to diminish in many patients on this program.

Results of Group Therapy

The statistical evaluation of therapeutic results of group work, as in all the therapies remains largely impressionistic. Unusually good results with analytical group therapy were secured by Schilder, who found 9 cured and 15 improved out of 31 neurotic patients treated. Improvement was obtained with hypochondriacal patients. A high degree of improvement was obtained with hysterical patients suffering from anxiety neuroses and obsessional and social neuroses. A recent study of 22 juvenile delinquents treated with interview and activity group therapy and of the same number of controls revealed statistically significant improvement in the experimental group as measured by psychometric tests, school achievement, and maturity tests as well as by Rorschach personality assessment technique. Also, neurotic depressions are said to respond well to group psychotherapy. Most therapists of well-constituted groups report results that compare favorably with those of individual psychotherapy.

BIBLIOGRAPHY

Abraham, K.: Selected Papers on Psychoanalysis. London, Hogarth Press, 1927.

Adler, A.: The Practice and Theory of Individual Psychology. New York, Harcourt, Brace & Co., 1927.

Alexander, F.: Psychoanalysis and Psychotherapy. New York, W. W. Norton & Co., Inc., 1956.

Idem: Principles and techniques of briefer psychotherapeutic procedures. Proceedings of Assoc. for Research in Nervous and Mental Diseases, Vol. XXXI, pp. 16–20. Baltimore, Williams & Wilkins Co., 1953.

Idem, and Ross, H. (Eds.): Dynamic Psychiatry. Chicago, The University of Chicago Press, 1952.

Appel, K. E. et al.: Long term psychotherapy. Proceedings of Assoc. for Research in Nervous and Mental Diseases, Vol. XXXI, pp. 21–34. Baltimore, Williams & Wilkins Co., 1953.

Idem: Principles and practice of psychotherapy. Am. J. Psychoanaly., 15:99–106, 1955.

Balser, B. H.: Psychotherapy of the Adolescent. New York, International Universities Press, 1957.

Barber, T. X.: Experiments in Hypnosis. Scientific American, 196:54–61, 1957.

Idem: The concept of "hypnosis." J. Psychol., 45:115–131, 1958.

Bernheim, H.: De la suggestion et ses applications à la thérapeutique. Paris, Octave Doin, 1886.

Blaine, Jr., G. B.: Short term psychotherapy with college students. New England J. Med., 256:208–211, 1957.

Brenman, M., and Gill, M. M.: Hypnotherapy. New York, International Universities Press, 1947.

Brill, A. A.: Freud's Contributions to Psychiatry. New York, W. W. Norton & Co., Inc., 1944.

Dorcus, R. M.: Hypnosis and Its Therapeutic Applications. New York, Blakiston, 1956.

Dubois, P.: The Psychic Treatment of Mental Disorders, 6th ed. New York, Funk and Wagnalls, 1909.

Foulkes, S. H.: Introduction to Group-Analytic Psychotherapy. New York, Grune & Stratton, 1949.

Frank, J. D.: The dynamics of the psychotherapeutic relationship. Psychiatry, 22:17–39, 1959.

Freud, S.: Collected Papers (5 Vols.). London, International Psychoanalytical Library, 1924–1950.

Idem: The Interpretation of Dreams. New York, The Macmillan Co., 1933.

Idem: Group Psychology and the Analysis of the Ego. London, Hogarth Press, 1948.

Fromm-Reichmann, F.: Principles of Intensive Psychotherapy. Chicago, The University of Chicago Press, 1950.

Idem: Notes on the personal and professional requirements of a psychotherapist. Psychiatry, 12:361–378, 1949.

Idem: Psychoanalytic and general dynamic conceptions of theory and of therapy. J. Am. Psychoanalyt. Assoc., 2:711–721, 1954.

Idem: Psychotherapy of schizophrenia. Am. J. Psychiat., 111:410–419, 1954.

Glover, E.: The indications for psychoanalysis. J. Ment. Sc., 100:393–401, 1954.

Greenacre, P.: The role of transference. J. Am. Psychoanalyt. Assoc., 2:671–684, 1954.

Hadden, S. B.: Treatment of neuroses by class technique. Ann. Int. Med., 16:33–37, 1942.

Idem: The utilization of a therapy group in teaching psychotherapy. Amer. J. Psychiat., 103:644–648, March, 1947.

Hampshire, A.: The use of groups in motivation for analytic group psychotherapy. Int. J. Group Psychotherapy, 4:95–102, 1954.

Hinckley, R. G., and Hermann, L.: Group Treatment in Psychotherapy. Minneapolis, University of Minnesota Press, 1951.

Hoch, P. H.: Aims and limitations of psychotherapy. Am. J. Psychiat., 112:321–327, 1955.

Hordern, A.: The response of the neurotic personality to abreaction. J. Ment. Sc., 98:630–639, 1952.

Janet, P.: Psychological Healing. New York, The Macmillan Co., 1925.

Jones, E.: Papers on Psychoanalysis, 4th ed. Baltimore, Wm. Wood & Co., 1938.

Jung, C. G.: Two Essays on Analytical Psychology. London, Ballière, Tindall and Cox, 1928.

Karush, A., and Ovesey, L.: Unconscious mechanisms of magical repair. Arch. Gen. Psych., 5:55–69, 1961.

Kelman, H., et al.: Goals in therapy. Am. J. Psychoanalysis, 16:3–23, 1956.

Knight, R. P.: Evaluation of psychotherapeutic techniques. Bull. Menninger Clin., 16:113–124, 1952.

Kolb, L. C.: Psychotherapeutic evolution and its implications. Psychiat. Quart., 30:579–597, 1956.

Kubie, L. S.: Practical and Theoretical Aspects of Psychoanalysis. New York, International Universities Press, 1950.

Linden, M. E.: Group psychotherapy with institutionalized senile women: Study in gerontologic human relation. Int. J. Group Psychotherapy, 3:150–170, 1953.

Idem: Transference in gerontologic group psychotherapy: Studies in gerontologic human relation, IV. Internat. J. Group Psychotherapy, 5:61–79, 1955.

Muncie, W.: Psychobiologic therapy. Am. J. Psychotherapy, 7:225–240, 1953.

Novey, S.: The technique of supportive therapy in psychiatry and psychoanalysis. Psychiatry, 22:179–187, 1959.

Nunberg, H.: Principles of Psychoanalysis; Their Application to the Neuroses. New York, International Universities Press, 1955.

Orne, M. T.: The nature of hypnosis: Artifact and essence. J. Abn. and Soc. Psychol., 58:277–299, 1959.

Orr, D. W.: Transference and Countertransference: A historical survey. J. Am. Psychoanalyt. Assoc., 2:621–670, 1954.

Powdermaker, F. B., and Frank, J. D.: Group Psychotherapy. New York, Commonwealth Fund, 1953.

Rickman, J.: The role and future of psychotherapy within psychiatry. J. Ment. Sc., 96:181–189, 1950.

Ross, T. A.: The Common Neuroses. Baltimore, William Wood & Co., 1937.

Ruesch, J.: Social Factors in Therapy in Psychiatric Treatment. Proceedings of the Association for Research in Nervous and Mental Diseases, Vol. XXXI, pp. 59–93, Baltimore, 1953.

Semrad, E. V., and Arsenian, J.: The use of group processes in teaching group dynamics. Am. J. Psychiat., 108:358–363, 1951.

Slater, R.: Interpretations. Am. J. Psychoanalysis, 16:118–124, 1956.

Slavson, S. R.: Analytic Group Psychotherapy with Children, Adolescents and Adults. New York, Columbia University Press, 1950.

Whitehorn, J. C.: Understanding psychotherapy. Am. J. Psychiat., 112:328–33, 1955.

Chapter Thirty-three

PHARMACOLOGICAL THERAPY

Following the introduction of the phenothiazine chlorpromazine in 1952 as a potent new pharmacological agent for the treatment of the psychosis, numerous analogues and other new compounds have been synthesized, tested, and placed in clinical usage. The effectiveness of the phenothiazine analogues and certain antidepressant agents has altered particularly the management of the psychoses. Their widespread prescription has superseded to a large extent the various forms of shock therapy and the use of psychosurgery.

These agents have the capacity of modifying affective states without seriously impairing cognitive functions. In the latter respect they differ from the sedative and hynotic drugs previously available. Since it is expected that the able psychiatrist comes to practice fully knowledgeable from his previous medical studies of the well-known properties and clinical indications of the long-known central nervous depressants such as the narcotics, anesthetics, hypnotics, and intoxicants, as well as the stimulants, consideration is not given to these drugs in this text. Their skillful prescription, often in conjunction with that of the new "neuroleptics," still is demanded in practice.

PHENOTHIAZINE DERIVATIVES

Chlorpromazine Hydrochloride

This is a synthetic drug, one of the series of alkyl amine derivatives of phenothiazine, its full chemical name being 10-(3-dimethylaminopropyl)-2-chlorphenothiazine hydrochloride. It was developed in the Rhone-Poulenc Specia Laboratories in France during research on potentiating agents in anesthesia. The first clinical investigations with the drug were carried out in that country in 1952 where, as in other European countries, it is marketed under the trade name Largactil. In this country it is marketed under the trade name of Thorazine.

Chlorpromazine is a white crystalline powder that is readily soluble in water. Since only a small part of the drug is eliminated by the kidneys, most of it is presumably metabolized in the body, although the route is unknown.

PHYSIOLOGICAL EFFECTS. One of the early effects of the administration of chlorpromazine is a fall in blood pressure according to dose and individual reaction. Other effects are slowing of the pulse and of respiration, lowering of temperature and of basal metabolic rate, and transient leukopenia. Also, it frequently causes dryness of the mucous membranes and nasal congestion. It has an antiemetic effect as well. In large doses, chlorpromazine produces motor retardation, muscular hypotonia, and an unsteady gait, and during the first two or three days of treatment, patients show a varying degree of somnolence but can be awakened without difficulty and are able to take food. However, as a rule, the increased need for sleep is reduced after a few days. Patients may complain of feeling faint, weak, cold, and drowsy, but the sensorium remains clear. The action of the drug is maximal at one hour after administration and appreciable effects continue for six hours. It potentiates the effects of barbiturates and of narcotics.

ADMINISTRATION. Chlorpromazine is available in 10-, 25-, 50-, 100- and 200-mg. tablets, and also in 25-mg. (1 ml.) and 50-mg. (2 ml.) ampules. There is no standard dose of the drug; this must be individualized. Chlorpromazine may be administered by oral or by intramuscular routes; however, it is so irritant that it should not be administered subcutaneously. Intramuscular injections should be given deeply in the upper and outer quadrant of the buttock, and when injected the solution supplied by the manufacturer should be diluted with physiological salt solution or a 2 per cent procaine solution and administered very slowly. Massaging the site of the injection for three or four minutes will help to reduce local irritation. Some physicians add hyaluronidase in order to facilitate absorption and prevent abscess formation. If quick action is desired, the patient may receive 25 mg. by deep intramuscular injection, and if this amount is not effective, an additional 25-mg. injection may be given within an hour unless contraindicated by marked hypotension. Subsequent intramuscular dosages may be increased gradually, even up to 400 mg. every six hours. The higher doses should be reached over a period of several days.

If, as frequently occurs, the acutely disturbed patient becomes quiet within 48 hours, oral doses (mg. for mg. or higher) may gradually replace intramuscular doses. Injections should not be continued for more than three or four days without beginning to replace them with oral therapy. It will not usually be necessary to increase oral administration to more than 800 mg. a day, but if sedation is not secured, the dosage may gradually be increased up to as much as 1200 mg. a day. Usually this amount is sufficient for a maximum dose, although some psychiatrists give a maximum of 2000 mg. in 24 hours. Amounts up to 4000 mg. have been given, but large doses cause confusion and are not to be recommended.

As the patient begins to grow quiet, the dose may gradually be reduced over a period of weeks or months. If signs of returning symptoms appear, the amount should be increased immediately and additional parenteral doses should be given if necessary. When the patient is no longer disturbed, the dose may usually be reduced gradually and then continued for an indefinite period, the amount being the smallest that will control symptoms. Usually in the chronically disturbed patient this will be approximately 600 to 800 mg. daily. If there has been no improvement in symptoms after the patient has received these amounts daily for two months, the drug should be gradually discontinued.

In the less acutely agitated patient, treatment may be begun with 50 mg. given orally three times a day. This should be increased gradually until an effective and tolerable level is reached. Frequently doses of 100 to 400 mg. daily, if continued over a long period, will maintain sedation.

The most obvious response to chlorpromazine is a somnolent effect varying from slight drowsiness to deep sleep. The somnolence is most marked within 15 to 20 minutes after an injection; however, even when the somnolence is deepest, it is possible to rouse the patient easily. He shows little or none of the residual clouding of consciousness that follows comparable barbiturate sedation. Acutely agitated, restless, or excited patients show a greater response than do less disturbed patients. The tranquilizing effect does not seem in any way related to the underlying nature of the excitement, whether schizophrenic, manic, or confusional. If the patient responds well to the drug, he develops an attitude of indifference both to his surroundings and to his symptoms. He shows decreased interest in and response to his hallucinatory experiences and a less assertive expression of his delusional ideas. Even though not somnolent, the patient may lie quietly in bed, unoccupied, and staring ahead. He may answer questions readily and to the point but offer little or no spontaneous conversation; however, questioning shows that he is fully aware of his circumstances.

INDICATIONS FOR USE. Chlorpromazine usually exerts a tranquilizing effect in a wide variety of disturbed psychiatric states—tension, psychomotor overactivity, agitation, impulsiveness, aggressive outbursts, destructiveness, and overtly anxious, antagonistic, paranoid reactions. It, therefore, has a wide field of usefulness in schizophrenia, both in acute reactions and in overactive chronic patients. The more destructive and aggressive the patient, the more likely is he to respond to chlorpromazine. In the acutely ill, schizophrenic hallucinations and delusional ideas frequently disappear within the first two weeks of treatment. Here, as elsewhere when rapid sedation is required, chlorpromazine is to be preferred to reserpine. The percentage of remissions or of improvements among schizophrenic patients who have been ill for less than six months is gratifyingly large and seems to be larger than in those who have received reserpine.

The longer the patient has been ill, the less are his chances of attaining a moderate or marked improvement. Of schizophrenics who receive chlorpromazine (or reserpine) relatively early in their illness, more become able to leave the hospital and make adequate social adjustment than has been the case with any previous method of treatment. Among them will be many who, despite electroconvulsive or insulin coma and other forms of treatment, have shown no improvement. Chronic psychotic patients should be treated for extended periods (6 to 8 months) before assessing the result. Best results are secured with patients who have not been ill for more than two years. Among these the results will depend largely on the clinical manifestations of the disorder, the degree of improvement being much greater in the overactive, disturbed patients.

Many patients previously so ill and preoccupied with the symptoms of their illness that they remained indifferent, or hostile, to attempts to alter their behavior, thinking, or emotional set become more amenable to therapy when taking chlorpromazine. Although many schizophrenics who have been hospitalized for years show some improvement, not more than 5 per cent of those hospitalized for five continuous years become able to leave the hospital. It will later become necessary that an appreciable number of them return to the hospital. The number of chronic schizophrenics who will be able to leave the hospital and remain in the community will depend on the understanding and tolerance of the patient's family and the guidance and supervision of the social worker, but it actually is not quite accurate to refer to the most favorable outcome of the chronic schizophrenic patient's illness as a cure.

From 30 to 35 per cent of the chronic schizophrenics who have long been hospitalized will not be materially improved by administration of chlorpromazine, yet the care of the approximately 60 per cent who do improve but are not able to leave the hospital is greatly eased. Delusions and hallucinations may persist but are usually no longer disturbing to the patient. The sullen, sarcastic, and antagonistic patient is less irritable and frequently becomes quiet, co-operative, and accessible, and there is a remarkable improvement in the atmosphere of the ward for disturbed patients. Many who long occupied seclusion rooms because of their assaultive and destructive tendencies may mingle with other patients and participate in occupational and useful activities. Even in patients whose response is less favorable, there is usually a lessening of tension and perhaps an attitude of quiet indifference. Although the withdrawn, inactive, unresponsive, regressed schizophrenic patient does not usually improve sufficiently to leave the hospital, he frequently is able to modify his behavior, discontinue soiling, and no longer discard his clothing. The relief from the anguish, bitterness, hostility, and despair from which many patients suffer is of incalculable value. The chronic schizophrenic who improves should continue on a carefully determined maintenance dose for an extended period.

In manic–depressive psychosis, chlorpromazine is not a substitute for electroconvulsive therapy, but in the early stages of the manic phase it is a useful adjunct if the patient is overactive and unmanageable and the period required for recovery is usually shortened. It is often desirable to administer the drug by intramuscular injections for two or three days and then to continue it by mouth in 50 per cent larger doses. If the depressed patient is agitated, chlorpromazine will usually relieve, or perhaps more accurately, mask the agitation. However, reactive depressions do not respond particularly well to chlorpromazine. Electroconvulsive therapy still remains the most effective means of treating depression.

The usually difficult problem of the restless or agitated patient suffering from senile dementia is often rendered much easier by the use of chlorpromazine. Sedation by means of the barbiturates may confuse him still further. Under chlorpromazine, in amounts of 25 to 50 mg. three times a day, he often becomes calm and manageable and can be cared for at home. Memory loss and disorientation are, of course, unaffected.

Occasionally, especially in institutions for their care, epileptic patients are subject to episodic or chronic disturbed states in which the patients may be hyperactive, noisy, hostile, aggressive, resistive, assaultive, destructive, and given to temper outbursts or furor states. A parenteral injection of 100 mg. of chlorpromazine is highly effective in quieting the acute, excited states. Most epileptic patients who exhibit chronic disturbed states are also quieted and relaxed by the drug. This may at first be given as 300 mg. daily and later reduced to 150 mg. Since chlorpromazine tends to potentiate the activity of barbiturates, it is well to reduce the dose of the latter drug during the administration of the former.

In relatively large doses, chlorpromazine is extremely helpful in the management of acute alcoholic states. It produces prompt control of motor excitement and of nausea and vomiting, permits restful, relaxed sleep, and contributes to the relief of tension and anxiety. Its sedative effect hastens recovery in delirium tremens. It is definitely beneficial in nearly all short-lived mental disturbances of a delirious type. The use of chlorpromazine should supplement and not replace the administration of glucose solution, of insulin, and of vitamin B complex. It is not, of course, of value in the treatment of the Korsakoff's syndrome or in the alleviation of chronic alcoholism.

UNTOWARD EFFECTS. Mention has already been made of some of the physiological effects of chlorpromazine. At times these side effects are troublesome but rarely lead to serious complications. Occasionally the somnolence may become excessive and require a reduction of dosage. Usually, however, it disappears after the first or second week of therapy. Not infrequently an unpleasant taste and a dryness of the mouth and "stuffiness" of the nose result in discomfort. Tachycardia, palpitation, persistent constipation even to the point of fecal impaction, headaches, pyrexia, and pains in the legs or abdomen may occur. A pale and "pinched" facial appearance is common in patients receiving full intramuscular doses.

Both chlorpromazine and reserpine cause hypotension of the orthostatic type.

This may lead to sensations of faintness or to actual fainting, especially on changing from a recumbent to a standing position. Both drugs should be given with great caution to patients suffering from atherosclerosis, cardiovascular disease, or other conditions in which a sudden drop in blood pressure may be undesirable.

Photosensitivity confined to areas exposed to sunlight may be produced by chlorpromazine. Usually this will result merely in redness and itching, but sometimes it will lead to edema and vesicle formation. Ordinarily interruption of the drug, the application of bland lotions, and the administration of antihistamines are sufficient treatment of the dermatological reactions. About 8 per cent of patients receiving chlorpromazine develop allergic skin reactions. One of the most frequent forms is a maculopapular, erythematous, pruritic eruption involving the trunk and arms.

Jaundice, usually appearing from the second to the eighth week after beginning the use of the drug, develops in approximately 4 per cent of the cases, and its duration is variable. Since there is no evidence of damage to the hepatic parenchyma, the jaundice is undoubtedly cholestatic in origin. The total bilirubin content of the blood is greatly elevated, and the alkaline cholesterol is much increased, as is the percentage of eosinophils. However, there is little or no disturbance of the cephalin flocculation and thymol turbidity. The obstruction is within the intralobular canaliculi and a result of a pericanalicular lymphocytic infiltration.

If the patient's mental state is such that he can note and report his observations, it is well to ask him if there has been any change in the color of his urine or stools, also if he has been aware of pruritus. As a precursory symptom of jaundice, this has been known to occur within two days after the administration of chlorpromazine. Since it is simple and can easily be done at the bedside as a screening measure, some internists advise doing a sodium bilirubinate test twice a week for three weeks after beginning the drug. If jaundice appears, the drug should be discontinued and glucose administered intravenously, if indicated. Vitamins should be given, also a high carbohydrate, high protein, and low fat diet. It is often difficult to determine whether the jaundice is caused by the drug or by extrahepatic obstruction. Surgery for supposed disease of the biliary tract should be avoided. Liver function tests should probably be continued until they show that normal function has been restored. To what extent, if any, the liver will suffer harmful effects as the result of long-continued administration of chlorpromazine is as yet unknown. Although the jaundice is apparently related not so much to dosage as to a special sensitivity on the part of the patient, the drug may be resumed after normal function has been restored. The beginning dosage should not exceed 25 mg. given three times a day and should be increased slowly thereafter.

Chlorpromazine depresses the production of leukocytes. Agranulocytosis is fortunately of low incidence, probably less than 0.3 per cent, and it occurs within three to six weeks after the beginning of treatment. It is more frequent in women, particularly in those between 40 and 60 years of age, and its onset is sudden. Patients should be asked to report at once the sudden appearance of sore throat or of lesions in the mouth. Any rise in temperature should also suggest an immediate blood count. These cannot be relied upon as the sole criterion for agranulocytosis. A weekly blood count is in order but is of little value is detecting an impending agranulocytosis. In case blood dyscrasia develops, chlorpromazine should be stopped at once and penicillin and the broad-spectrum antibiotics should be given immediately. Corticotropin (ACTH) is also usually employed, and transfusion is often advisable. In spite of active treatment, the outcome is often fatal.

Parkinsonism appears in about 10 per cent of the patients receiving full doses of chlorpromazine. The clinical picture is the usual one of muscular rigidity, slowing of movement, festinating gait, sialorrhea, and at times a pill-rolling tremor. The condition is always reversible and may be relieved with benztropine methanesulfonate (Cogentin), 1 mg. twice a day.

Miosis or blurring of vision is noted at times.

Occasionally nurses who administer chlorpromazine develop a troublesome contact dermatitis that clears when further exposure is avoided. The irritant qualities of the drug were dramatically illustrated in the case of one patient who rubbed an eye with a tablet of chlorpromazine. An extensive and violent inflammatory process resulted in loss of vision. A few patients have attempted suicide with large doses of chlorpromazine, but only one death has been reported.

Discontinuance. It is not difficult to decide when the administration of chlorpromazine should be discontinued in the case of acute, confusional excitement or in the case of acute manic episode of manic–depressive psychosis. In the former, its use may be terminated soon after the sensorium becomes fully clear. In the latter, the dose may be reduced as the symptoms subside, and the drug may be discontinued after mood and motor activity have been entirely normal for two weeks. Experience thus far suggests that in chronic schizophrenia the drug should be continued indefinitely in optimal individual dosage. Although undesirable side effects of the drug usually appear within two months after beginning its use, the patient who continues on a maintenance dose after leaving the hospital should report frequently to a physician.

Other Phenothiazines

The phenothiazine nucleus, from which the various analogues have been synthesized, consists of two benzine rings joined by a sulphur and nitrogen atom. By substitution of R_1 and R_2 of the formula given in the diagram, numerous deriva-

tives have been developed. From the attachment of a dimethylaminopropyl side chain at R_1 are derived chlorpromazine, promazine, and triflupromazine. Substitution of the piperazine side chain in this position leads to the development of perphenazine, prochlorperazine, and trifluoperazine. The piperidine side chain attached at R_1 evolves thioridazin and mepazine. Compounds in the piperazine substituted group are the most potent but also have the greater tendency to produce symptoms of extrapyramidal dysfunction.

The general indications for the prescription of the phenothiazine derivations are those for chlorpromazine. More than in their ability to modify selectively various "target symptoms" they differ in their toxic properties.

Promazine

This drug, sold commercially as Sparine, is identical chemically with chlorpromazine except for the absence of a chlorine atom on the ring structure. The general pharmacological properties are similar, also. Sparine has been recommended particularly for use for delirium tremens and in the treatment of the senile and arteriosclerotic brain syndromes, since it is claimed that it has less hypotensive effect than chlorpromazine. There is evidence that toxic manifestations, such as jaundice and hypoplastic anemia, are less likely to occur with its use. Transient leukopenia, agranulocytosis, and convulsive seizures have been reported but are infrequent in occurrence.

Promazine is available for both oral and parenteral administration. The tablets for oral use may be given in doses of 25 to 200 mg. every four to six hours, the dosage being varied according to the response of the patient.

Triflupromazine

Marketed as Vesprine or Vespral, this neuroleptic may be administered orally, as well as in emulsion or intravenously. The emulsion is useful for those patients with difficulty in swallowing and those who retain tablets in the mouth, such as the catatonics and senile psychotics. The daily oral dosage range generally used is from 20 to 200 mg.

Perphenazine

This drug, known commercially as Trilafon, combines the phenothiazine and piperazine rings. It is said to have fewer side effects than chlorpromazine. Photosensitivity has as yet to be reported, and for this reason it is a useful agent for those who are exposed much to the sun. Perphenazine is supplied in tablets of 2, 4, and 8 mg., and is recommended in oral doses of 6 to 16 mg. daily, although an amount as high as 64 mg. has been given. It is said to be useful for tension headaches, intractable pruritus, certain neurodermatoses, and chronic painful conditions, as well as the psychotic states.

Prochlorperazine

This drug, sold as Compazine, is recommended for use in the treatment of various neurotic conditions for the relief of anxiety. It has powerful antiemetic action and is useful in the control of nausea and vomiting associated with drug or alcohol withdrawal. It has been administered usefully in treatment of numerous psychosomatic conditions. Compazine is usually given by mouth in doses of 5 to 10 mg. three or four times daily.

Trifluoperazine

Better known under the trade name of Stelazine, this agent is said to be particularly useful in activation of the chronically apathetic, withdrawn, or depressed schizophrenic, in contrast to chlorpromazine, which often aggravates these types of behavior. The drug is prescribed for the psychotic in initial doses of 5 mg. three to four times daily, this dosage being increased by increments of 5 mg. until the patient is receiving 40 to 60 mg. daily. For office patients, 1 to 2 mg. given twice daily usually proves an effective dosage.

Trifluoperazine has been prescribed with chlorpromazine in the treatment of patients who fail to respond to one or the other drug alone, where motor activation is desirable, or as a means of avoiding toxic effects on high dosages of either drug when given alone.

Fluphenazine

Fluphenazine (Prolixin, Permitil) provides a sustained action over time and therefore may be used effectively in a single or double dose throughout the day. It is a powerful antiemetic but does not prolong barbiturate hypnosis. For psychotic behavior, the initial oral dosage is 0.5 mg.; this is then increased to 10 to 20 mg. daily. In the psychoneuroses, the effective daily dosage range is usually 0.5 to 3 mg. daily.

Thioridazine

This substituted piperidine derivative, marketed as Mellaril, has achieved wide usage as it appears to be as clinically effective as other phenothiazines but produces fewer side effects and toxic manifestations. In a few cases, however, it has led to a pigmentary retinopathy noted initially as diminishing vision, which has taken place between the twentieth and fiftieth day of administration.

The drug is highly effective in the treatment of the psychoses and also has been reported to relieve the symptoms of insomnia, fatigue, tension headaches, and anxiety associated with other psychophysiologic reactions. The usual daily oral dosage is 300 to 800 mg. for the psychoses, and 20 to 60 mg. in the neurotic and psychophysiologic reactions.

Methotrimeprazine or Levomepromazine

Sold as Nozinan, Veractel or Neurocel, this drug probably will receive wide usage as an analgesic. It is also reported to have antidepressive activity. It has been used successfully in the treatment of numerous chronic painful states, including posthepatic neuralgia, phantom limb pain, tabes dorsalis, and thalamic syndrome, and when given by injection it has been shown to be as effective as morphine in equivalent doses in acute postoperative and postpartum states. No addiction has been reported.

The effective dosage of levomepromazine for the chronic painful reactions ranges from 150 to 300 mg. daily. The drug is usually prescribed in 50 mg. doses three to five times each day. When relief of pain is obtained, the daily maintenance dosage often may be reduced.

Urine Test for Phenothiazines

Recently a simple test for detection of chlorpromazine and other phenothiazines in urine has been described. To a small amount of urine (1 ml.) is added an equal volume of a solution containing equal parts of 10 per cent H_2SO_4 and 5 per cent $FeCl_3$. The mixture is gently shaken. The presence of phenothiazines is indicated by the development of a violet color.

RAUWOLFIA DERIVATIVES

Reserpine

For centuries the root of the plant *Rauwolfia serpentina* Bentham, indigenous to India and known there as the "insanity herb," was used in that country for the treatment of a wide variety of diseases, including mental disorders. In 1953 Dr. R. A. Hakim of Ahrnabad, India, was awarded a gold medal for the presentation of a paper on the cure of schizophrenia with a compound, the major ingredient of which was this drug. Reference to its sedative effect had, however, been previously made by many Indian writers. In 1943 note was made in the *Indian Medical Gazette* of its increasing popularity in the treatment of mental disease, and report was made of improvement following use of the drug in manic–depressive psychosis, schizophrenia, and other forms of mental disorder. In 1953, prompted by Hakim's report, Kline, at the Rockland (N. Y.) State Hospital, began the experimental use of reserpine, a colorless, crystalline, ester alkaloid, the chief active principle of *Rauwolfia*, and concluded it is an effective sedative for use in mental hospitals.

Pharmacologically, the Rauwolfia derivatives have an effect on the metabolism of serotonin (5-hydroxytryptamine). Serotonin, a product of tryptophan metabolism, is produced by the argentaffin cells, which are dispensed throughout the body, particularly in the small intestine and nervous system tissues. The administration of Rauwolfia alkaloids liberates serotonin from the brain. This, it is believed, accounts for its tranquilizing effect. So far, no other tranquilizing drugs have shown this serotonin-releasing effect.

ADMINISTRATION AND DOSAGE. Reserpine (Serpasil) may be given intramuscularly or orally, and frequently in the early stages of treatment both methods are used simultaneously. However, the dosage must be individually adjusted in accordance with optimal results and the tolerance of the patient. Many physicians recommend 5 mg. intramuscularly once a day for 10 days and 1 mg. orally twice a day. If necessary, the oral dose may gradually be increased to 10 mg. and continued indefinitely. The maximum dose should not exceed 15 mg. in 24 hours. Sometimes the dose must be reduced to 2 mg. or 1 mg. because of side effects. Reserpine acts more slowly than does chlorpromazine. In the effect produced, 10 mg. of reserpine are equivalent to about 300 to 400 mg. of chlorpromazine. As with chlorpromazine, a confusional state may develop in case of overdosage; the optimal level of the dosage appears to be proportional to the intensity of the emotional disturbance. If a patient shows no improvement after two months of treatment, it is probably useless to continue the drug, but if improvement follows, treatment should be continued for at least three consecutive months. As is the case with chlorpromazine, it is usually desirable to continue reserpine indefinitely for the chronic psychotic patient who has improved with its use.

CLINICAL EFFECTS. Even though the chemical structures of reserpine and of chlorpromazine are completely different, they are used for almost identical purposes and their clinical effects are strikingly similar. Although the psychological effects of these drugs are subject to quantitatively large individual variations, they both usually have a definitely relaxing and quieting influence. Typically the patient receiving reserpine is somnolent and lethargic but is readily aroused and then seems quite alert. Recent studies of the effects of reserpine upon pathological activity suggest that these are less than were originally assumed, and that the apparent results are a result largely of the increased somnolence during the hours of the day when the patient would be normally awake. It is not certain that they are direct effects of the drug. Occasionally, from about two weeks to two months after beginning treatment, especially when receiving full doses of the drug, the patient may develop parkinsonism, usually of a more marked type than that produced by chlorpromazine.

Some patients receiving reserpine rapidly increase their tissue water, and this hydration may occasionally cause convulsions. Among other side effects occasionally observed are lactation in the non-pregnant woman and impotence in men. A serious drop in blood pressure occurs more frequently in the patient receiving reserpine than in the one receiving chlorpromazine. Reserpine also increases both the volume and acidity of gastric secretion and it is, therefore, contraindicated in patients with a known history of peptic ulcer. A rise of temperature occasionally occurs, as also does asthma. Clinical experience seems to show that, in general, the side effects of reserpine are less hazardous than those of chlorpromazine, yet deaths have occurred because of sudden and excessive drop of blood pressure.

CLINICAL USE AND SIDE EFFECTS. Although reserpine is of value in other disorders, its greatest use is in schizophrenia. In acute schizophrenia with ten-sion and anxiety or in milder chronic reactions, its use, as is true also of chlorpromazine, may shorten or prevent hospitalization. Perhaps one of its widest fields of use has been with the restless, combative, hostile, overactive, tense, and threatening patient. It has been extensively used also for the untidy, regressed patient who refuses to wear clothing and usually requires seclusion. The longer the patient has been ill, the less effective will be the treatment. The improvement in behavior in the overactive and aggressive patient is less marked than that observed following the use of chlorpromazine. There is usually an improvement in eating habits, toilet habits, and social participation. In some patients, the modified behavior following the administration of reserpine is maintained only as long as they are receiving the drug. In other cases, there is a prolonged improvement.

Experience has shown that reserpine may have a sedative effect in the irritable, quarrelsome, demanding, and hostile senile patient. Treatment may be begun with 0.5 mg. after each meal and 1.5 mg. at bedtime, given in tablet form. This may be increased every third day up to a maximum of 40 mg. a day if the patient does not become somnolent. As improvement occurs, the dosage may be reduced to a maintenance amount of 6 to 10 mg. daily by mouth. It is believed that the use of reserpine will enable many ambulant senile patients who would otherwise require institutional supervision to remain in the care of their families.

Both reserpine and chlorpromazine may exert a highly desirable sedative effect on the over-active, brain-injured child. It also often relieves the anxiety, fear, and restlessness frequently seen in the chronic asthmatic.

Reserpine may aggravate depressions and, in fact, has produced depression eventuating in suicide in the hypertensive patient. Such depressions are occasionally of such a severity that electroshock therapy is required for their relief.

There have been a few reports indicating that a combination of reserpine or chlorpromazine with electroconvulsive therapy may be dangerous.

Combined Use of Reserpine and Chlorpromazine

Because of the observation that chlorpromazine potentiated the effects of hypnotics and sedatives, the effect of combining reserpine and chlorpromazine was investigated. Consequently, it was found that the combined use of the drugs is sometimes more effective in chronically disturbed patients than is either drug alone.

Although the dosage scheduled in combined reserpine–chlorpromazine therapy may be varied, particularly with reference to the degree of the patient's disturbance, the following is recommended for the patient who is moderately disturbed. The patient is started on 3 mg. of reserpine and 25 mg. of chlorpromazine once a day. After 10 days, the chlorpromazine is increased to 25 mg. twice a day. At the end of three weeks, if the patient is not showing satisfactory progress, the amount of chlorpromazine is increased to 50 mg. twice a day, the dose of reserpine remaining at 3 mg. daily. If, after another three to four weeks, the patient is not improving satisfactorily, 5 mg. of reserpine given by intramuscular injection should be added daily for 10 days. If the patient still does not improve, the intramuscular dose may be increased to 10 mg. and continued until maximum results have been secured, when the intramuscular injections are gradually withdrawn but oral medication is continued indefinitely. In many patients receiving combined therapy, it is not necessary to add intramuscular injections of reserpine.

Patients receiving reserpine alone do not develop jaundice or agranulocytosis, but those receiving combined reserpine–chlorpromazine therapy may develop either of these toxic reactions.

Both chlorpromazine and reserpine have been used widely and, many believe, too indiscriminately in private office and in clinic practice in the treatment of psychoneurotic patients. They are much less effective in these disorders than in the active, grossly psychotic patient. Both drugs, if accompanied by psychotherapy, may be helpful in treating the early schizophrenic patient, and they also may make psychotherapy easier in anxiety reactions. They usually have little value in the treatment of obsessive–compulsive neuroses. Chlorpromazine sometimes seems to be helpful in phobic reactions, and patients with psychosomatic disorders accompanied by tension are often made more comfortable by these tranquilizing drugs. Sometimes in office or clinic practice the patient may be so alarmed by a feeling of strangeness and even of depersonalization that these drugs must be discontinued.

ANTIDEPRESSANT AGENTS

Following the observation of the mood-elevating capacity of iproniazid, a pharmacologic agent that suppresses the action of the enzyme monoamine oxidase, various other agents have been discovered with similar clinical effects and less toxic properties. Now widely used in the treatment of the various depressive reactions, these drugs have been designated by Delay as "psychoanaleptics." They are to be distinguished from the stimulants, such as the amphetamines, following the use of which mood elevation is transient and anorexic effects are common.

Those biological processes are unknown that modify the depressive affect and lead, probably secondarily, to relief of psychomotor retardation. One explanation proposed for the pharmacologic action of the antidepressants is the elevation of the cerebral amines, such as serotonin, norepinephrine, and others, due to suppression of the action of the enzyme monoamine oxidase. Although the inhibition of this enzyme has been found to correlate well with the antidepressant effect on clinical trial and thus to provide a means of selecting various newly produced hydrazines, other antidepressant agents, such as imipramine, do not have the property of inhibition of monoamine oxidase. Attempts to relate clinical antidepressant activity to stimulation or suppression of the reticular activating system also have failed to identify specific drug actions. Thus imipramine inhibits this system, while iproniazid leads to increased cortical electrical activity.

The antidepressant agents have proved useful in the treatment of manic–depressive reactions and are prescribed now as the initial form of therapy for the majority of patients suffering a depressive reaction. When delay in relief may be tolerated for several weeks and when suicidal drive is low, the antidepressants are preferable to electroshock therapy with its impairment of memory function, its other complications, and the greater demand for special equipment and nursing care.

Clinical trials have established as the preferred agents: the iminodibenzyl derivatives, imipramine (Tofranil) and amitryptyline (Elavil); the hydrazine monoamine oxidase inhibitors, isocarboxazide (Marplan), nialamide (Niamid), and phenelzine (Nardil). Unfortunately, good information is lacking to indicate the precise indications and the relative effectiveness of these agents. Although other antidepressants are on trial, they are excluded from consideration here, as neither their usefulness nor toxic effects are well defined.

Imipramine

Closely related to the phenothiazines, this drug, distributed under the name of Tofranil, was introduced for clinical use by Kuhn in 1957. It is similar to promazine, but a two-carbon chain replaces the sulfur in the latter.

PHYSIOLOGICAL EFFECTS. Imipramine reduces susceptibility to convulsions induced either by electroshock or metrazol. It depresses the action of the reticular formation and evokes on the electroencephalogram a sleep brain-wave pattern. Although it inhibits the lowering of brain serotonin by reserpine, it does not counteract the sedative action of that agent. It has anticholinergic effects and thus atropine-like side effects. Unlike chlorpromazine, it does not modify the conditioned escape–avoidance response in animals.

The oral route is preferred in the administration of the drug, although it may be given by intramuscular injection. The usual initial dosage range is 25 mg. given three or four times daily, the amount being increased to a total of 200 to 300 mg. within several days.

INDICATIONS. Imipramine has been more effective in the manic–depressive reactions, particularly those with retarded depression, than in other conditions. With the agitated depressions, it has not been effective, even when combined with the phenothiazines. Depressive reactions with organic brain syndromes have responded well, but its usefulness is limited with the neurotic depressive reactions and hypochondriacal states. In some patients with chronic pain, recurrent psychosomatic, and neurotic states, it has also been reported to be useful. Some of the apathetic patients with schizophrenia and catatonia have been mobilized with the drug, but, in general, it has not proved of value in the treatment of these reactions. Some physicians believe it is contraindicated.

The change in mood and behavior seldom become noticeable within the first week of administration, and maximum benefit accrues usually after two or three weeks of medication. Evidence of favorable response is shown with the patient first becoming less self-deprecatory and self-accusing and with reduction in his hypochondriacal complaints. Later there follow increased activity and socialization and improvement in general somatic functioning, including sleep.

Imipramine must be continued on a maintenance level after clinical improvement has taken place as symptoms recur with its withdrawal. Many recommend that the drug administration be continued three to six months following satisfactory change in affect. The drug should be gradually withdrawn.

UNTOWARD EFFECTS. The majority of

the side effects are minor, although they may impede acceptance of the drug by the patient. Dryness of the mouth is experienced by almost all who receive the drug and difficulties in accomodation in many. Perspiration is common, particularly about the head and neck, and by some it is thought to occur particularly in those who respond favorably. With it may occur flushing of the face. Dizziness, tachycardia, and postural hypotension are seen in the elderly and hypersensitive; thus the drug must be used with caution in patients with cardiovascular illness. With large doses, tremors may be induced. Impairment of urination has been observed. Photosensitivity occurs less frequently as a complication than it does with the use of the phenothiazines.

Insomnia is often noticed when the drug is first given. Hypomanic states have frequently followed its administration and require both its withdrawal and the use of a phenothiazine. Some patients suffer burning paresthesias in the forearms and hands and substernally. Rarely inco-ordination and convulsive attacks have been reported.

Although eosinophilia is common, leukopenia occurs much less frequently, and only a few instances of agranulocytosis have been seen.

Amitriptyline

Marketed as Elavil, this drug has similar actions, indications, and side effects as imipramine. The dosage range is 75 to 300 mg. daily, given by mouth. Knowledge of actions and toxicity now are less extensive than with imipramine. There is some evidence that its untoward actions are less than those of the latter drug.

MONOAMINE OXIDASE INHIBITORS

The capacity for iproniazid to produce euphoria in some persons was observed during its early usage in the treatment of pulmonary tuberculosis. It was found that the hydrazine iproniazid (Marsilid) had the property of preventing the breakdown of serotonin and epinephrine in the brain on administration of reserpine through its capacity to inhibit the enzyme, monoamine oxidase. Thus the cerebral levels of these amines rise. As mentioned elsewhere, it remains uncertain whether this biochemical process may be directly correlated with the action of these hydrazine agents to act as antidepressants.

These agents potentiate the effects of many other drugs. Thus the amphetamines may prove excessively stimulating when given to patients who are taking iproniazid. They also potentiate the sedative–hypnotic actions of alcohol and the barbiturates. All are characterized by latent periods extending from days to weeks before relief of depression is discernible. They share in common the side effects of hypotension expressed in dizziness, vertigo, and fainting. In the elderly, vascular collapse may occur when the patient is on high dosage. Constipation, vesical atony, peripheral edema, and such anticholinergic effects as dry mouth and blurred vision are seen. With central nervous activation there may occur hyperreflexia, tremors, insomnia, and restlessness. All may induce hypomanic episodes in the depressed individual when administered over time in high doses.

The agents described here are those now in general clinical usage and with limited toxicity in the prescribed effective dosage range.

Isocarboxide

Sold as Marplan, this drug is given by mouth in a dosage range of 10–30 mg. daily. It may induce hepatitis, blood dyscrasias, and skin disorders. It is as effective as iproniazid (Marsilid) but is regarded as less toxic than the latter, which has now been withdrawn due to the large number of cases of toxic hepatitis apparently induced by its usage.

Phenelzine

Known commercially as Nardil, this drug is usually administered in the dosage range of 40–60 mg. daily. It is considered by many clinicians to be as effective as iproniazid and more so than nialamide and is said to cause fewer hypotensive symptoms than other monoamine inhibitors. Cases of liver toxicity have not been reported.

Nialamide

Known commercially as Niamid, this drug is prescribed in the dosage range of 75 to 450 mg. daily. Generally clinicians have found it less effective as an antidepressant in severe states than other compounds in this group. It may produce toxic hepatitis but seems less likely to induce hypomanic episodes.

OTHER AGENTS

Meprobamate

Meprobramate, 2-methyl-2-propyl-l,3-propanediol dicarbamate, commercially sold as Miltown or Equanil in the United States, is known to synchronize selectively interneuronal electrical activity in the thalamic nuclei and to act as an anticonvulsant and muscle relaxant. It is said, in contrast to the previously described drugs, not to affect activity of the autonomic nervous system.

It is reported to be of value in anxiety and tension states, phobias, tension headaches, psychosomatic disorders, insomnia, premenstrual tension, and neurodermatitis. It often produces relief of headaches that are the result of constant, almost unremitting contraction of the posterior muscles of the neck.

Continued ingestion of large doses of meprobamate can create physical dependence, manifested on abrupt withdrawal of the drug by hyperirritability of the central nervous system and convulsions. The type of addiction caused by meprobamate resembles that caused by chronic intoxication with excessive amounts of barbiturates or alcohol. Especial care should be exercised in prescribing meprobamate for alcoholics or narcotic drug addicts.

A wide variety of side effects and untoward reactions has been reported. Among them have been dermal hypersensitivity reactions and acute nonthrombocytopenic purpura. Large doses taken with suicidal intent may produce complete respiratory and vasomotor collapse. The drug is not as effective in the treatment of the psychoses in the seriously disturbed as the phenothiazine derivatives.

It is available in tablets of 400 mg., which may be prescribed three to four times daily. Blood and urinary changes and local disturbances have not followed its prescription. In a few persons, allergic reactions have been noted with urticaria, erythematous rashes, and rarely fainting spells and bronchial spasm.

Chlordiazepoxide

This agent, marketed as Librium, has tranquilizing properties similar to those of the phenothiazines and reserpine. It is a muscle relaxant and anticonvulsant but exerts no autonomic blocking action. It produces stimulation of appetite and, in large doses, lowering of blood pressure and bradycardia. It affects the electroencephalogram as do the barbiturates.

In the clinic it has been used for relief of anxiety and tension in a wide range of psychiatric and medical conditions. Prescribed in 10-mg. capsules, the drug is given in a usual dosage range of 20 to 80 mg. daily. Common side effects are drowsiness and limitation of spontaneity, with impaired concentration. Ataxia, dysarthria, hyperactivity, and headache have been observed as well as some acute overactive behavioral disturbances.

BIBLIOGRAPHY

Brooks, G. W.: Withdrawal from neuroleptic drugs. Am. J. Psychiat., *115*:931–932, 1959.

Cole, J. O.: Progress in Drug Therapy. In Spiegel, E. A. (Ed.): Neurology and Psychiatry. New York, Grune & Stratton, 1959.

Forrest, I. S., Forrest, F. M., and Mason, A. S.: A rapid urine color test for imipramine. Am. J. Psychiat., *116*:1021–1022, 1960.

Idem: Review of rapid urine tests for phenothiazine and related drugs. Am. J. Psychiat., *118*: 300–307, 1961.

Freyhan, F. A.: The modern treatment of depressive disorders. Am. J. Psychiat., *116*:1057–1064, 1960.

Himwich, H. E.: Psychopharmacologic Drugs. Science, *127*:59–72, 1958.

Kalinowsky, L. B., and Hoch, P. H.: Somatic Treatments in Psychiatry. New York, Grune & Stratton, 1961.

Lasagna, L., and de Kornfeld, T. J.: Methotrimeprazine. J.A.M.A., *178*:887–890, 1961.

Norris, A. S., and Clancy, J.: Hospitalized depressions; drugs or electrotherapy? Arch. Gen. Psychiat., *5*:276–279, 1961.

Smith, J. K.: Spinal fluid changes during chlorpromazine therapy. Am. J. Psychiat., *115*:167–168, 1958.

Stein, L., and Seifter, J.: Possible mode of antidepressive action of imipramine. Science, *134*: 286–287, 1961.

Wilkens, B., and Malitz, S.: Some problems of dose variation in the use of tranquilizing drugs. Am. J. Psychiat., *117*:23–29, 1960.

Chapter Thirty-four

SHOCK AND OTHER PHYSICAL THERAPIES

The employment of the so-called shock therapies dates from 1933 when Manfred Sakel, then working in the Clinic of the University of Vienna, reported that deep hypoglycemic states produced by large doses of insulin produced a beneficial effect on the course of schizophrenia. With the subsequent introduction of other forms of shock therapy, attempts were made to establish a common denominator of action in them all. Not yet, however, has a theory been presented that satisfactorily explains the therapeutic action in any one of the forms of shock therapy, much less one that applies to all forms. There is now available a number of important follow-up studies that describe and delineate the nature of the therapeutic effect of these procedures over long periods of time, a necessity for the understanding of any treatment offered in the field of psychiatric therapy.

ELECTRIC CONVULSIVE THERAPY

In 1938 Cerletti and Bini described a method of producing convulsions by electricity and began its use in the treatment of schizophrenia.

The apparatus operates on 110-volt, 60-cycle, alternating current and contains mainly a variable transformer, ohm, volt, and ampere meters, and an automatic timer. The combined voltage and time settings constitute the "dose." Applications may range from 70 to 130 volts continuing from 0.1 to 0.5 second. Usually one starts with 80 volts for 0.2 second. If this fails to produce a convulsion, the voltage may be increased to 90 or 100 volts and the period of application increased. If this does not result in a seizure, no further application should be made until the following day. Only generalized seizures are productive of desired results. The operator will find that the dose must be determined by the convulsive threshold of the individual patient. This threshold is higher in female than in male patients, and higher in middle-aged than in younger persons. The threshold is raised after the first seizure.

The patient becomes unconscious immediately after the current is applied, even if no seizure follows. He will have no memory of a "shock." The convulsion conforms closely to those of spontaneous origin, with a tonic phase continuing for approximately 10 seconds followed by a

538

clonic phase of somewhat longer duration. The convulsion is accompanied by apnea.

Technique and Responses

In addition to the usual physical examination, including blood pressure, before the patient receives electric convulsive therapy, a roentgenogram should be made of the chest and of the lateral aspect of the spine; there should also be an electrocardiogram. An electroencephalogram is recommended. If the patient is to be treated in the morning, he receives either no breakfast or a glass of fruit juice and one slice of toast two hours before treatment. The patient should void, and dentures should be removed before treatment. If the patient suffers from nausea following the seizure, he may be given 50 mg. of Dramamine prior to the next treatment. He may receive the treatment either on a well-padded table or on a bed, the springs of which are supported by a board between spring and mattress. Compression fractures of vertebrae are occasional complications. Formerly it was believed that their frequency would be reduced if the spine were slightly overextended either by placing a firm pillow under the small of the back or by placing the patient on a Gatch bed during the treatment. This overextension is no longer generally recommended.

The patient is placed in a comfortable dorsal position, or the spine may be slightly flexed. The shoulders and arms are held lightly by a nurse to prevent extreme movements of the latter. Usually a restraint sheet is sufficient for the thighs, but if they are held, the control should not be too rigid lest fractures of an acetabulum or of a femur result. A padded tongue depressor or other resilient mouth gag is placed between the teeth to prevent biting the tongue or other injury. The assistant who holds the mouth gag in place holds the patient's chin firmly upon the gag so that the jaw cannot open too far and become dislocated. Electrode paste is rubbed into the skin on both sides of the forehead, and the electrodes, previously soaked in saturated salt solution, are applied to the prepared areas. The apparatus button is pressed and the patient becomes instantly unconscious. Following the clonic phase, there is a phase of muscular relaxation with stertorous respiration. It is well to roll the patient on his side to prevent inhalation of saliva. The patient remains unconscious for about five minutes, then slowly rouses during the next five to ten minutes.

After the treatment there is a period of confusion, during which the patient should be watched lest he fall out of bed. He should usually be permitted to lie for one-half to one hour after treatment. If left undisturbed, he may sleep an hour or more. In most cases there is no postconvulsive excited state, but a patient who is subject to this disturbance should receive 3 ¾ grains of sodium amytal intravenously just prior to application of the electricity.

There is insufficient evidence to show that unidirectional or brief stimuli techniques or the use of other types of currents or variant methods of application are superior to the ordinary form of treatment just described.

Frequency

Treatments are usually given three times a week. The period for which treatment should be continued depends largely upon the results obtained and upon the nature of the disorder treated. In depressive reactions, the patient may have received the maximum benefit after five to ten treatments. In disorders in which the patient is slowly but definitely improving, treatment may continue to 25 or 30 applications followed, if desirable, by maintenance treatments. Two treatments per day may be given for two or three successive days in the case of acutely disturbed patients who are threatened by psychotic exhaustion.

Indications

The greatest usefulness of electroconvulsive therapy is in depression. Its most frequent use, therefore, is in the treatment of involutional melancholia and of the depressive phase of manic–depressive psychosis. In case depression is an associated symptom in other disorders, this form of therapy may be followed by beneficial results. It is frequently used as a substitute for insulin shock therapy in acute and subacute schizophrenia reactions. Its use as a "maintenance" treatment in chronically disturbed schizophrenics and in the manic phase of manic–depressive psychosis are discussed in another section.

Contraindications

As experience with electroconvulsive shock therapy has increased, conditions regarded as contraindications have decreased. *Age*, in itself, is not considered a contraindication. The aged patient should, of course, be very carefully examined for physical abnormalities. Although the condition of the *cardiovascular system* should be carefully evaluated before electric convulsive therapy is given, the strain of the convulsion on that system has probably been exaggerated. Hypertension, abnormal electrocardiograms, or a history of angina pectoris or of coronary thrombosis are not in themselves contraindications to treatment if the patient has a good cardiac reserve.

Cardiac decompensation usually debars electroconvulsive therapy. The presence of aortic aneurysm also excludes the use of this treatment. If hypertension is largely caused by emotional factors, it need not be a cause for rejection of treatment but, on the contrary, may be an indication for its use. Vascular accidents as a result of electroconvulsive therapy are exceedingly rare. The use of electric convulsive therapy in the presence of myocardial disease depends upon its seriousness and the urgency of the need for treatment. If agitation is producing a constant strain on the heart, convulsive treatment may be used.

Generally speaking, *tuberculosis*, if there is a history of recent hemorrhage or evidence of high activity, excludes treatment, but the patient who is a feeding problem is often benefited through the resulting gain of weight. Latent tuberculosis is rarely activated. Except for recent fractures, *bone disease* is not a frequent contraindication to treatment. *Pregnancy* is not usually considered a contraindication. Electric shock is a safer form of therapy than insulin in the psychoses of pregnancy.

Complications

IMPAIRMENT OF MEMORY. Scarcely to be called a complication is the almost constant impairment of memory that accompanies electroconvulsive therapy. It may vary from a mild tendency to forget names to a severe confusion of the Korsakoff type. At first it tends to cover a long period prior to treatment, then gradually to diminish to events immediately before treatment. It is often distressing to the patient and may continue to some degree for several weeks or a few months following the termination of treatment. Full return of memory finally occurs. Psychological investigations indicate that electric convulsive therapy is not followed by any intellectual impairment.

FRACTURES AND DISLOCATIONS. The most frequent complications in electroconvulsive therapy are fractures and dislocations caused by muscular contraction. The fracture occurring most often is a *compression fracture of vertebrae*, in the dorsal area between the second and eighth, usually the third, fourth, or fifth vertebrae. Approximately 20 per cent of the patients suffer this injury, which occurs twice as frequently among men as among women. Apparently a majority of the fractures occur early in the course of treatment. They are not of major clinical importance and do not require special treatment. Many are found only on roentgenologic examination. Back pain may persist for a few days or weeks. Fractures of the femur, of the acetabulum, and of the neck of the humerus may occur. Dislocation of the jaw is frequent unless pressure is applied to prevent the opening of the mouth at the onset of the tonic phase.

APNEA. Apnea occurs physiologically in any general convulsive seizure, but in electroconvulsive therapy the respiratory arrest may be disturbingly prolonged. Some therapists use artificial respiration immediately after the convulsion as a safety measure. If apnea persists, artificial respiration should be continued. A metal airway should be available to prevent the tongue from falling back and to lead air through accumulations of saliva and mucus. Deaths as a result of electroconvulsive therapy are exceedingly uncommon.

"Softening" of Seizures

In order to avoid fractures or dislocations and to diminish the risk in elderly or infirm patients, convulsions may be modified by means of curare and other drugs. Curare inhibits the action of acetylcholine at neuromuscular junctions and softens the muscular contractions.

In recent years succinylcholine dichloride (Anectine) has largely supplanted curare preparations as a muscle relaxant because of less risk of respiratory paralysis attending its use. From 10 to 40 mg. of succinylcholine dichloride may be mixed in the same syringe with 0.8 mg. of atropine and 2 ml. of pentothal. At the end of the convulsion, oxygen under positive pressure is administered until the patient breathes spontaneously.

In approximately one in a thousand patients, prolonged apnea may occur after the use of succinylcholine. It has been suggested that those sensitive to this drug and its diethyl derivative, suxethonium, have inherited a less active variant of the enzyme pseudocholinesterase so that the drug action persists an undue length of time.

Usually a period of controlled respiration will terminate the apnea. Coramine (1 to 2.5 gm. in 4 to 10 ml.) may be given intravenously to counteract excessive barbiturate. If apnea persists for a half hour, edrophonium (Tensilon) should then be tried, and if this is unsuccessful, neostigmine (1.0 to 1.5 mg.) preceded by atropine (0.4 to 0.6 mg.) should be administered.

Results of Treatment

In the depressions of involutional melancholia and of manic–depressive psychosis, the improvement following electroconvulsive shock therapy is striking. In 80 per cent or more of these disorders, five to ten treatments are followed by full or social recovery. Prior to the treatment of involutional melancholia by electric shock therapy, protracted depression, sometimes lasting for years, was the rule. Early treatment of this disorder and of the depressions of manic–depressive psychosis by shock therapy will save many patients who would otherwise commit suicide.

Electroconvulsive shock therapy has no influence on the recurrence of manic–depressive episodes. Guilt and self-punishing, and self-accusatory trends are usually rapidly alleviated. In less than half of the cases of the paranoid type of involutional psychosis is treatment followed by much improvement, even though the maximum number of convulsions is induced. Senile depressions are usually relieved unless arteriosclerotic or senile brain changes have been important determinants.

The results of treatment of the manic phase of manic–depressive psychosis are less favorable than of the depressive phase but have been greatly improved by the practice of giving treatments more frequently. Best results are secured by giving two treatments a day for the first two or three days. These are usually followed by much confusion, but as this clears, the patient is found to be definitely improved.

The effectiveness of electroconvulsive treatment of schizophrenia has been the subject of much discussion. It is generally agreed that this form of treatment is beneficial in a large percentage of schizophrenics with affective features. It is also helpful in hastening a remission in early, acute forms of the disorder. It is of little value in hebephrenia or when the onset has been of a prolonged, insidious nature. The best results are secured in catatonic excitement. As with other shock therapies, this treatment is not followed by material improvement in the chronic, disorganized schizophrenic.

Electroconvulsive therapy is of little value in the treatment of psychoneuroses except in those manifesting depressive features and perhaps the anxiety states associated with gross stress reaction.

Ambulatory Treatment

For several years after the introduction of electroconvulsive therapy, it was considered essential that its application be limited to patients resident in a hospital. In more recent years there has been considerable relaxation in this practice. Whether, however, electric convulsive treatments are administered to patients continuously confined to a hospital or to those who are not hospitalized, they should be given only by a qualified psychiatrist well trained in the technique. Many patients, particularly those suffering from mild depressions, continue to reside at their homes but periodically visit a psychiatric or a general hospital to receive shock treatments. Later in the treatment day, after consciousness has become fully clear, the patient returns to his home. The degree of knowledge, understanding, and responsibility of relatives, and their ability to exercise constant supervision of the patient in his home, must be carefully determined. If treatment is undertaken in a general hospital or in a private office, provisions for dealing with postconvulsive confusion and excitement or with respiratory or other complications must be made. The patient should remain in the hospital or in the physician's office until there is no longer any danger of undesirable after effects. He should never be permitted to return home unaccompanied, and there should be reliable and instructed persons there to supervise him during the entire course of treatment. Some psychiatrists doubt the advisability of the use of electroshock on an ambulatory basis except in an out-patient clinic connected with a psychiatric hospital.

Mode of Action

The use of electroconvulsive shock is entirely empirical. Many theories, both psychogenic and physiogenic, have been suggested as explanations for its therapeutic action, but no one has offered a satisfactory explanation for the results obtained either by electroconvulsive or by insulin therapy. Some investigators suggest that cerebral anoxia, a result common to all the shock therapies, may somehow be the basis for the mental improvement. In both hypoglycemic and convulsive shock therapies, the brain is deprived by energy and oxidative metabolism to a degree that renders it inadequate to support cerebral function. The mechanisms producing these conditions are different, however. With hypoglycemia the brain is deprived of glucose and the cerebral metabolic rate is depressed. With electroshock, brain activity is raised to such a high pitch that cerebral function cannot be sustained by the oxygen and glucose coming to the brain in the blood.

INHALANT CONVULSIVE TREATMENT

Clinical trials have demonstrated that hexafluorodiethyl ether (Indoklon) given by a simple inhalation technique in doses of 4 to 6 ml. containing 0.05 of the agent per milliliter of solution is capable of inducing immediate convulsive responses.

This convulsant may be used as effectively as electroshock therapy for the same therapeutic purposes and is accepted more readily by some patients. Thus it may serve as an alternative procedure to electroshock treatment.

INSULIN SHOCK TREATMENT

In 1928 Sakel, believing that the nervous hyperactivity occurring in morphine addicts during withdrawal of that drug was caused by an excess of epinephrine, expressed the opinion that the excitement might be relieved by large doses of insulin. Later the similarity of the abstinence symptoms to other excited states suggested to Sakel that the latter also might be influenced by the same drug. He accordingly administered insulin to excited schizophrenic patients. After a period of experimental clinical work, he published his results in 1933. The basic features in the method developed by Sakel are still regarded as most effective. At first Sakel tried to avoid the development of deep hypoglycemic states but soon observed that better results occurred if coma was induced. He then increased the dose with the avowed intention of producing insulin shock.

Neurophysiology

Unlike other organs which can utilize carbohydrates, proteins, and fats for energy requirements, the brain is able to oxidize carbohydrates only. Since the rate of oxidation of carbohydrates is determined by the amount of insulin in the blood stream, the injection of a large amount of insulin into the body greatly reduces the sugar content of the blood. With a decrease in the amount of sugar available, the oxidative processes of the brain are so reduced that the effects are similar to anoxia of that organ, a condition known to lead to coma. The loss of consciousness in hypoglycemia is presumably caused by the fact that the brain cells are deprived of glucose, their principal fuel, without which the metabolic processes in the brain are progressively depressed.

According to the segmental-suprasegmental concept of evolutionary development of the central nervous system, there are ascending levels of integration both of structure and function. We may therefore think of successively higher levels, beginning with the lower medulla and culminating with the cerebral hemispheres. It has been shown that the rate of metabolism in each of the higher levels is greater than in that of the level immediately lower or older. The greatest susceptibility to low blood sugar exists, therefore, in the more complex and phylogenetically more recent areas of the forebrain. With the injection of large amounts of insulin, therefore, there is a step-like depression of function and there appear progressive neurological signs and symptoms corresponding to a phyletic regression or functional disturbance in the successively lower anatomical levels of cerebral cortex, diencephalon, midbrain, upper medulla, and lower medulla. There is a progressive dissolution of the functions of the brain, a dissolution that seems to turn back that organ through the path of evolution. As the blood sugar falls following the injection of a "coma dose" of insulin, various deficiency and release phenomena linked with functional patterns of different levels of the neuraxis become manifest in the signs and symptoms that characterize the successive stages of insulin coma. The symptoms and signs are listed in the table on page 545. The therapist must remember that the signs in Stage V are largely those of functional impairment of the cardiac, circulatory, and respiratory centers and therefore those of approaching danger.

All patients manifest in a general way the functional groups of signs listed in the table indicated. Each patient, however, presents an individual response, and there is often much overlapping of the stages. It is not uncommon, in fact, to see signs of various stages (such as II and IV) occurring simultaneously. This phenomenon is sometimes referred to as "irregular descent" and would seem to indicate that there is a variable resistance to hypoglycemia in various parts of the brain.

Preparation for Treatment

Although insulin shock therapy is a relatively safe procedure in the hands of a skilled therapist, most serious complications may occur with patients in whom an organic pathologic condition has been overlooked. In addition to careful and complete psychiatric, physical, and neurological examinations, such laboratory examinations should be made as will exclude the possibility of undertaking the treatment of a bad risk. It is generally agreed that there should be roentgenologic studies of the chest and of the lateral thoracic spine, a serological examination, urinalysis, blood count, and a determination of the fasting blood sugar. An electrocardiogram, especially in older patients, is highly desirable, even though the clinical examination is negative. It is advisable to discuss results and dangers with a responsible relative, also to secure written permission for treatment.

Contraindications to Treatment

The presence of any organic disease must be individually evaluated and its seriousness weighed against the urgency for treatment. The following disorders, however, are usually considered as contraindications: (1) any active infection, or any chronic or subacute infection that may be "lighted up" by treatment; (2) serious heart, liver, or kidney disease; (3) diabetes or other endocrine disorder; (4) skeletal pathology; (5) lack of adequate superficial veins; or (6) age under 16 or over 45 years. Some therapists, however, have successfully treated patients who were pregnant or had epilepsy, myxedema, or allergy.

Technique of Treatment

The patient usually receives his dose of insulin at about 7 a.m. while still fasting. He remains under vigilant nursing observation from the time the drug is given until after coma is terminated and consciousness fully regained. Because of the danger of "after-shock" or other complications, the patient should be under competent nursing supervision during the succeeding 24 hours. A physician trained and experienced in insulin therapy should watch him constantly from the time he becomes unconscious until consciousness is fully restored.

The original method of Sakel, still very widely followed, begins with the intramuscular injection of 15 to 25 units of insulin, which is increased by 10 to 15 units daily until the desired depth of coma is reached. This is usually not reached until the dosage is between 80 and 275 units and from 7 to 15 treatments have been given. After coma dose has been reached, the dosage may usually be reduced somewhat in the hope that

excessively deep reactions may be avoided, but it is adjusted daily for the remainder of the course of treatment. The dose of insulin required to produce coma is not related to the degree of hypoglycemia produced.

A technique in which rapidly increasing doses are administered was developed by Shurley and is often used. This method requires closer observation and greater skill than does the original Sakel technique but attempts to follow more closely what is known of the physiological principles of resistance and sensitivity to the drug. It seems, also, to have the advantage of shortening the induction phase, of producing a more rapid amelioration of symptoms, of reducing the amount of insulin required for the course of treatment, and of being safer for the patient. With this technique, the procedure begins with the administration to the fasting patient for five successive days of small doses of insulin increasingly graduated from 5 to 25 units. The purpose of this series of injections is to ascertain if the patient has a predisposition to allergic or hypoglycemic reactions. If there is no evidence of undue sensitivity, the course of treatment is begun.

The therapist seeks to produce the maximum physiological effect for the longest period of time permissible by the largest doses of insulin consistent with the patient's safety. Patients possess varying degrees of resistance to insulin. For that reason, the initial treatment dose does not exceed 50 units of U 100 ordinary insulin given by deep intramuscular injection. This dose is doubled each day until a clinical response is secured or a maximum dose of 1600 to 2200 units is reached. Some patients are extremely resistive to insulin. If in such cases coma does not occur within the dosage range stated, the maximum dose may be repeated for five or six days or the dose may be "zigzagged."

This procedure may be conducted in one of several ways. The most common method is first to give double the dose with which treatment was begun, the next day to give half the maximum dose,

HYPOGLYCEMIC SYMPTOMS

(Modified from Himwich)

STAGE	PSYCHOLOGICAL	MOTOR	SENSORY	AUTONOMIC

I
Depression of cerebral and cerebellar functions
	1. Gradually increasing clouding of consciousness with defects in:
	  a. orientation
	  b. attention
	  c. understanding
	  d. perception
	2. Wild excitement, with or without psychotic syndromes
	3. Sleep
		1. Muscular relaxation (hypotonia)
		2. Tremors
		  Imperfect voluntary acts (apraxia)
		4. Imperfect (incoherent) speech
			1. Visual disturbances	1. Parasympathetic overactivity
				  a. Watery sweat
				  b. Watery saliva
				  c. Bradycardia
				  d. Constricted pupil or
				2. Sympathetic overactivity
				  a. Viscid sweat
				  b. Viscid saliva
				  c. Tachycardia
				  d. Dilated pupil
				3. Vital signs vary within normal limits—temperature dropping

II
Release of sub-corticodien-cephalon
	1. Loss of environmental contact, i.e., coma	1. Stereotyped (primitive) movements
		  a. Involuntary grasping
		  b. Involuntary sucking
		  c. Protrusion of tongue
		  d. Kissing
		  e. Snarling
		  f. Grimacing
		2. Motor restlessness
		3. Choreiform, athetoid, and hemiballistic movements
		4. Fine myoclonic twitchings ——→clonic spasms——→ convulsions (release of subcortical motor nuclei)
			1. Increased sensitivity to external stimuli (release of the sensory thalamus)	1. Sympathetic overactivity in waves
				  a. Tachycardia
				  b. Dilated pupils (react to light)
				  c. Exophthalmos
				  d. Flushing
				  e. Viscid perspiration
				  f. Viscid salivation
				  g. Increased blood pressure and perspiration (release of hypothalamus)

III
Release of the midbrain
	1. Deep coma	1. Loss of primitive movements
		2. Increasing hypertonus
		3. Spasm
		  a. Tonic (flexion of upper extremities with extension of rest of body)
		  b. Torsion
		4. Dissociated eye movements
		5. Pathological pyramidal reflexes most easily elicited
			1. Decreased sensitivity to external stimuli	1. Parasympathetic signs, which are overcome periodically by sympathetic signs with each spasm (dilated pupils do not react to light)
				2. Paradoxical pupillary dilation and hippus
				3. Vital signs variable

IV Release of upper medulla	1. Deep coma	1. Recurrent extensor spasm in all extremities 2. Magnus and de Kleijn reflex	1. Loss of sensitivity	1. Sympathetic signs with each spasm (pupils dilate but do not react)

V
Release of lower medulla
	1. Deep coma	1. Muscular flaccidity
		2. Depressed reflexes
			1. Loss of all sensitivity
			2. Loss of corneal reflex
				1. Parasympathetic signs
				  a. Pallor
				  b. Pinpoint pupils (do not react)
				  c. Slow heart rate
				  d. Depressed respiration

and on the third day to repeat the maximum dose. If a patient does not respond to this routine, larger doses may be given or the route of administration may be changed to intravenous. When a clinical response is obtained, the rate of dose increase is reduced from a doubling of the amount to one of 10 to 20 per cent. When sensitization occurs as manifested by a deeper coma on the same or a smaller dose, by an earlier onset of coma, or by a somatic crisis or other complication, the dose is reduced rapidly (by halves) until one just sufficient to produce the desired depth of coma is reached. Thereafter the maintenance dose must be determined daily as indicated by the patient's response. The depth and duration of each coma will vary in accordance with the opinion and experience of the individual therapist.

Some physicians believe that Stage II is sufficiently deep to produce beneficial effects. Others insist on various combinations of Stages III, IV, or even V. Many allow a maximum of two hours of coma per day, reckoned from the time of loss of consciousness. The coma should be terminated when Stage V is reached or if some complication develops. It is generally agreed that 15 minutes of Stage V is the extreme limit of safety. Few therapists permit the patient to reach this depth of coma.

Termination of Coma

Hypoglycemic coma is terminated by giving an adequate amount of carbohydrates by one of three methods: orally, by gavage, or by intravenous administration. In emerging from the coma, the patient ordinarily re-traverses the phyletic stages through which he passed in developing coma. If he is able to drink, the patient is given eight ounces of a 50 per cent sugar solution. If he is unable to drink, the coma is terminated by tube-feeding or by glucose given intravenously. Each method has its proponents. Probably, however, a gavage of 500 ml. of a warm 50 per cent glucose solution is preferable, especially if the patient has had a convulsion, has been unco-operative upon waking, has inaccessible veins, or needs a reservoir of glucose during a prolonged coma. The intravenous method is always used in an emergency and routinely by many therapists.

When glucose is given intravenously, the patient receives from 20 to 50 ml. (sometimes more) of a $33\frac{1}{3}$ per cent solution. This method should be used also if the patient is not alert within 20 minutes after having received glucose by mouth. If he is suffering from simple hypoglycemia, he should respond to intravenous glucose within five minutes. If the coma is terminated intravenously, it is wise to give additional glucose by mouth lest there be a return of the hypoglycemic state. Following the termination of the coma, the patient should receive a substantial meal. It is important that he receive sodium chloride to replace that lost through perspiration.

Adjuncts to Treatment

Atropine sulfate (grains 1/150 to 1/75) is given routinely with the insulin dose and again before electroshock if that is used in conjunction with insulin therapy, to decrease vagotonia. Vitamins B_1 and C are given to supplement the deficiencies resulting from the intake of large quantities of vitamin-poor carbohydrates. Diphenylhydantoin sodium (Dilantin), $4\frac{1}{2}$ grains daily, may be given orally at the same time the patient receives insulin in order to prevent hypoglycemic convulsions. It should be gradually discontinued upon completion of the course of insulin therapy and should not be used if combined electric convulsive therapy is employed. Postural drainage and the insertion of gauze wicks should be used to prevent aspiration of the excessive amount of saliva. Care must also be exercised to prevent aspiration of vomited material. Airways, oxygen, and artificial respiration may aid in preventing serious complications.

Some therapists use potassium chloride prophylactically to correct electrolytic balance and to prevent prolonged comas. Its value is still undetermined. Hyaluronidase, in doses of 75 to 150 turbidity reducing units (T.R.U.) added to the insulin, has been found to be of value in reducing the amount of insulin required to produce coma, to increase the effective length of treatment levels, and to increase the number of therapeutically valuable reactions (comas). It is also said to diminish the frequency of aftershocks, as well as convulsions, restlessness, and exhaustion.

Duration of Treatment

Treatment is given five or six times a week for an average total course of 50 hours of coma. Although the number of treatment days may be somewhat smaller in acute cases and in those patients who have shown no benefit from treatment, the total number of hours should not be less than 30. More than 50 coma days are given by some therapists to patients who are continuing to show beneficial results. If a relapse takes place, it usually occurs within a month after discontinuance of treatment. The patient should therefore continue under observation for nearly that period of time.

Complications of Treatment

Since dangerous, and even fatal, complications may readily occur, it is essential that both physician and nurse possess sufficient experience and skill to enable them to recognize and deal immediately with emergency situations. Even though both possess these qualities, the mortality rate will be from 0.5 to 1 per cent.

PROLONGED COMA. Ordinarily there is a coincident termination of hypoglycemia and of coma following the administration of carbohydrates. Sometimes, however, the termination of hypoglycemia is not accompanied by a return to consciousness. If there is no evidence of returning consciousness within five minutes after intravenous administration of glucose or within 20 minutes after administration by gavage, one is confronted with a delayed awakening that may be the forerunner of prolonged or irreversible coma.

Treatment of delayed awakening consists of the intravenous administration of 100 ml. of 33⅓ per cent of glucose and 100 mg. of thiamine chloride. The latter stimulates the utilization of available glucose. If the patient has not already received intragastric glucose, he is given 500 ml. of warm 50 per cent glucose by gavage. If the patient does not respond within 15 minutes, it must be considered that prolonged coma exists. This is an emergency condition and accounts for over one-half of all deaths resulting from insulin coma. Persistent coma terminating in one to three hours is usually followed by complete recovery, but longer periods are dangerous.

Although not definitely proved, prolonged or irreversible coma is presumably caused by the nerve cells having become exhausted or otherwise irreversibly altered so that they are no longer able to utilize glucose, even though there is an ample supply present in the blood stream. In view of the marked diaphoresis that most patients manifest, there must be changes in water metabolism and also associated changes in electrolytic balance. The brain, following death from prolonged coma, shows either degenerative or hemorrhagic lesions to-

gether with cerebral edema. Even when prolonged coma is reversible, some patients are left with a permanent organic dementia. The hyperinsulism brings about a state of anoxia even in the presence of an abundance of oxygen. Histological examinations show that the cellular changes are identical with those alterations residual to severe degrees of cerebral anoxia in cases of carbon monoxide poisoning or mechanical strangulation.

If the patient is in Stage II or III and shows signs of cortical irritability, 50 ml. of 50 per cent sorbitol or sucrose are given intravenously as a dehydrating measure. If there is no response within 15 minutes, or if the patient is in deep coma (Stage IV or V), 50 ml. of doubly concentrated human plasma are given intravenously. If the patient shows motor excitement, he should be restrained. Narcotics and sedatives should be avoided. Oxygen by nasal catheter, even in the absence of cyanosis, is usually advisable. If the patient's temperature is over 103°F., he should receive alcohol sponges or an ice water enema. Circulation and respiration should be supported by Coramine, 2 to 5 ml., given intravenously every three to four hours until the patient awakes. Epinephrine and caffeine are not recommended.

If the patient has not responded within 30 minutes after having received plasma, the coma may continue for hours or days. Normal blood sugar level should be maintained by 10 per cent intravenous glucose drip. Blood sugar content should be checked every two to three hours. The administration of sucrose and of thiamine chloride should be repeated every two or three hours. Other measures previously described should be repeated as indicated. If treatment is begun again, it must be with a much smaller dose of insulin, since the patient will now be found to be very sensitive to the drug. In those who recover from prolonged coma, the episode is often followed by a dramatic improvement in the mental state.

A much less serious complication is the not infrequent and sometimes unavoidable secondary hypoglycemia or *"after-shock."* In this condition the patient has emerged from the coma in a normal manner but within 12 hours again develops signs and symptoms of hypoglycemia. It is usually prevented by giving an adequate amount of carbohydrates at the meal following emergence from coma, with interval nourishment during the afternoon and evening. It is readily controlled by the intravenous injection of 50 ml. of 33⅓ per cent solution of glucose. This may be followed by sweetened fruit juice and other carbohydrates if the patient can be encouraged to co-operate.

RESPIRATORY COMPLICATIONS. These are second in frequency as the cause of death in insulin therapy. A moderate degree of salivation is usual in insulin shock but may be so excessive that pneumonia may result from aspiration of saliva. It is therefore important that the patient's head be kept turned to the side during treatment and that secretions be aspirated or absorbed by a gauze wick. A lung abscess may follow regurgitation and aspiration of tube feeding by tube or by a poorly given gavage. If symptoms suspected to be due either to pneumonia or to abscess appear, the patient should receive antibiotics. Pulmonary edema is usually of cardiac origin and should be treated accordingly. Laryngospasm may be helped by atropine. Edema of the glottis may require tracheotomy. Hiccough, usually due to disturbing changes in the medulla, should be regarded as a dangerous symptom. Here, as in other complications, the patient should receive intravenous glucose.

CARDIOVASCULAR COMPLICATIONS. Such minor complications as tachycardia, bradycardia, or arrhythmias usually respond to glucose alone. More serious complications, such as myocardial failure, cardiac dilation, aortic insufficiency, or general vasomotor collapse, require intravenous glucose, Coramine, strophanthin, and the usual supportive measures.

CONVULSIONS. There are two types of convulsions, the early and the late. The former are of a grand mal type and usu-

ally occur in Stage II. These are not dangerous and are successfully controlled by intravenous injection of glucose and subsequent prophylactic use of anticonvulsants. Late convulsions occur in Stage IV and herald a critical condition for life. The late seizure is usually abortive or atypical, with apnea and cyanosis. If not followed immediately by death, it frequently eventuates in a prolonged or irreversible coma. The patient should receive intravenous glucose at once, also a similar injection of 2 to 4 ml. of Coramine. If there is respiratory embarrassment, oxygen and artificial respiration should be employed. After either type of convulsion, there should be a rest period of one to several days, following which the dosage of insulin should be reduced 10 to 20 per cent on again initiating treatment.

ALLERGIC REACTIONS. These may be either local or general. The former reaction is more common and is manifested by an itching, burning sensation at the point of injection, which becomes indurated and painful. The erythema and induration disappear after a few days of local treatment. The generalized allergic reaction is exhibited in the form of urticaria with much itching. It is relieved by an injection of epinephrine or other antihistaminic agents.

Results of Treatment

As already implied, the use of insulin shock therapy is limited to the treatment of schizophrenia. There is complete agreement among therapists that there is an inverse ratio between the duration of illness and the recovery rate. The best results are obtained with patients who have not been ill for more than one year. After an illness of two years, the percentage of recovery or of improvement falls rapidly. The highest recovery or remission rate is among patients in their twenties who previously had well integrated personalities, who have had a stormy onset of the illness, and have come to treatment within six months after its onset. Conversely, the results of treatment are poorer in the case of patients who have had limited personality resources, have long manifested schizoid traits, have had an insidious onset of their illness, and became overtly psychotic before 15 or after 40 years of age.

It is generally believed that patients showing tension or mixture of affective and of schizoid features have a more favorable outlook for recovery, also that patients who show a high resistance to insulin or fail to gain considerable weight during treatment do poorly. Much better results are secured with the paranoid and catatonic types of schizophrenia than with the simple and hebephrenic types, which respond very poorly.

There is admittedly a high rate of recurrence among schizophrenic patients treated with insulin therapy, but the remission or recovery rate for those who have been adequately treated with insulin is significantly higher than for a similar group of untreated patients. It has been said that over long periods of time recoveries are more stable in non-shock-treated patients than in those so treated. The use of insulin coma therapy is rapidly declining.

COMBINED INSULIN-CONVULSIVE THERAPY

Some psychiatrists prefer to combine insulin and convulsive therapies in the treatment of schizophrenia. The aim is to secure a summation of the therapeutic benefits of each procedure. Specific indications for the use of combined therapies are not precisely defined. However, these are commonly used: (1) when the patient fails to improve on either insulin coma therapy or electroshock therapy; (2) when the patient's improvement is unsatisfactory; (3) when he presents serious nursing problems, such as extremely overactive, unco-operative, assaultive, or regressive behavior, or suicidal tendencies; (4) if the patient is stuporous; or (5) if the patient shows definitely affective features.

METHOD. Various techniques are followed in the application of combined insulin-convulsive therapy. In the "block" method, the therapist gives short series (two to four treatments) of electroconvulsive therapy, widely spaced, throughout a course of insulin coma therapy. In the "alternating" method, electroconvulsive therapy is given on the days when no insulin shocks are given. In a "crossing" of the methods, a course of electroconvulsive therapy is given before or after a course of insulin therapy, or both. Commonly the most acute symptoms are relieved with electroconvulsive therapy prior to the use of insulin.

If indications for its use arise during a course of insulin therapy, convulsive treatment is added. It is considered advisable to defer the induction of convulsions until the patient is obtaining coma hours each day, since electroconvulsive therapy usually increases the insulin requirements and makes management difficult. It is therefore customary (except in the case of catatonic patients) for therapists to wait until the fifth or sixth week of an insulin shock course, or until a total of 15 to 30 hours of coma has been reached, before instituting both insulin and electric shock treatments. When the convulsive treatment is to be added, the patient receives 1/150 grains of atropine sulfate hypodermically, and the convulsion is induced 15 minutes later in Stage II of the insulin coma. At this point in the coma, the convulsive threshold is relatively low, muscular rigidity is not prominent, and the danger of fracture and of other complications is minimal. Despite the fact that at that time the dangers are greater and the response atypical, some therapists prefer to induce the convulsion during the deepest hypoglycemic coma in an attempt to intensify the therapeutic effects. The coma is terminated immediately following the convulsion by means of glucose given by vein, by stomach tube introduced before the convulsion, or by both routes. To continue the coma beyond this point places undue physical strain on the patient.

A course of electroconvulsive therapy during one of insulin shock is adapted to the needs of the individual patient and varies from one of a few treatments to one consisting of 20 to 25 treatments given three times a week. There is no evidence that risks are increased by combined treatment. It is a clinical impression that better results are secured in many cases by combined insulin-convulsive treatment, but such has not yet been statistically proved.

PSYCHOSURGERY

The operation of lobotomy, a surgical procedure consisting of a severance of the connection between the thalamus and frontal lobe, was developed by a Portuguese neurologist, Egas Moniz, and first performed by the neurosurgeon, Almeida Lima, in 1935. Moniz published his monograph in 1936, immediately following which the operation was introduced into United States by Dr. Walter Freeman and Dr. James Watts. In 1949 Moniz received the Nobel Prize in Medicine for his work in prefrontal lobotomy.

It is generally accepted that the dorsomedial nucleus of the thalamus is the physical substratum of emotion. It is known that fibers run from this nucleus to the frontal poles, and it is believed that the stimuli that pass along these radiations are concerned with the conscious experience of emotion. It is postulated that a cutting of these fibers so alters affective responses that tensions do not accumulate and that therefore regressive, reparative behavior is no longer necessary. Abundant experience has now shown that a severing of these fibers contributes greatly to the control of pathological emotional states. It is the aim of the neurosurgeon to sever the thalamofrontal radiation in such a manner that the emotional component of the neurosis or psychosis can be reduced to the point where the ideas no longer dominate the behavior of the patient, yet that the incisions leave sufficient quantities of the frontal lobes to permit the patient to retain the capacity for productive work and to make a satisfactory adaptation in a social environment. Following the section of the thalamocortical fibers, there is a retrograde degeneration of the dorsomedial nucleus.

Techniques

Several types of operation have been derived from the original prefrontal leukotomy developed by Moniz. One of the most widely used techniques is the modification developed by Freeman and Watts. This is a "blind" procedure performed through small lateral burr holes. The white matter in both frontal lobes is cut in the plane of the coronal suture. Unless the patient is disturbed, the operation is performed under local anesthesia. The burr holes are made in both sides of the skull at a point 6 cm. above the zygomatic process and 3 cm. behind the lateral rim of the orbit. A leukotome is introduced through the burr holes and section of the frontal white matter in both hemispheres is made. The cortex is not cut except in a small area for the introduction of the leukotome. The exact plane of the cortical incision is of great importance. If the incision is too far anteriorly, the results of the operation are negligible; if it is made too far posteriorly, apathy, inertia, and some degree of dementia may follow.

In order that he might operate with the advantage of clear vision, Lyerly, in 1947, devised an "open" procedure permitted by the use of an osteoplastic flap. By a superior approach, he separated the frontal lobe fibers, and by means of a lighted speculum, he worked under direct vision.

Another technique developed in 1948 by Scoville is known as *cortical undercutting*. In this operation, a line of cleavage is made at the junction of the gray and white matter in the prefrontal cortex, the underlying long association fibers thus being severed.

A few neurosurgeons have limited frontal lobe operations to a full sectioning of the white matter on either the right or the left side, but not on both.

In 1948 Pool, Mettler and a group of workers from Columbia University and from the New Jersey State Hospital at Greystone Park developed an operation called *"topectomy,"* consisting of the removal of symmetrical areas of the frontal cortex, especially of Brodmann's areas 9 and 10. In this study, an attempt was made to evaluate the ablation of various selected areas. Apparently the therapeutic results are not determined so much by the excision of any one specific area as by the amount of brain substance removed. Topectomy does not seem to be followed by the unpleasant personality changes often seen in prefrontal lobotomy. It is, however, followed more frequently by convulsions than are other operative procedures. For this reason the operation is now rarely employed.

Spiegel and Wycis conceived the idea of interrupting the frontothalamic connections not by cutting the radiations but by coagulating the dorsomedial nucleus of the thalamus. By elaborate technique they accurately locate this nucleus, in which they then produce a lesion by electrolysis or by electrocoagulation. This procedure is known as *thalamotomy*.

In 1937 Fiamberti of Vareze, Italy, developed a different technique for severing the thalamofrontal radiations. In 1946 Freeman introduced this technique into the United States where it has become extensively employed. In this operation, known as *transorbital lobotomy*, the frontal lobes are entered through the bony cavity above the eye and the thalamofrontal radiations severed just lateral to the anterior horn of the lateral ventricle. The superior part of these radiations is supposed to underlay areas 9 and 10 of Brodmann. The severance of the connections of these areas with the thalamus is, as in other forms of lobotomy, supposed to dissociate by surgical means the pathological thinking from its emotional reverberations and permit reorganization of more nearly normal patterns of cerebral activity. In carrying out the technique of transorbital lobotomy, a general anesthetic is not given. Anesthesia is secured by the administration of two electroshocks within one or two minutes of each other. The lobotomy is then performed while the patient is in the postconvulsive coma. A slender, sharply pointed instrument is inserted in the conjunctival sac and driven through the skull at a point opposite the pupil and 2 cm. posterior to the frontal sinus. The base of the frontal lobe is penetrated about 3 cm. lateral to the midline and 2 cm. behind the frontal pole. The total depth of penetration from the tip of the instrument to the edge of the upper eyelid is 7 cm. Connections of this part of the frontal lobe with the thalamus are severed on an arc of 30 degrees by moving the handle of the instrument laterally about 15 degrees and medially the same distance. When the handle of the instrument, the leukotome, is in the lateral position at the 7 cm. mark, a deep frontal cut is made. The handle of the leukotome is strongly elevated until the shaft lies as nearly parallel as possible to the orbital plate. From this position the handle is then returned to the parasagittal plane and withdrawn. Following the completion of the operation on one side, the patient receives a third electroshock treatment, or, if he becomes restless, a fourth shock before the operation is performed on the second side. There are no important structures such as vessels, nerves, or glands in the path of the instrument. No preparation of the operative field is necessary, since the conjunctival sac is normally sterile.

Advocates of transorbital lobotomy stress that complications are less frequent and mortality less than in other forms of psychosurgery. Among the advantages claimed are: (1) ease of performance; (2) economy of time; (3) minimal hospitalization and nursing care; (4) minimal expense to patient and institution; (5) the apparent fact that undesirable personality traits following operation are less frequent; and (6) postoperative hemorrhage and seizures are less frequent.

Although the operation of transorbital leukotomy appears to be relatively simple and does not require the accouterments of major neurological surgery, most neurosurgeons hesitate about the blind passing of an instrument through the orbit into the brain with the possibility of damage to paranasal sinuses, and without full neurosurgical facilities for dealing with complications that may arise.

In 1951 Greenblatt, Solomon, and Levine introduced what is known as the *bimedial* operation. This, too, is a bilateral prefrontal lobotomy carried out in the frontal or coronal plane. Instead, however, of all the white matter in both frontal lobes being cut, the bimedial operation is restricted to cutting only the medial half of the white matter in each frontal lobe. Reports suggest that this operation is followed by a greater relief of anxiety, tension, hostility, and disorganization than are the full bilateral or unilateral operations.

Acute Effects of Operation

Immediately after prefrontal lobotomy, the patient loses his nervous tension and may appear stuporous or confused for a few days to a week. He remains indifferent to his surroundings, pays no attention to excretory functions, has to be fed and moved about in bed, is somnolent, and may vomit. He may confabulate and deny that he has had an operation. A few patients are noisy and manifest a repetitious, destructive overactivity. In many instances the success of the operation depends upon the supervision the patient receives for several weeks following. He must be forced out of bed, taken to the toilet at regular intervals, and made to bathe, dress, and feed himself. An excessive appetite is common and may result in a great gain in weight. In even the simplest matters the patient should be specifically instructed and guided for a considerable time. It is usually desirable that the patient go home as soon as possible after the operation in order that the constant social pressure of the home may stimulate more adequate social behavior. It is highly important that the operation be followed by an active rehabilitation program, which should include retraining and re-educational measures and a system of graded privileges.

The chief complication of lobotomy is the development of convulsive seizures. These are usually of the gland mal type and can be controlled by anticonvulsive medication.

Indications

Prefrontal lobotomy is a radical procedure that will be undertaken only after other forms of treatment, including tranquilizing drugs and some form of shock therapy, have failed. Its use since the introduction of the tranquilizing drugs has greatly decreased. Patients are selected for operation on the basis of symptoms rather than of diagnosis. The best results are secured in patients who show tension, agitation and distress, depression, worry, emotional aggressiveness, hostility, and excited, impulsive behavior. Such symptoms as phobias, obsessions, hallucinations, and delusional experiences are relieved if they have not existed for extended periods, although the basic pathology of the thought process is not affected. Cruelty, avoidance of responsibility, and excessive use of alcohol before the development of the psychosis are contraindications.

In *schizophrenia* prefrontal lobotomy has no effect on the fundamental disease process, but in well selected cases may be followed by a great improvement in adjustment. The better organized the prepsychotic personality, the better the results, provided deteriorated, psychotic habits have not existed for several years. In general, lobotomy may be recommended after a two-year illness if the patient has, in the meantime, received active treatment with tranquilizing drugs, insulin, and electroconvulsive therapy without beneficial results. If the patient is a chronically deteriorated, inactive *hebephrenic* whose affect has been "burned out," little benefit is to be expected from operation. On the other hand, the behavior of the over-active, resistive, excitable, destructive, restless, unmanageable schizophrenic may be greatly improved. Such a patient may become quiet and somewhat sociable, and perhaps later he may be able to leave the hospital and even become self-sustaining. Not a few patients become free, cheerful, relaxed, interested in events of the day, and able to carry on a conversation on various topics. Sometimes activity may be so reduced that the patient sits about in a lethargic state.

Lobotomy is rarely undertaken in acute *manic–depressive* psychosis, since most cases yield either to electroconvulsive therapy or to tranquilizing drugs. It may be advisable in prolonged depressive states with tension that have not yielded to electric convulsive therapy. It has not usually been of value in chronic manic states. Since the recovery rate in *involutional melancholia* following convulsive therapy is high, lobotomy is rarely used in this disease. There are, however, some cases of rut depression and rumination on abnormal ideas, or cases with schizophrenic features that do not respond to convulsive therapy. In such cases and in the paranoid type of involutional psychosis lobotomy may be a beneficial procedure.

In severe obsessive-compulsive, obsessive-ruminative, and hypochondriacal types of *psychoneuroses* that have not been benefited by psychotherapy the disabling tension and anxiety states may be relieved by lobotomy. Obsessive ideas may continue, but the relief from tension may permit the patient to pursue his normal activities. In general, previous conflicts remain, but the quantity of emotional charge is reduced. Probably the best results in lobotomy are secured in agitated depressions and in severe obsessive–compulsive reactions accompanied by so much tension that the patient is incapacitated. One should, however, be conservative in recommending lobotomy for the treatment of psychoneuroses.

The success of prefrontal lobotomy in controlling emotional disturbance and overactivity arising from it as seen in some chronic manic and schizophrenic states suggested that the operation might be of benefit in the treatment of severe behavior disorders following acquired brain disease or in pathological personalities. The results, however, have been poor and the operation is not considered justifiable.

Explanation for Beneficial Effect

Any explanation for the beneficial effect produced by prefrontal lobotomy in relieving tension and anxiety remains speculative. It has been suggested that the operation may act in one of three ways: (1) the relay to the frontohypothalamic mechanism of the nervous activities engendered by the mental conflict is prevented; (2) the intensity of the mental conflict loses its force when no longer stimulated by this mechanism; or (3) the mechanism of a mental conflict at a cortical level is highly complex and may be directly interfered with by the operation to such an extent that it can no longer develop the intensity required to stimulate the emotions.

Unpleasant Sequences

Observation of patients who have been subjected to prefrontal lobotomy suggests that the function of the "silent" regions of the frontal lobe is to elaborate and integrate affective responses with the other modes of response of the individual to the environment so as to secure an emotionally harmonious life. A change in personality with an accentuation of previous unpleasant traits is not uncommon but is by no means true in all cases. The patient's relatives must expect him to show an absence of self-consciousness, a facetiousness, and childlike pleasure in simple things. Sarcastic remarks and undesirable behavior must be overlooked. Not for several months, if ever, should most patients be permitted to assume financial responsibilities or to attempt unusual social adjustments. Long and persistent re-educating and rehabilitating efforts should be continued. With the best results, the patient loses his anxiety, becomes cheerful and friendly, takes an interest in matters about himself, and even works regularly but without ambition.

Even in cases in which results are otherwise good the patient's sense of responsibility and his feeling for others may be impaired. Frequently there is a reduction in depth of feeling, in sensitivity, and in richness of inner life. Affect is more shallow than before the illness, and the patient usually lacks former sympathies and altruistic motives. There is an increase in self-esteem, tactlessness, and lack of self-criticism and of restraint. Imaginative foresight is usually less than normal. "He doesn't care whether school keeps or not." With less desirable results the patient may be lazy, tactless, suggestible, and childish, and manifest a silly euphoria. He may be unrestrained in word and action, careless in eating habits and personal appearance, and perhaps vulgar and profane. In the usual case, the outstanding change is in affect and not in intellect. The careful long term follow-up of Smith and Kinder on patients subject to topectomy have shown significant losses in their performance on various psychological tests. Some patients, particularly those schizophrenics who have led a purely vegetative existence without active mental conflict, may show no improvement and even exhibit an organic dementia also. Patients whose prepsychotic tendencies were characterized by active aggressiveness may, after operation, manifest an undesirable lack of restraint of these impulses.

Results of Operation

The percentage of improvement is highest in patients who are operated upon as soon as all other measures have been tried and failed. Not even a tentative evaluation of the results should be made for at least six months after the operation, and usually a period of at least one year should be allowed for the attainment of the patient's best level. In the bilateral sectioning of all white matter in suitable patients on whom operation has not been unduly deferred, approximately one-third will leave the hospital and make a tolerable or better adjustment. In some instances the degree of recovery is dramatic, the patient re-gaining a completely successful social, occupational, and economic adjustment. Another third will show a significant improvement. Some of them can be cared for at home, and the institutional adjustment of the remainder will be improved. A third of those operated upon will show no improvement. Paul, Fitzgerald, and Greenblatt report that in a 5-year follow-up of patients who had received a bimedial operation, 65 per cent showed a significant improvement.

BIBLIOGRAPHY

Alexander, L.: Treatment of Mental Disorders. Philadelphia, W. B. Saunders Company, 1953.

Bond, E. D.: Results of treatment in psychoses—with a control series. Am. J. Psychiat., *110*:881–887, 1954.

Cerletti, U.: Old and new information about electroshock. Am. J. Psychiat., *107*:87–94, 1950.

Idem, and Bini, L.: L'Elettroshock. Arch. Gen. di Neurol., Psichiat., e Psicoanal., *19*:266–268, 1938.

Committee on Public Health Relations. New York Acad. of Med.: Electroshock therapy. New York State J. Med., *51*:653–655, 1951.

Courville, C. B.: Late cerebral changes incident to severe hypoglycemia (insulin shock). Arch. Neurol. & Psychiat., *78*:1–14, 1957.

Ebaugh, F. E., et al.: Fatalities following electric convulsive therapy. Arch. Neurol. & Psychiat., *49*:107, 1943.

Ferraro, A., and Roizin, L.: Cerebral morphologic changes in monkeys subjected to a large number of electrically induced convulsions. Am. J. Psychiat., *106*:278–284, 1949.

Foldes, F. F., Rendell-Baker, L., and Birch, J. H.: Causes and prevention of prolonged apnea with succinylcholine. Current Res. Anesth. & Analg., *35*:609–633, 1956.

Freeman, W.: Prefrontal lobotomy: final report of 500 Freeman and Watts' patients followed for 10 to 20 years. South. Med. J., *51*:739–745, 1958.

Idem, and Watts, J. W.: Psychosurgery in the Treatment of Mental Disorders and Intractable Pain, 2nd ed. Springfield, Illinois, Charles C Thomas, 1950.

Fulton, J. F.: Frontal Lobotomy and Affective Behavior. A Neurophysiological Analysis. New York, W. W. Norton & Co., Inc., 1951.

Idem, Aring, C. D., and Wortis, S. B.: The Frontal Lobes. Proceedings of Assoc. for Research in Nerv. and Ment. Dis., Vol. XXVII. Baltimore, Williams & Wilkins Co., 1948.

Grassi, J. R.: Impairment of abstract behavior following bilateral prefrontal lobotomy. Psychiatric Quart., *24*:74–88, 1950.

Greenblatt, M., and Solomon, H. C.: Psychosurgery. New England J. Med., 248:19–27, 59–67, 1953.

Group for the Advancement of Psychiatry: Report No. 15, Revised Electroshock Therapy Report. Topeka, Kansas, 1950.

Himwich, H. E.: Brain Metabolism and Cerebral Disorders. Baltimore, Williams & Wilkins Co., 1951.

Impastato, D. J., and Berg, S.: Methods of administration of succinylcholine dichloride in electroshock therapy with a description of a simple and modified technique and a succinylcholine dichloride test. Am. J. Psychiat., 112:893–897, 1956.

Kalinowsky, L. B., and Hoch, P. H.: Somatic Treatments in Psychiatry. New York, Grune & Stratton, 1961.

Kurland, A. A., Cuervo, R., and Krantz, J. C.: Hexafluorodiethyl ether as a convulsant in psychiatric treatment. J. Neuropsychiat., 1:260–265, 1960.

Liddell, J., et al.: Physical separation of pseudocholinesterase variants in human serum. Lancet, 1:463–464, 1962.

Maclay, W. S.: Death due to treatment. Proc. Roy. Soc. Med., 46:13–20, 1953.

Moniz, E.: Tentatives Opératoires dans le Traitement de Certaines Psychoses. Paris, Masson et Cie., 1936.

Overholser, W. (Ed.): Proceedings of the Third Research Conference on Psychosurgery. Washington, Public Health Service Publications, No. 221, 1954.

Paul, N. L., Fitzgerald, E., and Greenblatt, M.: The long-term comparative results of three different lobotomy procedures. Am. J. Psychiat., 113:808–814, 1957.

Prout, C. T., and Hamilton, D. M.: Results of electro-shock therapy in patients over 60 years of age. Bull. New York Acad. Med., 28:454–461, 1952.

Regan, P. F.: Effective utilization of electric convulsive treatment. Am. J. Psychiat., 114:351–356, 1957.

Sakel, M.: The Pharmacological Shock Treatment of Schizophrenia. New York, Nervous and Mental Diseases Publishing Co., 1938.

Sargant, W., and Slater, E.: An Introduction to Physical Methods of Treatment in Psychiatry, 3rd ed. Baltimore, Williams and Wilkins Co., 1954.

Scheflen, A. E., Reiner, E. R., and Jetter, W. W.: Fatalities in insulin therapy of the psychoses. Arch. Neurol. & Psychiat., 67:32–43, 1952.

Shurley, J. T., and Bond, E. D.: Insulin Shock Therapy in Schizophrenia. Washington, Veterans Administration Technical Bulletin, 10–501, 1948.

Smith, A., and Kinder, E. F.: Changes in psychological test performances of brain-operated schizophrenics after 8 years. Science, 129:149–150, 1959.

Solomon, H. C., and Greenblatt, M.: Frontal Lobes and Schizophrenia. New York, Springer, 1953.

Spencer, A. M.: Posthypoglycemic encephalopathy in Sakel's insulin treatment. J. Ment. Sc., 94:513–554, 1948.

Stengel, E.: The patients' attitudes to leucotomy and its effects. J. Ment. Sc., 98:382–388, 1952.

Tooth, G. C., and Newton, M. P.: Leucotomy in England and Wales, 1942–1954. Ministry of Health Reports on Public Health and Medical Subjects, No. 104. London: Her Majesty's Stationery Office, 1961.

Tyndel, M.: Hyaluronidase as an adjuvant in insulin shock therapy. J.A.M.A., 162:32–34, 1956.

Chapter Thirty-five

PSYCHIATRY AND THE LAW

Both psychiatry and the law—the former to a large degree, the latter to an important but lesser extent—deal with human behavior. Psychiatry seeks to ascertain the forces that result in behavioral deviations and how they may be re-directed to lead to greater intrapersonal serenity and to more constructive and socialized purposes. The law deals largely with the social control of behavior. Although these two disciplines deal with two quite different aspects of behavior, they have many contacts, and since they approach problems of behavior from quite different points of view, it is not surprising that differences of emphasis and of opinion sometimes exist.

HOSPITALIZING MENTALLY ILL PERSONS

One of the important differences between the psychiatrist and the lawyer is in their respective attitudes toward the admission of the mentally ill person to a hospital. The psychiatrist urges that the dignity of the patient be respected and that the obstacles to his admission be no greater than those experienced by the physically sick person. The laws of many states still contain much archaic legal phraseology carrying connotations of criminal prosecution and guilt in their provisions for the hospitalization of the mentally ill. Since in many instances the mental patient does not recognize that he is ill, he does not seek treatment and may even resist measures designed to provide it, and since the Constitution of the United States provides that a person may not be deprived of his liberty without adequate notice and a chance to be heard, the law insists on a punctilious observance of what it regards as human rights.

A few years ago a special committee of the American Bar Association, in referring to the formal legal procedures of commitment of the mentally ill person, stated that these are "fundamental principles of justice which cannot be ignored. Without them, no citizen would be safe from the machinations of secret tribunals, and the most sane member of the community might be adjudged insane and landed in a madhouse." Although it is perhaps theoretically possible that a sane person might be "railroaded" into an institution, it probably rarely occurs now in this country, certainly not in a public mental hospital. The lawyer should not be criticized too severely for his vigilant solicitude for the legal rights of the individual. The physician believes, however, that one's medical rights are no less fundamental than his legal rights, and that the sick person should not be subjected to heartless and harmful mental torture incident to commitment. Until very recently one state in the United States required that a mentally sick person must, except for temporary commitment, have a "trial by jury." (A jury trial is now optional.)

All but six states have laws that permit a mentally ill person to apply for treatment in a public mental hospital. Such laws frequently state that the applicant must be mentally competent to make application and must give a certain number of days' notice in writing if he desires to leave. The extent to which persons apply for admission under the provisions of such a statute varies greatly among the states. For many reasons the number who apply for admission is usually not large.

In addition to any laws providing for the voluntary admission of patients, every state has various laws governing the commitment of mentally ill persons. Frequently the patient with mental disorder caused by, or associated with, impairment of brain tissue function is not mentally competent to make application for his admission to a hospital. Among such persons may be those suffering from acute brain disorders associated with intoxication or infection, or from chronic brain disorder associated with cerebral arteriosclerosis or senile brain disease. The laws of four states wisely permit the legal guardian or close relative of such an incompetent person to arrange for his admission. "A person who is a fit subject for mental treatment should not be denied the easy method for admission merely because he may be too indecisive, weakminded or incompetent to sign his own papers."*

Many states provide for the emergency commitment of a patient. These commitments are temporary, and commitment for an indeterminate period must be completed before the expiration of

* Addendum, Law of Maryland, March, 1944, page 63, 34A.

the period for which the emergency commitment is permitted. The procedure to be followed in an emergency commitment varies greatly. In some states the law merely requires that a petition be filed with the hospital to which commitment is desired, together with a certification of one physician that the patient is in need of immediate hospital care.

In most states the law provides in general that when an involuntary commitment for an indeterminate period is contemplated, a petition for the patient's commitment must be filed with a judicial agency, that the patient be notified of the proposed judicial hearing on his mental state, and that he be examined by two physicians who will certify that he is suffering from mental disease. The judge presiding at the hearing is the commiting agent, although in 21 states the hearing may be held before a jury if requested by the patient.

In a few states the law permits, without a judicial hearing or order, the superintendent of a mental hospital to receive a mentally sick person and detain him for an indeterminate period. Usually in such a case a relative or other responsible person submits to the superintendent a petition for the patient's admission. This petition contains a sworn statement setting forth reasons why the petitioner believes the patient is mentally ill. Accompanying the petition is a certification by two physicians that they have, within a prescribed period, examined the patient and that in their opinion he is mentally ill and in need of care and treatment in a hospital for the mentally sick. In one state most patients are admitted under the provisions of such a statute. It has been operative in practically the same form for over 70 years and has proved eminently satisfactory.

British Mental Health Act, 1959

The laws governing commitment are, however, gradually becoming more liberal and reflect the need to preserve the psychiatrically ill from humiliating publicity and deprivation of his rights as well as to open more easily to him treatment on the same grounds as those with predominantly physical illnesses. Nowhere is this trend more advanced than in England, where a new Mental Health Act became law in July, 1959, and went into effect on November 1, 1960. Today in England non-statutory admissions are allowed to the mental hospitals; the patient may enter informally if he so desires without the signature of papers by himself or others and thus he receives treatment under the same circumstances as those with medical or surgical problems.

In cases in which compulsory admission is required to safeguard the patient or the community, this is recognized solely as a medical decision and not a civil or judicial one. The authorization for admission consists of the recommendation of two physicians, one of whom must be experienced in the treatment of mental disorders. In cases of emergency, the patient may be admitted and detained three days on the application of a mental welfare officer or any relative on the recommendation of one physician.

Discharge from the hospital also may be carried out informally on the decision of a physician, or at the request of the patient or relative on three days' written notice. When the patient is considered too disturbed to be discharged, he may be detained on medical recommendation, but he has recourse to appeal to the newly established Mental Health Review Tribunals. Such tribunals are composed of legal and medical members as well as persons qualified in administration of social service. The tribunals are independent local bodies of skilled persons which evaluate the patient's mental condition and his need for continuing hospital care. If he is found to be without illness or unlikely to endanger himself and others, his discharge must be ordered. Each adult patient may apply to the tribunal once in the six months following his initial admission and once in each succeeding year of detention.

Special provisions are established for such groups as the psychopath. This act

guaranties certain rights to the hospitalized patient. It establishes, as well, new systems for the management of criminal cases. Thus the courts may order hospitalization instead of imprisonment for the convicted mentally ill persons who are suitable for treatment when facilities exist for such care.

To many, the British Mental Health Act of 1959 represents the penetration of a new frontier in the treatment of those with serious behavior disturbances. It reflects as well a profound concern with the development of community resources for their care. Its operation in these forthcoming years will be observed with deep interest throughout the world; its social pioneering may well establish the model for new humanitarian health legislation in other countries in the future.

Model Act Governing Hospitalization of the Mentally Ill*

As previously indicated, each state has its own laws governing the commitment of the mentally ill. Because of this, there is great disparity among the states as to legal procedure in commitment. In many states, too, these procedures subject the patient to indignities and humiliations. For this reason, the National Advisory Mental Health Council in 1949 requested the United States Public Health Service to develop what might be considered as a model act. Very few states have enacted a law patterned on this "Model Act" but presumably, as states gradually modify their commitment laws, there will be a tendency to incorporate into concrete legal procedure the modern thinking reflected in the provisions of this suggested act. The act will not be quoted but attention is called to some of its most important features.

Voluntary Hospitalization

The proposed act is so drawn as to facilitate voluntary admissions but pro-

* A *Draft Act Governing Hospitalization of the Mentally Ill*, U. S. Federal Security Agency, Public Health Service, Publication No. 51, U. S. Government Printing Office, 1951.

vides that upon the patient's written request he shall be forthwith discharged. If, however, in the opinion of the head of the hospital the release of the patient would be dangerous to himself or others, this official may notify the court and the patient's discharge may be postponed for as long as the court deems necessary for the commencement of proceedings for judicial hospitalization, but in no event for more than five days.

Involuntary Hospitalization

The draft of the proposed act distinguishes between involuntary hospitalization and compulsory hospitalization. Commitment proceedings may be involuntary in the sense that they are initiated by someone other than the patient himself, but the patient accepts the judgment of the physician and his family. In that case, there is no judicial hearing, and the commitment procedure consists merely of the filing of a request for the patient's admission and the certification of two qualified physicians that they have examined the individual and that in their opinion he should be hospitalized. It is presumed that most patients would be admitted on this medical certification were statutes based on the "Model Act" adopted.

Compulsory Hospitalization

If the patient refuses hospitalization, a judicial hearing is necessary before the commitment may be made compulsory. In such a case, a petition for the patient's commitment may be filed with the court. This petition must be accompanied by a certificate of a physician stating that he has examined the patient and is of the opinion that he is mentally ill and should be hospitalized. Upon receipt of the application, the court gives notice thereof to the patient and appoints two physicians to examine him. If the examiners report that the patient is mentally ill, the court sets a date for a hearing at which the patient is afforded an opportunity to appear. If, upon completion of the hearing, the court finds that the patient is in need of custody and treatment, it orders

his hospitalization for an indeterminate period or for a temporary observational period not to exceed six months.

The "Model Act" also has humane provisions for the emergency commitment of a patient pending opportunity to initiate proceedings for an indeterminate commitment.

The proposed draft contains various provisions designed to promote the welfare and protect the rights of the patient requiring hospitalization. Among these is one that, pending his removal to a hospital, a committed patient shall not, except because of and during an extreme emergency, be detained in a non-medical facility used for the detention of individuals charged with or convicted of penal offenses. As is already provided in many states, the "Model Act" would, except under unusual circumstances, permit the patient to communicate with official agencies inside or outside the hospital; to receive visitors and confer with counsel; to exercise all civil rights, including the right to dispose of property, execute instruments, make purchases, enter contractual relationships, and vote, unless he has been adjudicated incompetent. The act also greatly restricts the information that may be divulged concerning a patient except with the permission of either himself or his guardian.

Observation Commitment

Several states have legal provision whereby a person charged with, or under indictment for, a criminal offense, or if having been found guilty is awaiting sentence, may be committed to a public mental hospital for a limited period of observation. Following the examination of the prisoner, the hospital submits a report to the court. The hospital does not, of course, express any opinion as to the guilt or innocence of the prisoner. If he is found to be psychotic, commitment will usually be recommended. Frequently the report may include a statement as to whether or not the prisoner's mental condition is such that he is capable of conferring with counsel and preparing his defense. Some courts, especially juvenile courts, may, if the hospital has thoroughly investigated the social situation of the patient, welcome suggestions as to disposition of the prisoner. A juvenile court is, however, more an administrative than a judicial tribunal. Courts are, to an increasing extent, committing prisoners for observation before trial or sentence. Many criminal courts in large cities now employ a full time or part time psychiatrist. Occasionally a prisoner, while serving a sentence, develops a psychosis under the stress of confinement. He will then be transferred to a mental hospital, where he will remain until his recovery or until his sentence expires.

Commitment, Competency, and Civil Rights

Commitment does not in itself automatically adjudicate incompetency; in most states, in fact, a mentally ill patient is not by his commitment adjudged incompetent or deprived of his "civil rights." If, at the time of his commitment, the patient is formally adjudged as "insane" by judicial action, he is thereby rendered incompetent and deprived of certain civil rights. He may not buy or sell property or sign legal papers; he may not vote or hold office; it suspends his driver's license; it usually vacates his license to practice medicine, law, or other learned profession; takes away from him the right to consent to or refuse to consent to the adoption of a child; it casts doubt on his right to make a will; and it impairs his right to marry, although usually, if he does marry while psychotic, the marriage will be valid unless specifically set aside. In most states he cannot start a divorce action.

The methods of erasing the adjudication and of restoring legal competency vary from state to state. Generally speaking, if commitability and incompetency are determined by separate procedures, then discharge (not leave-of-absence or parole) will vacate the commitment order but have no effect on the finding of incompetency. Another court action will be necessary to declare the patient competent and to discharge a guardian.

Habeas Corpus

A right that the psychotic person preserves, even though he has been legally adjudicated as insane, is that of applying for a writ of habeas corpus. This writ has for its object the speedy release by judicial decree. Under American and English law, this writ may be sued out on behalf of anyone who claims he is being restrained of his liberty illegally. Since a commitment may continue only so long as the patient needs care and custody, he may at any time petition for the issuance of such a writ on the ground that he is now sane and so entitled to release. At the hearing on the petition, the sanity of the patient is inquired into, and if the court finds him sane, he may be discharged. In some jurisdictions the court impanels a jury to determine the issue of sanity. In only a few jurisdictions are there any restrictions imposed on the frequency with which application for a writ may be made.

PRIVILEGED COMMUNICATIONS

In nearly all jurisdictions, a physician on the witness stand is not allowed, without the patient's consent, to disclose any information acquired in attending the patient in a professional capacity. It is generally held that the confidentiality of a patient's relations with his psychiatrist is peculiarly close, even more so than in ordinary medicine, and is not subject to violation even on a court summons. Usually courts have held that relations between a patient committed to a mental institution and a staff doctor are likewise of a privileged professional nature and are therefore protected from disclosure on a witness stand. The privilege has, in fact, been extended so far beyond the premise of protecting confidential communications that courts assume without argument that all statements of inmates to hospital doctors come within the rule.

Yet psychiatrists should be aware that the right of medical privileged communication exists only by statute. In some state jurisdictions, patients do not possess the right of privilege. It is therefore important that all psychiatrists ascertain the status of privilege in the state or states in which they practice. Where the patient does not have the legal right of a privileged communication and does not understand the consequences of waiving his right, it is imperative that the psychiatrist advise him of the legal limits of confidentiality and privilege in that particular community.

Physicians in public mental hospitals receive so many requests for information about their patients that they frequently forget the extent to which the hospital records are really of a privileged nature. They should therefore be guarded lest they divulge more information concerning patients than is permissible.

Marriage

In most states the criterion of legal capacity to marry is the ability to understand the nature of the marriage contract and the duties and obligations such a contract entails. The statutes are of little help in defining the degree of mental unsoundness that will suffice to void a marriage. If it is clear that one party was so psychotic, drunk, or defective at the time of marriage that he or she did not understand the obligations assumed by the marriage contract, an annulment will usually be decreed. In general, however, courts are reluctant to declare a marriage void. Many states have laws forbidding mentally ill persons to marry. The objective of such laws is presumably to prevent the procreation of defective children. If such is the case, the law is not based on any scientific proof of the inheritability of the disorder. Usually the courts will not annul a marriage on the grounds of fraud if a concealment of previous mental disease is the basis of the charge. Concealment of previous commitment to a mental hospital is not a ground for annulment on the basis of fraud unless the party concerned affirmatively stated that he never was in a mental hospital.

Divorce

In most states insanity is not a ground for divorce; however, in some states divorce will be granted if the insane spouse has been committed to a hospital for mental diseases for a period of years. The statutes in some states specify that the spouse must be "incurably insane." The psychiatrist is reluctant to testify that any mental illness is absolutely incurable. Perhaps he can say that in the light of present-day medical knowledge it is his opinion that the patient's disorder is incurable. He will remember that at the beginning of the present century he would have testified that general paresis, even in its early stage, was incurable. He certainly would not do so now.

Wills

A person's competency to make a will is known as testamentary capacity. This capacity must meet three criteria. The testator, or a person making a will, must (1) know that he is making a will, (2) know the nature and extent of his property, and (3) know the natural objects of his bounty. Expressed a little more simply, the person signing a will must know clearly what he is doing when he signs it. Although it is not necessary that he know the minutest details concerning his property, he must have a substantially accurate knowledge of what he owns. By "natural objects of his bounty" is meant the members of the testator's family, his warm friends, others to whom he feels especially grateful, or institutions or organizations in which he has felt an interest. Although he must know who are his living near relatives, the law does not require that he bequeath them anything. The failure of a testator to include a member of his family because of paranoid delusions of a psychotic intensity concerning the relative would probably render the will invalid, since the delusion would affect his understanding of the natural objects of his bounty. Statutes sometimes state that the testator must be of "sound mind and memory." This phrase means, in effect, that the testator must possess the testamentary capacity just described. The fact that the testator was psychotic or was committed to a hospital for mental disorders when he made the will does not necessarily mean that he lacked mental capacity to make a will or renders it invalid. The psychiatrist must at all times bear in mind the three basic criteria as to testamentary capacity.

Since it is often difficult to draw a line between simple senility and senile dementia, the question of testamentary capacity of the elderly person may arise. Even though the testator's mental processes be slow, the courts will consider him competent if he can call to mind his property and the natural objects of his bounty. Senile persons may suffer not only impairment of mind and memory but also increased suggestibility and therefore be subject to undue influence. Many aged individuals are easy prey to the flattery of younger persons. The courts will hold invalid a will obtained by deception, threat, or the persistent suggestion of a domineering relative or of a flattering confidant.

Occasionally the psychiatrist will be requested to testify in court concerning the testamentary capacity of a testator, now deceased, at the time he made his will. In such a case the attorney will ascertain from witnesses every possible fact concerning the testator's behavior that will be helpful to the psychiatrist in forming an honest opinion concerning the testator's capacity on the day he made his will. These facts will be assembled in the hypothetical question describing the testator's behavior. At times a lawyer will request that his client be examined as to his competency at the time a testator prepares his will. The psychiatrist's examination will then be directed with special reference to the three basic criteria of testamentary capacity. He will secure from the testator a description of his property and its estimated value. He will ask the patient to name the members of his family and indicate their relationships. As he secures a description of each relative, the physician will note the nature of the emotional response evoked by the respective discussions concerning each. The physician's report to the lawyer should contain such verbatim statements made by the patient as will later suggest his testamentary capacity.

Competency and Contracts

Every person of legal age is presumed to be mentally competent, i.e., to have the mental capacity to carry on his everyday affairs. The burden of proof is, therefore, on one who would declare the adult incompetent. To determine that a person is incompetent, it must be shown that he has a mental disorder, that this mental disorder causes a defect in judgment, and that this defect in judgment renders him incapable of managing his property, the prudent making of contracts, or the taking of some other specific action.

The establishment of a mental disorder is not sufficient to warrant a finding of incompetency. It must also be shown that the mental disorder causes an impairment of judgment. No valid generalization can be made on the relationship of the various mental disorders to competency. The diagnostic label attached to the disorder is not as important as the degree to which judgment is impaired. Consideration must also be given as to whether the condition is static, progressive, or improving. A progressive organic disease of the brain is typically a disorder that renders a patient incompetent, but many patients suffering from psychogenic disorders, such as manic–depressive psychosis, schizophrenia, or paranoid disorders, suffer from such seriously impaired judgment that they are rendered incompetent.

If a person is considered incompetent and he has business affairs that require attention, a petition for the appointment of a guardian will be filed with the appropriate court. The issue of incompetency is usually tried before either a probate or a county court, without a jury. In several states a jury is still used. Usually a member of the patient's family is the petitioner, but anyone who has an interest in preserving the patient's estate may petition the court for the appointment of a guardian. Notice of a hearing on the petition must be given to the person, and in many states to certain others, such as his next of kin. A few states provide not only that the person is entitled to be present if he desires but that his presence is required. It must be shown, usually by medical evidence, that there is danger that in the absence of a guardian for the person's estate he will dissipate his property or become the victim of designing persons. Some courts require personal testimony by a physician, while others will accept a certificate of incompetency in lieu of personal testimony. If the person is declared incompetent, the court will decide whether his interests are best served by the appointment of a friend, relative, stranger, or corporation as the guardian. In some states the fact of commitment automatically adjudges the patient as incompetent. In such a case the appointment of a guardian is merely an administrative matter and requires no judicial hearing. Usually a guardianship obtains only in respect to the patient's estate and does not, unless so specified, include guardianship of his person.

CONTRACTS. Courts will usually rule that a contract or other legal transaction will not be set aside on the grounds of mental incompetency if the person had sufficient mental capacity to understand the nature and effect of the particular transaction. A higher degree of mental capacity may be required to understand a complex instrument or transaction than a simple one. The degree of judgment needed may vary greatly. It is sometimes claimed that a contract was executed during a lucid interval of a person admittedly disordered. Psychiatrists are inclined to question whether in most cases the patient's lucidity during such intervals was not more apparent than real. It is the prevailing theory that where the incompetency of one party was not known to the other party, where no advantage was taken of the incompetent, and where the contract has been executed and the parties cannot be put back *in status quo* the contract is binding and cannot be voided on the grounds of incompetency.

Criminal Responsibility

The concepts of mind held by psychiatry and by the law are so disparate that it is difficult for the two professions to agree as to responsibility for behavior, especially criminal behavior. According to the concept held by law, the mind is dominated by reason and full will, and behavior results from a consciously determined intent. The law does not recognize partial responsibility, although to the psychiatrist responsibility does not have definable boundaries and degrees. Law confines its exploration of behavior to conscious data and assumes that a disorder of the cognitive faculty (knowledge) is the only basis for the determination of responsibility for behavior termed criminal. Psychiatry, on the other hand, assumes that mental processes are controlled by both conscious and unconscious factors, the latter playing a very important part; that behavior is an expression of the personality as a whole as determined by a multiplicity of complex factors, including the unconscious effect of early experiences, later pressures, and emotional needs. To the psychiatrist, the unlawful act may not be the result of a consciously determined "intent" but the surface manifestation of a more profound psychic disturbance, an indicator of breakdown in a system of psychic adaptive defenses erected to balance inner conflicts. The psychiatrist would go beyond the act itself and evaluate the total personality, both in its conscious and unconscious aspects. He recognizes the role of the intellect, but would give to emotions and the unconscious a greater weight in the balance of forces in mental life.

The difference in these concepts is a logical result of the gradual development of psychological knowledge. In ancient times lunatics were not regarded as suffering from disease but were believed to be possessed of demons and were beaten, kept in chains, and not uncommonly sentenced to death by burning or hanging. Even if the alleged lunatic had committed some crime, there was no consideration as to the offender's responsibility.

Gradually, however, rules to determine criminal responsibility were formulated. Since American law is based largely on English law, it is of interest to note the early application of responsibility tests in the laws of England. In 1723 an English court declared that for an accused to escape punishment he must "not know what he is doing, no more than . . . a wild beast." This requirement, that to qualify for immunity the accused shall know no more than a wild beast, was altered and moderated somewhat about 1760 when the terms "right and wrong" were substituted for "good and evil." Slightly earlier, however, an accused person was executed after it had been determined that he had not shown a "*total want of reason.*"

The American law generally prevalent at this time stems directly from the famous M'Naghten case. In 1843 Daniel M'Naghten was tried for the willful murder of Edward Drummond, the private secretary of Sir Robert Peel. For several years M'Naghten had suffered from delusions of persecution. He had attempted to escape from his persecutors by leaving Scotland and going to England or to France. On many occasions he had complained to his father and to various public authorities. He became increasingly embittered and finally determined to right his imaginary wrongs by killing Sir Robert Peel. With this object in mind, he watched Peel's house. Seeing Drummond come out, he followed and shot him under the belief that he was shooting Peel. At M'Naghten's trial, his counsel entered a plea of "partial insanity." He was declared of unsound mind and committed to an institution for the criminally insane.

This case caused a great sensation in England, with the result that a few days after the trial a discussion took place in the House of Lords that proposed five questions to the fifteen Judges of England regarding the law of insanity. The answers of the Judges can be reduced to two rules to determine the responsibility of a person who pleads insanity as a defense to a crime:

(1) "To establish a defense on the ground of insanity it must be clearly proved that, at the time of committing the act, the party accused was laboring under such a defect of reason, from disease of the mind, as not to know the nature and quality of the act he was doing, or if he did know it, he did not know he was doing what was wrong."

As a rule, the defendant "knows" the facts concerning the particular criminal act that he has committed, knows its harmfulness ("quality"), and its unlawfulness and consequences, but does not know the unconscious basis for it.

(2) "Where a person labors under partial delusions only and is not in other respects insane" and commits an offense in consequence thereof, "he must be considered in the same situation as to responsibility as if the facts with respect to which the delusion exists were real."

It should be borne in mind that the M'Naghten Rules are not a test of sanity and were not formulated as such. They are a test of responsibility in law for acts done. In 28 states the M'Naghten formula is the sole test of responsibility, and in 17 others and in American Military Law it is still the main test supplemented by the "irresistible impulse test."

In 1922 the Lord Chancellor of England appointed a committee to consider and report upon what changes, if any, were desirable in the existing law, practice, and procedure relating to criminal trials in which the plea of insanity as a defense was raised. The committee approved of the M'Naghten Rules and held they should be maintained. It recommended an addition to the effect that "a person charged criminally with an offense is irresponsible for his act when the act is committed under an impulse which the prisoner was by mental disease in substance deprived of any power to resist." As indicated, the laws in 17 states of the United States exempt from criminal responsibility persons suffering from irresistible or uncontrollable impulse. To most psychiatrists, however, the word "impulse" is unsatisfactory for it covers only a small and very special group of those who are mentally ill. It suggests some sudden episode, yet in many cases the sufferer acts, not suddenly or impulsively, but coolly and with ingenious calculation. This is characteristic of many who suffer from paranoid schizophrenia or paranoid psychosis. Although courts have hung tenaciously to the M'Naghten "right and wrong test," it has been severely criticized, and increasingly, not only by psychiatrists but also by many eminent lawyers. In 1953 Justice Felix Frankfurter stated in testifying before the British Royal Commission on Capital Punishment: "The M'Naghten Rules were rules which the Judges, in response to questions by the House of Lords, formulated in the light of the then existing psychological knowledge. . . . I do not see why the rules of law should be arrested at the state of psychological knowledge at the time when they were formulated."

The above statement, quoting the opinion of one of the most eminent American jurists, reflects the view of an increasing number of lawyers.

In 1869, influenced by Dr. Isaac Ray, doubtless the most enlightened American psychiatrist in the medical jurisprudence of insanity, the Supreme Court of New Hampshire handed down an opinion sweeping aside the M'Naghten Rules. The court recognized simply that an accused person is not criminally responsible if his unlawful act was the result of mental disease or mental defect. Under this decision, insanity is no longer defined as a matter of law; instead, it is made a question of fact to be determined by the jury like any other fact. This determination rests upon testimony of the psychiatric expert respecting the latest knowledge of human behavior and his interpretation of such knowledge in terms of his observations of the accused. If the accused has a mental disease and if the criminal act is the product of it, he is found not guilty by reason of insanity.

In 1954, the case of Durham v. United States, the Court of Appeals for the District of Columbia Circuit handed down a decision adopting in substance the same rule as the New Hampshire one. This case involved a defendant, Durham, who had been convicted of housebreaking. He had previously been committed to a hospital for mental diseases. At Durham's trial the issue of responsibility was raised. A psychiatrist testified that he thought Durham was of unsound mind but that he might give the correct answer if a question of right or wrong were put to him. The appeal court ruled that the trial court was in error in declaring Durham sane on an obsolete test of responsibility. The essence of the decision is contained in the following passage:

"We find that as an exclusive criterion the right–wrong test is inadequate in that (a) it does not take sufficient account of psychic realities and scientific knowledge, and (b) it is based upon one symptom and so cannot validly be applied to all circumstances. We find that the 'irresistible impulse' test is also inadequate in that it gives no recognition to mental illness characterized by brooding and reflection and so relegates acts caused by such illness to the application of the inadequate right–wrong test. We conclude that a broader test should be adopted. . . .

"The rule we now hold must be applied on the retrial of this case and in future cases is not unlike that followed by the New Hampshire court since 1870. It is simply that an accused is not criminally responsible if his unlawful act was the product of mental disease or mental defect."*

In 1957 the Vermont legislature adopted the following test of insanity when this is used as a defense in criminal cases:

"1. A person is not responsible for criminal conduct if at the time of such conduct as a result of mental disease or defect he lacks adequate capacity either to appreciate the criminality of his conduct or to conform his conduct to the requirements of law.

"2. The terms 'mental disease or defect' do not include an abnormality mani-

* Durham v. United States: 59 App. D. C. 144 (1929).

fested only by repeated criminal or otherwise anti-social conduct. The terms 'mental disease or defect' shall include congenital and traumatic mental conditions as well as disease.

"3. The M'Naghten test of insanity in criminal cases is hereby abolished."

This statute seems to reflect the increasing dissatisfaction with the M'Naghten Rules as a test of criminal responsibility.

When testifying at a trial, the psychiatrist should remember that the determination of responsibility is a legal issue. The psychiatrist's function is to present the data; the application of the law to the facts is for the court and the jury. He will therefore not express any opinion as to whether or not the defendant can distinguish between right and wrong. Any testimony beyond professionally recognized medical data descriptive of the defendant's mental status, and informative to the court and jury, is therefore beyond the province of the psychiatric expert. All expert testimony should be free of moral and value statements. The psychiatrist will be wise not to attempt to scale degrees of responsibility in terms of symptoms.

If a person charged with crime is found not guilty by reason of insanity, he may, in some states, at the discretion of the court be committed to a state hospital for mental diseases. In other states the law is mandatory that he be committed. In some states the patient may, upon recovery, be discharged by the court that ordered his commitment; in other states, if regarded as no longer dangerous if allowed at large, he may be discharged by the governor. In one state the patient may be discharged only by act of legislature.

Patients are not tried or executed while insane. The issue in such a case is not the patient's ability, or lack of it, to distinguish between right and wrong, but his ability to confer with counsel and prepare his defense.

In one state, Massachusetts, the law (the so-called Briggs Law) provides that a person who commits a capital offense or commits more than one felony, or who commits the same crime more than once must be referred for examination by experts appointed by the State Department of Mental Health. The examinations are usually made at the jail where the defendant is being held. The psychiatrist's report is filed with the clerk of the court and is accessible to the court, to the district attorney, and to the counsel for the accused. If the examiner reports that the prisoner is suffering from mental disease, he is not directly asked to say whether the patient is able to distinguish between right and wrong, or whether he is able to refrain from doing wrong because of an irresistible impulse, but he is asked whether the patient suffers from a mental illness sufficiently severe to affect his responsibility and to require treatment in a mental hospital. It is apparently assumed that the examiner bases his opinion on the right–wrong test and the irresistible impulse test, but the reports submitted to the courts neither ask nor answer the question in these terms.

Under this law, juries have shown a commendable tendency to take the word of the impartial examiner as against that of psychiatrists hired by either side. The "battle of experts" has become almost unknown in Massachusetts.

BIBLIOGRAPHY

Alexander, J. E.: Commentaries on the Law of Wills. San Francisco, Bender-Moss Co., 1918.

Barrow, R. L., and Fabing, H. D.: Epilepsy and the Law. New York, Paul B. Hoeber, 1956.

Davidson, H. A.: Forensic Psychiatry. New York, Ronald Press, 1952.

Diamond, B. L.: Isaac Ray and the trial of Daniel M'Naghten. Am. J. Psychiat., 112:651–656, 1956.

G. A. P. Report No. 26: Criminal Responsibility and Psychiatric Expert Testimony. Topeka, Kansas, 1954.

G. A. P. Report No. 45: Confidentiality and Privileged Communication in the Practice of Psychiatry. New York, 1960.

Glueck, S.: Mental Disorder and the Criminal Law. Boston, Little, Brown & Co., 1925.

Guttmacher, M.: The quest for a test of criminal responsibility. Am. J. Psychiat., 111:428–433, 1954.

Idem, and Weihofen, H.: Psychiatry and the Law. New York, W. W. Norton & Co., Inc., 1952.

Hall, J.: Mental disease and criminal responsibility—M'Naghten versus Durham and the American Law Institute's tentative draft. Indiana Law J., 33:212–225, 1958.

Maclay, W. S.: The new Mental Health Act in England and Wales. Amer. J. Psychiat., 116: 777–781, 1960.

Mental Health Act., 1959. London, Her Majesty's Stationery Office, 1961.

Overholser, W.: The place of psychiatry in the criminal law. Psychiatric Quart., 10:197–223, 1936.

Ray, I.: A Treatise on the Medical Jurisprudence of Insanity. Boston, Charles C. Little & James Brown, 1838.

Sobeloff, S. E.: From M'Naghten to Durham and beyond. Psychiatric Quart., 29:357–371, 1955.

Tracey, J. E.: The Doctor as a Witness. Philadelphia, W. B. Saunders Company, 1957.

Usdin, G. L.: The physician and testamentary capacity. Am. J. Psychiat., 114:249–256, 1957.

Weihofen, H.: The Urge to Punish. New York, Farrar, Strauss & Cudahy, Inc., 1956.

Willcox, B. F., and Roemer, R.: Hospitalization under the British Mental Health Act, 1959. Am. J. Comparative Law, 9:606–633, 1960.

INDEX